Paediatric Radiology Rapid Reporting

Michael Paddock • Caoilfhionn Ní Leidhin
Amaka C. Offiah

Paediatric Radiology Rapid Reporting

Second Edition

Springer

Michael Paddock
Medical Imaging Department
Perth Children's Hospital
Nedlands, WA, Australia

Caoilfhionn Ní Leidhin
Medical Imaging Department
Perth Children's Hospital
Nedlands, WA, Australia

Amaka C. Offiah
Division of Clinical Medicine
School of Medicine and Population Health
University of Sheffield
Sheffield, South Yorkshire, UK

ISBN 978-3-031-48254-0 ISBN 978-3-031-48255-7 (eBook)
https://doi.org/10.1007/978-3-031-48255-7

This Springer imprint is published by the registered company Springer Nature Switzerland AG
The registered company address is: Gewerbestrasse 11, 6330 Cham, Switzerland

Paper in this product is recyclable.

To Luke, 我的小宝宝*—for putting me back together*
MP

To Sumanth, Ciara, bump & Muintir Uí Leidhin ar fad—for your love and support
CNL

To Nkechi—Laru k'oke, ka mmunwa laru ka ngwele
ACO

Foreword to the First Edition

I was delighted to be asked to prepare a foreword for this book written by my colleagues, Dr. M Paddock and Dr. AC Offiah. As the Training Programme Director for South Yorkshire, it is wonderful to see an enthusiastic radiology trainee producing high-quality teaching material, supported by an established consultant expert in their field of interest. Passing down knowledge continues the important cycle of learning and teaching with benefit to future generations of radiologists.

Reading this book is a must for any specialist trainee in radiology preparing for the final FRCR examination. Paediatric radiology is often an area that is neglected during revision when the RCR curriculum requires a very wide breadth of knowledge. Many trainees have limited exposure to paediatric radiology during their training, and there may have been an interval between a paediatric attachment and preparing for the FRCR 2B examination. Paediatric imaging does however form part of all FRCR examinations, and you will be assessed in this area. I have been an examiner at the Royal College of Radiologists for many years, and there is a recognised reduced performance in questions related to paediatric imaging.

This book consists of cases set out in the style of the FRCR 2B Rapid Reporting examination. The high-quality images and attached notes are beautifully presented in a format that is easy to read. Your knowledge will be enhanced with what I think you will find to be an enjoyable learning experience. The carefully selected cases are either commonly seen in daily practice or are important to be aware of. This book will help you prepare for all components of the FRCR 2B examination (not just the Rapid Reporting element) and your future career as an independent practitioner.

Happy reading and good luck!

The Royal Hallamshire Hospital
and Sheffield Children's Hospital
Sheffield, UK

Ruth Batty

Foreword to the Second Edition

Preparing for the final Fellowship examination is a monumental undertaking and every candidate seeks the best possible assistance for each subspecialty. Paddock and Offiah's *Paediatric Radiology Rapid Reporting for FRCR Part 2B* has already proven itself as an invaluable resource, and careful study of this fully revised second edition will maximise candidates' chances of success.

Although the tests are set out in the style of the FRCR Part 2B Rapid Reporting examination, there is a comprehensive coverage of the field. The concise explanations of each case, along with the recommended further reading, provide a depth of knowledge that furthers its utility for other components of the FRCR Part 2 examination. For example, one of the specimen questions for the Part 2A Single Best Answer test asks:

'An athletic 13-year-old boy presents to the emergency department with a painful right hip. Pelvic x-ray demonstrates an irregular shaped bone [fragment] adjacent to the anterior inferior iliac spine. The avulsion of which muscle is most likely to have caused this injury?' If you go to the explanations for Test 4, you will find a list of all the pelvic and proximal femoral avulsion fractures that you need to know.

The material covered in this book is universal and so would also be useful for candidates preparing for Fellowship (or Board) examinations in other training systems. Of course, once all the tests are passed, the candidate will emerge into a new life as a consultant radiologist and the knowledge gleaned from this book will stand them in good stead throughout their career. The much-lauded first edition of this book has cemented its place amongst radiologists and all those involved in the interpretation of paediatric radiographs. The addition of three new tests, as well as meticulous revision of the original ten tests, will send it even further down the road to classic status.

Perth Children's Hospital
and The University of Western Australia
Perth, Australia

Derek Roebuck

Preface to the First Edition

Firstly, congratulations on passing the FRCR Part 2A—well done! Now to the FRCR 2B examination where the fun can really begin…

All three components of the 2B examination may contain a significant proportion of paediatric imaging. Candidates 'struggle with interpretation of paediatric imaging—even for common paediatric pathologies' as identified in the Royal College of Radiologists Examiners' report. Better preparation in this component will also help you when faced with paediatric cases in the long case reporting and viva sections, and you will definitely get some!

The amount of paediatric radiology training up and down the country is variable, and some candidates may not feel adequately prepared to tackle paediatric imaging in the Rapid Reporting section of the examination. The reality is that the majority of radiologists will go on to work in District General Hospitals (DGHs) where paediatric imaging can feature prominently in the day-to-day workload of the department. Most children will initially present to and be imaged in DGHs, given that most do not live next to a dedicated paediatric tertiary centre.

The examiners need to make sure that you are a safe radiologist and that you are able to provide a sound radiological opinion which may contribute to effective patient management and care. This is what the 2B examination is assessing—your ability to use your knowledge and skills effectively and your preparedness to practise radiology safely as an independent practitioner.

We felt that there was a lack of dedicated paediatric radiology revision resources for the 2B examination, and we wrote this book to address that need. All radiographs are from standard day-to day practice and have been collected over a 3-year period by one of the authors: the images range from the obvious buckle fracture to the subtle metaphyseal fracture (specific to physical child abuse) which is easily missed.

Following the answer key for each test, we have expanded on certain abnormal findings or normal variants to further enhance your learning. We have purposefully not used arrows or line diagrams to show you where or what the abnormality is—abnormal radiographs do not come with this in the examination or in real life. As clinical radiologists, we have described the abnormality, and where subtle, it has been magnified as you would do in the examination and in clinical practice. Being a text comprised of paediatric radiographs, the image quality is dependent on the limited dose used to acquire the images. Thus, the quality of some of the magnified images in the explanations may be degraded but still remain adequate to sufficiently demonstrate the pathology. Where relevant, we have included tips for the viva examination. The references also include excellent pictorial reviews and links to educational websites so that you can get the most out of your revision.

We emphasise that the best practice for the Rapid Reporting section of the examination is to report paediatric radiographs and get them checked by your local paediatric radiologists. This book can be used to supplement your learning during normal working hours.

We are extremely grateful to Dr. Jonathan M. Smith and Dr. Robin Dale, specialty trainees on the Sheffield radiology training scheme, for their insight and feedback throughout the preparation of this book.

Finally, we wish you the best of luck in all components of the examination and your future careers. We hope that you will use this book as a future reference text, even after the examination. We welcome any comments, suggestions or feedback, and if you have any queries, please email us on paedsradrapidreporting@gmail.com.

Good luck!

Sheffield, UK

Michael Paddock
Amaka C. Offiah

Preface to the Second Edition

Following the international success of the first edition, we were delighted to be asked to prepare a second edition of this text. The content of the first edition has been fully revised and, with the addition of three new tests, this comprehensive resource now includes nearly 400 practice paediatric radiographs providing an unrivalled educational resource to aid candidates in their examination preparation. It has always been our goal to provide an accessible and valued paediatric radiology text to bridge the gap in knowledge for those candidates preparing for the FRCR 2B examination, and indeed for any healthcare professional reviewing and reporting paediatric radiographs.

Since the publication of the first edition in 2019, the world has been impacted significantly by the COVID-19 pandemic. This has also extended to the delivery of the FRCR 2B examination which has evolved to computer-based assessment of the reporting components and the oral component being delivered via video conferencing at selected venues. Given these changes, candidates are strongly advised to read all relevant information pertaining to the delivery and format of the examination on the Royal College of Radiologists' website prior to their examination sitting for any further changes.

Whilst most of the images included in this text reflect the format of the examination, i.e. those that would be expected to be encountered in a typical Emergency Department reporting session or referred by a General Practitioner, we have also included a handful of neonatal radiographs which demonstrate important pathology. There is a notable decreased performance of candidates in relation to paediatric imaging, and we hope that inclusion of these images and their accompanying explanations will enable candidates to maximise their revision given that these cases may be tested in the other components of the examination.

As with any printed text there will always be some loss of image quality, even more so with paediatric radiographs given the lower dose used to acquire the images and the technical challenge that comes with imaging children who do not want to be imaged! An electronic version of this book is also available which candidates are encouraged to use: this format not only replicates an authentic examination experience but will also help to remediate any perceived decrease in image quality.

We are incredibly grateful to the clinical radiology speciality registrars, Dr. Katherine Hocking (South Yorkshire radiology training programme, UK) and Dr. Tony Bose, Dr. Nihar Jha and Dr. Roger Smyth (Western Australia radiology training programme, Australia), whose insight and feedback were invaluable to ensure the ongoing relevance and high-impact educational value of this revised edition.

Finally, we welcome and thank Dr. Caoilfhionn Ní Leidhin for joining the authorship. Her invaluable contributions in revising the first edition and co-authoring the three new tests have been instrumental in making the second edition a richer and more impactful text for which we are indebted.

We hope that you enjoy using this text as much as we have enjoyed preparing it. We wish you the very best of luck in the examination and your future careers.

Perth, WA, Australia Michael Paddock
Caoilfhionn Ní Leidhin
Sheffield, UK Amaka C. Offiah

Testimonies for the First Edition

Excellent resource for the paediatric components of the FRCR exam, highly recommend! The authors are experts in their field and deliver some excellent cases – 5.*
Dr. Vartan Bailan FRCR

Unlike the online rapids packets I used, this book offers explanations which are really helpful for confidently identifying abnormalities and discounting normal findings unique to paediatric radiology. The discussions are also great for viva preparation. It definitely helped me to pass the FRCR 2B examination.
Dr. Robin Dale FRCR

Large number of paediatric cases covering an extensive range of pathologies. Extremely well-written explanations to complement the cases means this book is not only helpful in preparing for the Rapids but also for the long reporting and viva components of the FRCR 2B examination. Very helpful in my exam preparation as other resources cover very little paediatric content.
Dr. Thomas Geh FRCR

Most UK registrars will know that perhaps the easiest way to fail the 2B exam is to lose points on the Rapid Reporting section. Equally, an 8 on the Rapids will really take the pressure off for the remaining components of the exam. An outsized portion of the Rapids exam consists of paediatric MSK films, and seeing a good number of these is hardest during a normal working week. This book is an excellent resource to get good at paediatric MSK and to make sure that you don't drop points on the Rapids.
Dr. Nathan Jenko FRCR

I recently sat the final FRCR and found this book to be invaluable. The case selection is perfect and really reflects the topics that come up in the exam. Where the book really excels is in the explanations following each case. They manage to be detailed enough while not being too long. I've seen some other reviews critiquing the image quality. From my experience of using multiple revision books for this exam there is always some degradation in image quality when printed. I do not think the image quality is any worse than the other books I have used, and they are in fact better than some of the most popular 2B books. Overall, I think this book is a must have for the exam. Paediatrics is always a difficult area and many UK trainees have minimal experience in this area. I would highly recommend this book and I think the authors should be commended!

Dr. Matthew S. Kinsella FRCR

Whilst a challenging topic at FRCR 2B level, after reading this book I significantly improved my confidence when assessing paediatric plain films, which helped me in both the Rapid Reporting and viva components of the exam. Highly recommended to anyone studying for the FRCR 2B exam or any practicing radiologist wishing to familiarise themselves with paediatric plain film interpretation.

Dr. Sam Kular FRCR

Great book and very useful in 2B prep.

Dr. Christine McMullin FRCR

This book is a great resource for the FRCR 2B Rapid Reporting component and also for the viva component. The image quality is very good and far superior compared to other books. I highly recommend this book for the FRCR 2B. I sat the exam recently and passed. Paediatric imaging, mainly plain films, is an essential component of the exam. This book will enable you to ace the paediatric plain films when encountered in the exam.

Dr. Yousef A Shahin FRCR

Excellent resource for Registrars doing paediatric radiology rotations and for revising for the FRCR 2A or 2B exams, or general consultants who want to keep up to date. The image quality is good and the cases are suitably challenging but the book really comes into its own with the detailed explanations of findings and pathology. This should be in every radiologist's collection.

Dr. Lisa Shannon FRCR

I used this book in the run up to sitting the Final FRCR Part B examination in autumn 2018 and I believe it played an important role in obtaining a high score in the Rapid Reporting element. Most practice exam sets include a few paediatric radiographs, but no other resource on the market provides a concentrated bank of paediatric radiographs with which you can hone your skills. This makes it particularly useful for candidates like me, who had completed their paediatric rotation a long time before sitting the exam, or for those candidates who are not very confident in paediatric reporting. The explanations are thorough and provide some useful tips for the viva component of the exam, also.

Dr. Jonathan M. Smith FRCR

Excellent book covering an often-challenging area for the final FRCR exam: paediatric imaging, in particular Rapid Reporting. Clear and concise explanations. Good image quality.

Dr. Daniel Ward FRCR

Introduction

Purpose of the Rapid Reporting Component of the FRCR 2B Examination

Emergency Department imaging constitutes a significant proportion of most radiologists' workload. The Rapid Reporting component of the FRCR 2B examination assesses candidates' ability to decide rapidly if an image is normal or abnormal, and where abnormal, provide a diagnosis. This component of the examination tests your ability to confidently state when an abnormality is present and exclude it when it is not.

The examination contains 30 radiographs to be reported with no other imaging modality examined. The majority of the images are trauma cases, primarily musculoskeletal/extremity radiographs, in addition to some chest and abdominal radiographs, as would be expected in a typical emergency department reporting session or those referred by a general practitioner. We have replicated this brief, except that all the radiographs are paediatric, ranging from neonates to adolescents, recognising the inherent challenges of interpreting radiographs of the developing skeleton. In this second edition, we have also included a handful of neonatal radiographs of important pathologies to allow prospective candidates to maximise their revision time for other components of the 2B examination.

Structure

Candidates will have 35 min to report 30 images and denote each image as either normal or abnormal. Approximately 45–50% of the cases will be normal. Each image contains one significant diagnosable abnormality which is *not* complex; as such, differential diagnoses should not be offered. Images will be viewed on a single monitor. In the examination, some cases may show either a single or several projections.

Any anatomical variants, including those which do not cause symptoms, may be examined and should be denoted as 'normal'. Those normal variants which may cause symptoms will *not* be included, e.g. accessory navicular, supracondylar spur. Minor age-related change should also be recorded as 'normal'.

Candidates should keep their comments short and precise regarding the site and nature of the abnormality. For those radiographs that demonstrate a well-recognised fracture pattern in which two fractures would be expected to occur together, e.g. fractures of the distal radius *and* ulna, you will be expected to identify and write down *both* fractures to get the mark. Candidates will lose marks where responses are incomplete, e.g. 'Monteggia' instead of 'Monteggia fracture-dislocation left forearm', or inaccurate.

Scoring

Since the publication of the first edition, the Royal College of Radiologists (RCR) has updated the scoring system for this component of the examination. Candidates report 30 radiographs and have the opportunity to attain two marks per image for a maximum of 60 marks. The scoring system used is taken directly from the RCR website and is outlined below:

Image type	Candidate response	Mark
Normal image	Correctly classified	+2
	Incorrectly classified (false positive)	+2
	No answer given	0
Abnormal image	Correctly classified and correctly identified	+2
	Correctly classified with partially correct answer	+1
	Correctly classified but incorrectly identified	0
	Incorrectly classified (false negative)	0
	No answer given	0

Subsequently, the total marks obtained in the Rapid Reporting component are converted into an overall mark between 4 and 8:

Total marks	Overall mark
00–48	4
49	4.5
50–51	5
52–53	5.5
54	6
55–56	6.5
57–58	7
59	7.5
60	8

This score is combined with the converted overall scores from the long case reporting component and the *viva voce* examination (which comprises two stations taken over 1 h). Candidates will be given a score of 4–8 in each of the four components, of which the pass mark in each section is 6, giving an overall pass mark of 24.

Additionally, candidates must obtain a mark of 6 (or above) in *at least* two of the four sections to pass the FRCR 2B examination overall.

All candidates should aim for a minimum score of 54/60 (90%) in the Rapid Reporting component to achieve a converted overall mark of 6. Whilst this component is thought of as the most difficult, it is possible for candidates to score full marks and receive a converted overall mark of 8. This can contribute significantly to the final overall score when combined with the scores from the long case reporting and *viva voce* examination stations, emphasising the importance of scoring highly in the Rapid Reporting component.

We encourage candidates to read *all* available Examiners Reports in preparation for their upcoming examination sitting, in particular, the Spring 2021 report which provides example answers. Candidates must be aware of the need to supply **full and accurate descriptions** so that full marks can be awarded for their responses:

https://www.rcr.ac.uk/exams-training/rcr-exams/clinical-radiology-exams/examiners-reports-radiology/

The latest information pertaining to all examination components, the format, the scoring system, allocation of marks, along with general candidate guidance can be found on the RCR website which should be checked regularly for updates. This is particularly important in light of the introduction of computer-based assessment and video conferencing for the reporting and oral components of the examination, respectively.

Hints and Tips

Revising for the FRCR 2B examination seems like a daunting task, but, as with anything, organisation and preparation are key. Below are a few hints and tips to help prepare you for your up-and-coming examination sitting:

- Treat the examination as if you were at work and report the radiographs as you would in daily practice.
- Before the exam, report as many radiographs as possible and get them checked by consultant radiologists. This is the only way to receive feedback on your practice and to identify areas for development. Where areas for improvement have been identified, report more of these radiographs and get them checked.
- Best practice, both in the examination and in clinical practice, is to state the side of the abnormality. Given the time limitations in the examination, L and R can be typed in place of 'left' and 'right', respectively. Additionally, typing # in place of 'fracture' is acceptable and will also save time.
- Develop review areas for each body part: there are a number of resources and 'checklists' available online.
- If unsure, denote the radiograph as 'normal'.
- Completing each test in this book within the allotted 35 min (be strict with the timing) will give you the realistic practice needed to succeed in this component of the examination.

Good luck!

Further Reading

The Royal College of Radiologists, accessed February 2023:

- Final FRCR Part B Examination. https://www.rcr.ac.uk/exams-training/rcr-exams/clinical-radiology-exams/frcr-part-2b-radiology-cr2b/
- Final FRCR Part B Examination–Purpose of Assessment Statement. https://www.rcr.ac.uk/exams-training/rcr-exams/clinical-radiology-exams/frcr-part-2b-radiology-cr2b/frcr-part-2b-radiology-purpose-of-assessment-statement/
- Final Examination for the Fellowship in Clinical Radiology (Part B)–Guidance Notes for Candidates. https://www.rcr.ac.uk/exams-training/rcr-exams/clinical-radiology-exams/frcr-part-2b-radiology-cr2b/frcr-part-2b-radiology-guidance-notes-for-candidates/
- Final Examination for the Fellowship in Clinical Radiology (Part B)–Scoring System. https://www.rcr.ac.uk/exams-training/rcr-exams/clinical-radiology-exams/frcr-part-2b-radiology-cr2b/frcr-part-2b-radiology-cr2b-scoring-system/
- Final FRCR Part B Examination Board–Examiners Reports. https://www.rcr.ac.uk/exams-training/rcr-exams/clinical-radiology-exams/examiners-reports-radiology/

Contents

About the Authors

Michael Paddock is a Fellow in Paediatric Radiology at Perth Children's Hospital, Australia, and a Senior Clinical Lecturer at the University of Sheffield and the University of Western Australia (UWA).

He completed an EPSRC-funded Biomedical Imaging MSc during his undergraduate medical training at Guy's, King's & St Thomas' School of Medicine at King's College London. He went on to clinical paediatric training on the North-West London rotation including a post at Great Ormond Street Hospital for Children.

Subsequently, he completed an NIHR Academic Clinical Fellowship in Clinical Radiology at the University of Sheffield conducting research into fetal brain development using *in utero* MRI whilst successfully completing his postgraduate clinical radiology training and attaining the FRCR. He has numerous first author publications and has won several national and international research awards. He is currently working towards a PhD in the radiological investigation of suspected physical child abuse supervised by Professor Amaka C. Offiah.

He holds postgraduate certificates in Clinical Research, Medical Education and Advanced Child Protection Studies, alongside the Diploma in Legal Medicine from the Faculty of Forensic & Legal Medicine of the Royal College of Physicians. He is one of only a handful of individuals internationally to have been awarded the inaugural European Diploma in Paediatric Radiology administered by the European Society of Paediatric Radiology, and is a Fellow of both the Higher Education Academy and the Academy of Medical Educators.

Caoilfhionn Ní Leidhin is a Fellow in Paediatric Radiology at Perth Children's Hospital, Australia.

She received her undergraduate medical degree from University College Dublin, Ireland. Following several years of postgraduate clinical work, she obtained a role as a Lecturer/Registrar in Radiology with Trinity College Dublin. During this time, she conducted research on arterial spin labelling magnetic resonance imaging leading to an MD (Res). She completed her first 4 years of specialist training in clinical radiology at St. James's Hospital, Dublin, successfully completing the FFR RCSI examinations, which was followed by a final year of subspecialty paediatric radiology training at Children's Health Ireland.

She has several first author publications and has delivered numerous national and international presentations. She has previously served as Vice-Chair of the Faculty of Radiology Trainee Committee, Ireland.

Amaka C. Offiah is Chair of Paediatric Musculoskeletal Imaging at the University of Sheffield and an Honorary Consultant Paediatric Radiologist at Sheffield Children's NHS Foundation Trust.

After completing radiology training in Sheffield, she worked at Great Ormond Street Hospital for Children where she obtained her PhD in the imaging of suspected inflicted injury at the Institute of Child Health, University College London. She returned to Sheffield as a HEFCE-funded Clinical Senior Lecturer and was promoted to Professor in 2020. She is a Fellow of the Higher Education Academy.

In addition to over 200 original scientific publications, over 35 peer-reviewed review articles and 15 book chapters, she has co-authored two 'Highly Commended' textbooks: *A Radiological Atlas of Child Abuse* and *Fetal and Perinatal Skeletal Dysplasias: An Atlas of Multimodality Imaging*.

She is currently Managing Editor (Outside Americas) for *Pediatric Radiology*, the leading international peer-reviewed paediatric radiology medical journal, and was the first female and first paediatric radiologist to be appointed the Royal College of Radiologists Roentgen Professor. She is Chairperson of the ESPR Child Abuse Taskforce, Convenor for the Skeletal Dysplasia Group for Teaching and Research and has been an expert witness for the courts in over 500 cases of suspected child abuse.

Abbreviations

ABC	Aneurysmal bone cyst
ACJ	Acromioclavicular joint
AFP	Alpha-fetoprotein
AIIS	Anterior inferior iliac spine
ALL	Acute lymphoblastic leukaemia
ALTE	Apparent life-threatening event
AP	Anteroposterior
ARCO	Association Research Circulation Osseous
ARPKD	Autosomal recessive polycystic kidney disease
ASIS	Anterior superior iliac spine
AVN	Avascular necrosis
BBI	Button battery ingestion
BRUE	Brief resolved unexplained event
β hCG	Beta human chorionic gonadotropin
CCAM	Congenital cystic adenomatoid malformation
CDH	Congenital diaphragmatic hernia
CF	Cystic fibrosis
CHD	Congenital heart disease
CLE	Congenital lobar emphysema
CLO	Congenital lobar overinflation
CMCJ	Carpometacarpal joint
CML	Classic metaphyseal lesion
CMV	Cytomegalovirus
CPAM	Congenital pulmonary airway malformation
CRMO	Chronic recurrent multifocal osteomyelitis
CSF	Cerebrospinal fluid
CT	Computed tomography
CTPA	Computed tomography pulmonary angiogram
DA	Ductus arteriosus
DDH	Developmental dysplasia of the hip
DGH	District General Hospital
DIOS	Distal intestinal obstruction syndrome
DJ	Duodenojejunal
DRUJ	Distal radioulnar joint

ED	Emergency Department
ESWL	Extracorporeal shock wave lithotripsy
ETT	Endotracheal tube
FCD	Fibrous cortical defect
FDG	Fluorodeoxyglucose
FGFR3	Fibroblast growth factor gene 3
FOOSH	Fall onto an outstretched hand
FRCR	Fellowship of the Royal College of Radiologists
GAS	Group A *Streptococcus*
GCT	Giant cell tumour
GI	Gastrointestinal
GP	General practitioner
HIV	Human immunodeficiency virus
HMD	Hyaline membrane disease
HME	Hereditary multiple exostoses
IJV	Internal jugular vein
IO	Intraosseous
ITU	Intensive therapy unit
IV	Intravenous
IVC	Inferior vena cava
LCH	Langerhans cell histiocytosis
MCDK	Multicystic dysplastic kidney
MIBG	Metaiodobenzylguanidine
MPR	Multiplanar reconstructions
MPS	Mucopolysaccharidosis
MRI	Magnetic resonance imaging
NAI	Non-accidental injury
NEC	Necrotising enterocolitis
NGT	Nasogastric tube
NICE	National Institute for Health and Care Excellence
NICU	Neonatal Intensive Care Unit
NOF	Non-ossifying fibroma
NRSTS	Non-rhabdomyosarcoma soft-tissue sarcoma
NSAID	Non-steroidal anti-inflammatory drug
OA	Oesophageal atresia
OCD	Osteochondral defect
OI	Osteogenesis imperfecta
OPG	Orthopantomogram
ORIF	Open reduction and internal fixation
PACS	Picture archiving and communication system
PDA	Patent ductus arteriosus
PET-CT	Positron emission tomography-computed tomography
PPB	Pleuropulmonary blastoma
pPNET	Peripheral primitive neuroectodermal tumour
PSIS	Posterior superior iliac spine

PUJO Pelviureteric junction obstruction
RCR Royal College of Radiologists
RDS Respiratory distress syndrome
RTA Road traffic accident
SCBU Special Care Baby Unit
SCFE Slipped capital femoral epiphysis
SDD Surfactant deficiency disorder
SH Salter-Harris
SLE Systemic lupus erythematosus
SPA Suspected physical abuse
SPNBF Subperiosteal new bone formation
ssp. subspecies
SUFE Slipped upper femoral epiphysis
TEF Tracheo-esophageal fistula (in the USA)
TFCC Triangular fibrocartilage complex
TOF Tracheo-oesophageal fistula (in the UK)
TORCH Toxoplasmosis; Others (HIV, syphilis); Rubella; Cytomegalovirus; Herpes Simplex
UAC Umbilical arterial catheter
UBC Unicameral bone cyst
UK United Kingdom
UVC Umbilical venous catheter
VACTERL Vertebral anomalies; Anorectal anomalies; Cardiac anomalies; Tracheo-oesophageal fistula; Renal/radial ray anomalies; Limb anomalies
VP Ventriculoperitoneal
VR Volume rendered
VSD Ventricular septal defect

Test 1

1

M. Paddock et al., *Paediatric Radiology Rapid Reporting*,
https://doi.org/10.1007/978-3-031-48255-7_1

1.1 Images

Image 1

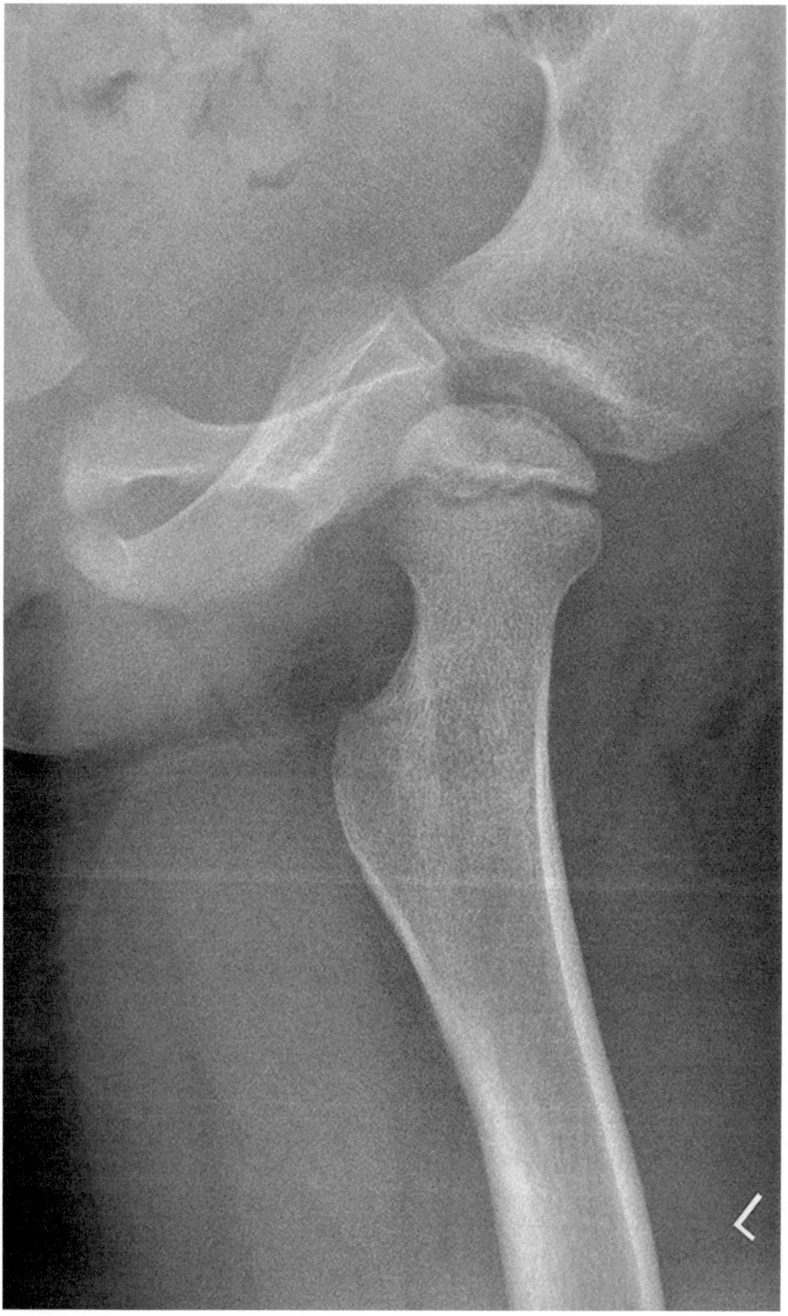

Image 2

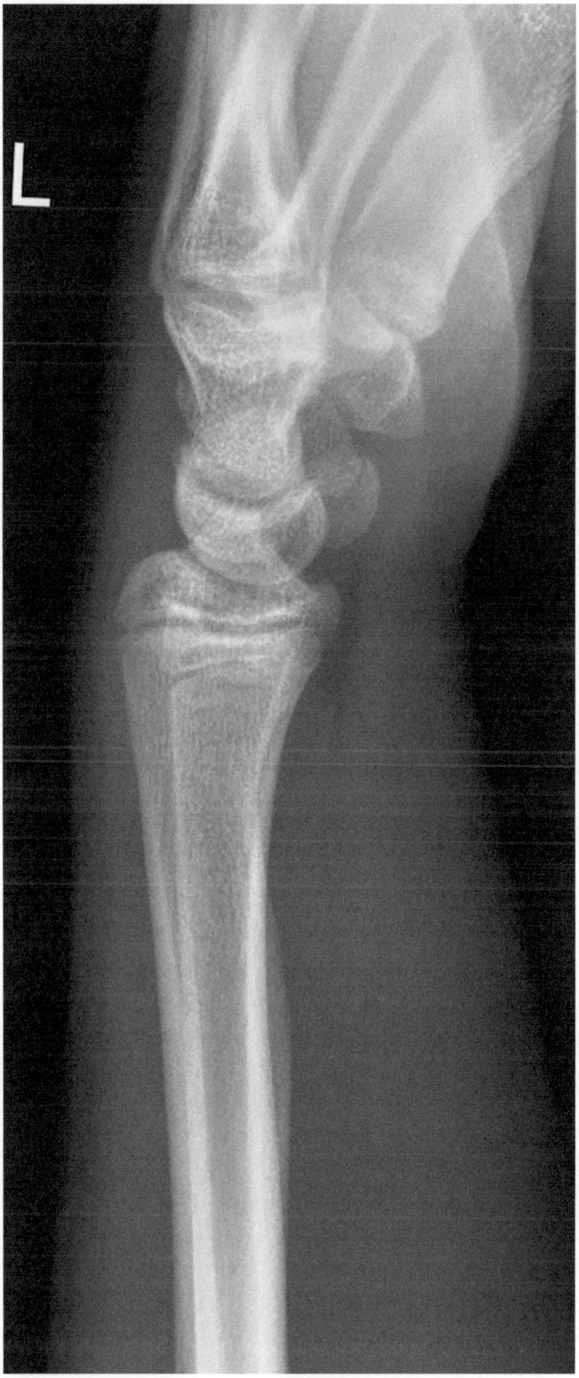

Image 3

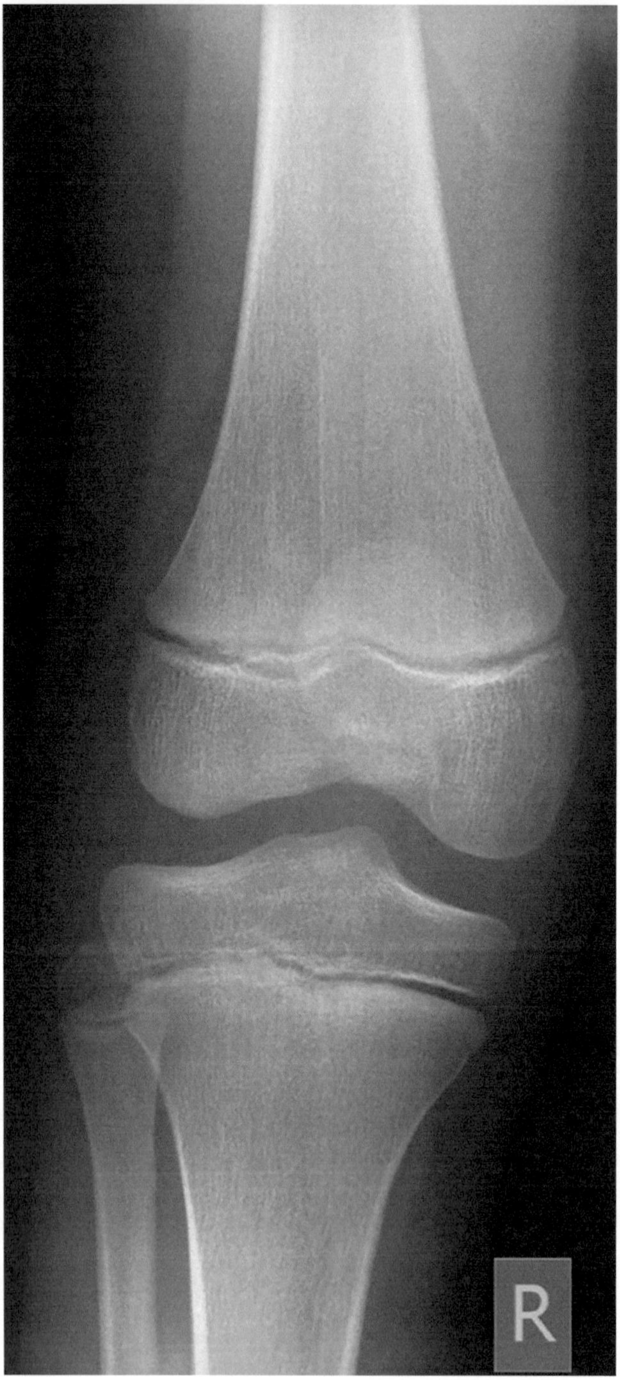

Image 4

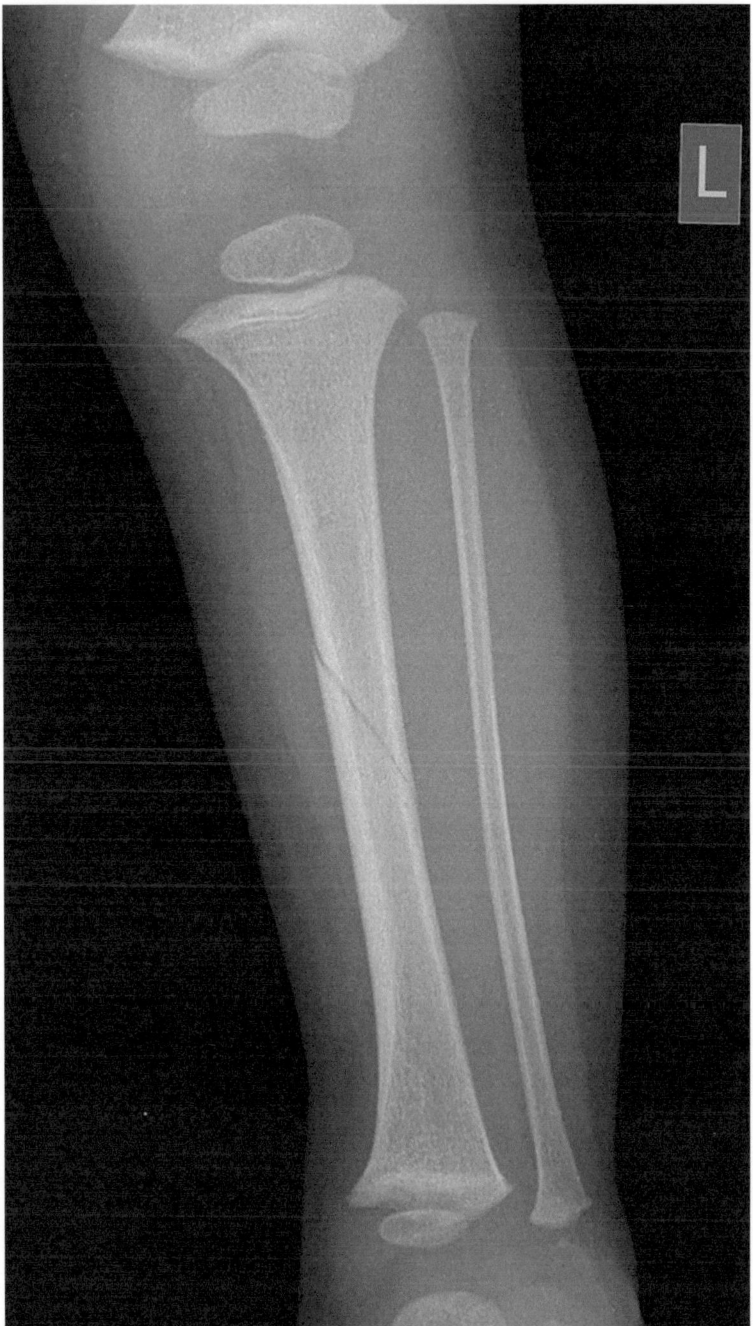

Image 5

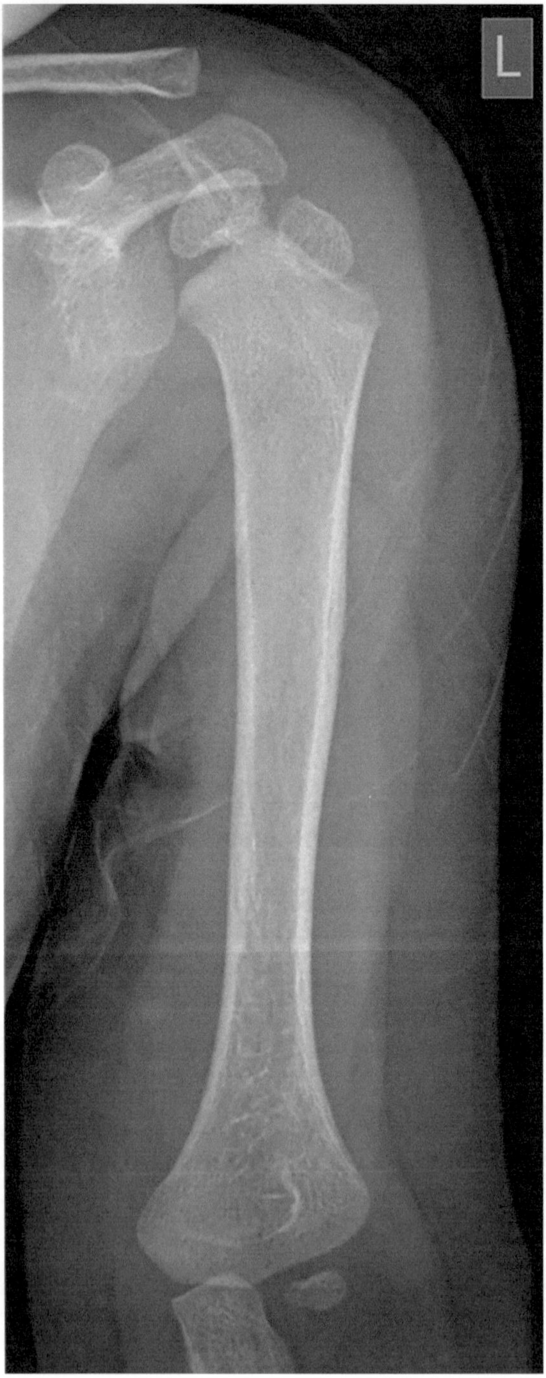

Image 6

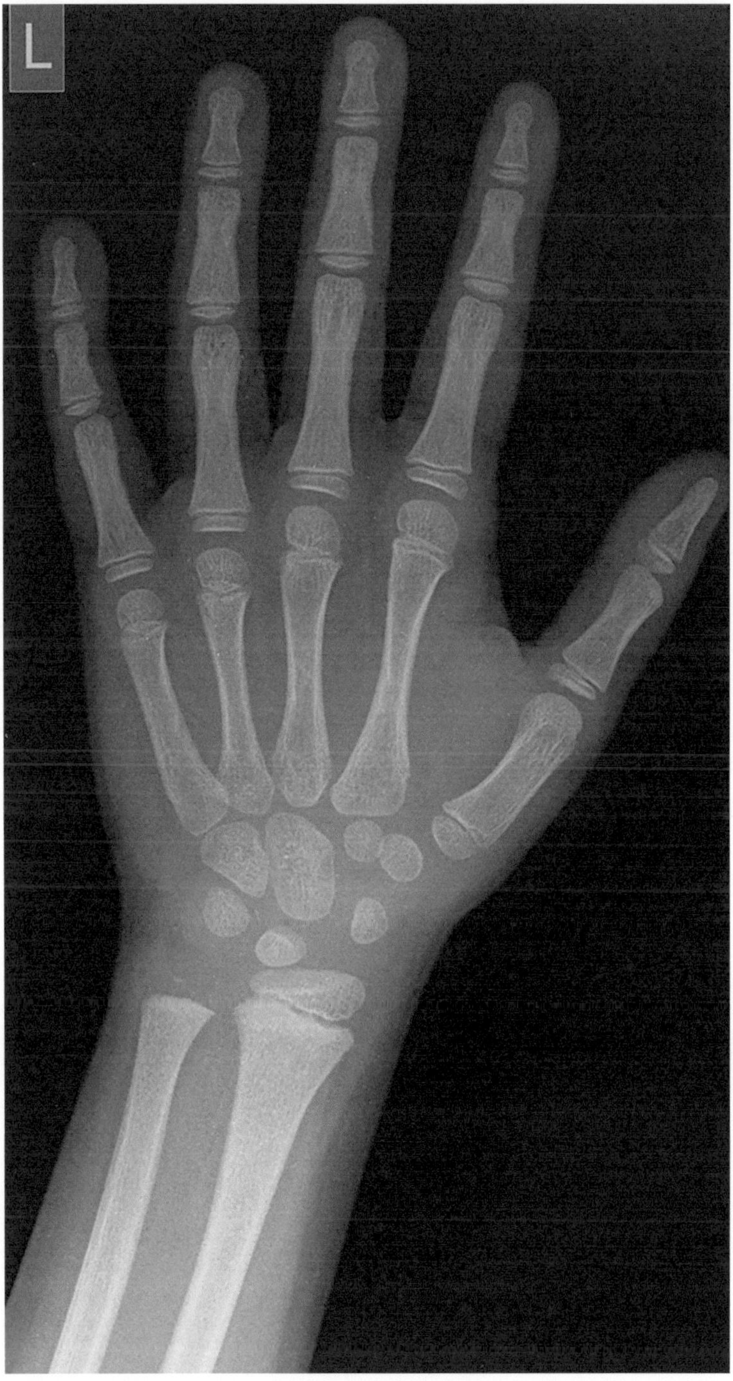

Image 7

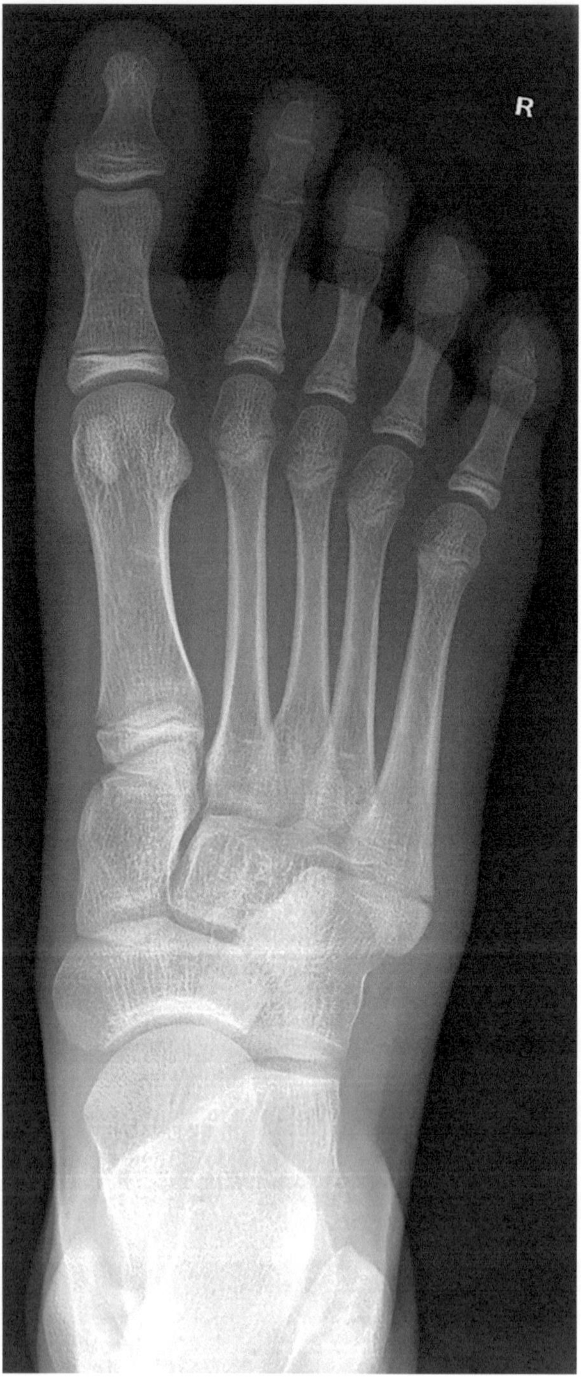

Image 8

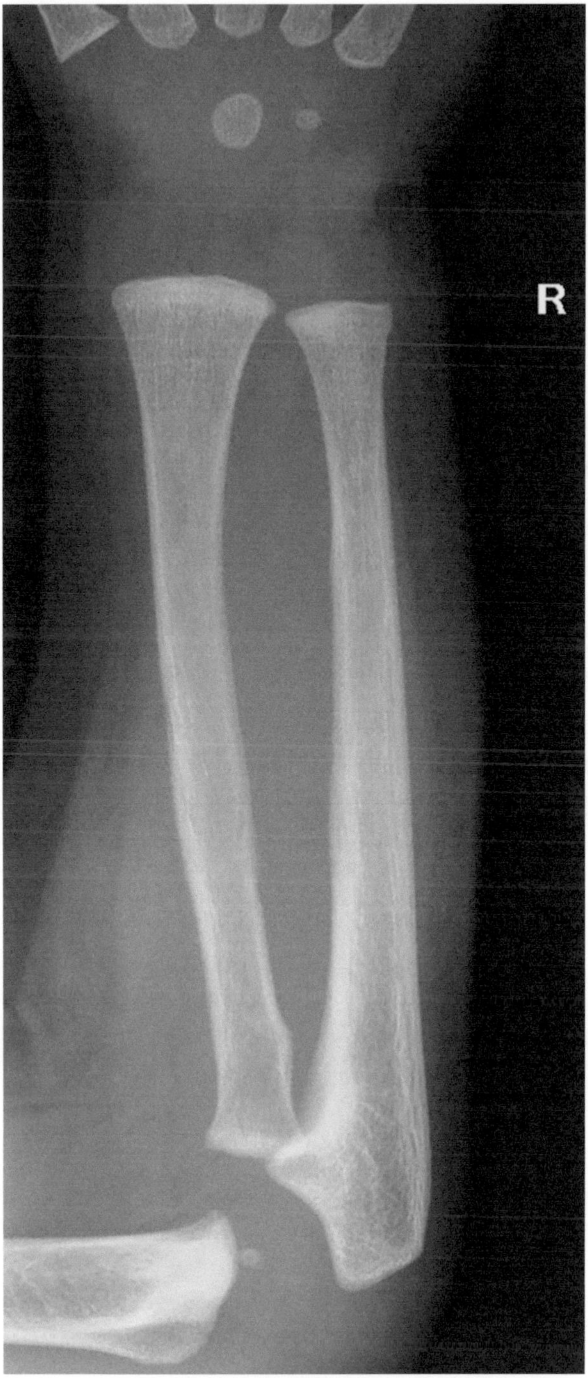

Image 9

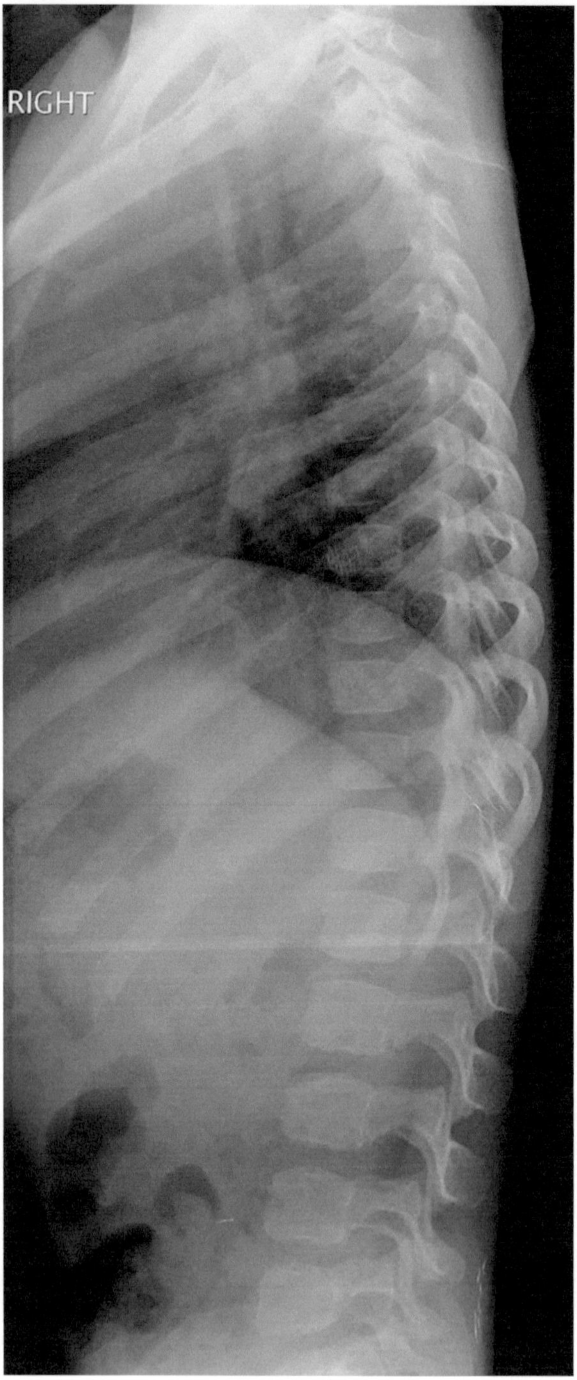

Image 10

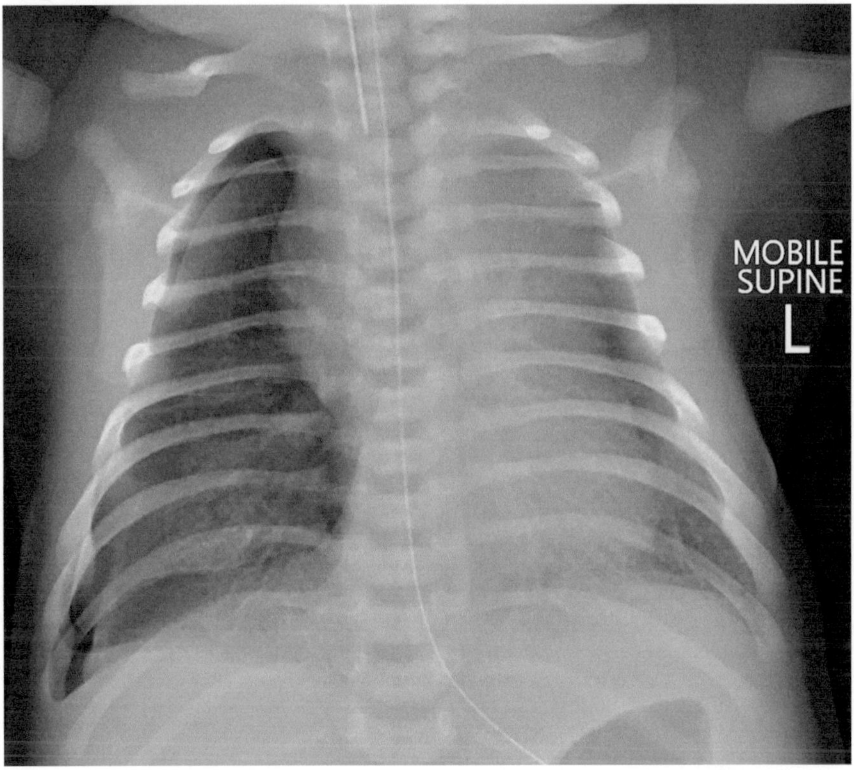

Image 11

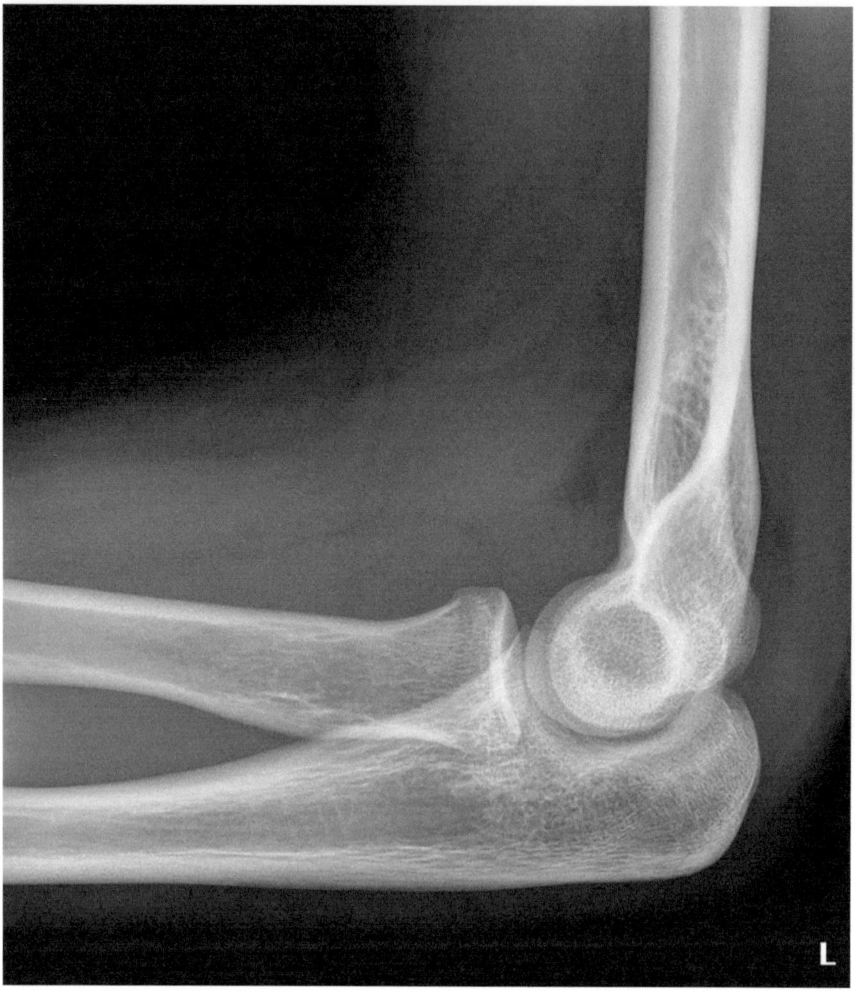

Image 12

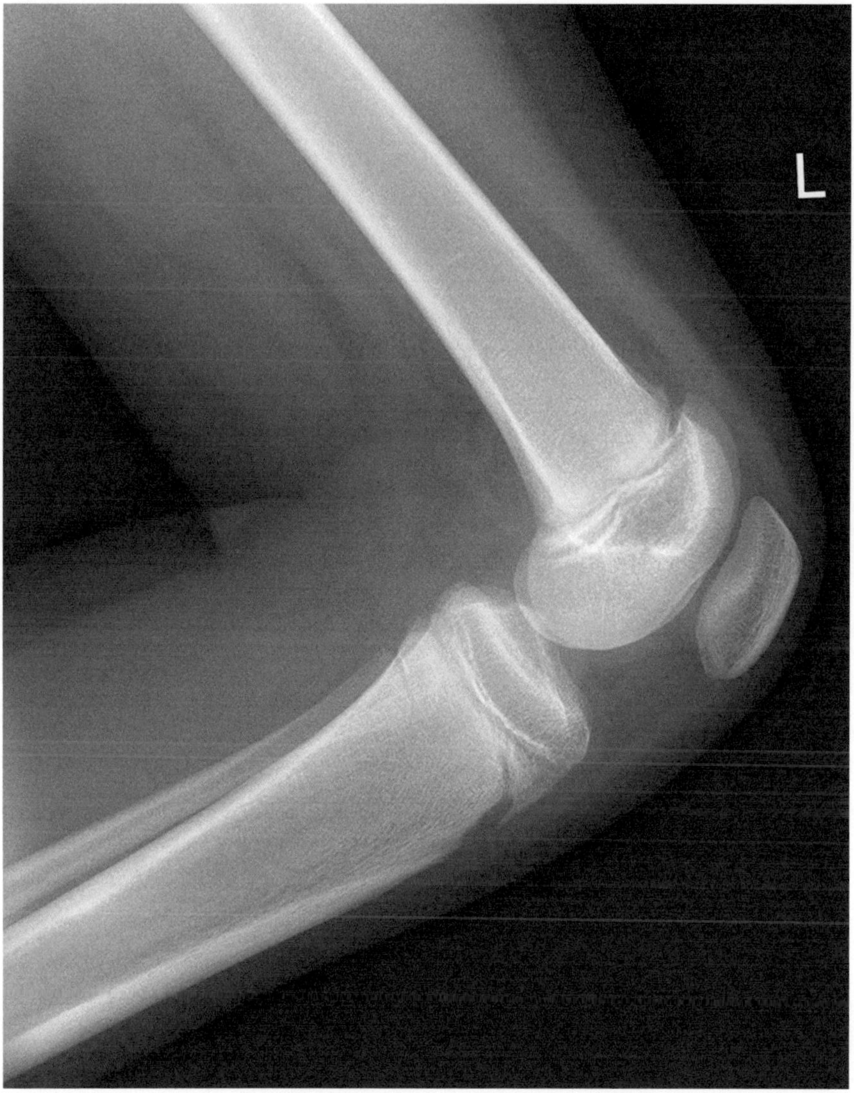

Image 13

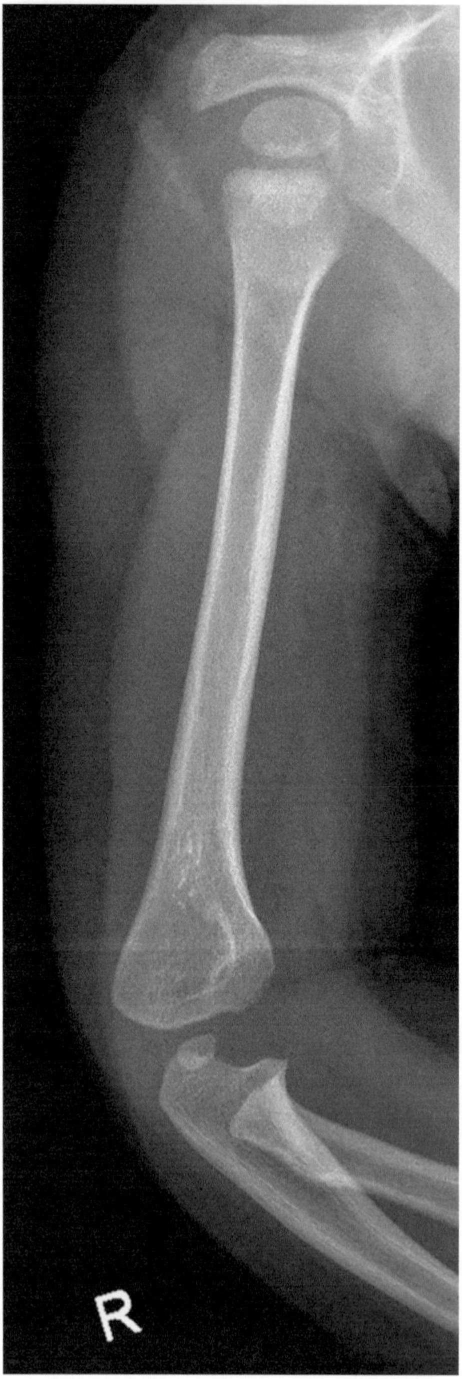

Image 14

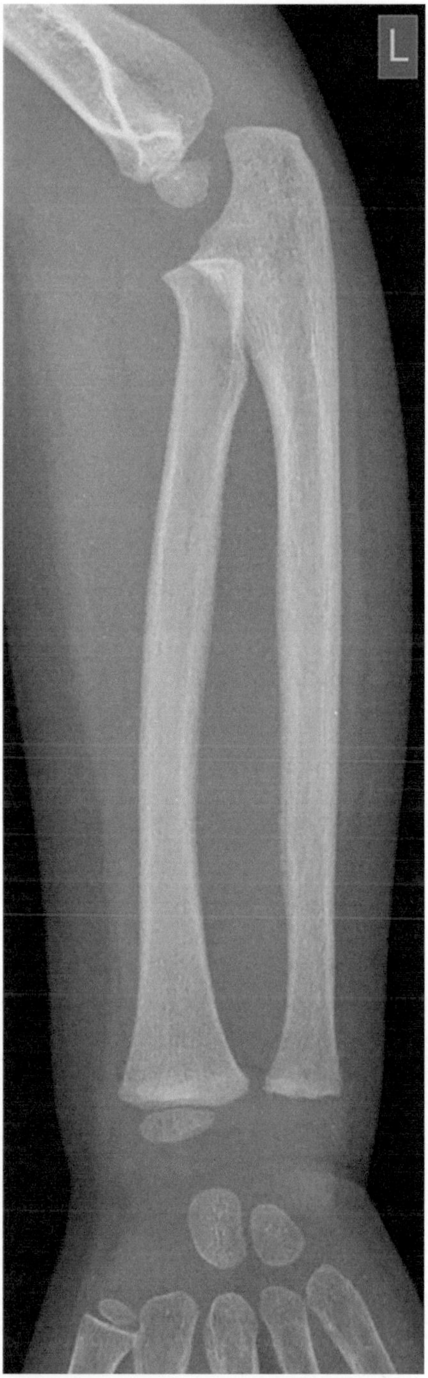

Image 15

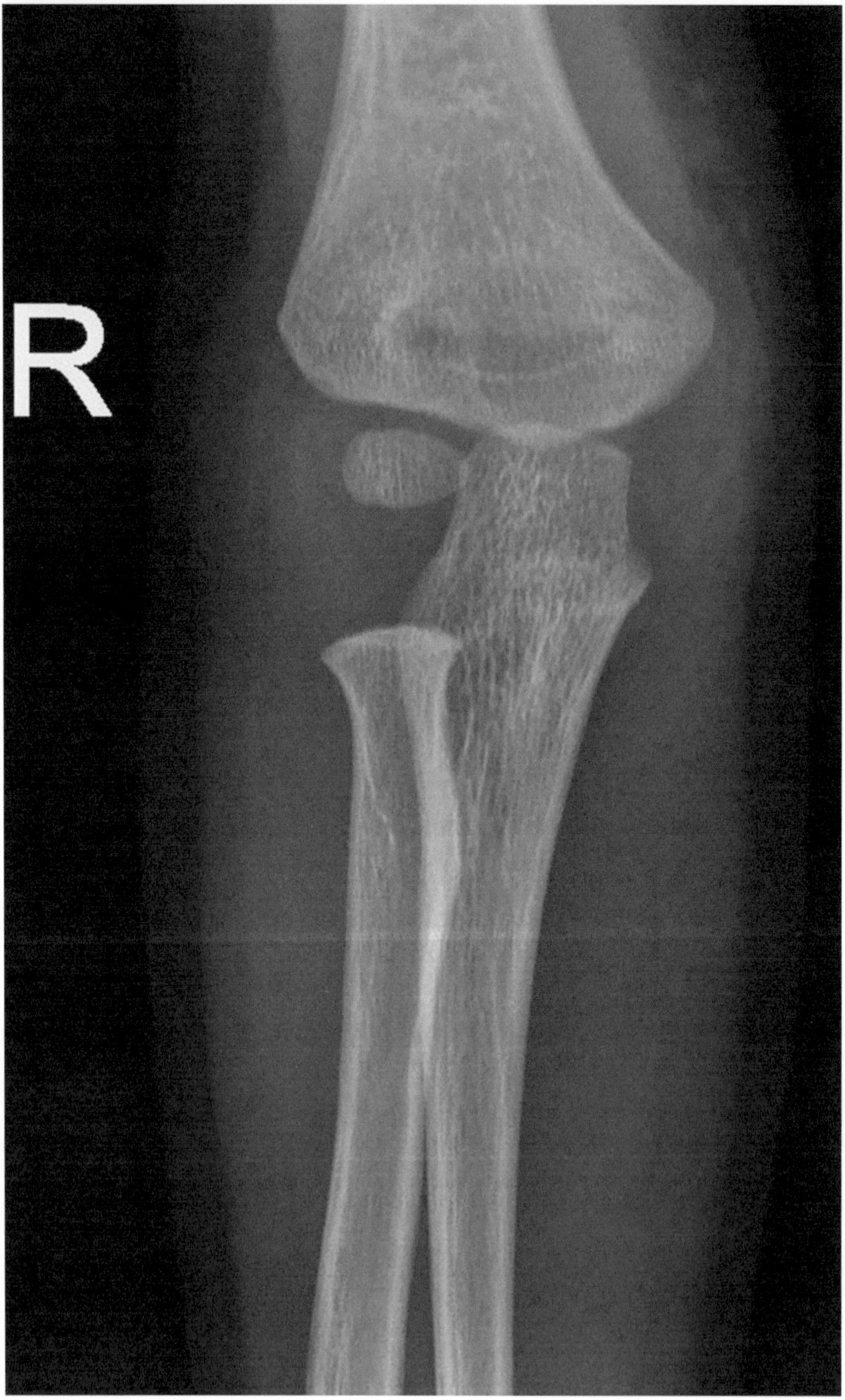

Image 16

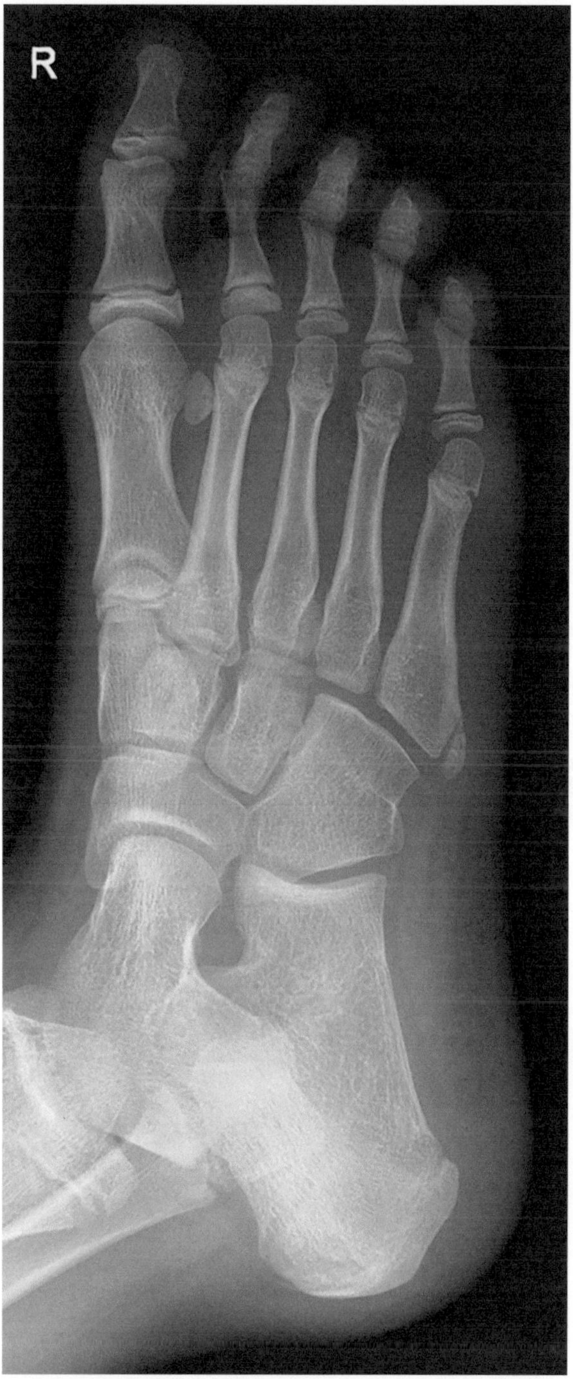

Image 17

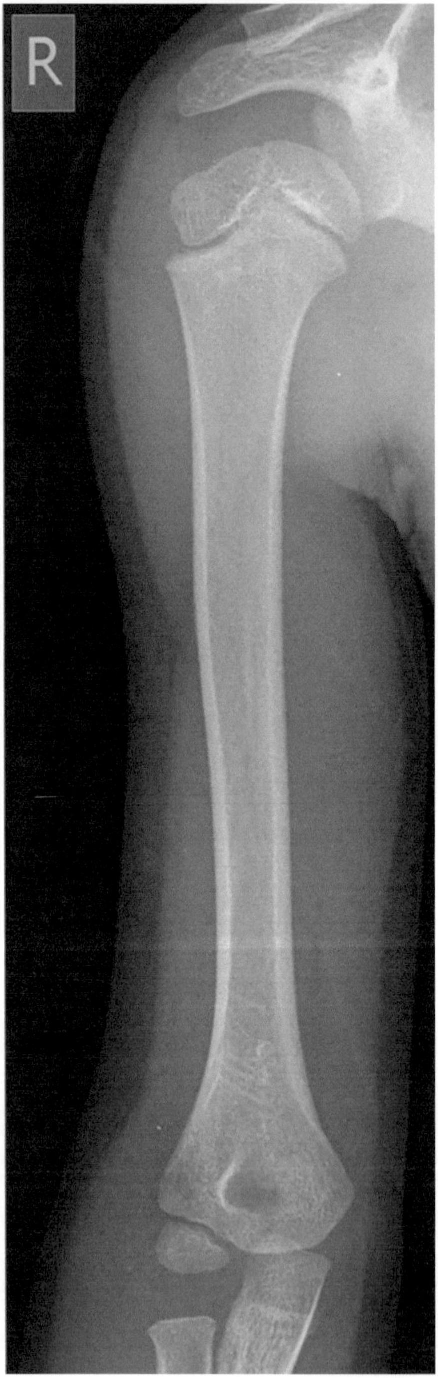

Image 18

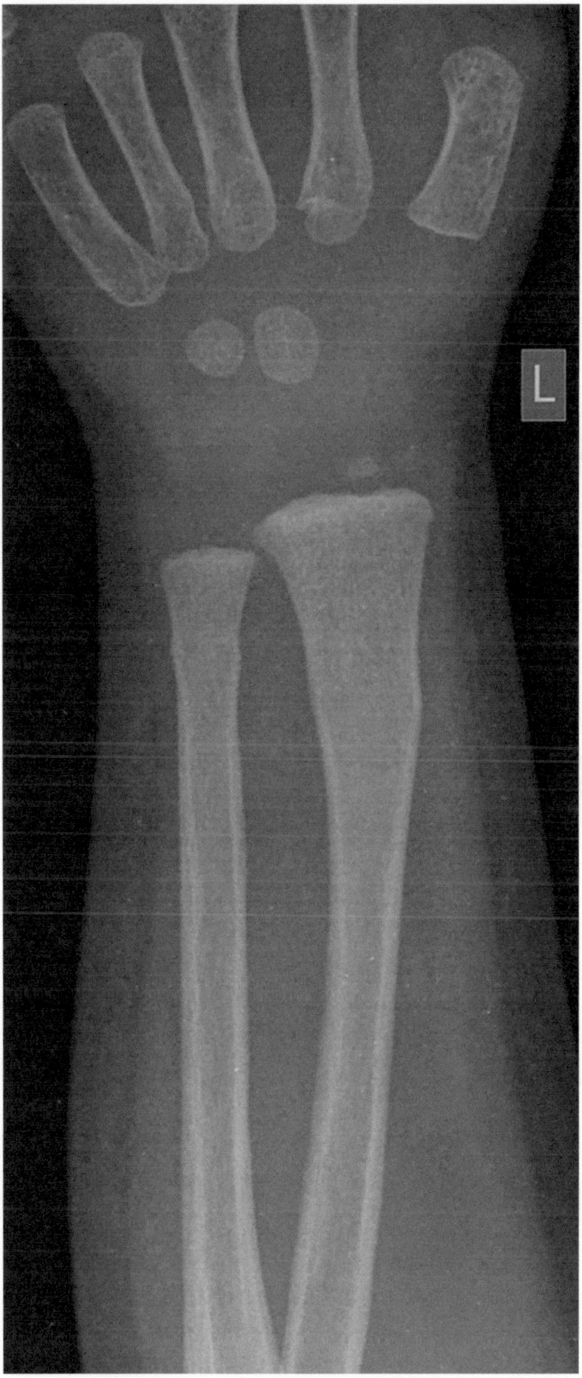

Image 19

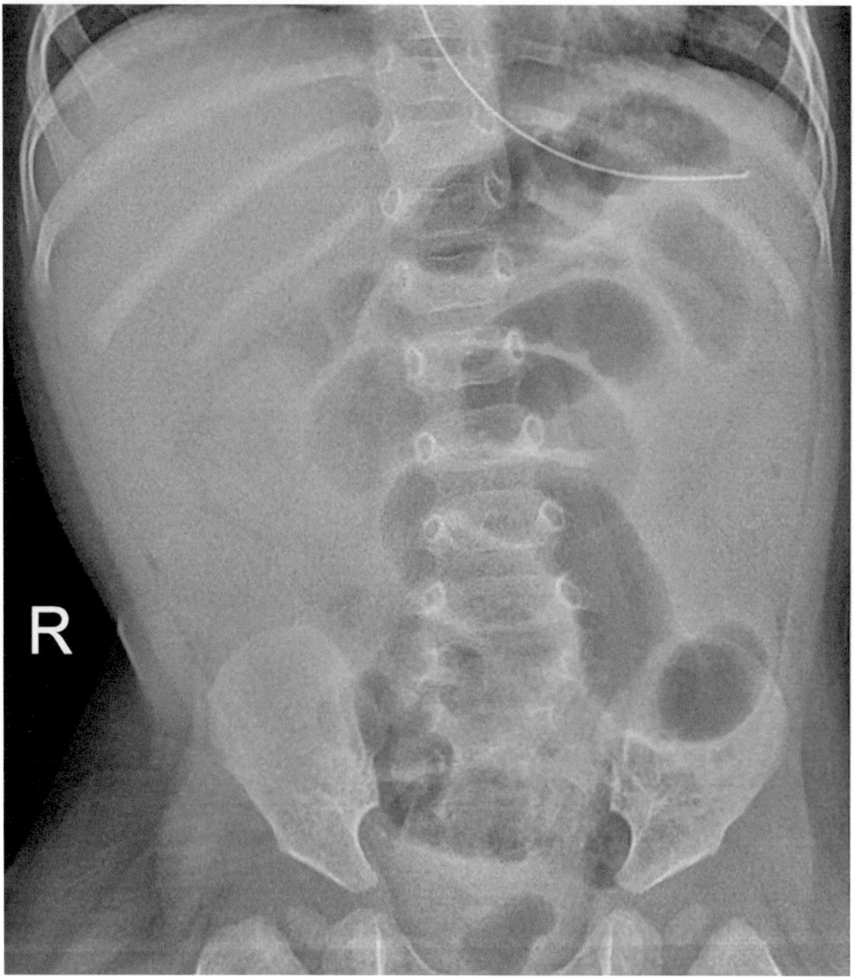

Image 20

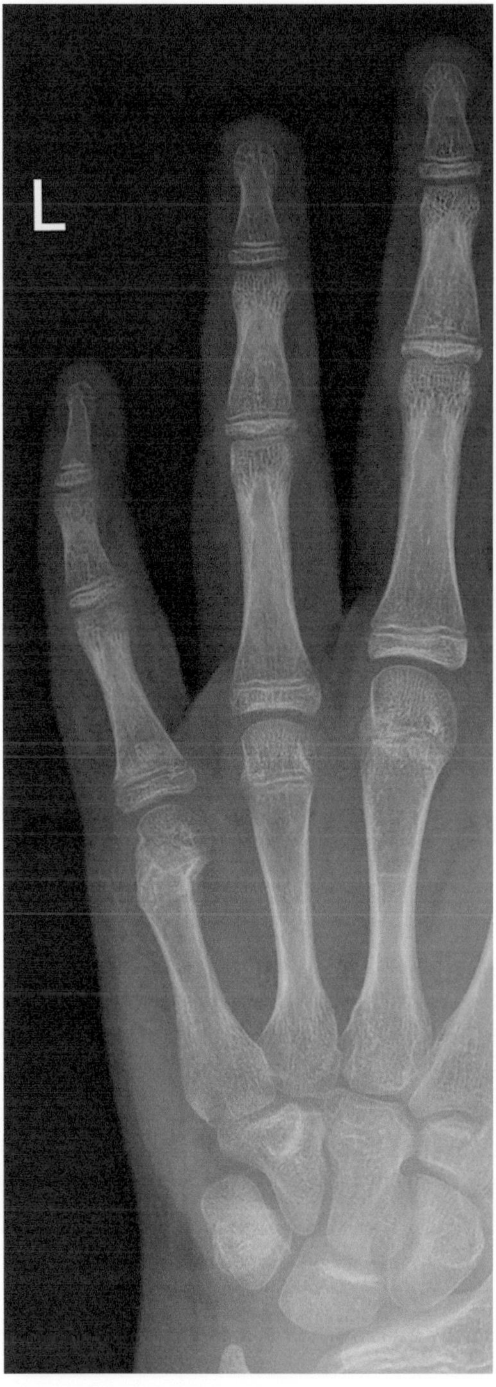

Image 21

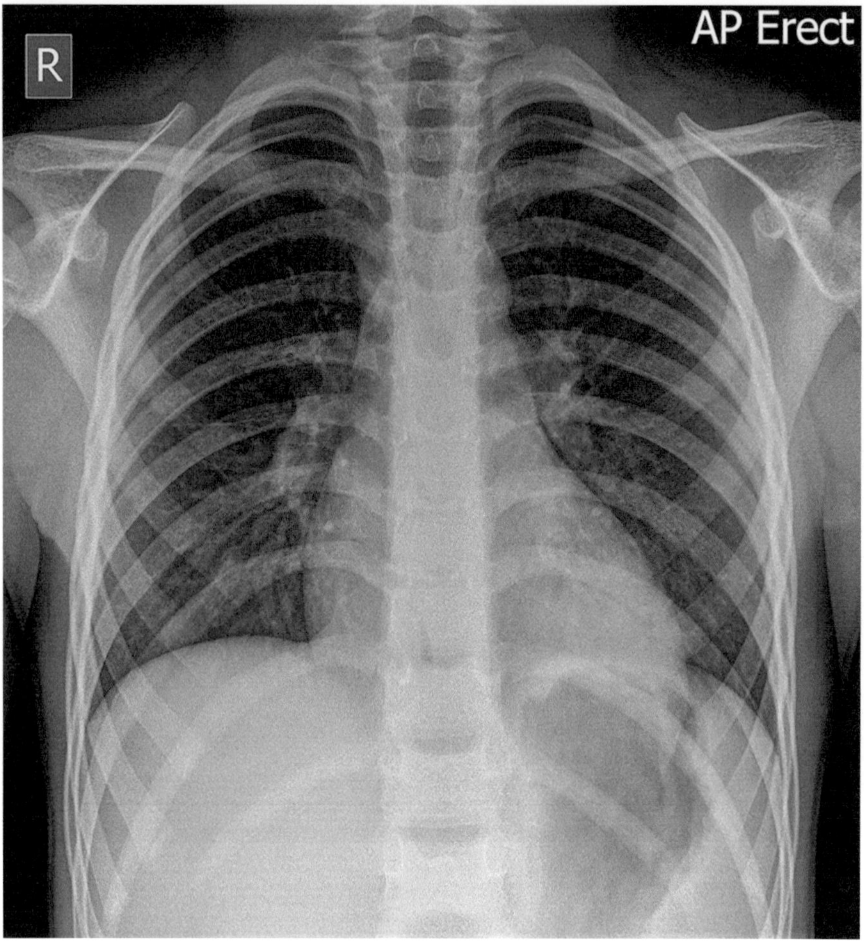

Image 22

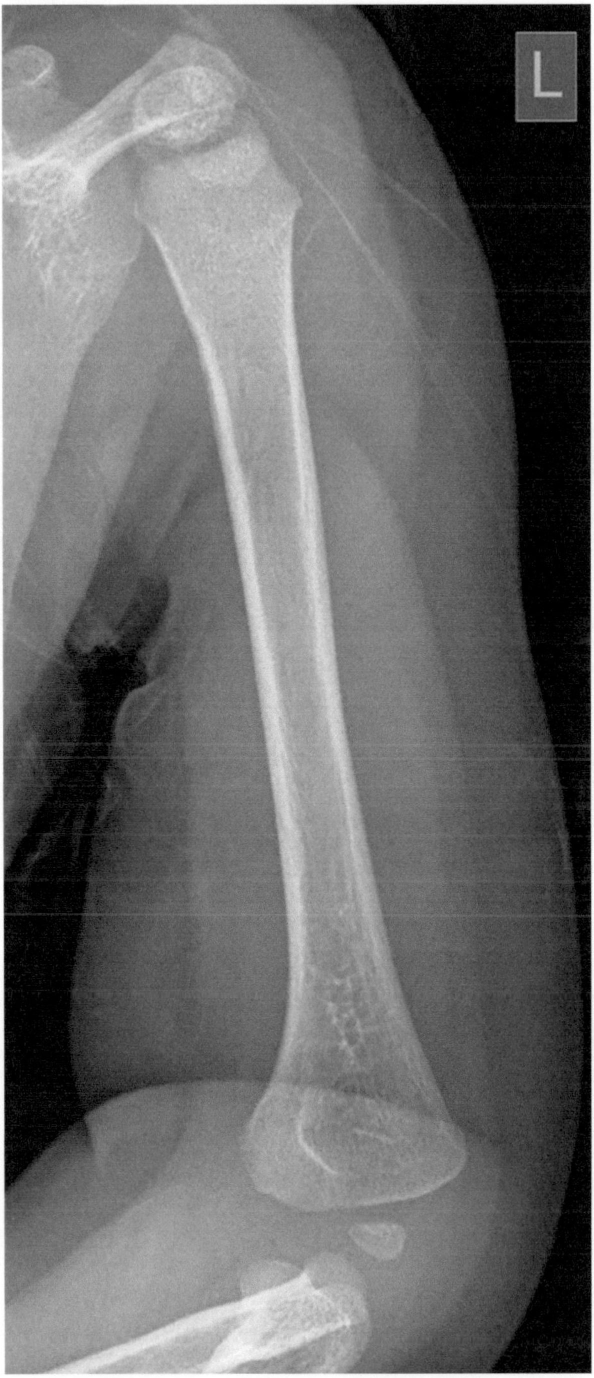

Image 23

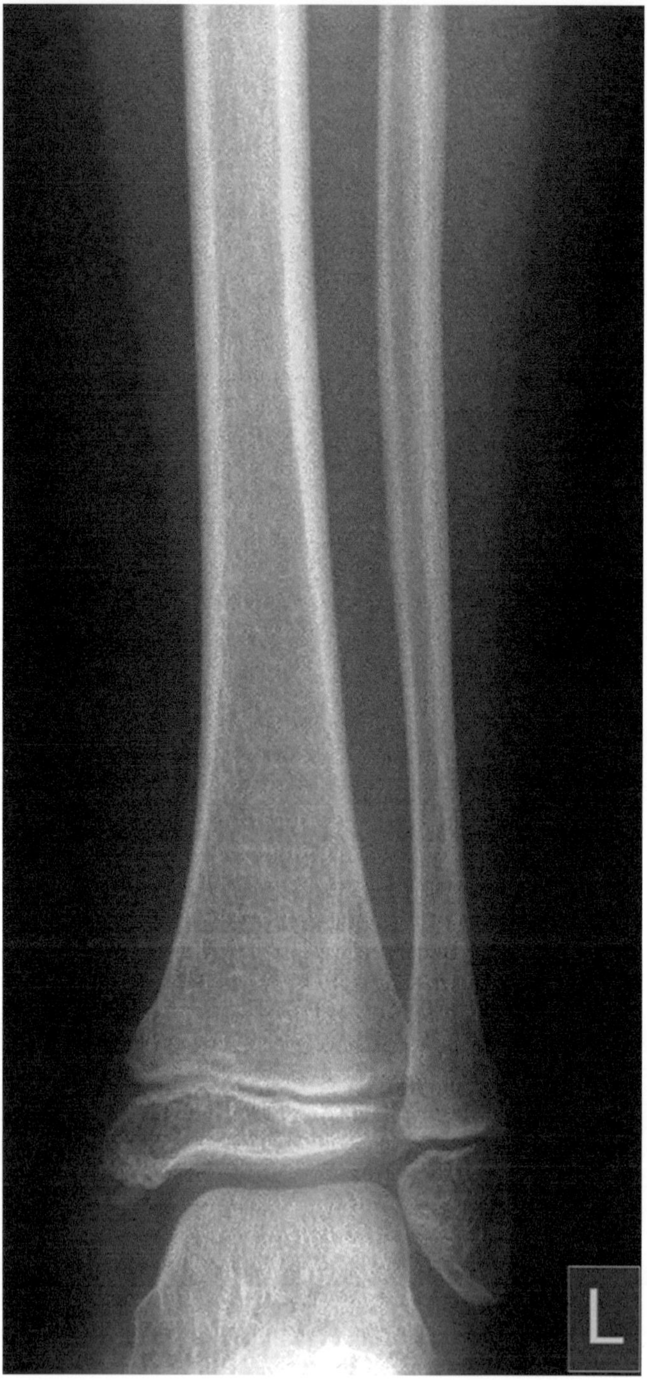

Image 24

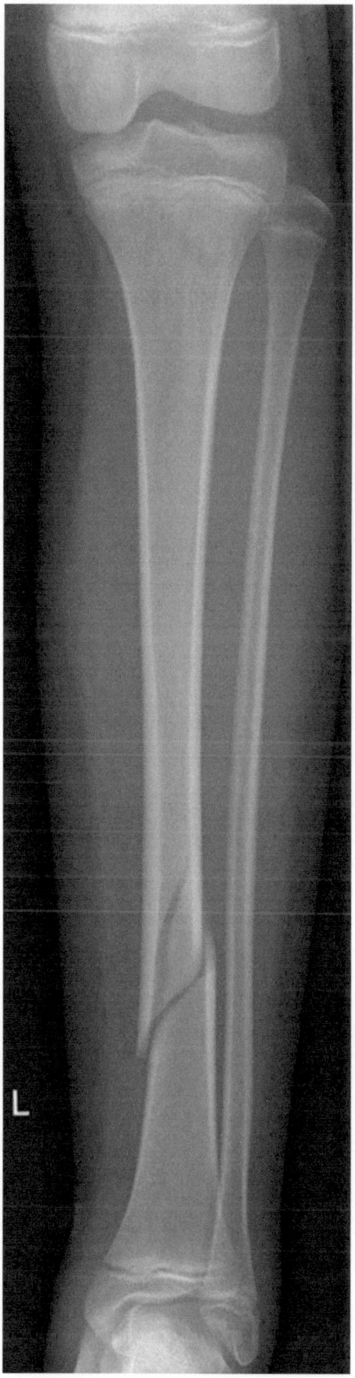

Image 25

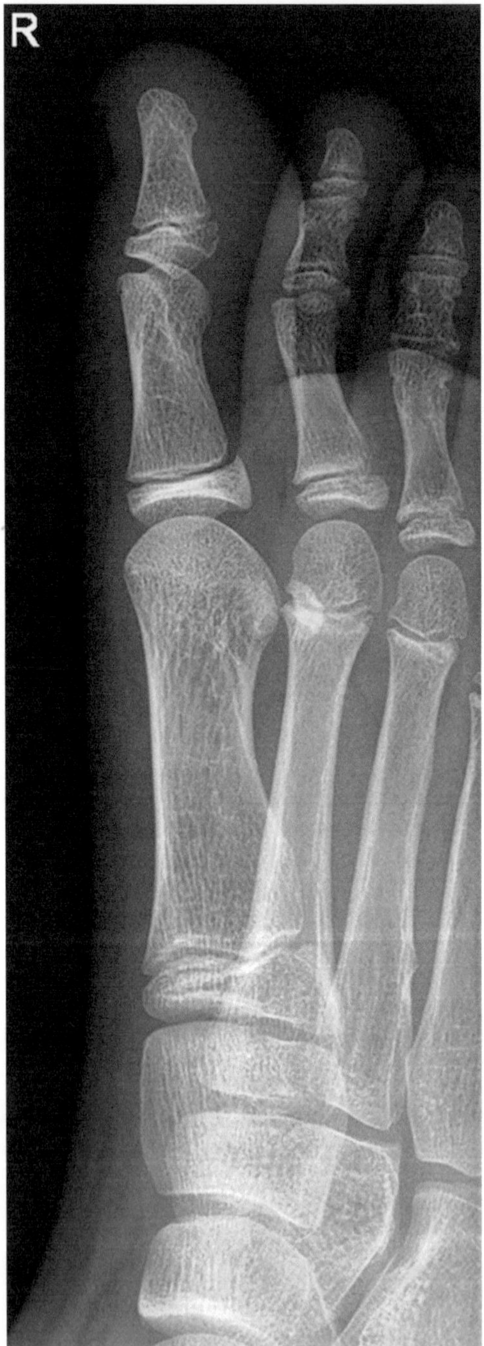

Image 26

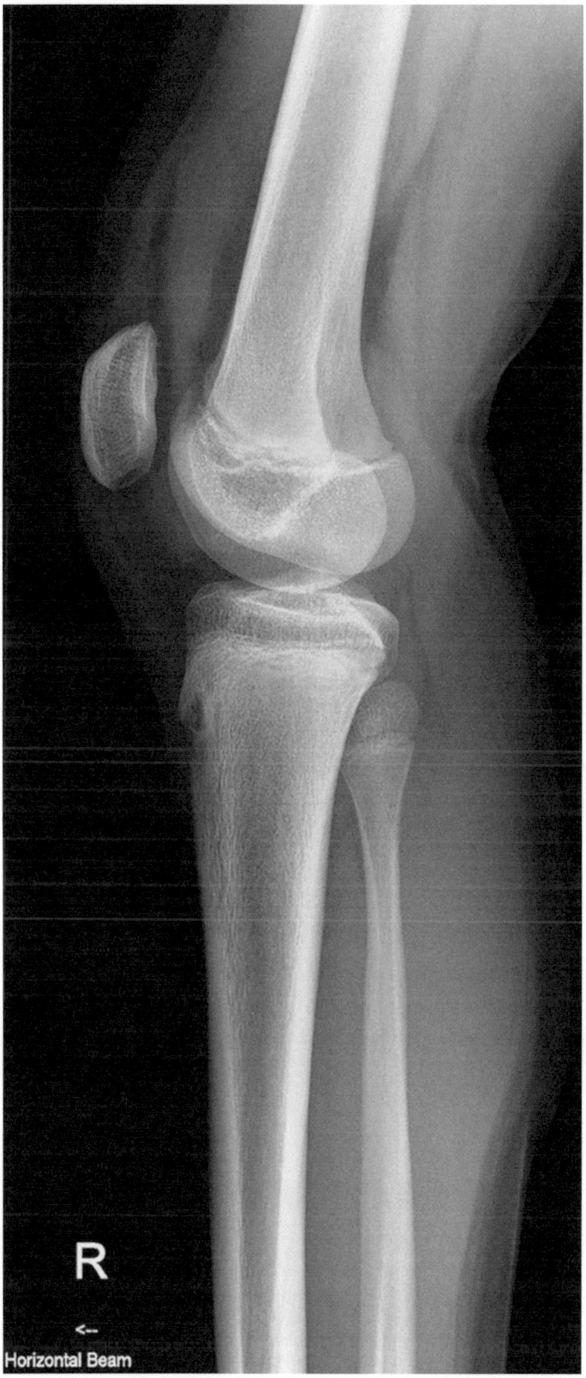

Image 27

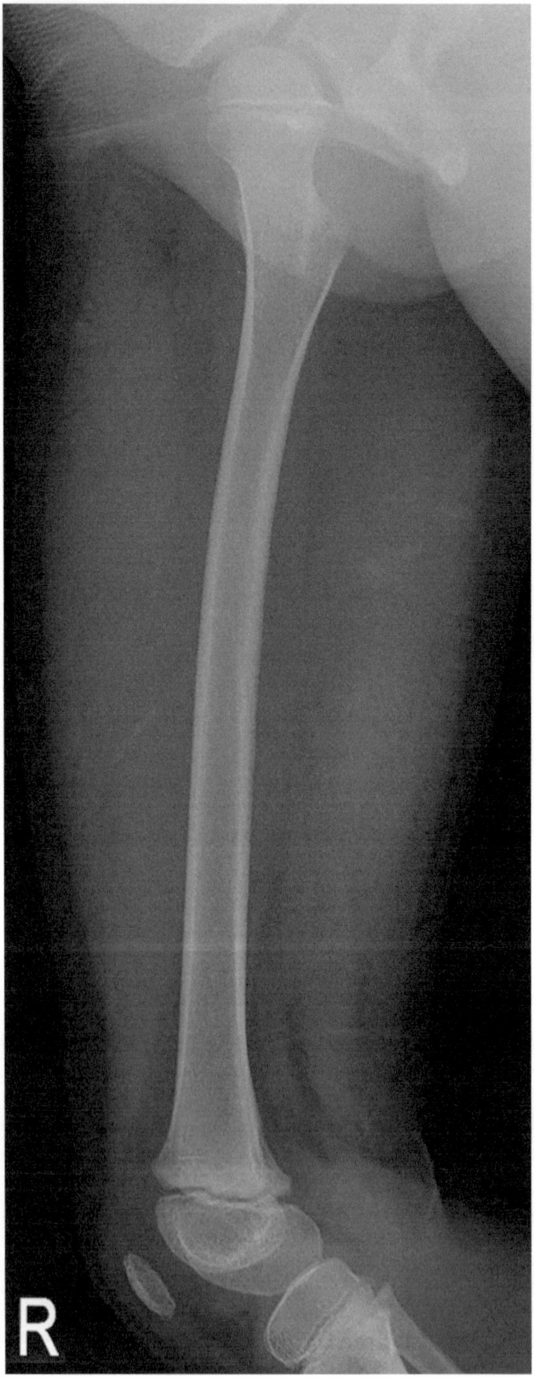

Image 28

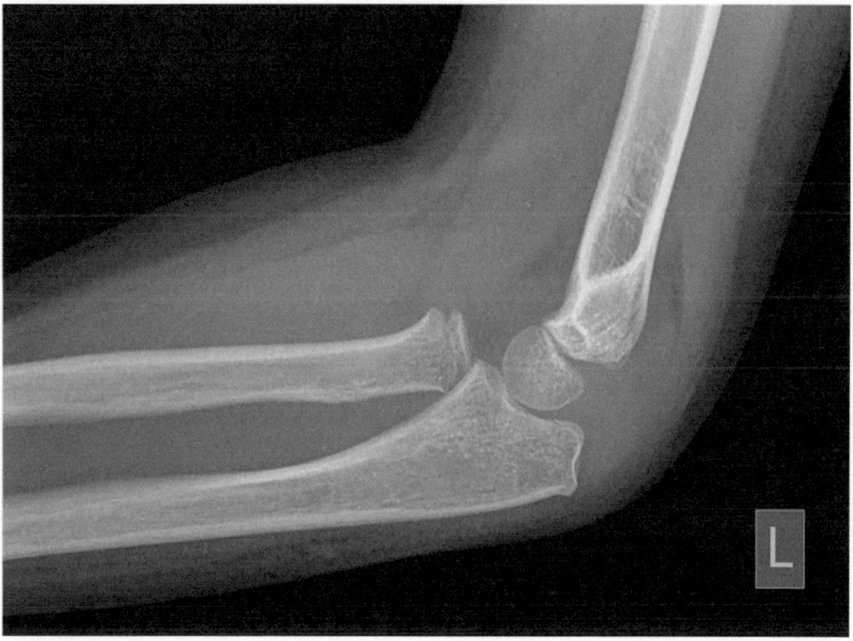

Image 29

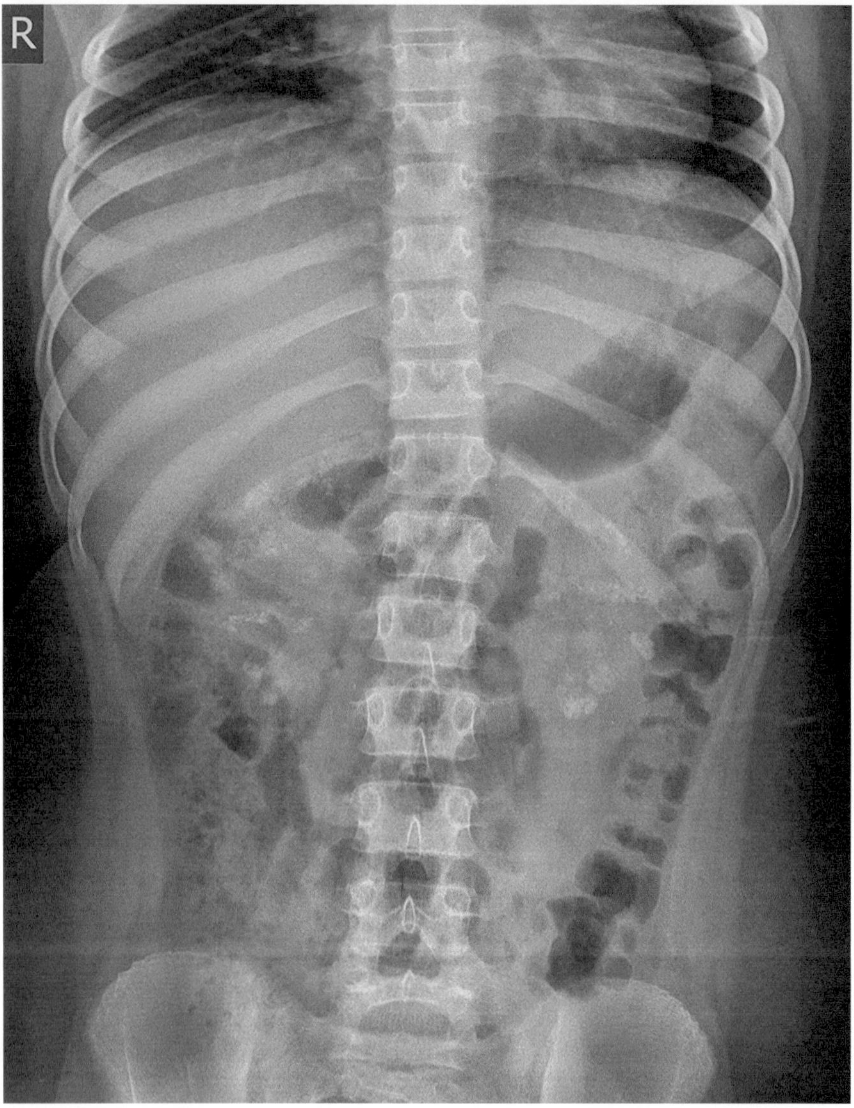

Image 30

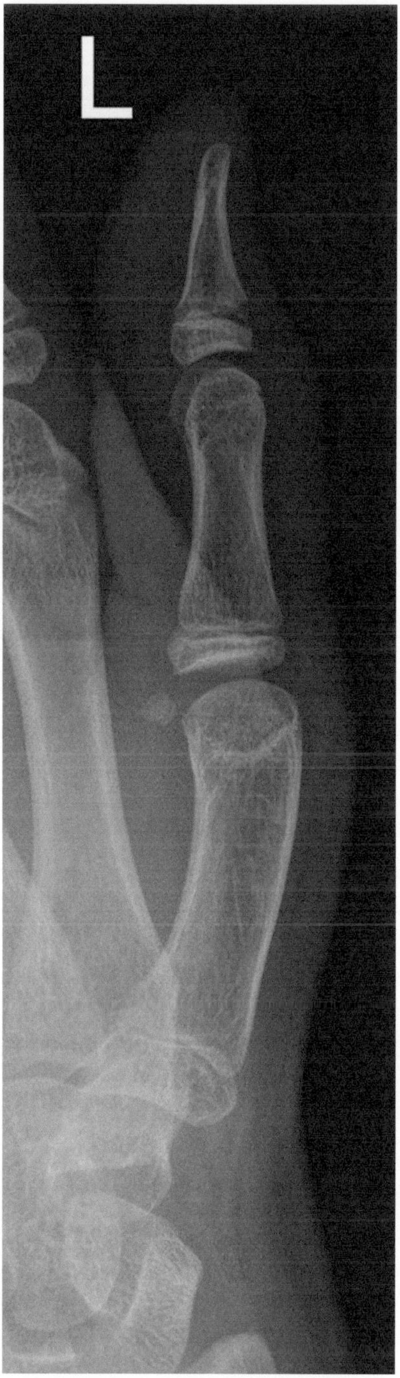

1.2 Answers

Image	Normal	Abnormal	Diagnosis/abnormality (only if abnormal)
1		✓	AVN L proximal femoral epiphysis
2	✓		
3	✓		
4		✓	Oblique # L tibial diaphysis
5	✓		
6	✓		
7		✓	# R fifth metatarsal base
8	✓		
9	✓		
10		✓	R pneumothorax
11		✓	Joint effusion L elbow
12	✓		
13	✓		
14	✓		
15		✓	# R supracondylar humerus
16	✓		
17	✓		
18		✓	Buckle #s L distal radius and ulna
19		✓	Bowel obstruction
20		✓	# L little finger metacarpal neck
21		✓	Round pneumonia L lower lobe
22	✓		
23		✓	Buckle # L distal tibial metaphysis
24		✓	#s L distal tibial diaphysis and L proximal fibular metaphysis
25	✓		
26		✓	Lipohaemarthrosis R knee
27	✓		
28		✓	Dislocation L radial head
29		✓	Bilateral nephrocalcinosis
30		✓	SH2 # L thumb distal phalanx

1.3 Explanations

1. **Avascular necrosis L proximal femoral epiphysis**
This radiograph demonstrates the subchondral lucency 'crescent sign' of avascular necrosis (AVN) in the anterolateral aspect of the left proximal femoral epiphysis. This sign heralds imminent articular collapse and represents stage 3 (of 4) in the Ficat and Arlet radiographic staging of AVN.
The cause of AVN in this case was idiopathic. Such cases are commonly known as Perthes (or Legg-Calvé-Perthes) disease, the eponymous name for idiopathic AVN of the proximal femoral epiphysis. In the examination, it would be more accurate to write 'avascular necrosis left proximal femoral epiphysis' rather than 'Perthes disease' because you will not know the underlying aetiology in the absence of clinical history.
Perthes disease is five times more common in boys with a peak incidence of around 6 years of age and it can affect children from as young as 2 years old to those aged 14 years. The majority of children present with a painful hip or limp in the absence of trauma and it is a diagnosis of exclusion. *Both* proximal femoral epiphyses may be affected in up to approximately 15% of cases but usually asymmetrically, with one side affected before the other.
The differential diagnosis of AVN is wide and is summarised by the mnemonic **PLASTIC RAGS**:
   - **P**ancreatitis; **P**regnancy.
   - **L**upus (Systemic lupus erythematosus, SLE).
   - **A**lcohol.
   - **S**teroids.
   - **T**rauma.
   - **I**diopathic; **I**nfection.
   - **C**aisson disease: also known as decompression syndrome or 'the bends'. The rapid or uncontrolled ascension from a high-pressure environment or deep-sea depth can result in the formation of intravascular nitrogen gas bubbles leading to arterial occlusion and osteonecrosis; **C**ollagen vascular/**C**onnective tissue disease.
   - **R**adiation; **R**heumatoid arthritis.
   - **A**myloid arthropathy.
   - **G**aucher disease: an autosomal recessive lysosomal storage disorder arising from a deficiency of glucocerebrosidase, which results in the accumulation of glucocerebroside within the lysosomes of macrophages in the liver, spleen, and bone marrow. As such, its most common form (type 1) presents with hepatosplenomegaly and skeletal manifestations such as pain, pathological fractures, and osteonecrosis. Consider this as a cause of AVN in the context of hepatosplenomegaly—remember to look for the Erlenmeyer flask deformity in the femur (relative constriction of the diaphysis and flaring of the metaphysis).
   - **S**ickle cell disease.

The Steinberg staging of AVN may also be used, which quantifies the extent of proximal femoral epiphyseal involvement (mild, moderate or severe). Magnetic resonance imaging (MRI) is used to assess the extent of disease, femoral head deformity, and the degree of subluxation, whilst also allowing for an assessment of vascularity on dynamic contrast enhanced sequences. The Mitchell classification of AVN assesses the T1- and T2-weighted signal characteristics within the centre of the lesion. The revised ARCO (Association Research Circulation Osseous) classification uses both radiographs and MRI.

Tip for the viva:

- Cases of AVN are common exam fodder; the causes are myriad and should be learned *ad nauseum*! Remember the 2B viva adage: *common pathologies in uncommon places.*

4. **Oblique # L tibial diaphysis**
   An oblique/spiral fracture of the left tibial diaphysis in an ambulant toddler is also known as a 'toddler's fracture', a common accidental injury. Children may be presented to the Emergency Department (ED) with either refusal to walk/bear weight or noted to not use/move their leg. Often, there is no memorable history of injury. Occasionally, a definitive fracture line may not be visualised if the fracture is not displaced. If the initial radiographs are normal but there is a high clinical suspicion of bony injury, follow-up radiographs may be performed 7–10 days later to assess for healing (periosteal reaction).

   An isolated oblique/spiral fracture of the tibial shaft should not be regarded as suspicious if present in the appropriate age group and clinical context (remember that toddler's fractures are not always witnessed). As such, the absence of a history of impact/injury does not necessarily imply an abusive aetiology. However, the same fracture in a *pre-ambulant* infant (i.e. one who is not yet independently walking) is highly suspicious for an inflicted injury and (radiographic) evidence of other physical abuse should be sought.

7. **# R fifth metatarsal base**
   It is important that you are familiar with the normal appearance of the base of the fifth metatarsal apophysis. This apophysis is normally aligned to the vertical (longitudinal) plane, i.e. parallel to the orientation of the metatarsals and is usually best appreciated on oblique projections. The normal apophysis appears at approximately 10 years of age and can be angulated or fragmented before fusing between 2 and 4 years later. Conversely, fractures of the base of the fifth metatarsal are horizontally (transversely) orientated, as demonstrated in this radiograph, and there will be associated focal soft tissue swelling indicating an acute injury.

   Tip for the viva:

   - Apophysis = ossification centre which is the site of ligamentous attachment or tendinous insertion, e.g. base of fifth metatarsal apophysis which is the site of the peroneus brevis insertion.
   - Epiphysis = ossification centre that contributes to the formation of a joint, e.g. proximal radial head epiphysis.

8. *Normal right forearm radiograph*
   This radiograph is normal. The rectangular 'bump' along the ulnar aspect of the distal ulna represents the subperiosteal bone collar which is found at the end of long bones. This is a normal finding and does not represent a buckle fracture.

10. **R pneumothorax**
    This radiograph demonstrates the deep sulcus sign at the right costophrenic angle. Remember that in neonates who are imaged supine (labelled in the top left corner of the image) in their cots or incubators, a pneumothorax will collect anteriorly/in the most non-dependent pleural space at the lung base (as opposed to apically in an upright patient) deepening the costophrenic angle. Further evidence confirming the presence of a pneumothorax in this radiograph is the crisp mediastinal and diaphragmatic margins, and depression of the right hemidiaphragm. Also note the clear visualisation of the margin of the right lung due to apical extension of the pneumothorax.

    Do not fall into the trap of 'satisfaction of search': once you have identified one pneumothorax, check that there is not one on the other side. Whilst not present in this example, do not forget to look for pneumomediastinum. Note the prominence of the superior mediastinum, which is consistent with thymus and is normal. The endotracheal tube (ETT) and nasogastric tube (NGT) are appropriately positioned.

    Tip for the viva:
    - Look for pneumothoraces (and pneumomediastinum) on supine radiographs (which will usually be labelled as such) obtained in the special care baby unit (SCBU)/neonatal intensive care unit (NICU) or resuscitation room, typically in the context of the patient becoming increasingly difficult to ventilate and/or increasing airway pressures. The same radiographic principles discussed above will apply, and apply to supine radiographs in adult patients. When present, assess all lines and tubes for satisfactory or malposition.

11. **Joint effusion L elbow**
    The presence of an intra-articular fracture is inferred by the elbow joint effusion. Commonly, only elevation of the anterior fat pad is seen but if the posterior fat pad is also elevated/visualised, then a joint effusion is *definitely* present. Once a joint effusion has been identified, you must look for the associated fracture. However, sometimes, the fracture may not be identified and is radiographically occult. In this radiograph, both the anterior and posterior fat pads are elevated in keeping with a right elbow joint effusion but no acute bony injury is demonstrated. The child will still be clinically managed as for fracture.

    Alignment should be assessed on *every* elbow radiograph, including any contemporaneous orthogonal projection. Both the anterior humeral and radiocapitellar alignment must be assessed on every lateral elbow radiograph. An imaginary line drawn along the radial neck should bisect the capitellum ossification centre on both the AP and lateral elbow projections—this is known as the radiocapitellar line, and is visualised as the orange line in the normal left anteroposterior (AP) and lateral elbow radiographs below in a different child:

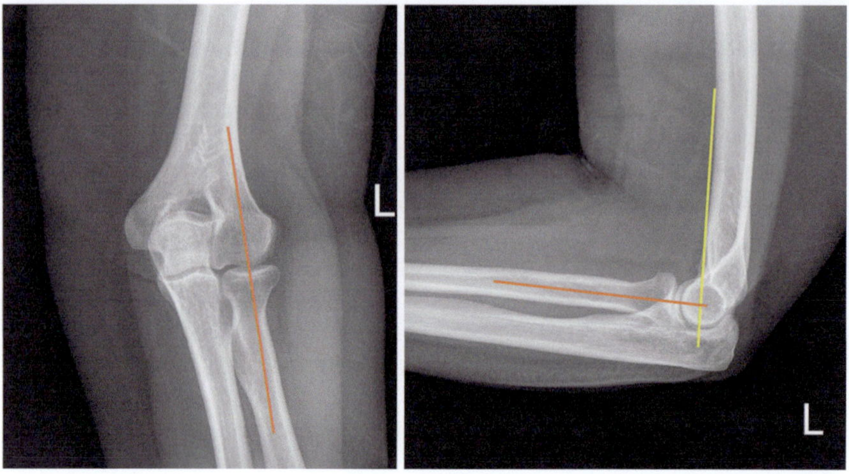

If this is not the case and the radiocapitellar line is 'disrupted', there is a radial head subluxation/dislocation. A line drawn along the anterior surface of the humerus should intersect the middle third of the capitellum—this is known as the anterior humeral line, and is visualised as the yellow line in the above lateral elbow radiograph. If the line passes *anterior* to the middle third of the capitellum, a supracondylar fracture should be suspected.

Children usually present with an unwillingness to use their arm following a fall onto an outstretched hand (FOOSH). This history should prompt the search for ancillary features of elbow trauma such as a joint effusion, radial head subluxation/dislocation and any concomitant soft tissue swelling.

Tip for the viva:

- In children, the commonest intra-articular elbow fractures are supracondylar humeral followed by radial head/neck. These areas should be carefully examined on every elbow radiograph, particularly once an elbow joint effusion has been identified.

12. *Normal lateral left knee radiograph*
Note the indentation at the anterior aspect of the lateral femoral condyle which is normal. This should not be confused with the deeper 'lateral femoral notch sign' which is suggestive of an osteochondral fracture and may be associated with anterior cruciate ligament injury.

15. **# R supracondylar humerus**
A horizontally oriented supracondylar fracture line is visualised with associated soft tissue swelling indicated by the 'blurring' of the supracondylar fat-muscle planes over the radial aspect of the fracture. The fracture is better visualised in the magnified image below:

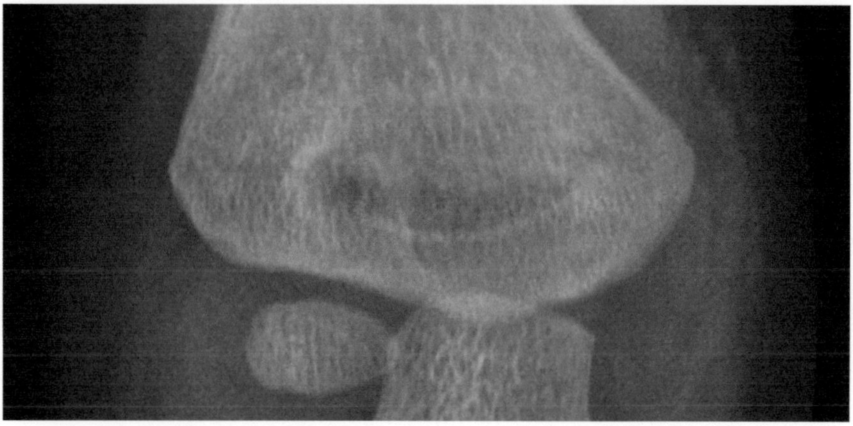

Whilst humeral supracondylar fractures are usually well visualised on lateral projections, this case reinforces that the AP projection should also be thoroughly evaluated.

16. *Normal right foot radiograph*
Note the normal base of the fifth metatarsal apophysis which is aligned longitudinally (vertically) to the metatarsals. Compare this image to the fracture in Image 7 of this test.

18. **Buckle #s L distal radius and ulna**
Buckle (or torus) fractures (from the Latin *torus*, meaning 'protuberance') are very common in children. They result from trabecular compression due to an axial loading force along the long axis of the bone. Buckle fractures of the radius and ulna commonly occur together, usually following a FOOSH. A discrete fracture line is not visible but the cortex of the bone bulges outwards, with or without angulation. These fractures are often incomplete but are stable and typically heal without complication.
In the examination, there will usually be only one significant diagnosable abnormality per radiograph. However, in those radiographs which demonstrate a well-recognised fracture pattern in which two fractures frequently occur together, you would be expected to identify and write down *both* fractures to get the mark as explained in the Introduction section.

19. **Bowel obstruction**
This 10-month-old infant was presented to the ED with vomiting and was found to have a 'firm abdomen' on examination. The radiograph shows several dilated loops of bowel in the central abdomen with a paucity of bowel gas elsewhere consistent with bowel obstruction. Note the tip of the enteric tube projected over the stomach.

It can be difficult to differentiate between dilated small- and large-bowel loops on radiography in neonates and young infants. Often it is more helpful to describe the relative number of dilated loops, their position, and whether the imaging appearances are more in keeping with a proximal (high) or distal (low) obstruction. In this case, the number and calibre of the dilated bowel loops, and their central position, indicate that the obstruction is of the small bowel. An intussusception was confirmed on ultrasound.

The aetiology of bowel obstruction in children is age dependent. A neonate (from the Latin *neonatus*, meaning 'newborn') refers to a baby in their first 28 days of life. An infant (from the Latin *infans*, meaning 'unable to speak' or 'speechless') generally refers to a young child from 1 to 11 months of age. The term toddler is used for those who are walking unsteadily, i.e. 'toddling', from the age of 12 to 36 months. Thereafter, the terms young and older child can be used. A 'school-aged child' is usually one from the age of 5 years onwards.

Neonatal bowel obstruction can be categorised by proximal (high) or distal (low):

- Proximal: the 'double bubble sign' describes the appearance when the stomach and first part of the duodenum are distended with gas and no other gas is visualised distally, indicating duodenal atresia. Where gas is visualised distal to the first part of the duodenum, other causes of proximal obstruction need to be considered, including: duodenal web; duodenal stenosis; jejunal atresia; and annular pancreas. An upper gastrointestinal (GI) contrast examination is the investigation of choice alongside close liaison with paediatric surgical colleagues—it is often helpful if they observe the contrast examination in real time.
- Distal: the causes can be remembered using the mnemonic, **HAMM**:
  - **H**irschsprung's disease: also known as colonic aganglionosis. Usually a short segment, it affects the rectum and distal sigmoid in approximately 75% of cases. It almost always affects *term* neonates (especially in boys) and is the most common cause of neonatal bowel obstruction (20% of cases). The affected segment is narrow in calibre, often with an abnormal fasciculated/sawtooth contour on lower GI contrast examination, and the proximal bowel is dilated. This typically results in an abnormal rectosigmoid ratio (<1) where the rectum is abnormally narrower than the dilated proximal sigmoid/descending colon. While lower GI contrast examination may be helpful, ultimately, biopsy is required for diagnosis. Treatment typically involves surgical resection of the affected segment and/or a pull-through procedure (where the normal ganglionic bowel is connected to the anus). The type of surgery will depend on the extent of the aganglionosis.
  - **A**tresia: ileal; anal. Associated with **V**ertebral anomalies, **A**norectal anomalies, **C**ardiac anomalies, **T**racheo-o**E**sophageal fistula, **R**enal/**R**adial ray anomalies, and **L**imb anomalies (**VACTERL**) syndrome.
  - **M**econium ileus: the meconium is abnormal and inspissated (meaning thickened in consistency) becoming impacted in the distal ileum, resulting in obstruction. Approximately 20% of infants with cystic fibrosis present with meconium ileus at birth.

- **M**econium plug syndrome: also known as small left colon syndrome (i.e. there is a left microcolon resulting from never having been used). This is a functional obstruction secondary to a meconium plug. Lower GI contrast enema examination can be both diagnostic and therapeutic, facilitating the passage of *normal* meconium (cf. meconium ileus where the meconium is abnormal).

- Necrotising enterocolitis (NEC) is a consideration in premature infants. Obstruction can result from strictures as a long-term complication in those infants in whom NEC has been medically managed. Prematurity is a significant risk factor for the development of NEC with approximately 90% of cases occurring in premature infants, reducing in prevalence with increasing age—the more premature the infant, the higher the risk and mortality. NEC may occur in term infants, albeit uncommonly, and is associated with congenital heart disease (CHD); those with more complex CHD have a higher risk of developing NEC.

Bowel obstruction in older infants and children is more likely to be secondary to an acquired aetiology. Late presentations of those entities occurring in the neonatal period should also be considered in the appropriate clinical context. **AAIIMM** is a mnemonic which can be used to remember the common causes of bowel obstruction in children:

- **A**ppendicitis.
- **A**dhesions: from previous surgery.
- **I**ntussusception.
- **I**ncarcerated inguinal hernia.
- **M**eckel's diverticulum: do not forget the '*Rule of 2's*':
  - 2% of the population.
  - 2 inches (5 cm) long.
  - 2 feet (60 cm) from the ileocaecal valve.
  - 2/3rds contain ectopic mucosa.
  - 2 types of ectopic tissues are commonly present (gastric and pancreatic).
  - 2 years old at presentation.
  - 2% become symptomatic.
  - 2 times more common in boys.
- **M**alrotation/midgut volvulus.

Tip for the viva:

- Midgut volvulus should be excluded in *any* neonate with *bilious* vomiting. The normal position of the duodenojejunal (DJ) flexure lies at/above the level of the pylorus to the left of the spinous process. With malrotation, an upper GI contrast study demonstrates an abnormal position of the (duodenum and) DJ flexure which does *not* lie at the normal position stated above. In the setting of midgut volvulus, a corkscrew appearance of the distal duodenum and jejunum may be seen. Ultrasound may demonstrate the 'whirlpool' sign of a twisted mesentery.

20. **# L little finger metacarpal neck**
It is important that you trace the outline of every single bone—doing so reveals the fracture of the left little finger metacarpal neck. Note the subtle periosteal reaction around the radial aspect of the fracture in keeping with bony healing.

Be sure to carefully inspect the alignment of the carpometacarpal joints (CMCJ) on every hand radiograph in the context of blunt trauma; in particular, to exclude dorsal subluxation of the little finger CMCJ, which is commonly overlooked. It can occur as part of a fracture-dislocation complex (also known as a reverse Bennet fracture-dislocation), which is the commonest base of metacarpal fracture complex. It is an unstable injury with subluxation resulting from the unopposed action of the extensor carpi ulnaris on the fracture fragment. Delayed or missed diagnoses can result in pain, stiffness, and impaired function/weakened grip, which can be avoided (or improved) following prompt diagnosis and treatment with/without surgical stabilisation.

21. **Round pneumonia L lower lobe**
There is a rounded area of left lower lobe opacification. The presence of an air bronchogram helps to establish the radiological diagnosis of consolidation as opposed to a solid pulmonary mass. In round pneumonia, the consolidation is usually well circumscribed, appearing 'roundish', but it may also have irregular margins. The border/dome of the left hemidiaphragm is obliterated, localising the pathology to the left lower lobe. The appearance is typical of infective consolidation in children.

The rounded appearance of the consolidation results from the not-yet-developed collateral airways in the paediatric lung (the pores of Kohn and the canals of Lambert) and is commonly identified in young school children aged between 5 and 8 years. When the collateral airways are not yet fully established the spread of infection is limited, resulting in a 'more compact' consolidation and the subsequent rounded radiographic appearance. As the airways develop with advancing age, this finding becomes less common and older children will develop a more 'lobar' pattern of consolidation due to lateral air drift via the collateral airways between subsegments in the same lobe.

Follow-up chest radiographs are less commonly obtained in children compared to adults. Given that most cases will have resolved on follow-up imaging, some centres *only* perform a further radiograph in those children who have either not improved clinically or have deteriorated (consider empyema and lung necrosis in the appropriate clinical context).

Tip for the viva:

- You may be asked why this pattern of consolidation develops (rounded versus lobar), which is why you should understand the pathology behind this radiographic appearance. Discuss the radiographic follow-up of round pneumonia with your local paediatric radiologists. If questioned, you can state what you do locally.

23. **Buckle # L distal tibial metaphysis**
The buckle fracture is seen as an acute 'step' in the medial cortex of the left distal tibial metaphysis as visualised in the magnified image below:

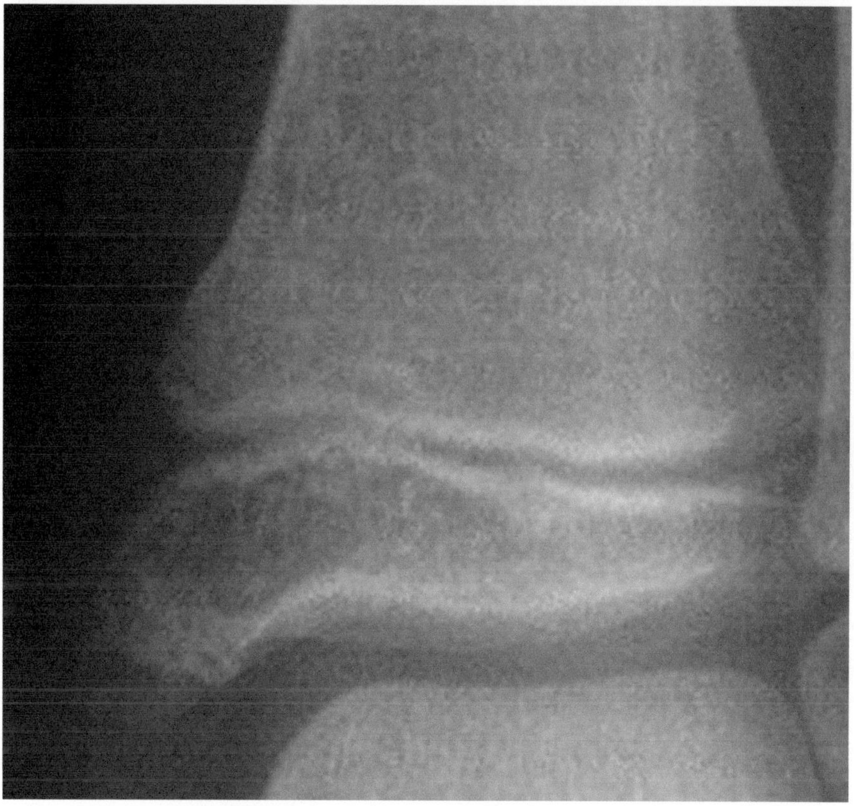

In the examination, as in real life, you will be able to magnify the images and it is recommended that you do so when assessing for subtle cortical abnormalities. The fragmentation of the medial aspect of the distal tibial epiphysis/medial malleolus is normal: remember that epiphyseal ossification can have variable appearances at all ages.

24. **#s L distal tibial diaphysis and L proximal fibular metaphysis**
Did you also identify the proximal fibular fracture? Whilst there is a spiral fracture of the left distal tibial diaphysis, there is also a buckle fracture of the proximal fibular metaphysis. Compare the original image with the magnified image below:

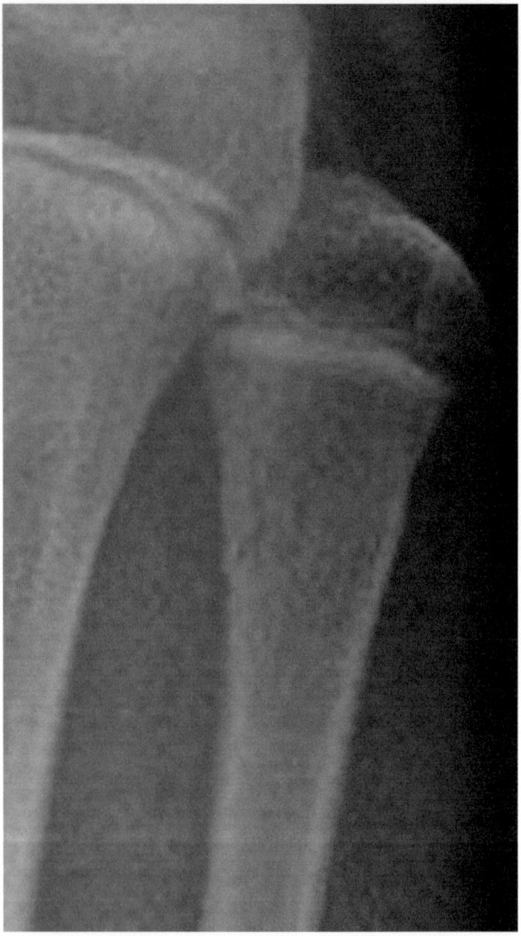

Do not suffer 'satisfaction of search': once you have recognised the relatively obvious tibial fracture, you must carefully examine every other bone for a further/associated fracture. Whilst spiral tibial fractures occur more often in isolation, they can occur together with proximal fibular fractures because the force is transmitted from the tibia (the weight-bearing bone) along the interosseous membrane to the proximal fibula where the force is dissipated. You would be expected to identify *both* fractures to get full marks for this question in the examination—see the Introduction section.

Note that this is *not* the Maisonneuve fracture complex, which is the combination of a proximal fibular fracture (usually the proximal third) and a distal tibial fracture (usually of the medial malleolus/deltoid ligament) with widening of the distal tibiofibular syndesmosis.

26. **Lipohaemarthrosis R knee**
A lipohaemarthrosis is an important radiographic sign indicating an intra-articular fracture, which may be radiographically occult. It represents a fat-fluid level in the suprapatellar bursa, resulting from the fatty marrow, which is less dense, floating on top of haemorrhage. When identified, it should prompt the search for a fracture of the tibial plateau or tibial spine, a distal femoral fracture, an osteochondral defect or less commonly, a patella fracture. Importantly however, the absence of a lipohaemarthrosis does *not* exclude the presence of an intra-articular fracture.

Tip for the viva:
- A lipohaemarthrosis can be identified on other imaging modalities: look for the fat-fluid level.

28. **Dislocation L radial head**
In the presence of a joint effusion, a bony injury should be sought and alignment should be thoroughly assessed. In this radiograph, the anterior humeral alignment is normal but the radiocapitellar alignment is not, consistent with dislocation of the left radial head. See the explanation for Image 11 of this test.

Tip for the viva:
- In the presence of a radial head dislocation, a concomitant ulnar shaft fracture should be sought as part of the Monteggia fracture-dislocation pattern, and vice versa. Formal forearm radiographs (which should include both the wrist and elbow joints) should be recommended if they have not yet been obtained.

29. **Bilateral nephrocalcinosis**
The renal outlines, and those of the other intra-abdominal organs, should not be overlooked on the abdominal radiograph. Nephrocalcinosis is categorised depending on where the calcium salts are deposited in the renal parenchyma: medullary, being the more common and representing 95% of cases; or cortical, comprising the remainder. Both conditions are associated with nephrolithiasis (renal calculi), which may be present anywhere along the urinary tract.

The aetiology of nephrocalcinosis can be best remembered using the following mnemonics:

Medullary–HAM HOP

- **H**yperparathyroidism.
- (Renal tubular) **A**cidosis.
- **M**edullary sponge kidney: a condition affecting the formation of the medullary and papillary renal collecting tubules resulting in cystic dilatation. Given that patients may be asymptomatic, the diagnosis may only be made incidentally when the renal tract is imaged for other reasons. However, patients may present with a complication such as urinary tract infection, haematuria, or nephrolithiasis, the latter occurring in the majority (approximately 80%) of cases.
- **H**ypercalcaemia/**H**ypercalciuria.
- **O**xalosis.
- **P**apillary necrosis: think of this in patients (children and adults) with a longstanding history of pain and associated non-steroidal anti-inflammatory drug (NSAID) use; in the setting of infection (pyelonephritis, tuberculosis); or in those with sickle cell disease.

Cortical–COAG

- **C**ortical necrosis.
- **O**xalosis.
- **A**lport syndrome: an X-linked recessive disease affecting type IV collagen production. Type IV collagen is found in the eyes, ears, and kidneys and explains why patients present with ocular anomalies, high frequency sensorineural hearing loss, and basement membrane glomerulonephritis.
- (chronic) **G**lomerulonephritis.

In this case, the underlying cause was medullary sponge kidney which was diagnosed following recurrent presentations of abdominal pain and urinary tract infection.

Tip for the viva:

- Whilst not present in this case, search for additional radiographic features of the underlying cause of nephrocalcinosis, e.g. in the context of hyperparathyroidism, look for osteopenia, rugger jersey spine (i.e. endplate sclerosis), subchondral resorption of the sacroiliac joints, or Brown's tumours. Cases of hyperparathyroidism from renal osteodystrophy (secondary hyperparathyroidism in patients with chronic renal failure) are particularly common in the examination setting.

30. **Salter-Harris 2 # L thumb distal phalanx**
The Salter-Harris classification is the most widely used system to describe physeal (growth plate) fractures and can be remembered using the mnemonic, **SALTER**:

- **S**lipped, type 1: the fracture passes through the physis *only* and not through the adjacent bone. There may be an associated shift (slip) about the physis with widening of its medial or lateral aspect with focal overlying soft tissue swelling at the level of the physis. These fractures do *not* occur if the growth plate is fused.
- **A**bove, type 2: the fracture passes through and *above* the physis into the metaphysis. These are the most common injuries and account for approximately 75% of all physeal injuries.
- **L**ower/be**L**ow, type 3: the fracture passes through and *below* the physis into the epiphysis.
- **T**hrough **E**verything/**T**og**E**ther, type 4: the fracture passes through *everything*–the metaphysis, physis, and the epiphysis.
- **R**ammed/c**R**ush, type 5: the physis is damaged by *direct compression* from the metaphysis and epiphysis. These injuries are uncommon and account for <1% of physeal fractures.

It is important that the physis and adjacent metaphysis and epiphysis are scrutinised for a Salter-Harris injury on *every* skeletal radiograph. The prognosis worsens progressively from Salter-Harris type 1 to 5. See the references for illustrative figures of the above classification.

Tip for the viva:

- Do not forget that a slipped upper femoral epiphysis (SUFE) is a Salter-Harris 1 injury and that Tillaux and triplanar fractures of the distal tibia are Salter-Harris 3 and 4 fractures, respectively.

Further Reading

Image 1

Bomer J, Holscher H (2015) Hip pathology in children. https://radiologyassistant.nl/pediatrics/hip/hip-pathology-in-children. Accessed Feb 2023

Knipe H et al (2023) Gaucher disease. https://radiopaedia.org/articles/gaucher-disease. Accessed Feb 2023

Munir MA et al (2020) Avascular necrosis causes (mnemonic). https://radiopaedia.org/articles/avascular-necrosis-causes-mnemonic. Accessed Feb 2023

Sharma R et al (2022) Caisson disease. https://radiopaedia.org/articles/decompression-sickness. Accessed Feb 2023

Worsley C et al (2022) Erlenmeyer flask deformity. https://radiopaedia.org/articles/erlenmeyer-flask-deformity-1. Accessed Feb 2023

Image 4

Bauer JM, Lovejoy SA (2019) Toddler's fractures: time to weight-bear with regard to immobilization type and radiographic monitoring. J Pediatr Orthop 39:314–317

Image 7

Gu Y, Ren H (2022) Proximal fifth metatarsal fracture involving both zones 1 and 2. Asian J Surg 21:S1015-9584(22)01406-3

Image 10

El-Ali AM, Strubel NA, Lala SV (2022) Congenital lung lesions: a radiographic pattern approach. Pediatr Radiol 52(4):622–636

Yoon H (2016) Interpretation of neonatal chest radiography. J Korean Soc Radiol 74(5):279–290

Image 11

El-Feky M et al (2022) Anterior humeral line. https://radiopaedia.org/articles/anterior-humeral-line. Accessed Feb 2023

Jones J et al (2021) Paediatric elbow radiograph (an approach). https://radiopaedia.org/articles/paediatric-elbow-radiograph-an-approach. Accessed Feb 2023

Knipe H et al (2022) Radiocapitellar line. https://radiopaedia.org/articles/radiocapitellar-line. Accessed Feb 2023

Image 18

Little JT, Klionsky NB, Chaturvedi A et al (2014) Pediatric distal forearm and wrist injury: an imaging review. Radiographics 34(2):472–490

Image 19

Bomer J, Stafrace S, Smithuis R et al (2020) Acute abdomen in neonates. https://radiologyassistant.nl/pediatrics/abdominal-masses/acute-abdomen-in-neonates. Accessed Mar 2023
El-Feky M et al (2022) Double bubble sign (duodenum). https://radiopaedia.org/articles/double-bubble-sign-duodenum. Accessed Feb 2023
El-Feky M et al (2023) Meconium plug syndrome. https://radiopaedia.org/articles/meconium-plug-syndrome. Accessed Feb 2023
Foster T et al (2020) Meconium ileus. https://radiopaedia.org/articles/meconium-ileus. Accessed Feb 2023
Hull NC, Kim HHR, Phillips GS et al (2022) Neonatal and Pediatric Bowel Obstruction: Imaging Guidelines and Recommendations. Radiol Clin North Am 60(1):131–148
Nguyen HN, Navarro OM, Bloom DA et al (2022) Ultrasound for midgut malrotation and midgut volvulus: *AJR* Expert Panel Narrative Review. AJR Am J Roentgenol 218(6):931–939
Nikjenad M et al (2018) Hirschsprung disease. https://radiopaedia.org/articles/hirschsprung-disease. Accessed Feb 2023
Reid JR (2012) Practical imaging approach to bowel obstruction in neonates: a review and update. Semin Roentgenol 47(1):21–31
Vadera S et al (2022) Rule of 2s in Meckel diverticulum. https://radiopaedia.org/articles/rule-of-2s-in-meckel-diverticulum-1. Accessed Feb 2023
Worsley C et al (2021) Necrotising enterocolitis. https://radiopaedia.org/articles/necrotising-enterocolitis-1. Accessed Feb 2023

Image 20

Cobb WA, Dingle L, Adami RZ et al (2018) Management of fracture-dislocations of the little finger carpometacarpal joint: a systematic review. J Hand Surg Eur 43(5):530–538
Lustosa L et al (2022) Reverse Bennett fracture-dislocation. https://radiopaedia.org/articles/reverse-bennett-fracture-dislocation-2. Accessed Feb 2023

Image 21

McCrossan P, McNaughten B, Shields M et al (2017) Is follow up chest X-ray required in children with round pneumonia? Arch Dis Child 102(12):1182–1183
Uçan B, Gökçe Çınar H (2022) Radiological features of round pneumonia in children: 10 years of experience. J Health Sci Med 5(2):523–527

Image 24

Allen D (2022) Monteggia fracture—pediatric. https://www.orthobullets.com/pediatrics/4015/monteggia-fracture%2D%2Dpediatric. Accessed Mar 2023
Vanmarsnille T, Laloo F, Herregods N et al (2021) Pediatric imaging of the elbow: a pictorial review. Semin Musculoskelet Radiol 25(4):558–565

Image 29

Yap J et al (2018) Medullary nephrocalcinosis. https://radiopaedia.org/articles/medullary-nephrocalcinosis-mnemonic. Accessed Feb 2023
Yap J et al (2023) Cortical nephrocalcinosis. https://radiopaedia.org/articles/cortical-nephrocalcinosis-mnemonic. Accessed Feb 2023

Image 30

Chong JCF (2017) Salter-Harris fractures. https://www.emnote.org/emnotes/salter-harris-fractures. Accessed Feb 2023
Murphy A et al (2023) Salter-Harris classification. https://www.orthobullets.com/pedia. Accessed Feb 2023

Test 2

2

M. Paddock et al., *Paediatric Radiology Rapid Reporting*,
https://doi.org/10.1007/978-3-031-48255-7_2

2.1 Images

Image 1

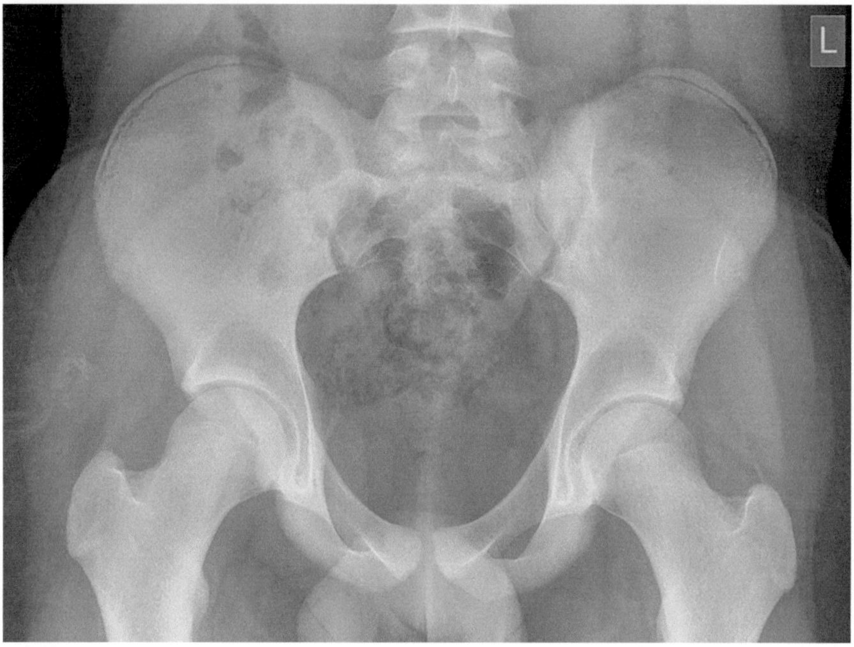

Image 2

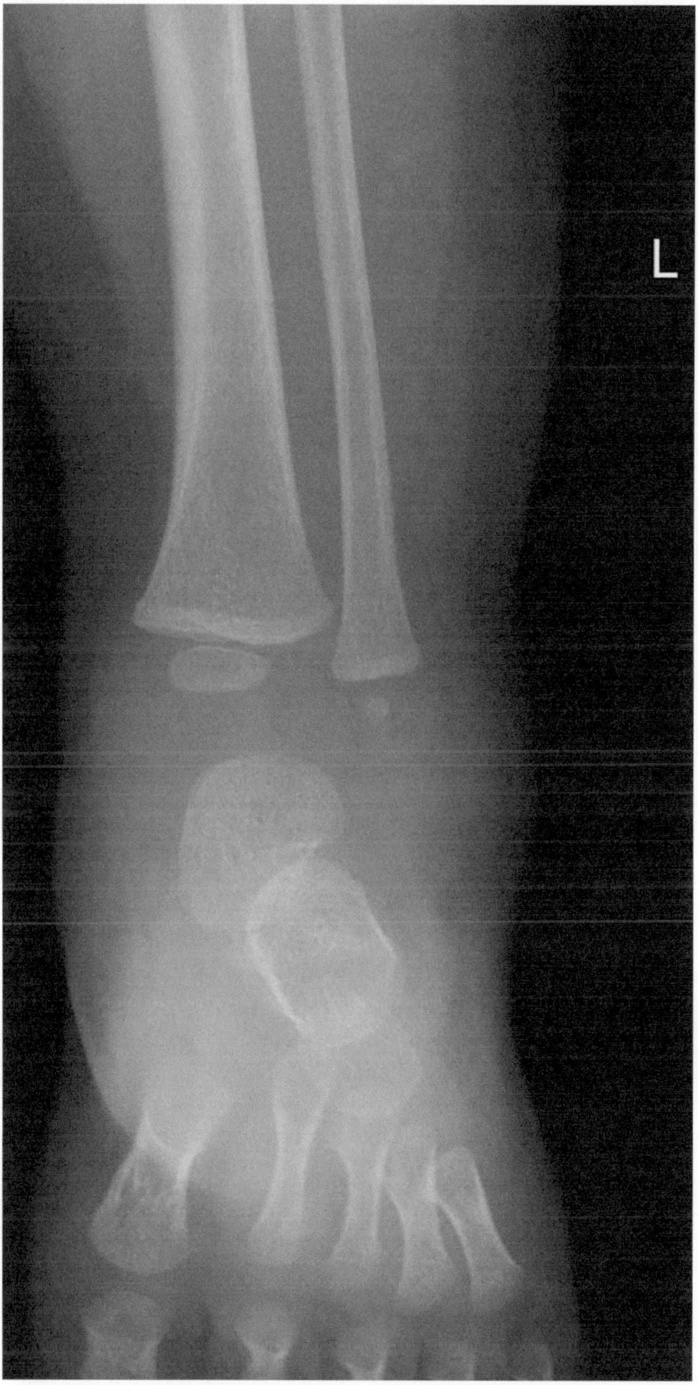

Image 3

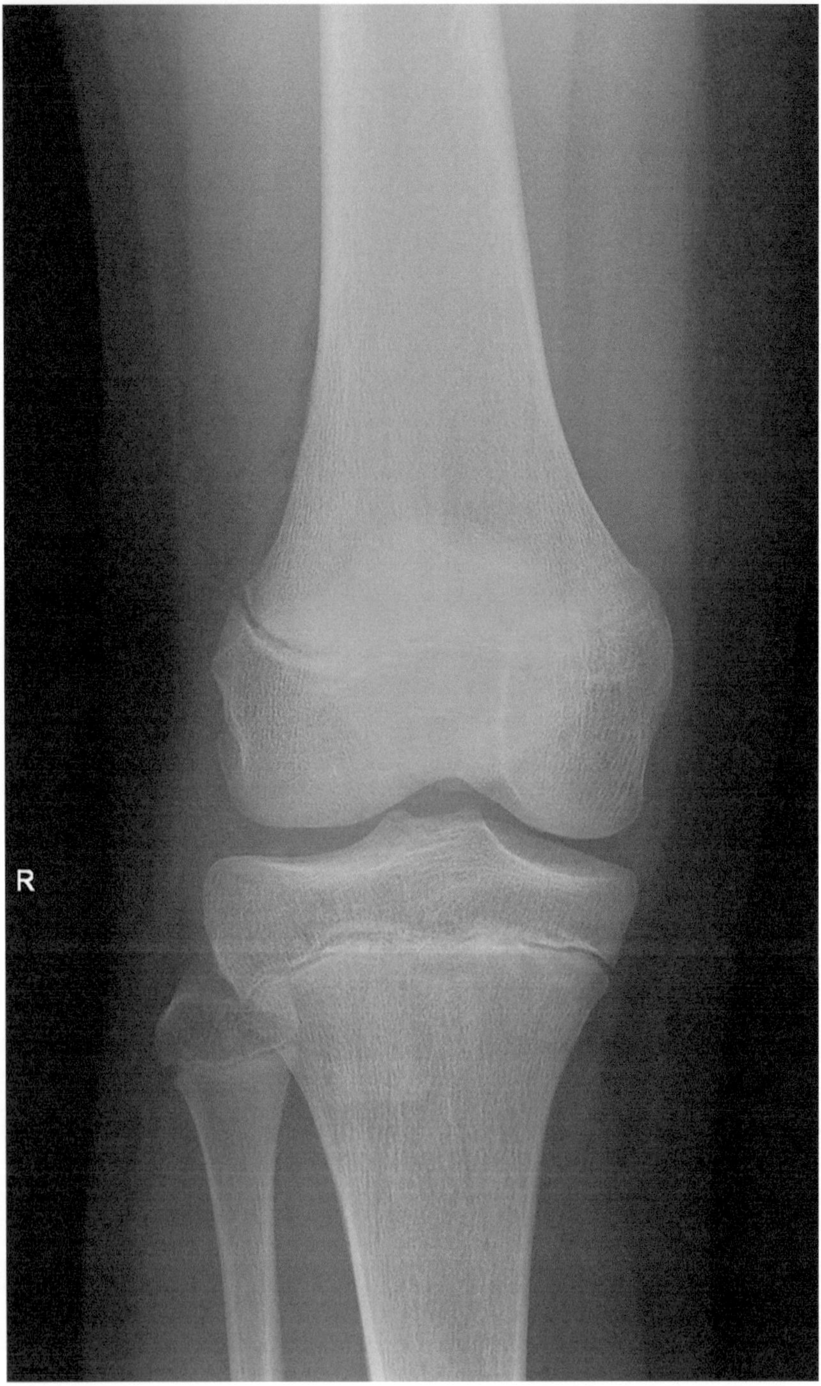

Image 4

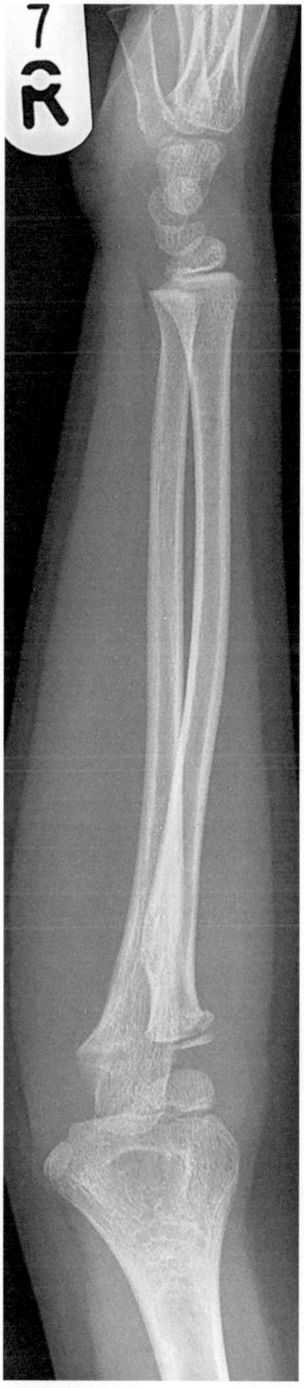

Image 5

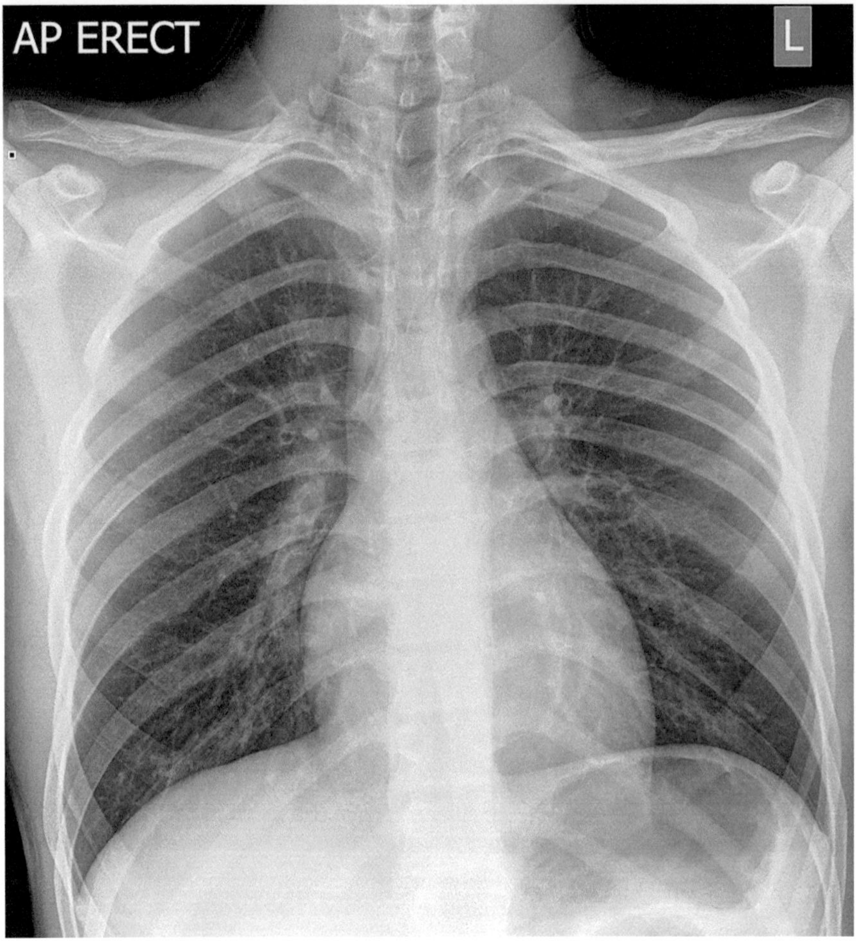

Image 6

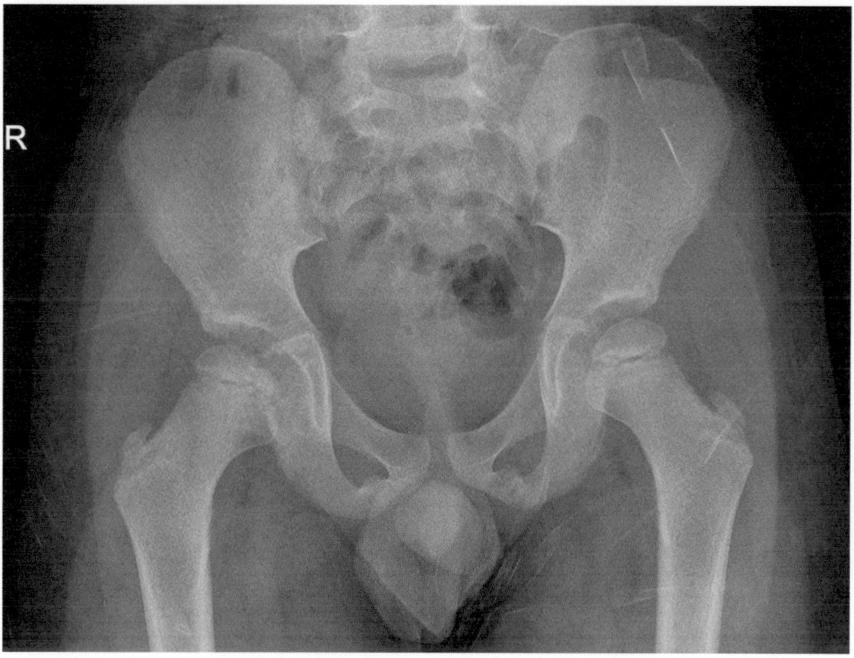

Image 7

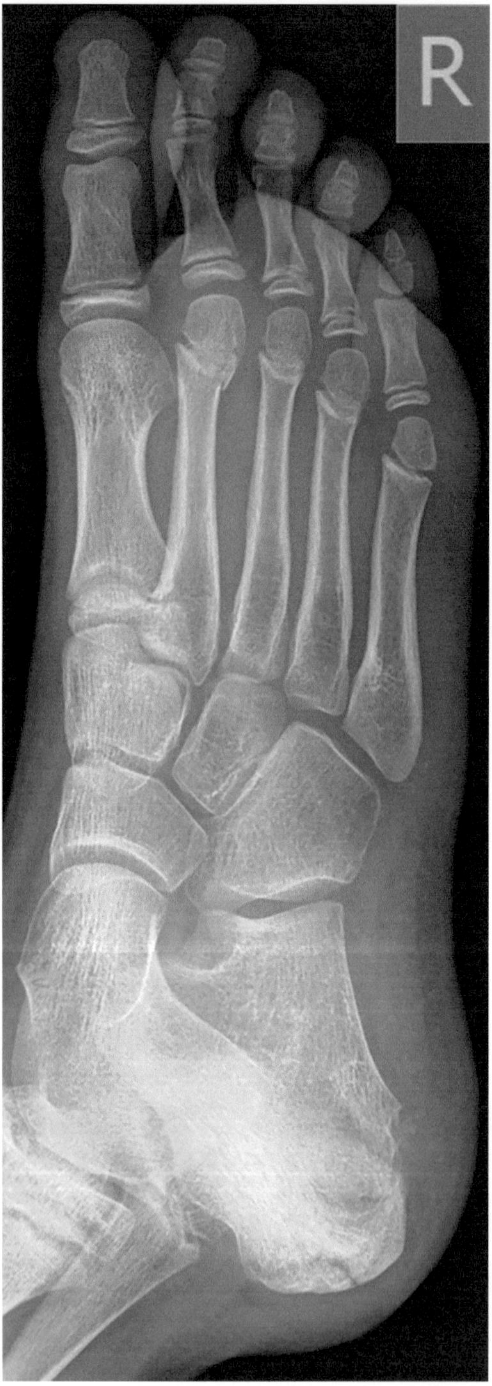

Image 8

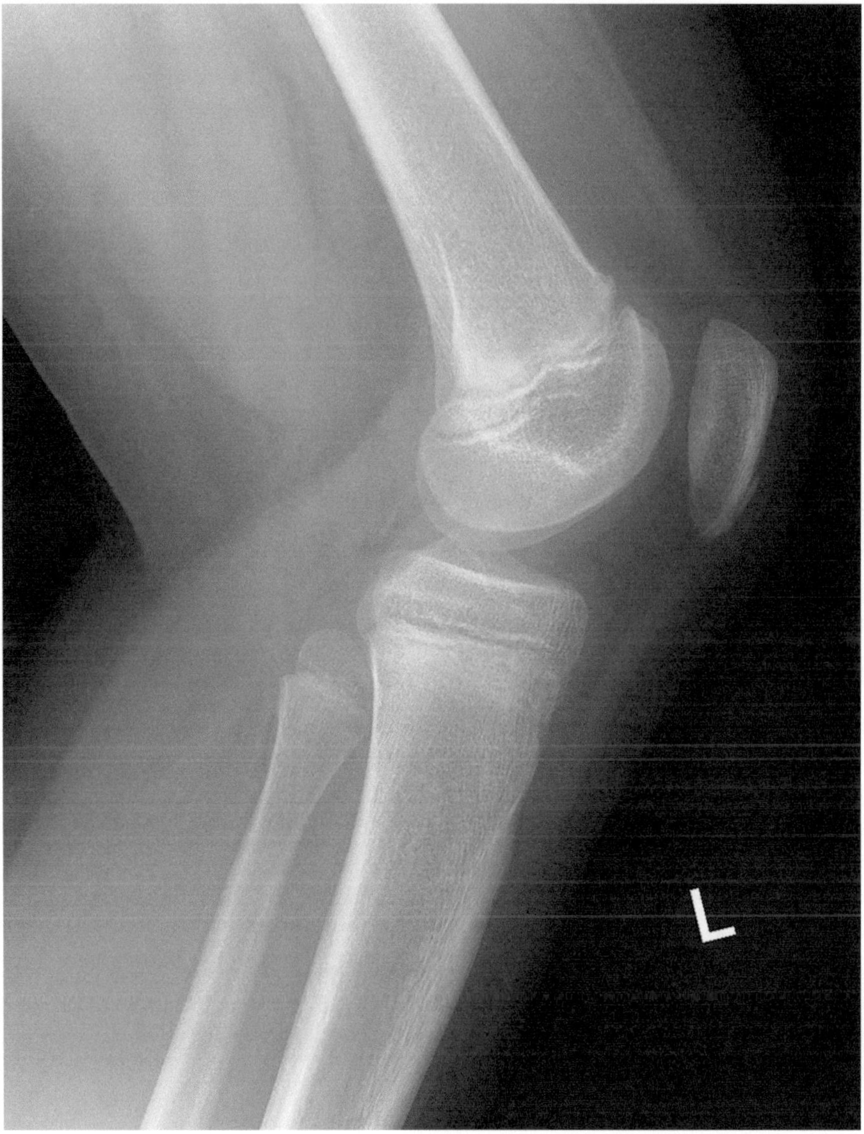

Image 9

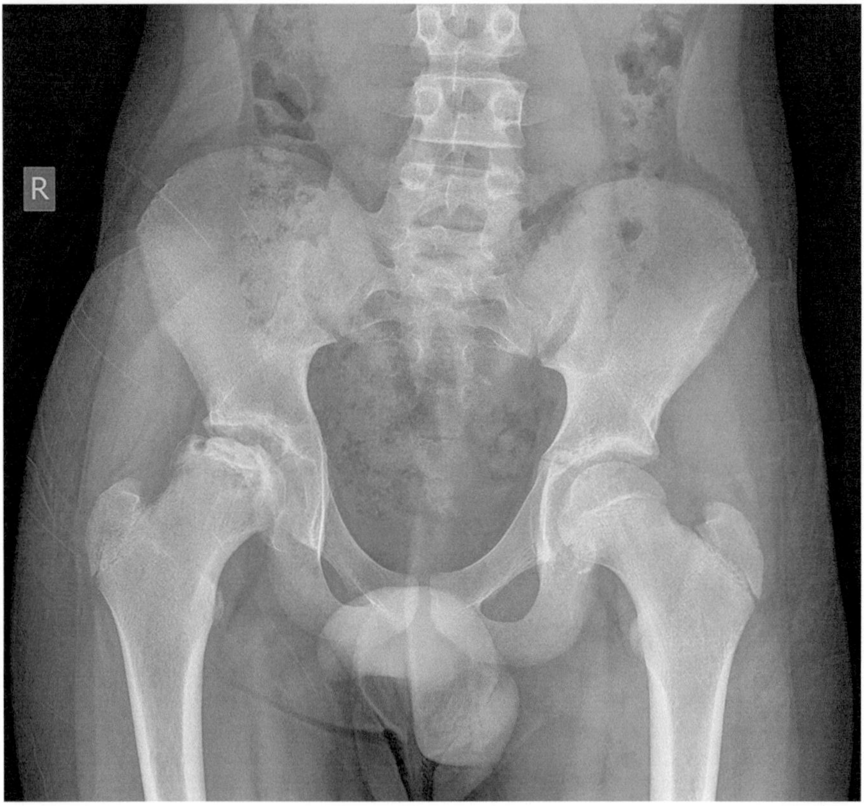

Image 10

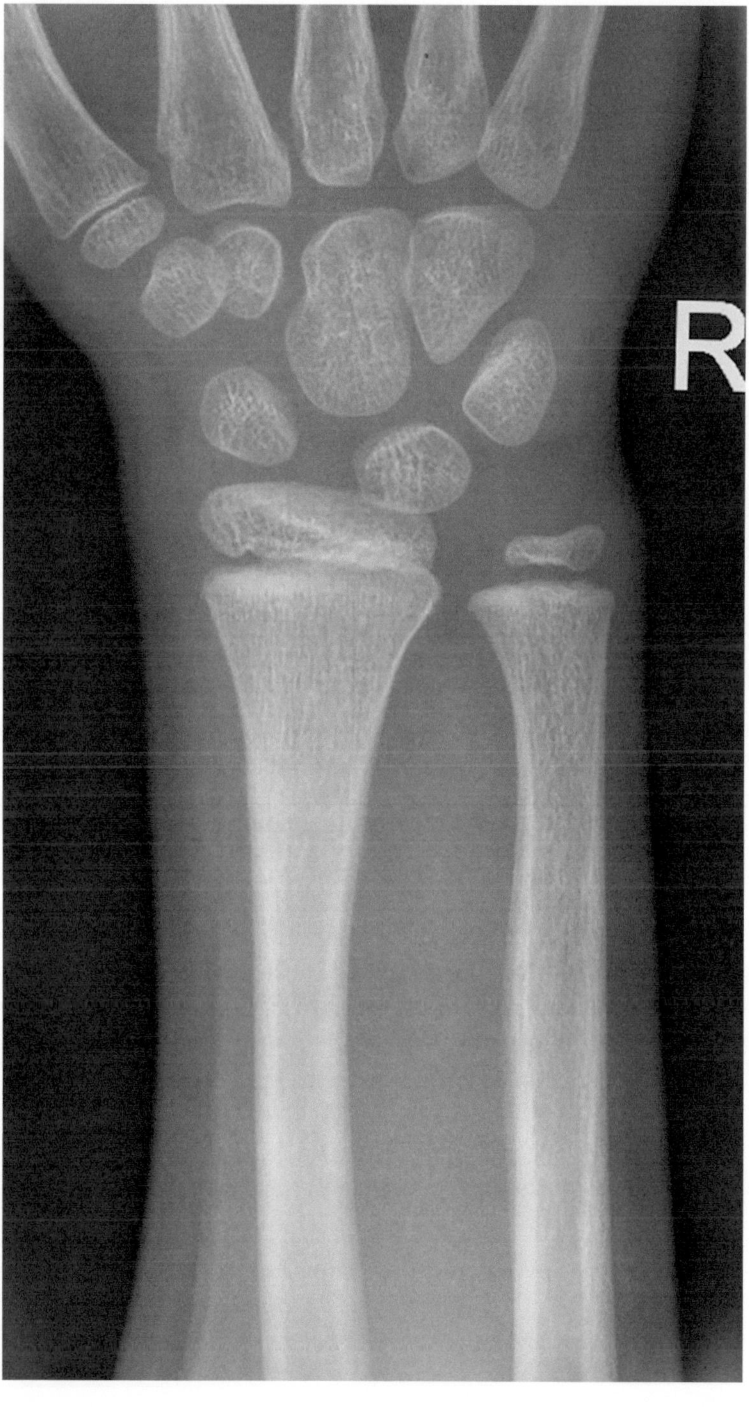

Image 11

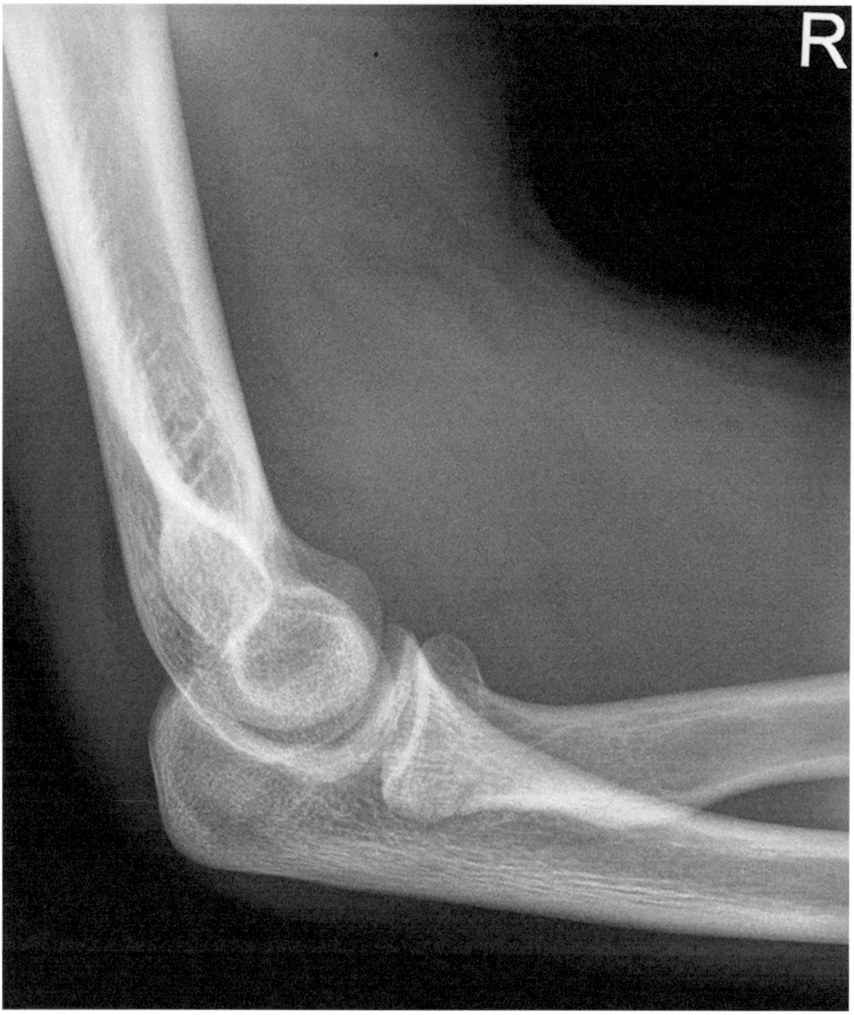

Image 12

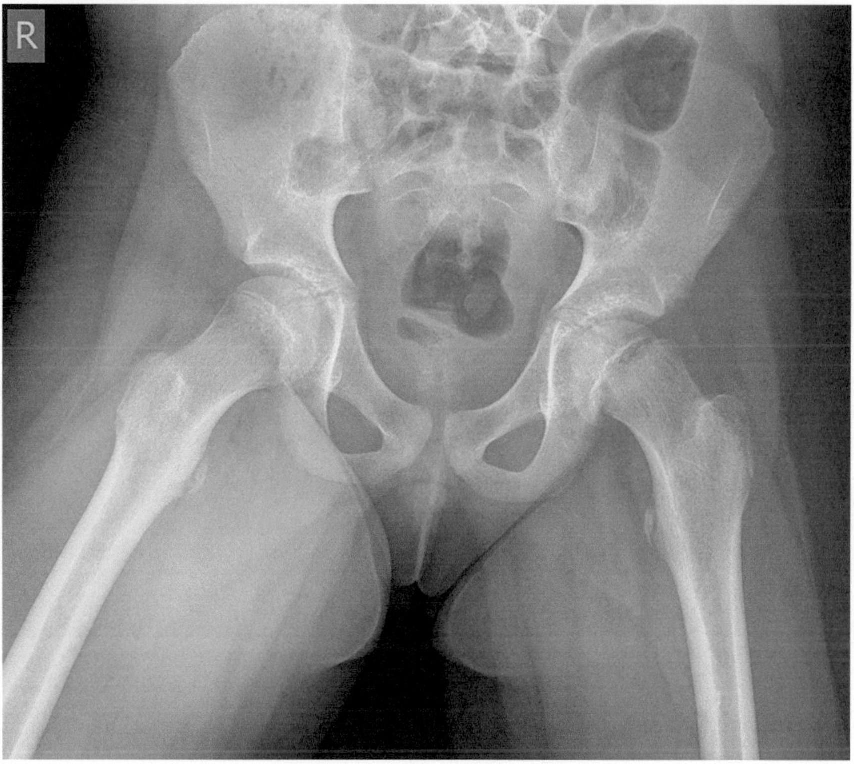

Image 13

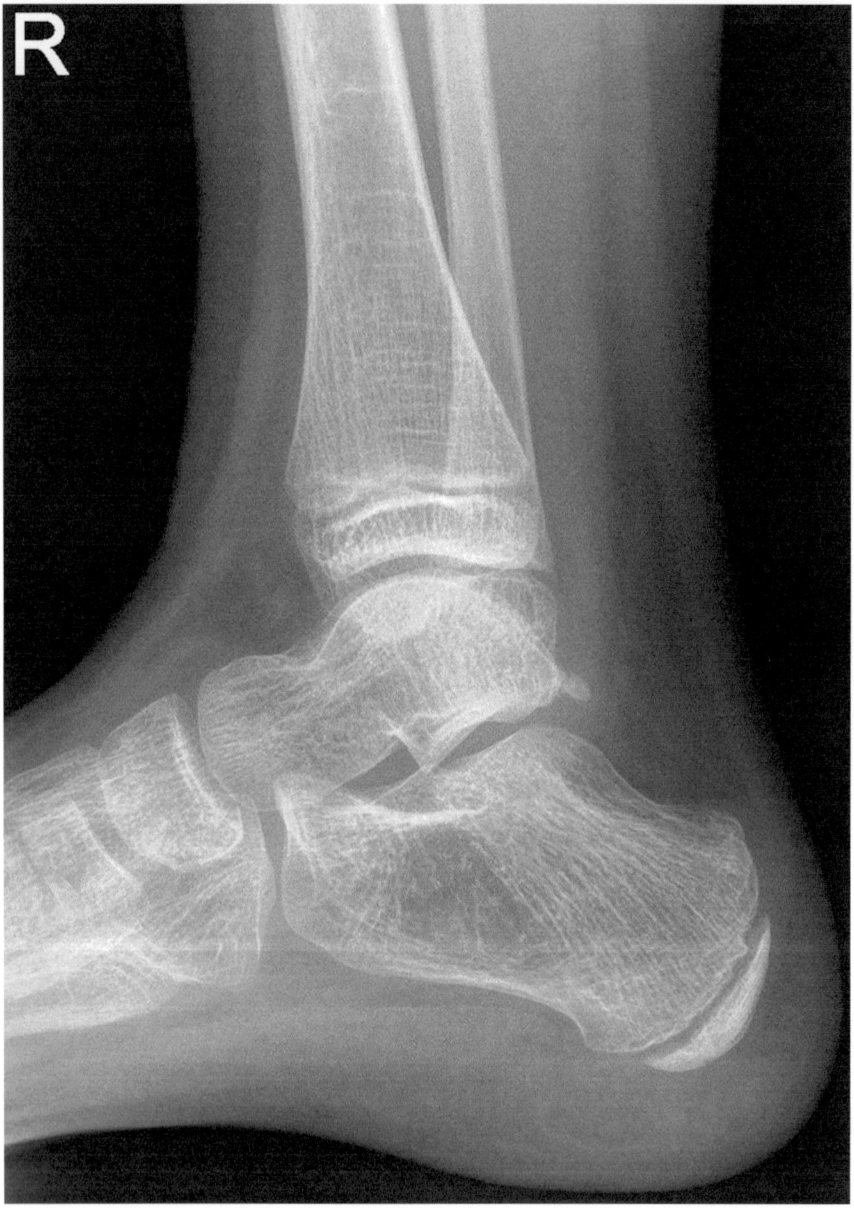

Image 14

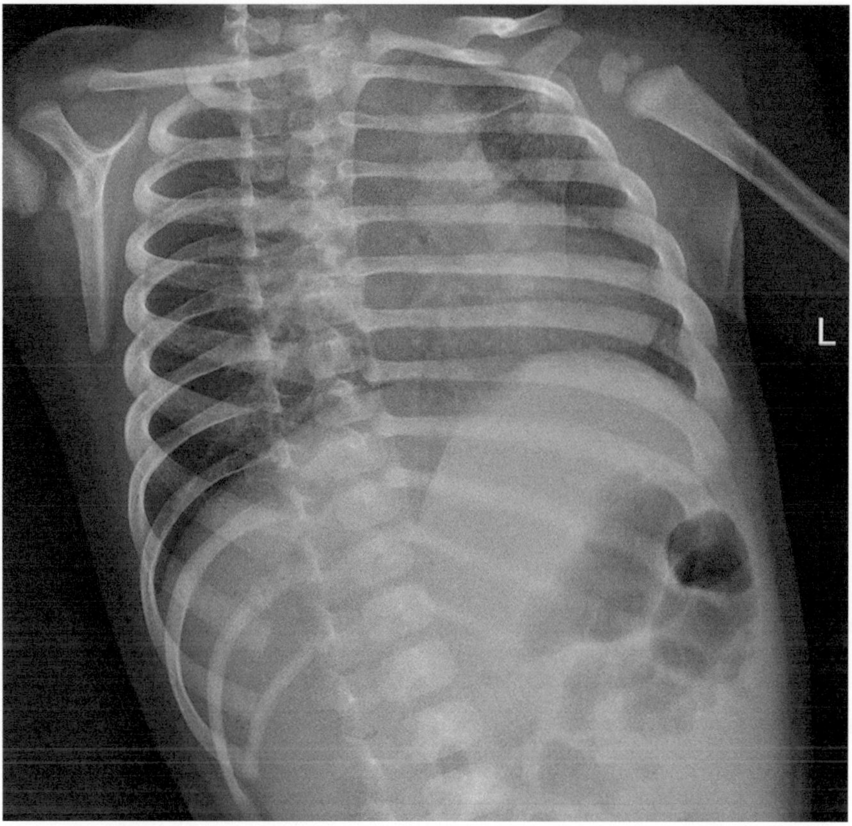

Image 15

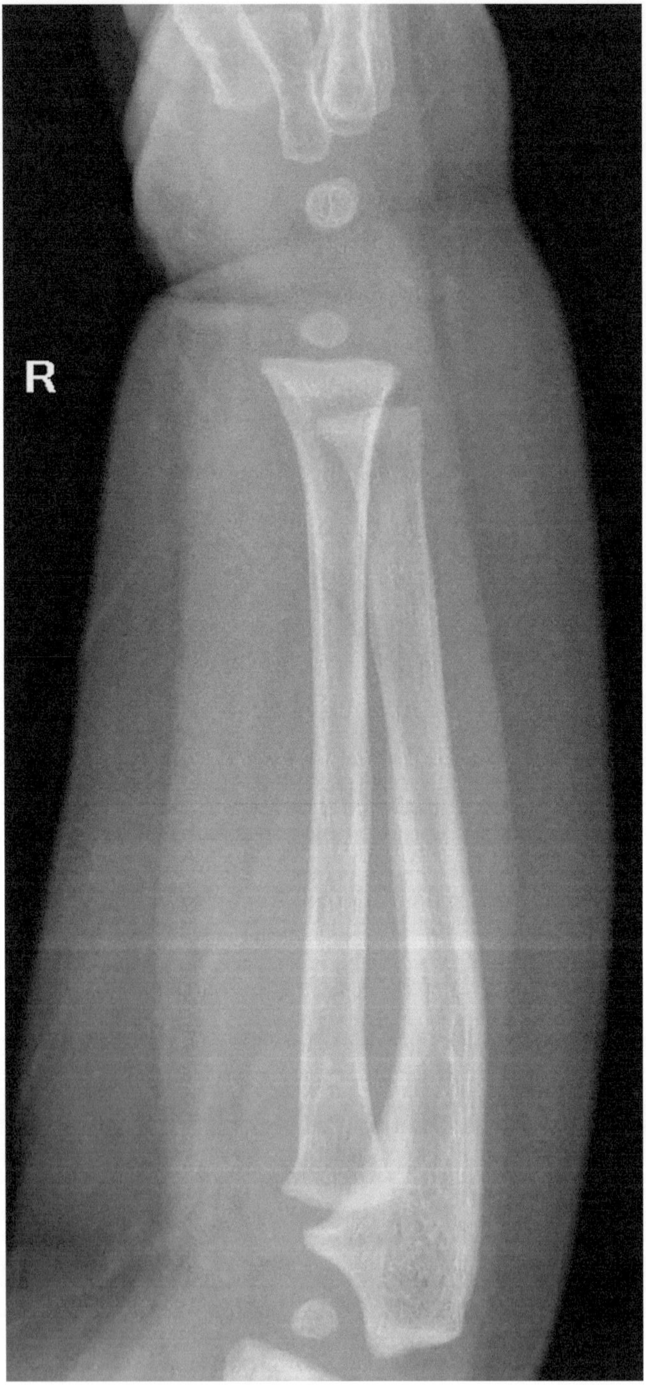

Image 16

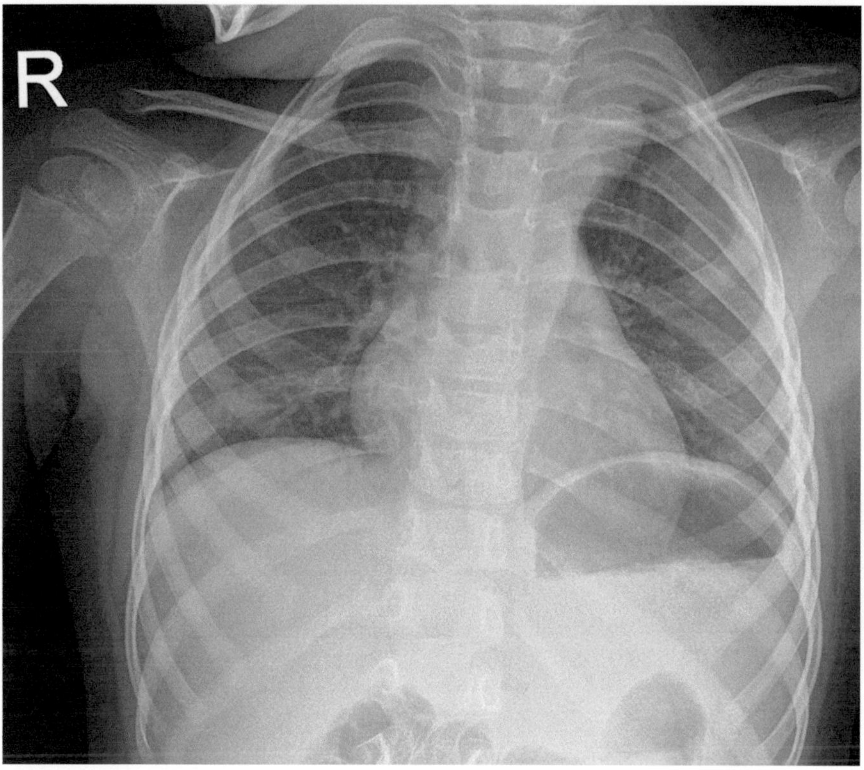

Image 17

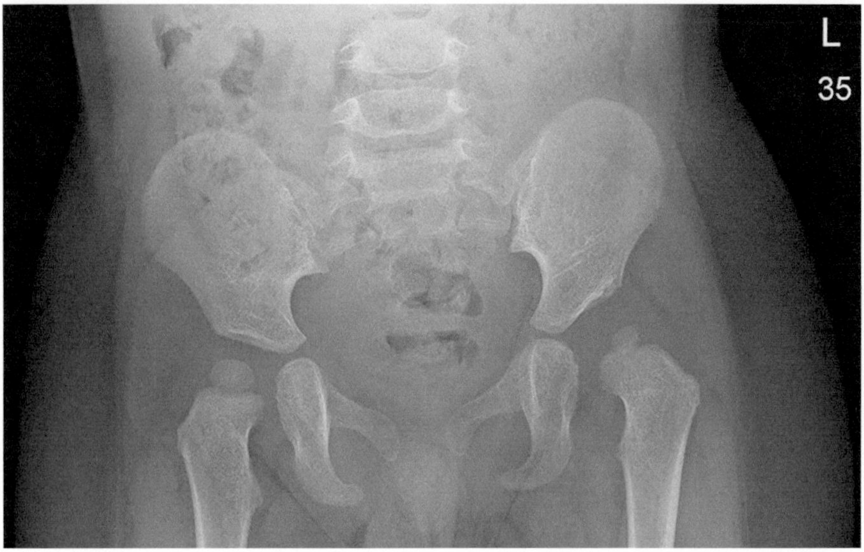

Image 18

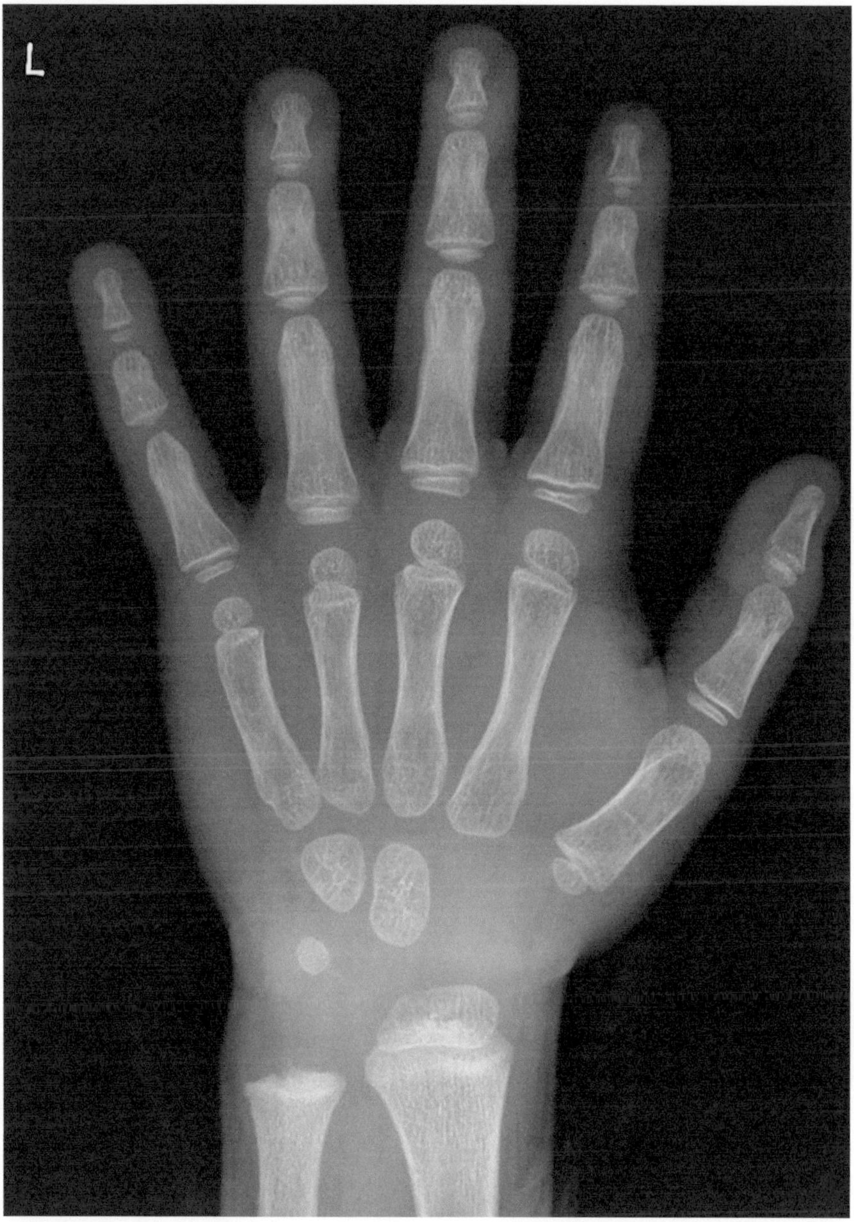

Image 19

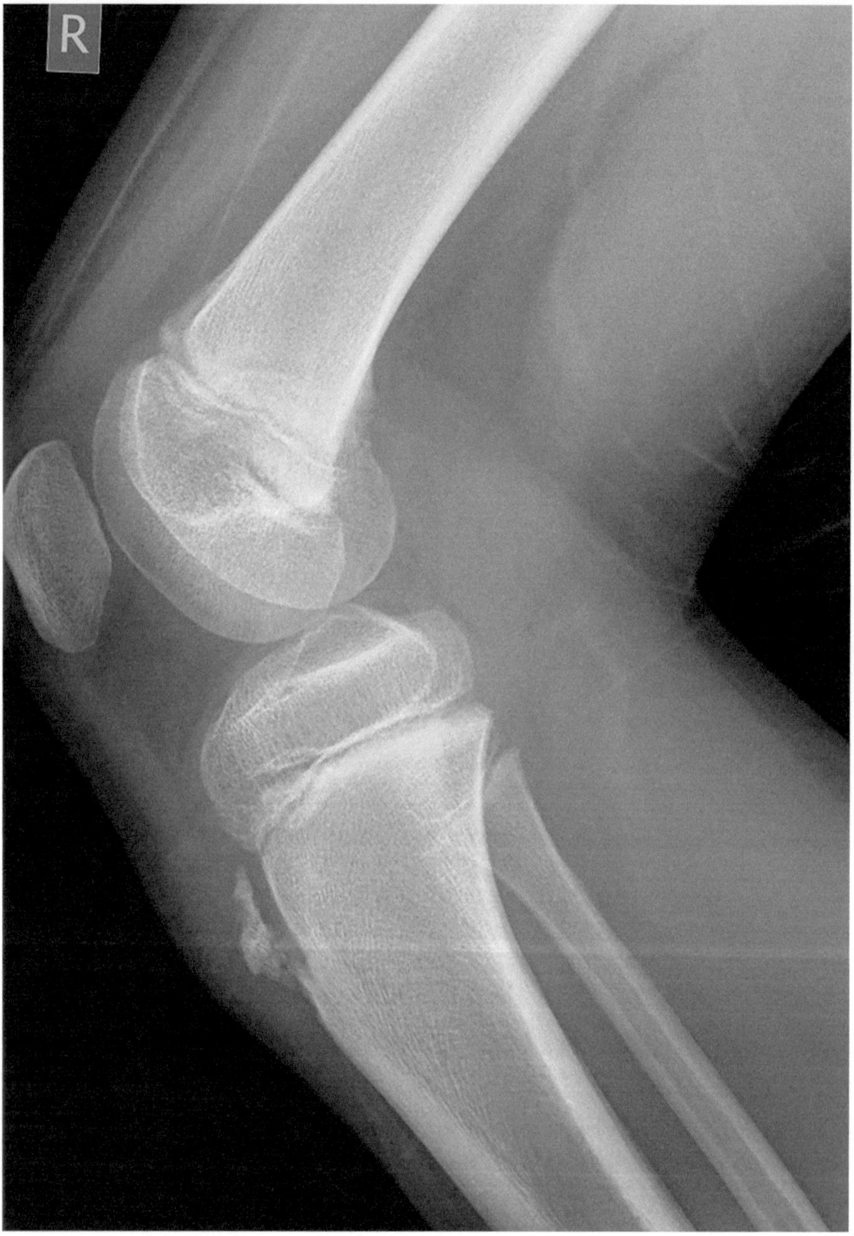

Image 20

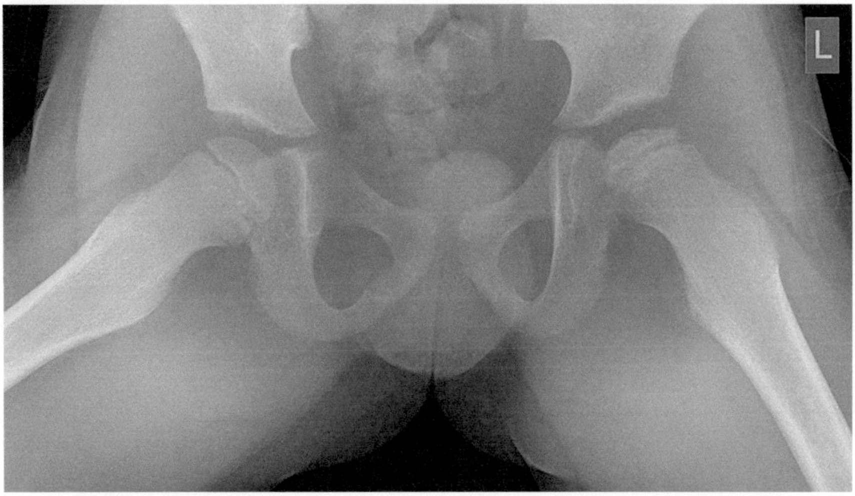

Image 21

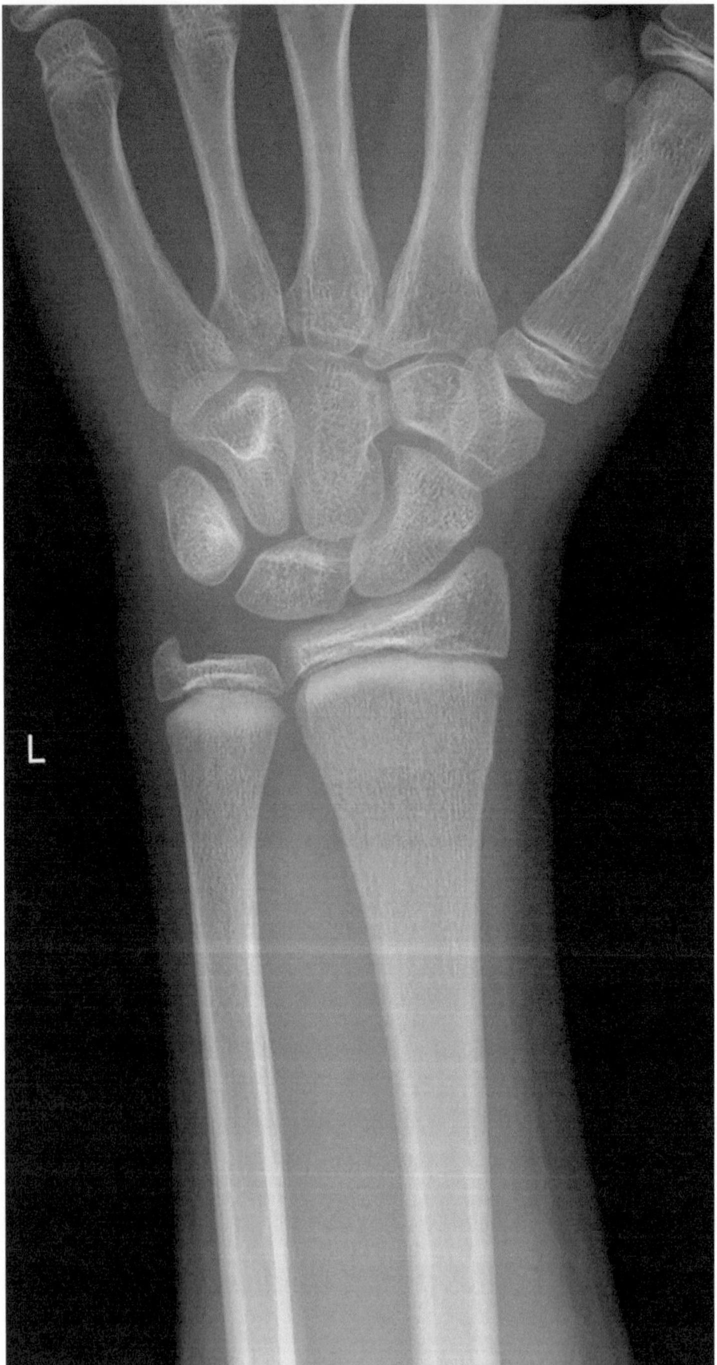

Image 22

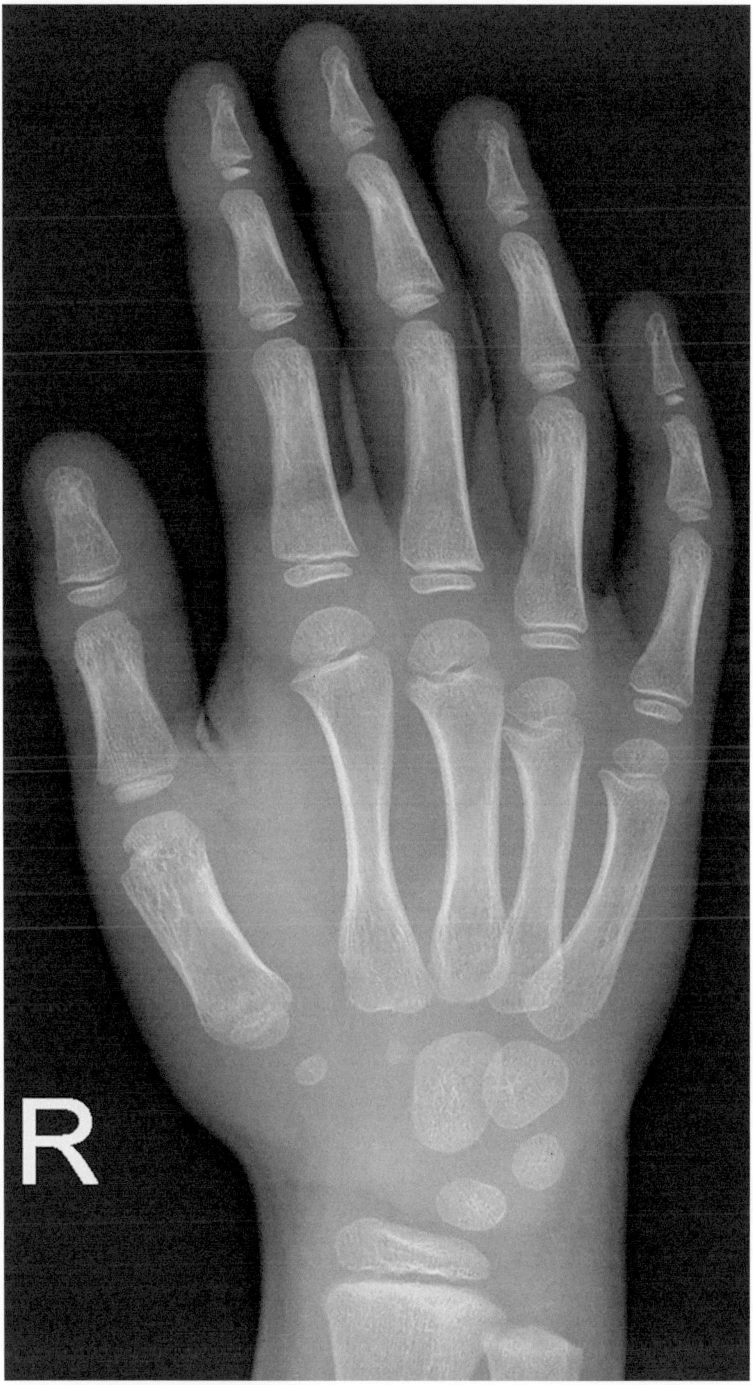

Image 23

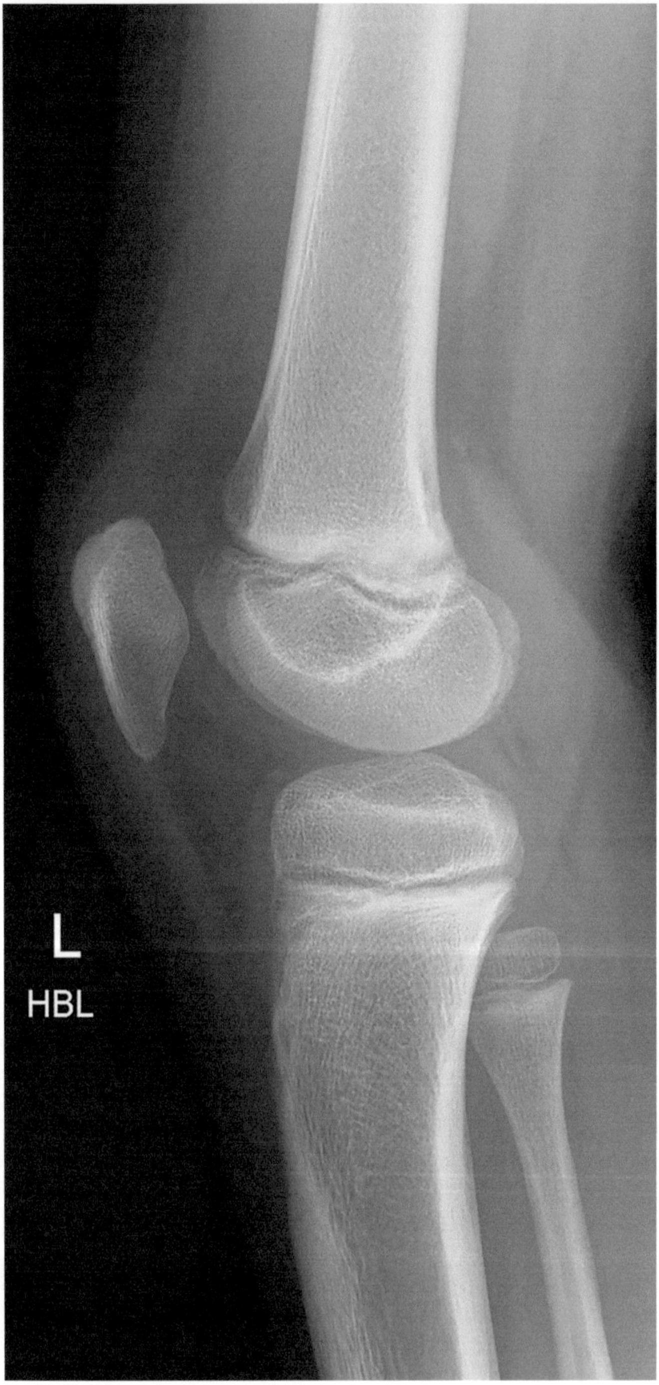

Image 24

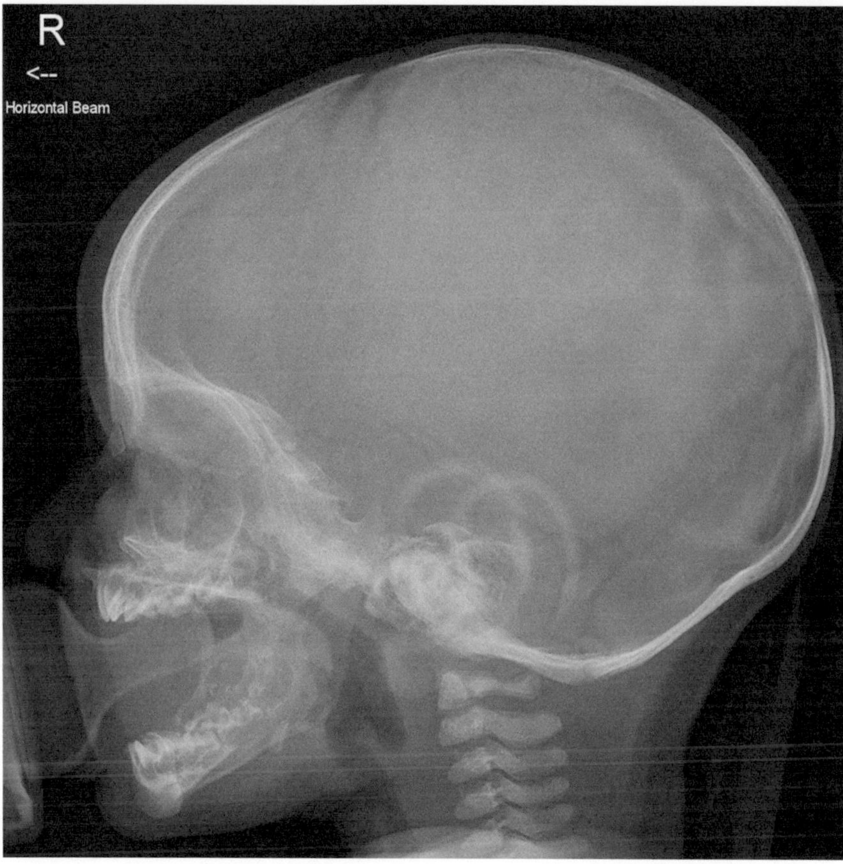

Image 25

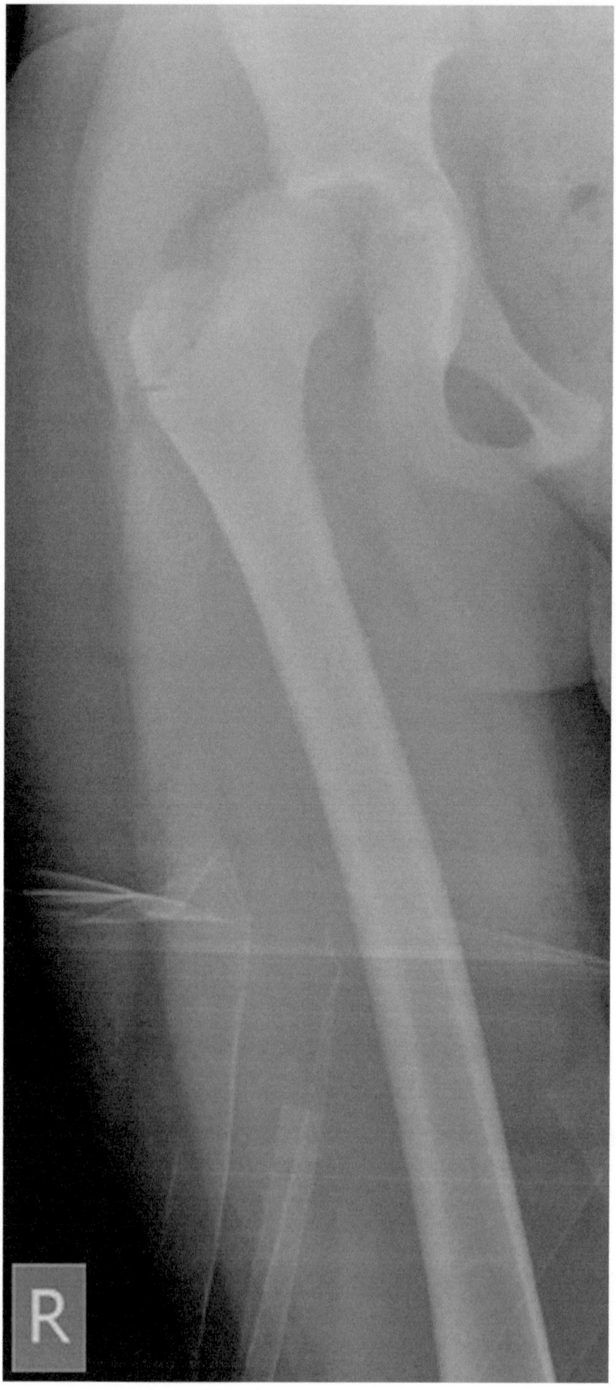

Image 26

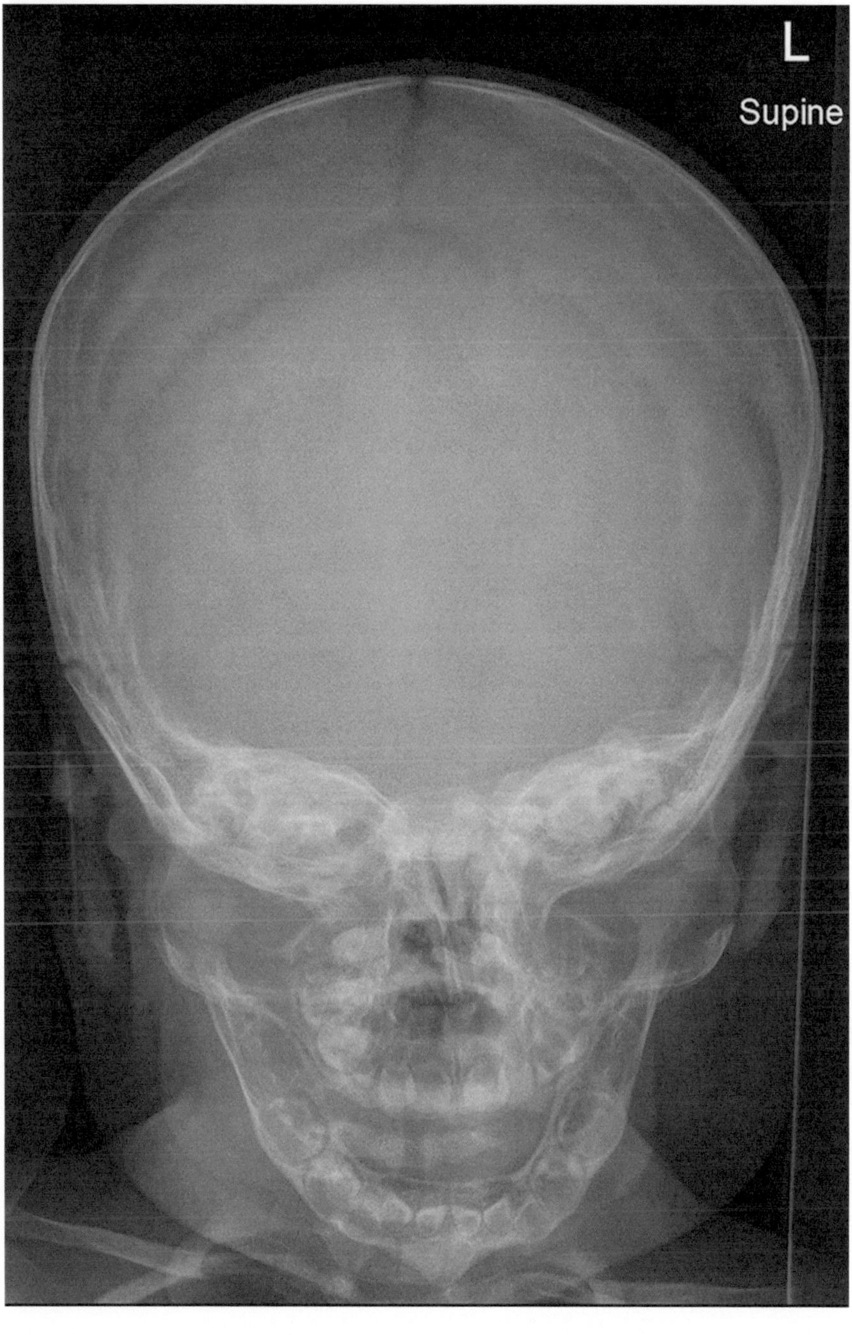

Image 27

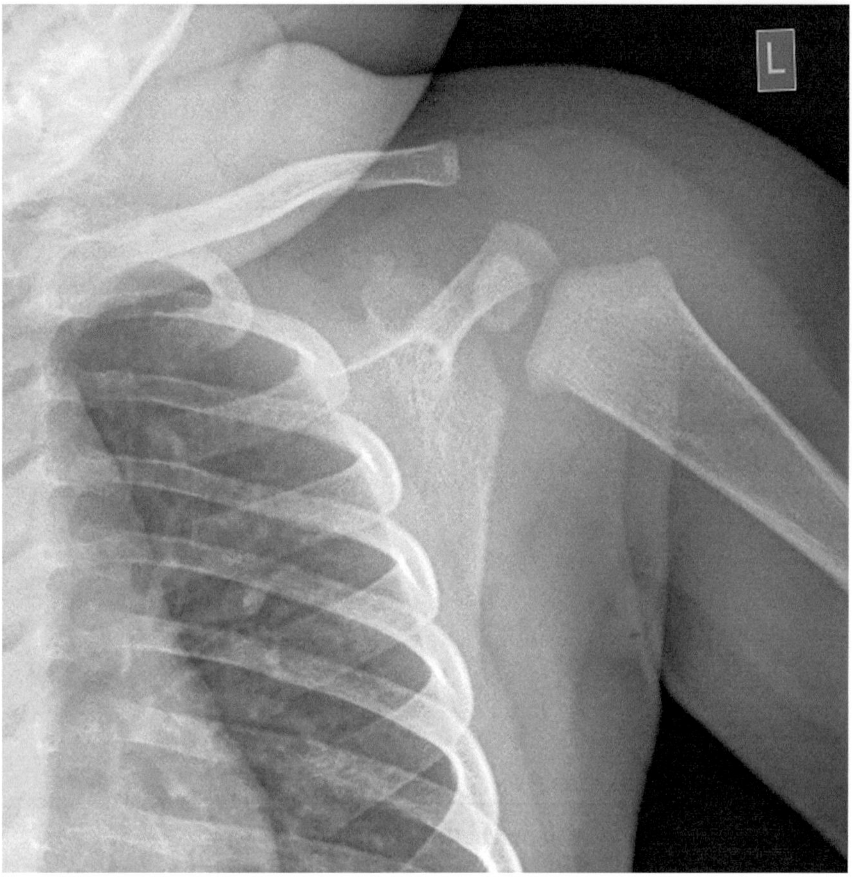

Image 28

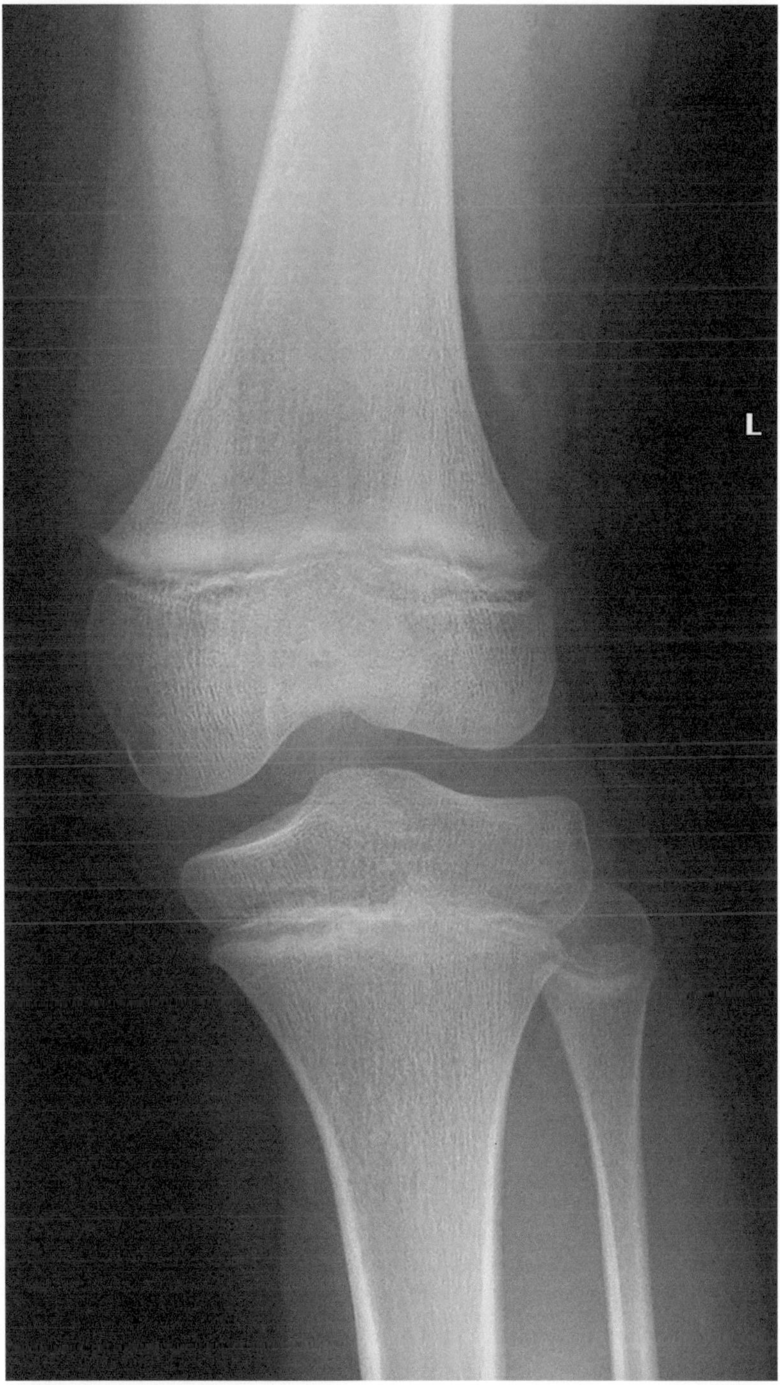

Image 29

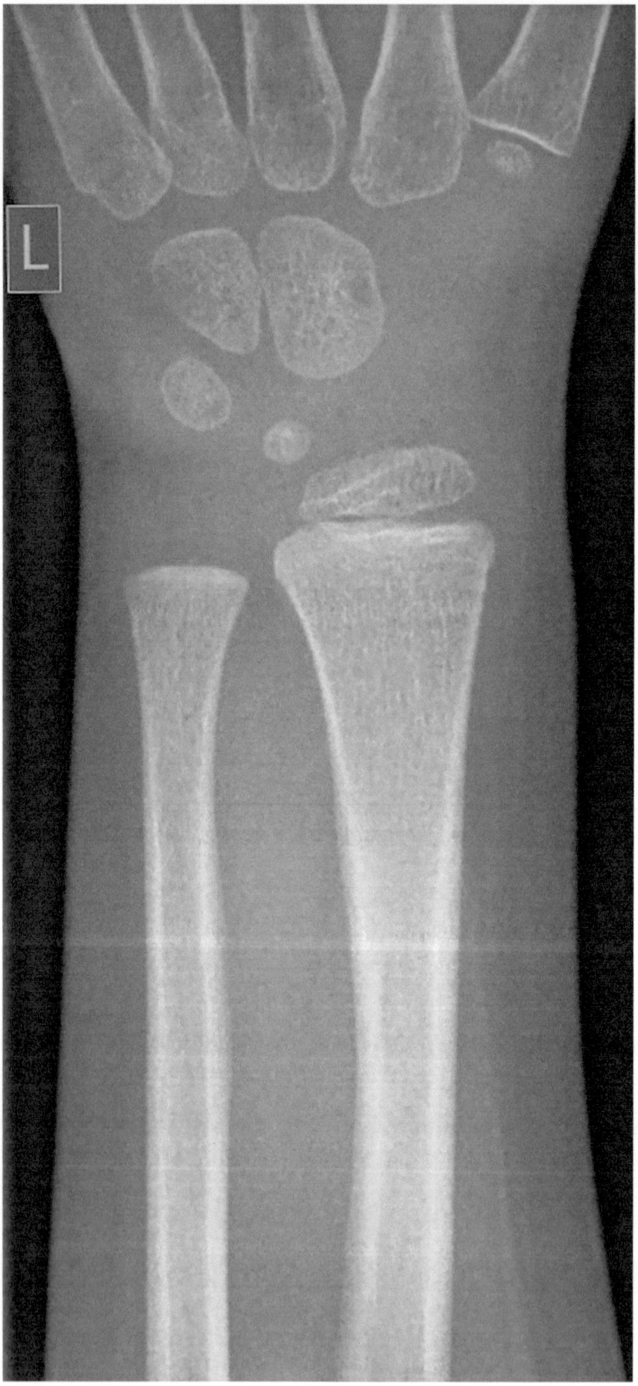

Image 30

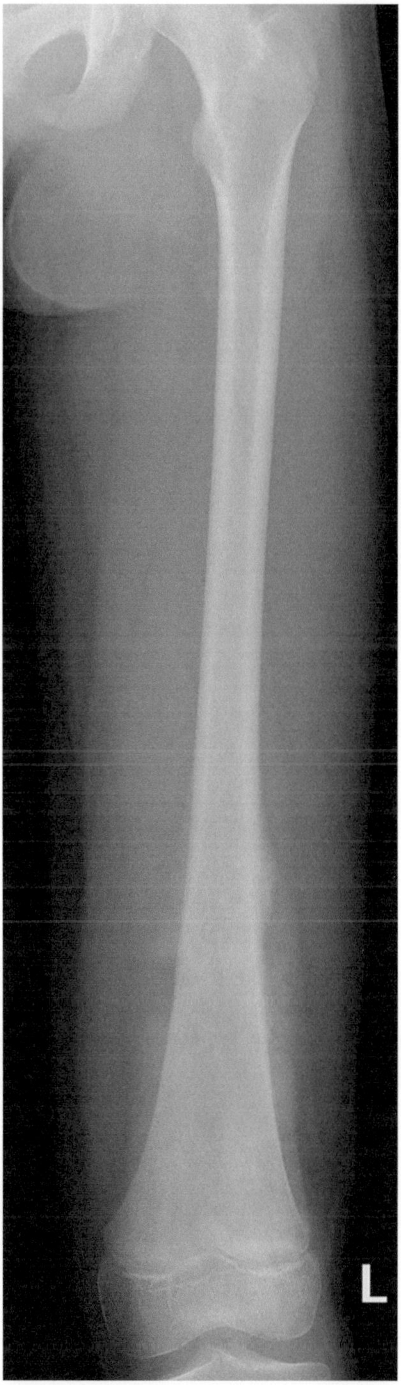

2.2 Answers

Image	Normal	Abnormal	Diagnosis/abnormality (only if abnormal)
1	✓		
2	✓		
3	✓		
4		✓	SH2 # R radial neck
5		✓	Pneumomediastinum
6		✓	AVN R proximal femoral epiphysis
7		✓	SH2 # R second metatarsal neck
8	✓		
9		✓	AVN R proximal femoral epiphysis
10		✓	Healing stress # R distal radial diaphysis
11		✓	# R radial neck
12		✓	L SUFE
13	✓		
14		✓	Healing # R 11th posterior rib
15	✓		
16		✓	L paraspinal mass
17		✓	L DDH
18	✓		
19		✓	Osgood-Schlatter disease R knee
20		✓	AVN L proximal femoral epiphysis
21		✓	Buckle #s L distal radius and ulnar metaphyses
22	✓		
23	✓		
24	✓		
25		✓	R posterior hip dislocation
26	✓		
27	✓		
28	✓		
29	✓		
30		✓	Aggressive bone lesion L distal femur

2.3 Explanations

1. *Normal pelvic radiograph*
   Note the iliac crest apophyses which have not yet fused and are normal. The iliac crest apophyses ossify lateral to medial, i.e. from the anterior superior iliac spine (ASIS) to the posterior superior iliac spine (PSIS).
   The Risser classification is a system which grades skeletal maturity based upon the degree of ossification and fusion of the iliac crest apophyses. This can be used as a surrogate marker for skeletal maturity and the ossification of the vertebrae, which generally parallels that of the iliac crest. The higher the Risser grade, the greater the skeletal maturity. As such, this can be used to predict the progression of scoliosis based on the amount of skeletal maturation that remains and may be used when planning corrective spinal surgery. The Risser classification is comprised of the following stages:
   - Stage 0: no ossification of the iliac crest apophysis.
   - Stage 1: apophysis <25% of the iliac crest.
   - Stage 2: apophysis 25–50% of the iliac crest.
   - Stage 3: apophysis 51–75% of the iliac crest.
   - Stage 4: apophysis 76–100% of the iliac crest.
   - Stage 5: complete ossification and fusion of the iliac crest apophysis.

2. *Normal left ankle radiograph*
   The relatively dense 'rectangles' at the left distal tibial and fibular metaphyses are the normal subperiosteal bone collars which are commonly found at the end of long bones. See Image 8 in Test 1 for similar appearances of the right distal radius and ulnar metaphyses.

3. *Normal right knee radiograph*
   The subtle lucency over the proximal tibial metaphysis represents the incompletely fused tibial tuberosity ossification centre which is imaged *en face* on anteroposterior (AP) projections. See the contemporaneous orthogonal projection below which confirms this normal developmental appearance (and not a lucent lesion):

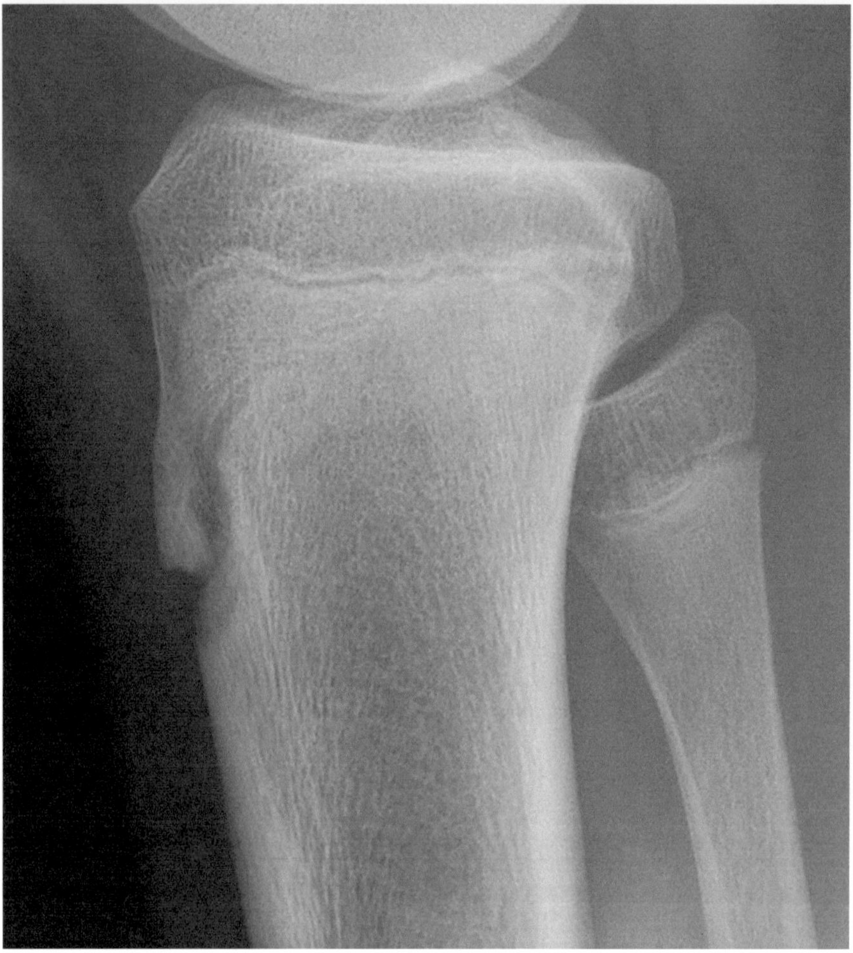

4. **Salter-Harris 2 # R radial neck**
The outline of every bone must be traced for cortical irregularity. Whilst there is no appreciable elbow joint effusion, scrutiny of the right radial neck reveals an acute fracture which is magnified below:

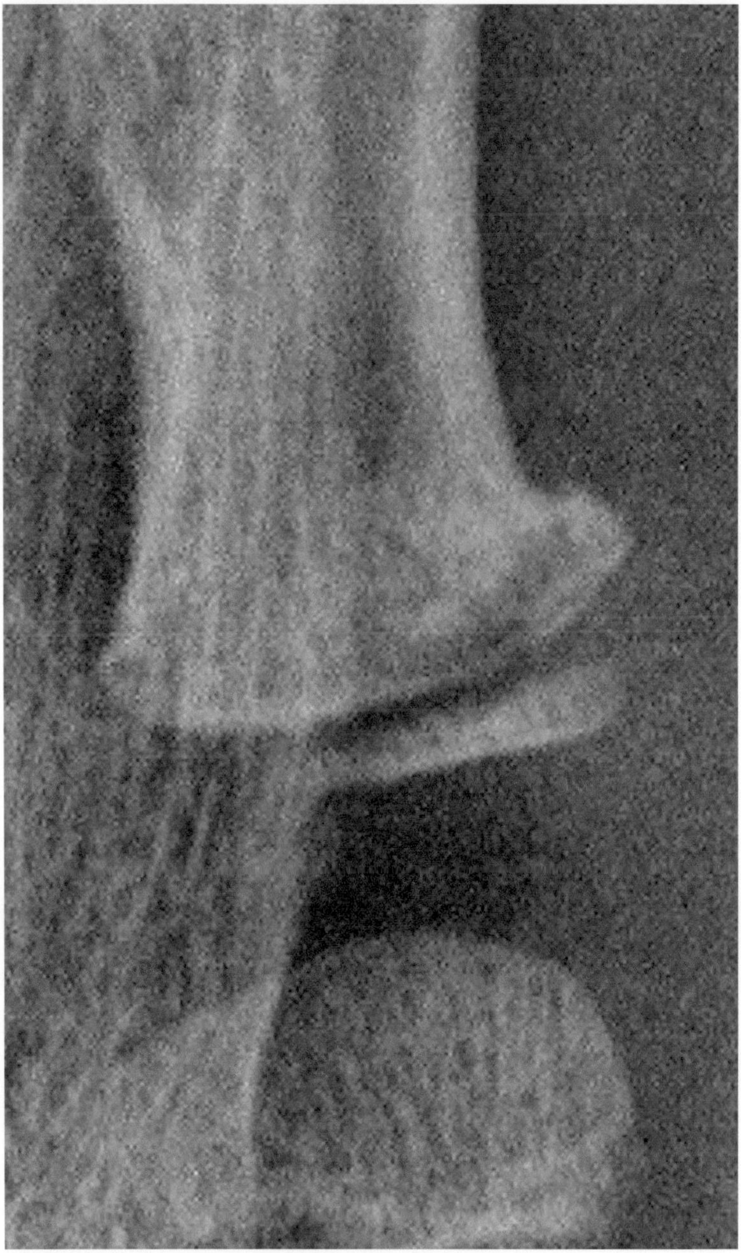

5. **Pneumomediastinum**
   This is a subtle but important finding. Note the streaky linear paratracheal lucencies projected at the level of the lower cervical spine/thoracic inlet, superior mediastinum and at the level of the carina/right main bronchus. This child with a known history of asthma (the cause of the pneumomediastinum) presented with chest pain. He was managed conservatively and a follow-up chest radiograph performed several days later demonstrated near-complete resolution of the pneumomediastinum.

   The examination is made more difficult by the absence of clinical information. However, this is not unlike actual clinical practice! Therefore, you must ensure that you adopt a structured approach to your radiographic interpretation to ensure that important findings are not overlooked.

   Tip for the viva:
   - Once a pneumomediastinum has been identified, look for an associated pneumothorax (uni- or bilateral) and vice versa, particularly in the context of wheeze, chest pain, or when provided with a history of asthma.

6. **Avascular necrosis R proximal femoral epiphysis**
   Note the increased sclerosis and loss of height of the right proximal femoral epiphysis compared to the left. See the explanation for Image 1 of Test 1.

7. **Salter-Harris 2 # R second metatarsal neck**
   This minimally displaced fracture reinforces the point that the physis *and* the adjacent metaphysis and epiphysis must be scrutinised on every radiograph. See the explanation for Image 30 of Test 1 for a discussion of the Salter-Harris classification.

   Tip for the viva:
   - When presented with an extremity/skeletal radiograph, you must ask for the contemporaneous orthogonal projection to complete your imaging evaluation.

8. *Normal accessory ossification centre inferior pole left patella*
   The patella can have variable ossification at all ages: it can appear fragmented and may have multiple centres of ossification resulting in a bi- or multi-partite patella. An accessory ossification centre at the inferior pole of the patella is a well-recognised normal variant which in the examination should be denoted as 'normal' (see the Introduction section). Furthermore, secondary signs of injury are absent with no overlying soft tissue swelling, effusion, or lipohaemarthrosis.

Tip for the viva:

- If presented with a similar appearance *plus* associated soft tissue swelling and/or other acute findings, consider these diagnoses:
  - **Patella sleeve fracture**: also known as an osteochondral avulsion fracture. Accompanied by an appropriate history, this is an acute avulsion injury at the inferior pole of the patella at the origin of the patella tendon. This injury results from a forceful contraction of the quadriceps tendon in a flexed knee. These fractures may be difficult to discern on radiography given the sometimes variable (but normal) patellar ossification. Moreover, this fracture is extra-articular, and so a joint effusion may not be present. Evaluation with magnetic resonance imaging (MRI) is essential to assess the extent of the osteochondral defect, the extensor mechanism of the knee, and the presence of anterior soft tissue swelling (which may not be apparent radiographically).
  - **Sinding-Larsen-Johansson syndrome**: also known as 'jumper's knee'. This is often thought of as the 'Osgood-Schlatter equivalent' at the inferior patellar pole and represents a chronic traction injury. Children usually present with focal soft tissue swelling and point tenderness. If radiography is performed, appearances may be normal, i.e. normal radiographic appearances do not exclude this diagnosis. When present, positive findings include soft tissue swelling, thickening of the proximal portion of the patella tendon, stranding of the infrapatellar fat pad (of Hoffa), and irregular/dystrophic calcification at the inferior patellar pole.

9. **Avascular necrosis R proximal femoral epiphysis**

This 12-year-old boy was referred for radiography by his General Practitioner (GP) for long-standing atraumatic right hip pain. He walked into the radiology department with a painful limp but was otherwise fit and well. Children are usually quite robust and may tolerate significant symptom burden before being presented. Perthes disease may present at any time, and if not investigated promptly, children can present late with significant changes, as in this case. The radiographic changes include:

- Subarticular collapse of the right proximal femoral epiphysis which is flattened and sclerotic.
- Subsequent widening of the right hip joint space with associated acetabular remodelling and sclerosis.
- The right proximal femoral metaphysis is starting to flatten/widen (coxa magna) and there is lateral uncovering of the proximal femoral epiphysis.

One must always assess the contralateral hip, given that Perthes disease affects *both* hips in approximately 15% of cases. In this image, the left proximal femoral epiphysis is enlocated and is normal in size, morphology and radiographic density. See the explanation for Image 1 of Test 1 for a comprehensive discussion of avascular necrosis (AVN).

Tip for the viva:

- *Both* proximal femoral epiphyses must be carefully inspected on *every* paediatric pelvic radiograph for early radiographic changes of AVN.
- In the appropriate clinical context, the late sequelae of septic arthritis could have similar radiographic appearances.
- Bilateral symmetrical 'Perthes' should raise the suspicion of multiple epiphyseal dysplasia.

10. **Healing stress # R distal radial diaphysis**

This image was obtained in a 7-year-old female gymnast who was presented with recurrent right wrist pain. The findings in this radiograph include sclerosis, cortical thickening, and associated subtle benign/non-aggressive periosteal reaction of the right distal radial diaphysis in keeping with a healing stress fracture. If you had been presented with these findings in the second metatarsal on an oblique foot radiograph, you would not hesitate in reporting a healing stress fracture.

Stress fractures result from incongruity between bone strength and the chronic mechanical stress placed upon it, i.e. abnormal stress on normal bone. Compare with the normal stress placed on abnormal bone in the case of insufficiency fractures or pathological fractures in the presence of an underlying bone lesion.

Radiographs have poor sensitivity initially and may appear normal. The radiographic features of healing become more apparent over time and include: subtle loss of cortical definition; increased sclerosis and/or cortical thickening; periosteal reaction; and a fracture line (which is not always visualised). Subperiosteal new bone formation (SPNBF; also known as periosteal reaction) may take up to 14 days after the injury to be detected radiographically, but is usually present from day 7, and most often by day 10.

MRI is the most sensitive modality for diagnosis: in this case, MRI demonstrated the fracture line which is not apparent radiographically.

Tip for the viva:

- Remember the 2B viva adage: *common pathologies in uncommon places.*

11. **# R radial neck**

Note the acute cortical step in the volar aspect of the radial neck with an associated elbow joint effusion.

12. **L slipped upper femoral epiphysis**

Slipped upper femoral epiphysis (SUFE), also known as Slipped Capital Femoral Epiphysis (SCFE), is one of the more common hip pathologies in adolescence. As a Salter-Harris 1 injury, it is thought to result from repeated biomechanical stress or trauma but it may also occur acutely. It is more common in boys than girls, with boys typically presenting later (10–17 years) than girls (8–15 years), and also more common in Afro-Caribbean children than Caucasians. Obesity is a significant risk factor and there may be a predisposing endocrine condition (e.g. hypothyroidism, hyperparathyroidism).

As the slip is *posteromedial* (often more posterior than medial), the most sensitive radiographic projection is the frog-leg lateral projection and it is often the only projection performed; the AP projection rarely adds any further diagnostic information. Early radiographic changes include widening, blurring, and increased lucency of the physis. Klein's line (a line drawn along the lateral femoral neck) fails to traverse the proximal femoral epiphysis, which it would do in a normal hip.

As the changes progress, the metaphysis may be displaced laterally such that it no longer overlaps the posterior lip of the acetabulum—this is known as the metaphyseal extrusion sign. Additionally, there may be increased density over the metaphysis due to resultant overlapping of the 'slipped' epiphysis—this is known as the metaphyseal blanch/steel sign. As the changes become more chronic, the physis becomes sclerotic with metaphyseal widening/flattening, resulting in coxa magna (enlargement and deformation of the femoral head and neck) on the affected side(s). The chronic changes are sequelae of AVN.

Tip for the viva:

- In this case, the SUFE is evident on the left but careful evaluation of the right hip is required because *both* hips can be affected in up to 20% of cases. Discuss the imaging protocol used (frog-leg lateral and/or AP projections) with your local paediatric radiologists.

13. *Normal right ankle radiograph*

This radiograph is normal. The ill-defined lucency in the calcaneus represents a normal variant termed pseudotumour of the calcaneus. Recognition of this normal appearance is important so that it is not overcalled as pathology. If the lucency is well-defined with a sclerotic margin, an intraosseous lipoma or bone cyst should be considered. The axial projection of the calcaneus can be extremely helpful in excluding a tumour.

In this radiograph, there is an ossicle posterior to the talus—if this does not fuse with the lateral tubercle of the posterior talar process, it persists as an *os trigonum*.

14. **Healing # R 11th posterior rib**

Posterior rib fractures, along with complex skull and metaphyseal fractures, are highly specific for physical abuse in infants and young children below the age of 2 years. Suspected physical abuse (SPA) is also termed suspected inflicted injury and was (but often still is) ubiquitously known as non-accidental injury

(NAI). In this case (and indeed, on every paediatric radiograph), every rib and bony structure must be assessed for evidence of acute or healing fracture(s). The healing fracture is magnified below (note the callus formation around the fracture line and compare to the adjacent normal right 10th and 12th ribs):

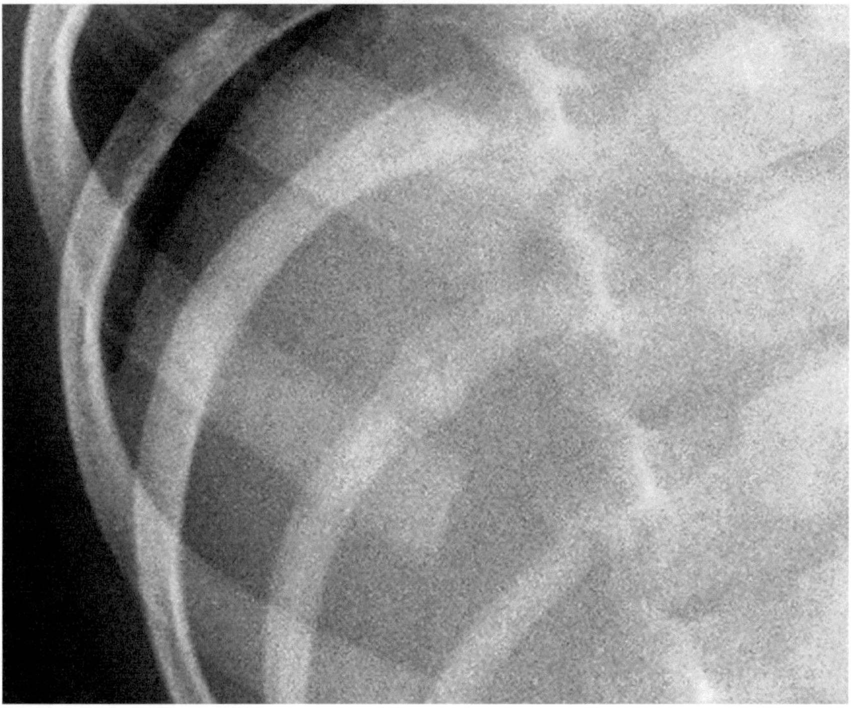

Oblique left and right chest radiographic projections increase the conspicuity of rib fractures as they allow visualisation of the ribs in two further planes. They form part of the radiographic skeletal survey which is the standardised series of radiographs performed in the investigation of SPA. Candidates should be familiar with the United Kingdom (UK) national guidance on the radiological investigation of SPA in children published by the Royal College of Radiologists (RCR). There are also key pictorial reviews in the references which provide a comprehensive overview of the radiographic findings of SPA, which you are strongly encouraged to read, not only for the examination, but for your future clinical practice.

Tip for the viva:

- Given that oblique chest radiographs obtained in infants and young children are specifically acquired to better visualise the ribs, look very carefully for acute/displaced or healing rib fractures when presented with these projections.

16. **L paraspinal mass**

The left apical mass in this image traverses the thoracic plane (of Ludwig) which is the imaginary line that separates the superior and inferior mediastinum at the level of the T4 vertebral body/manubriosternal joint. The mass extends above the superior aspect of the (left) clavicle (the imaginary border of the anterior mediastinum), which is known as the positive *cervicothoracic sign*. As such, it must lie either in the neck and/or the posterior mediastinum. Furthermore, the left hilar vessels are visualised (the hilum overlay sign) along with the left heart border, thereby excluding its presence in the middle mediastinum. As such, the mass lies in the posterior mediastinum in addition to traversing the 'border' of superior/inferior mediastinum.

In the examination, you will have approximately 1 min to decide whether an image is normal or abnormal. Although 'left posterior mediastinal mass' is more accurate, 'left paraspinal mass' would be sufficient.

Lateral radiographs to confirm/further localise a mediastinal mass are not routinely obtained in children (and diminishingly so in adults), both to reduce radiation burden and because a suspected mediastinal mass will require investigation with computed tomography (CT). However, this does not preclude the examiner from presenting you with one in the viva examination! If one has been obtained and is presented to you, the examiner will expect you to be able to interpret it before moving on to the inevitable CT.

In children, the most common mediastinal masses (all compartments) are:

- Neurogenic tumours: comprising the majority of cases, these arise from the sympathetic ganglia (neuroblastoma) or nerve roots (schwannoma or neurofibroma).
- Malignant germ cell tumours: teratomas account for the majority of tumours in the anterior mediastinum. These are a type of germ cell tumour which may contain several different types of tissue including fat, soft tissue, calcification (including teeth) and cystic spaces (which may contain fluid, mucous or a combination of both). These tumours can range from the more benign, mature, well differentiated cystic lesions to those which have undergone malignant transformation to immature, poorly differentiated tumours with solid components. Correlation with serum tumour markers is required (remember that *both* alpha-fetoprotein (AFP) and beta human chorionic gonadotropin (β-hCG) are elevated in germ cell tumours).
- Foregut duplication cysts: these may be bronchogenic which are usually mediastinal in location (but can also be intrapulmonary) and are often asymptomatic and do not communicate with the tracheobronchial tree; or oesophageal, which may be symptomatic resulting in dysphagia due to compression of the oesophagus. These cysts can be lined by gastric mucosa and are prone to infection, perforation, and haemorrhage. Rarely, these cysts may also be neurogenic in origin (<1%) resulting from incomplete resorption of the neurenteric canal.

- Extramedullary haematopoiesis: this is the deposition of normal blood cells outside the bone marrow resulting from a failure of erythropoiesis. Consider this in patients with thalassemia, sickle cell disease, or myelofibrosis in the context of smooth, well defined, and lobulated paraspinal masses, which may be unilateral or bilateral.

In this case, CT confirmed the presence of a posterior mediastinal mass, iodine-123 metaiodobenzylguanidine (MIBG) scintigraphy demonstrated corresponding high uptake, and CT guided biopsy confirmed the suspected radiological diagnosis of thoracic neuroblastoma. The majority of neuroblastomas (approximately two-thirds) arise from the adrenal glands and the retroperitoneum with posterior mediastinal thoracic neuroblastoma comprising approximately 20% of cases.

Tip for the viva:

- If presented with a suspected mediastinal mass on chest radiography, you must first localise the lesion *to*, and then *within*, the mediastinum. You may be presented with some clinical information following your initial interpretation which is often necessary to contextualise the radiographic findings to order/narrow the differential diagnosis.
- If no history has been provided, and in the context of a mediastinal mass, remember to look for 'H-shaped' vertebrae, AVN of the humeral head(s), and/or cardiomegaly as clues to a diagnosis of sickle cell disease.

17. **L developmental dysplasia of the hip**

The appearances in this radiograph are consistent with developmental dysplasia (DDH) of the (left) hip. The key radiographic features are:

- A small left ossific nucleus.
- A shallow and dysplastic left acetabulum.
- Lateral subluxation of the left hip joint.
- Broadening/widening of the left proximal femoral metaphysis.

DDH describes an abnormally developed hip joint with a subsequent abnormal relationship between the proximal femoral epiphysis and the acetabulum. It is thought to result from abnormal positioning *in utero*. Oligohydramnios and breech positioning during pregnancy are associated risk factors alongside a previous positive family history. There is also a female predominance with it being approximately eight times more common than in males.

DDH is suggested clinically by asymmetric thigh creases and a positive Barlow manoeuvre (hip adduction followed by posterior/downward force to dislocate the femoral head posteriorly) and Ortolani test (flexing then gently abducting the hips to relocate the [possibly dislocated] femoral head anteriorly into the acetabulum with a positive 'clunk').

Ultrasound is the modality of choice in infants under the age of 6 months given that the proximal femoral epiphyses are not yet ossified. After this age, radiographic evaluation is usually required to assess the hip joints which includes:

- Symmetry, size, shape, and radiographic density of the proximal femoral ossific nuclei—a delay in ossification i.e., a smaller and more lucent proximal femoral epiphysis, is a feature of DDH.

- Acetabular morphology—a shallow or dysplastic acetabulum is more likely to sublux/dislocate.
- A subluxed (as in this case) or frankly dislocated joint.

It is important to remember that DDH is a dynamic disease which is not always present or clinically apparent at birth. The pelvis and both hip joints should be evaluated on every radiograph (including abdominal radiographs which may also include the pelvis), particularly if performed for an unrelated clinical indication.

Tip for the viva:

- Careful evaluation of *both* hips is required given that DDH can be bilateral in *up to one-third of cases.*

18. *Normal left hand radiograph*
The tiny focus of ossification adjacent to the centre of the left distal ulnar metaphysis represents the start of the left distal ulnar epiphyseal ossification. Note also the subperiosteal bone collar at the left distal ulnar metaphysis, which is normal. See Image 2 of this test and Image 8 of Test 1 for further examples of this normal appearance.

19. **Osgood-Schlatter disease R knee**
This is a chronic traction apophysitis of the distal portion of the patellar tendon at its insertion onto the tibial tuberosity apophysis. It is more commonly seen in young active adolescent boys who kick and jump, typically affecting those aged 10–15 years. It can be bilateral in up to 50% of cases and affected children typically present with focal soft tissue swelling and point tenderness over the tibial tuberosity, which is exacerbated by exercise.
As this is a clinical diagnosis, it does not require investigation with radiography. However, if radiography is performed, there is typically fragmentation of the tibial tuberosity with focal overlying soft tissue swelling. However, it is important to note that fragmentation is a normal finding in the asymptomatic adolescent knee and represents normal ossification of the apophysis (secondary ossification centre). Thus, the radiological diagnosis of Osgood-Schlatter disease should not be made on the basis of fragmentation alone and explains why the diagnosis is largely clinical. The condition typically resolves once the tibial tuberosity physis has fused.

20. **Avascular necrosis L proximal femoral epiphysis**
See the explanation for Image 1 of Test 1.

21. **Buckle #s L distal radius and ulnar metaphyses**
Buckle fractures of the distal radius and ulna commonly occur together. Whilst the radial fracture is more obvious, the buckle fracture of the distal ulna is a genuine finding and is seen along the radial aspect in the magnified image below:

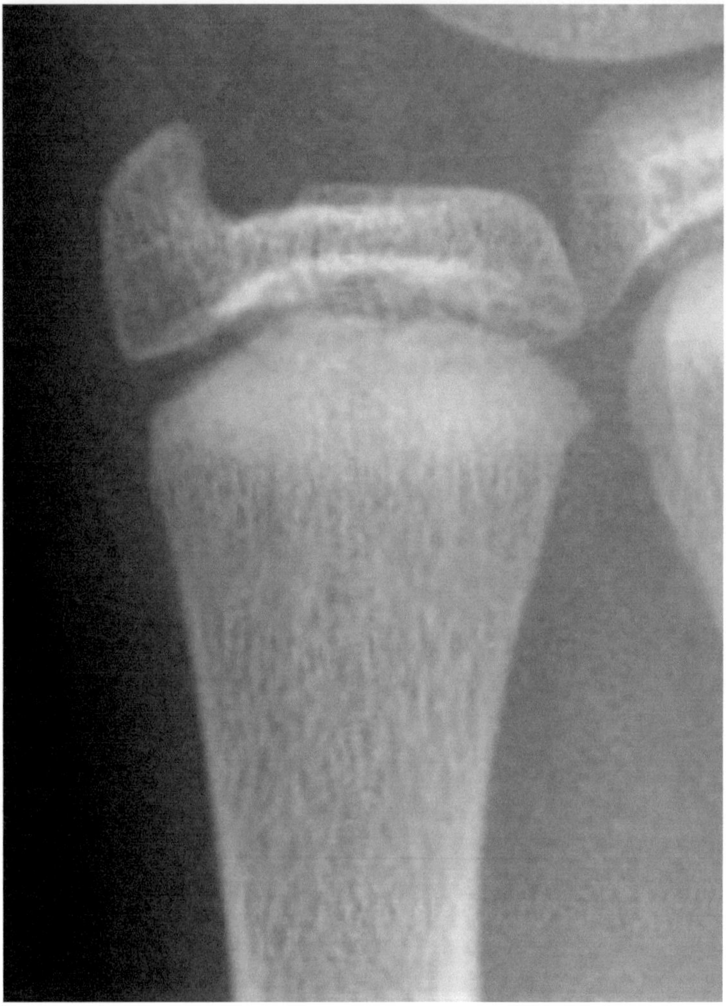

23. *Normal left knee radiograph*
The smooth elongation of the inferior left patella pole is an anatomical variant and should be denoted as 'normal' in the examination. If there is associated cortical irregularity, fragmentation and/or dystrophic calcification (which may progress to heterotopic ossification), overlying soft tissue swelling and a supportive clinical history (point tenderness in active adolescents typically between the ages of 10 and 14 years), a diagnosis of Sinding-Larsen-Johansson disease (chronic traction injury of the patella tendon at its insertion on the inferior patellar pole) should be considered. See the explanation for Image 8 of this test.

25. **R posterior hip dislocation**
Significant force is required to displace the femoral head from the normal hip joint. As such, traumatic hip dislocations are uncommon in the paediatric population and are only usually seen in the context of high energy impact trauma, e.g. road traffic accident (RTA). This child fell off a trampoline and landed awkwardly; the contemporaneous lateral projection confirmed the dislocation.

Tip for the viva:
- In the context of an acute traumatic subluxation/dislocation (any joint), do not forget to evaluate any contemporaneous orthogonal projection(s) for an associated fracture.

26. *Normal skull radiograph*
See the references for an annotated presentation of the radiological anatomy of the normal paediatric skull sutures and the craniosynostoses.

30. **Aggressive bone lesion L distal femur**
There is a permeative ('moth-eaten') appearance of the left distal femoral diaphysis and metadiaphysis with a wide zone of transition. There is aggressive spiculated/'hair-on-end' periosteal reaction and Codman triangle on the lateral aspect of the distal femoral diaphysis. The latter results from the fact that the periosteum does not have time to ossify given the aggressive nature of the lesion, so only the edge of the raised periosteum ossifies. There is also associated mild soft tissue swelling. The contemporaneous (magnified) lateral projection better demonstrates the spiculated/'hair-on-end' periosteal reaction, and the destruction of the anterior distal femoral cortex with lamellated periosteal reaction:

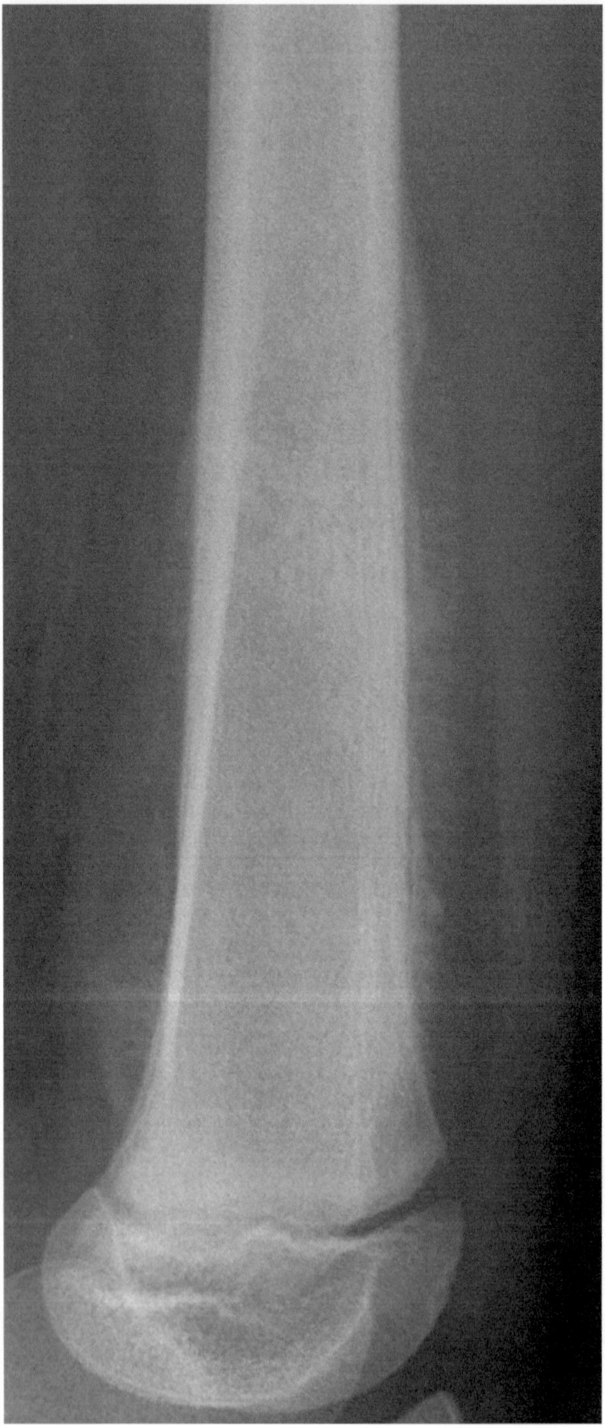

This 8-year-old girl was diagnosed with primary osteosarcoma. The imaging evaluation for suspected (and confirmed) osteosarcoma includes: MRI of the affected limb/area to assess the primary tumour (its location, size, extent and adjacent structures) and for "skip" lesions, i.e. lesions within the same bone but separate from the primary tumour; a feature of osteosarcoma; technetium-99m (m for metastable, denoting an intermediate energy state) bone scintigraphy to assess for distant sites of bony disease; and CT thorax to evaluate for metastases (the most frequent site of metastases is pulmonary, which may or may not be calcified).

Tip for the viva:

- Patients should be referred to a specialist paediatric orthopaedic centre experienced in managing suspected cases of primary bone malignancy: any biopsy tract will need to be carefully planned and included in any subsequent resection to reduce the risk of malignant seeding. Preoperative chemotherapy may help to downstage the tumour prior to resection.

Further Reading

Image 1

Cheung JPY, Luk KD (2017) Managing the pediatric spine: growth assessment. Asian Spine J 11(5):804–816
Glick Y et al (2022) Risser criteria. https://radiopaedia.org/articles/risser-classification. Accessed Feb 2023
Hacquebord JH, Leopold SS (2012) In brief: the Risser classification: a classic tool for the clinician treating adolescent idiopathic scoliosis. Clin Orthop Relat Res 470(8):2335–2338

Image 4

El-Feky M et al (2021) Patella sleeve fractures. https://radiopaedia.org/articles/patellar-sleeve-fracture-1. Accessed Feb 2023
Niknejad M et al (2022) Sinding-Larsen-Johansson disease. https://radiopaedia.org/articles/sinding-larsen-johansson-disease. Accessed Feb 2023
Pai DR, Strouse PJ (2011) MRI of the pediatric knee. AJR Am J Roentgenol 196(5):1019–1027

Image 10

Knipe H et al (2022) Stress fracture. https://radiopaedia.org/articles/stress-fracture-2. Accessed Mar 2023

Image 12

Hesper T, Zilkens C, Bittersohl B et al (2017) Imaging modalities in patients with slipped capital femoral epiphysis. J Child Orthop 11(2):99–106
Lustosa L et al (2023) Slipped upper femoral epiphysis. https://radiopaedia.org/articles/slipped-upper-femoral-epiphysis. Accessed Feb 2023
Sparks C, Phillips L, Kucera JN (2021) Imaging findings in pediatric hip pain: a pictorial review. J Rad Nu 40(4):345–352. https://www.sciencedirect.com/science/article/abs/pii/S1546084321001450, https://doi.org/10.1016/j.jradnu.2021.09.007

Image 13

Lustosa L et al (2023) Intraosseous lipoma. https://radiopaedia.org/articles/intraosseous-lipoma. Accessed Feb 2023
Thurston M et al (2017) Pseudotumour of the calcaneus. https://radiopaedia.org/articles/pseudotumour-of-the-calcaneus. Accessed Feb 2023
Yap J et al (2022) Os trigonum. https://radiopaedia.org/articles/os-trigonum. Accessed Feb 2023

Image 14

Bennett CE, Christian CW (2021) Clinical evaluation and management of children with suspected physical abuse. Pediatr Radiol 51:853–860
Gunda D, Cornwell BO, Dahmoush HM et al (2019) Pediatric central nervous system imaging of nonaccidental trauma: beyond subdural hematomas. Radiographics 39(1):213–228
Marine MB, Forbes-Amrhein MM (2021) Fractures of child abuse. Pediatr Radiol 51(6):1003–1013
Paddock M, Sprigg A, Offiah AC (2017) Imaging and reporting considerations for suspected physical abuse (non-accidental injury) in infants and young children. Part 1: initial considerations and appendicular skeleton. Clin Radiol 72(3):179–188
Paddock M, Sprigg A, Offiah AC (2017) Imaging and reporting considerations for suspected physical abuse (non-accidental injury) in infants and young children. Part 2: axial skeleton and differential diagnoses. Clin Radiol 72(3):189–201

Image 16

Baba Y et al (2022) Neuroblastoma. https://radiopaedia.org/articles/neuroblastoma. Accessed Feb 2023
Bhalla S, Hazewinkel M, Smithuis R (2007) Masses differential diagnosis. https://radiologyassistant.nl/chest/mediastinum/masses-differential-diagnosis. Accessed Feb 2023
El-Feky M et al (2018) Anterior mediastinal germ cell tumours. https://radiopaedia.org/articles/anterior-mediastinal-germ-cell-tumours. Accessed Feb 2023
Hacking C et al (2018) Thoracic plane. https://radiopaedia.org/articles/thoracic-plane. Accessed Feb 2023
Khedr DKM et al (2018) Extramedullary haematopoiesis. https://radiopaedia.org/articles/extramedullary-haematopoiesis. Accessed Feb 2023
Murphy A et al (2022) Bronchogenic cyst. https://radiopaedia.org/articles/bronchogenic-cyst. Accessed Feb 2023
Ranganath SH, Lee EY, Restrepo R et al (2012) Mediastinal masses in children. AJR Am J Roentgenol 198(3):W197–W216
Sreedher G, Tadros SS, Janitz E (2022) Pediatric mediastinal masses. Pediatr Radiol 52(10):1935–1947
Vadera S et al (2022) Spinal neurenteric cyst. https://radiopaedia.org/articles/spinal-neurenteric-cyst. Accessed Feb 2023

Image 17

Barrera CA, Cohen SA, Sankar WN et al (2019) Imaging of developmental dysplasia of the hip: ultrasound, radiography and magnetic resonance imaging. Pediatr Radiol 49(12):1652–1668
Rasuli B et al (2018) Developmental dysplasia of the hip. https://radiopaedia.org/articles/developmental-dysplasia-of-the-hip. Accessed Feb 2023
Robben S, Smithuis R (2018) Developmental dysplasia of the hip—ultrasound. http://www.radiologyassistant.nl/en/p54ba2c50995c5/developmental-dysplasia-of-the-hip-ultrasound.html. Accessed February 2023

Image 19

Lam JJH, Venkatesh SH, Ho CL et al (2019) Clinics in diagnostic imaging (202). Osgood-Schlatter disease (OSD). Singapore Med J 60(12):610–615

Merrow AC, Reiter MP, Zbojniewicz AM et al (2014) Avulsion fractures of the pediatric knee. Pediatr Radiol 44(11):1436–1445

Sørenson LB, Rathleff MS, Dean BJF et al (2021) A systematic review of imaging findings in patients with Osgood-Schlatter disease. Transl Sports Med 4(6):772–787

Thapa MM, Chaturvedi A, Iyer RS et al (2012) MRI of pediatric patients: part 2, normal variants and abnormalities of the knee. AJR Am J Roentgenol 198(5):W456–W465

Image 24

Eley KA, Johnson D, Sheerin F (2018) Cranial sutures & craniosynostosis. https://www.bir.org.uk/media/76496/cranial_sutures___craniosynostosis_-_ka_eley__f_sheerin__d_johnson__final_.pdf. Accessed Feb 2023

Image 30

Alhusseiny K et al (2023) Osteosarcoma. https://radiopaedia.org/articles/osteosarcoma. Accessed Mar 2023

Goyal N, Kalra M, Soni A et al (2019) Multi-modality imaging approach to bone tumors—state-of-the art. J Clin Orthop Trauma 10(4):687–701

Nguyen JC, Baghdadi S, Pogoriler J et al (2022) Pediatric osteosarcoma: correlation of imaging findings with histopathologic features, treatment, and outcome. Radiographics 42(4):1196–1213

van der Woude HJ, Smithuis R (2018) Bone tumor—systematic approach and differential diagnosis. http://www.radiologyassistant.nl/en/p494e15cbf0d8d/bone-tumor-systematic-approach-and-differential-diagnosis.html. Accessed Feb 2023

Test 3

3

M. Paddock et al., *Paediatric Radiology Rapid Reporting*,
https://doi.org/10.1007/978-3-031-48255-7_3

3.1 Images

Image 1

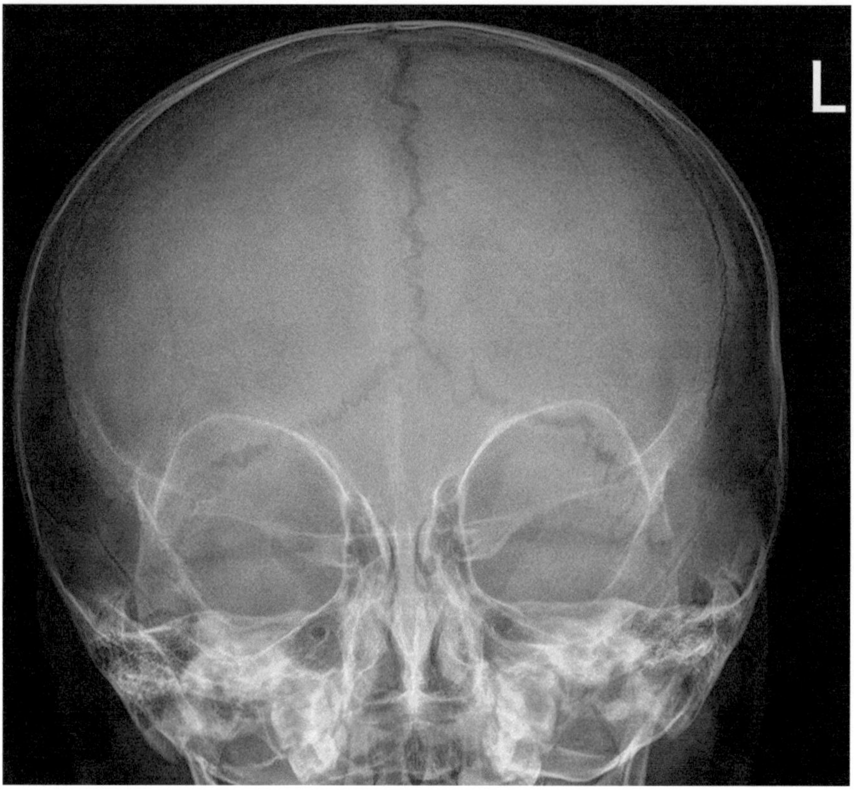

Image 2

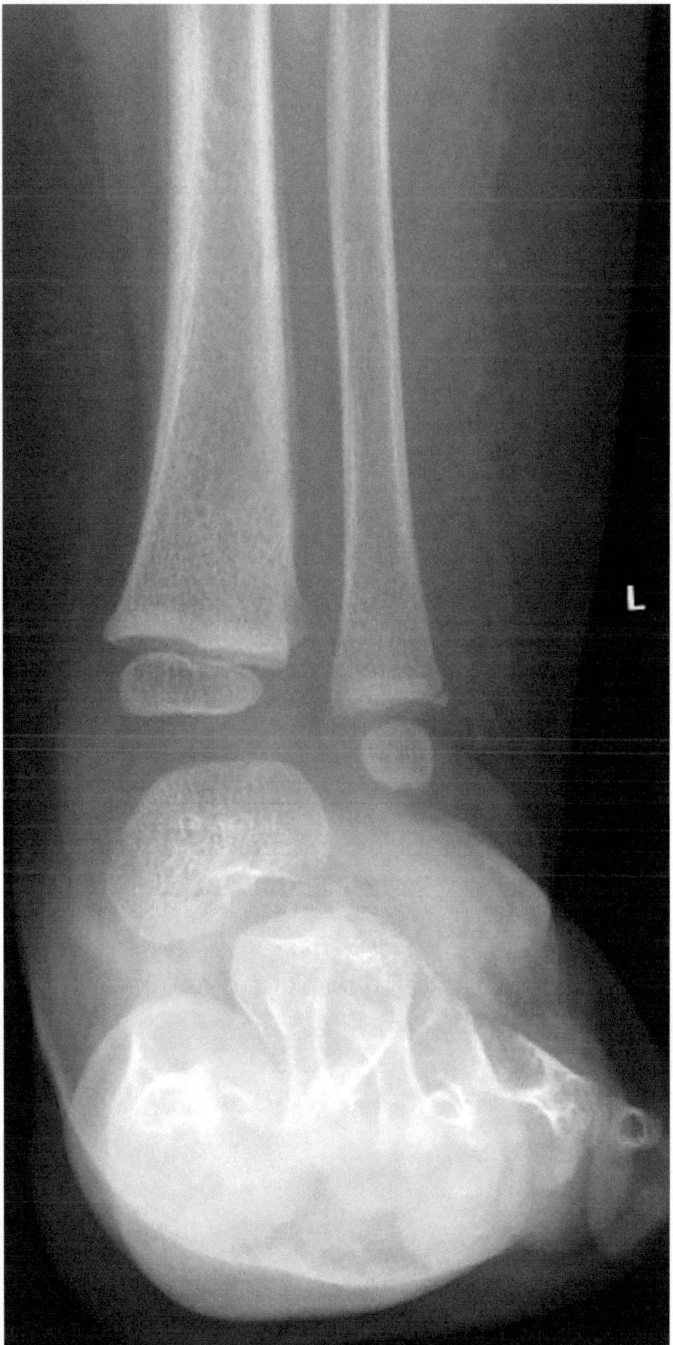

Image 3

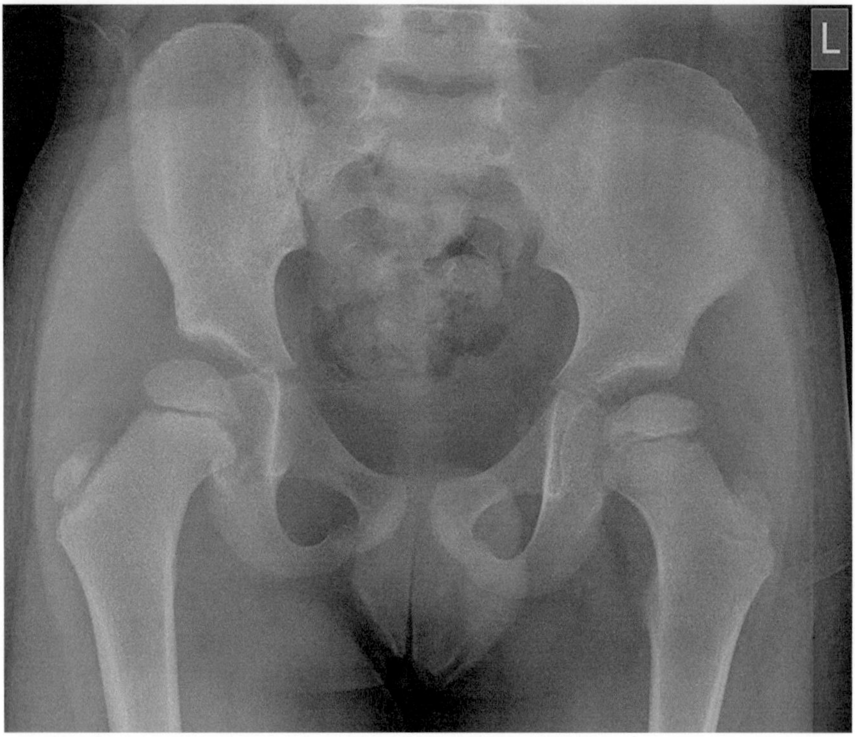

Image 4

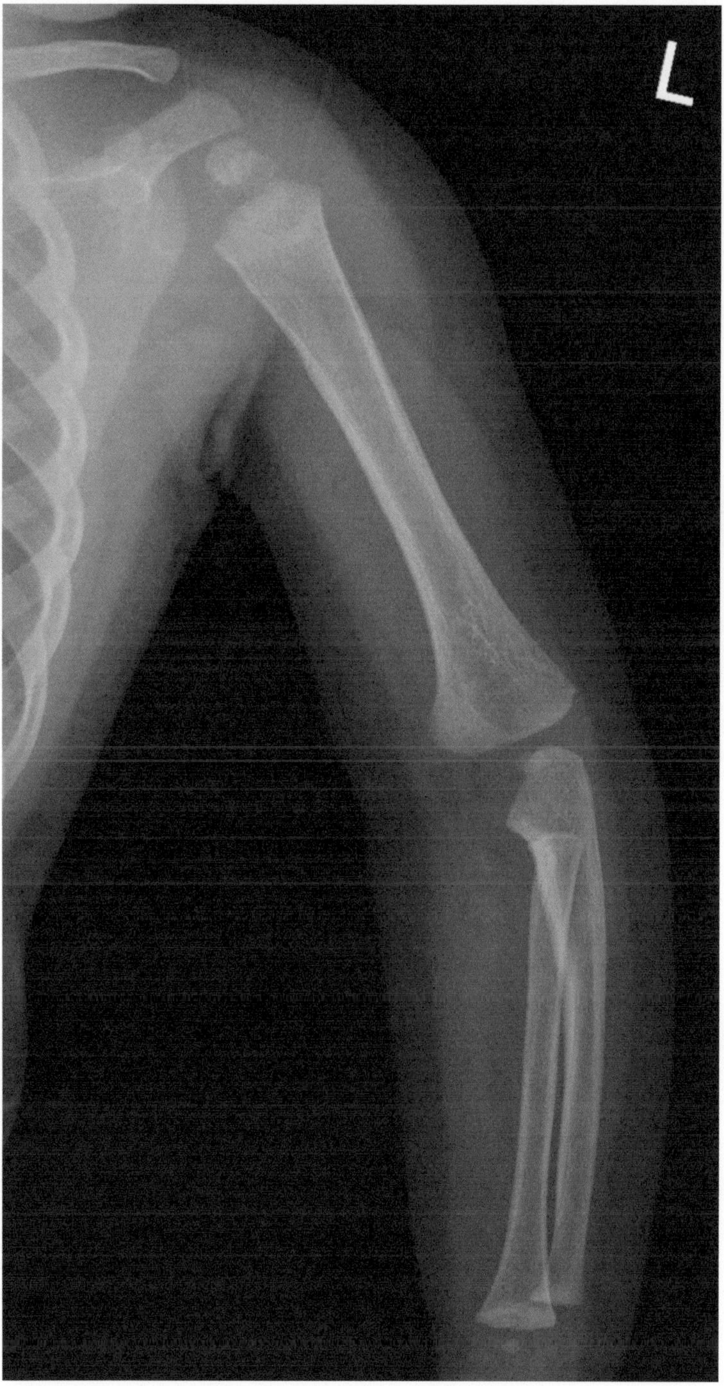

Image 5

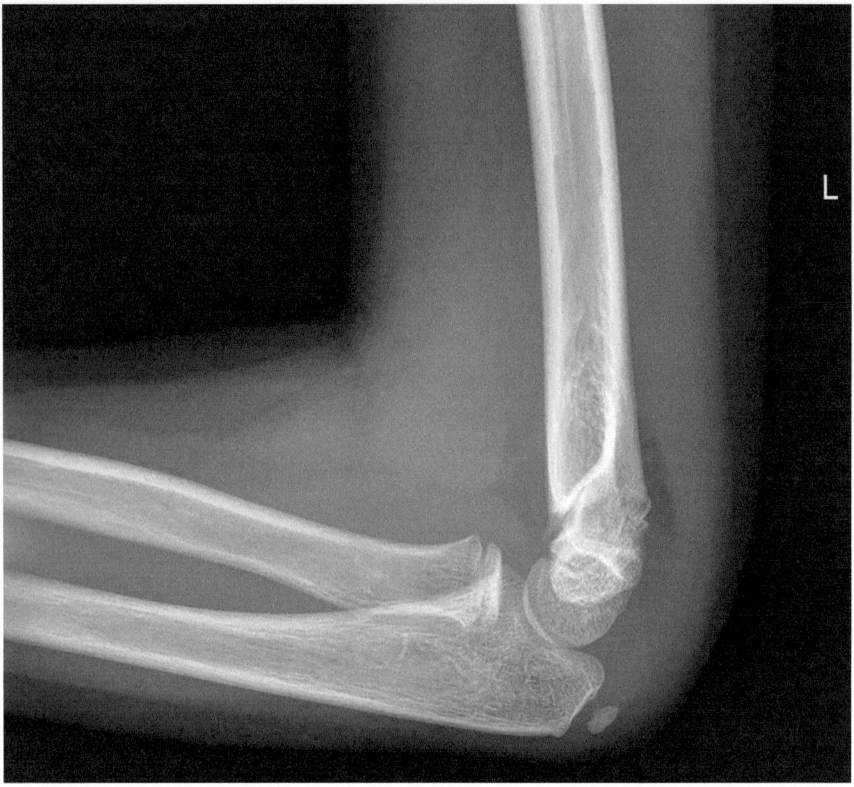

Image 6

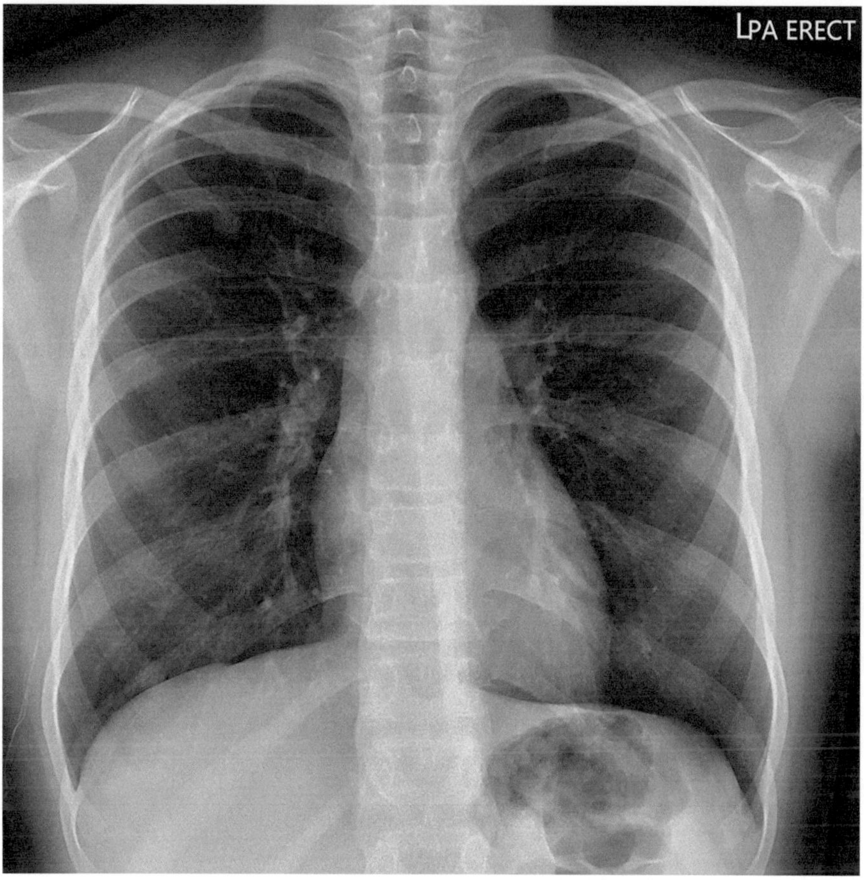

Image 7

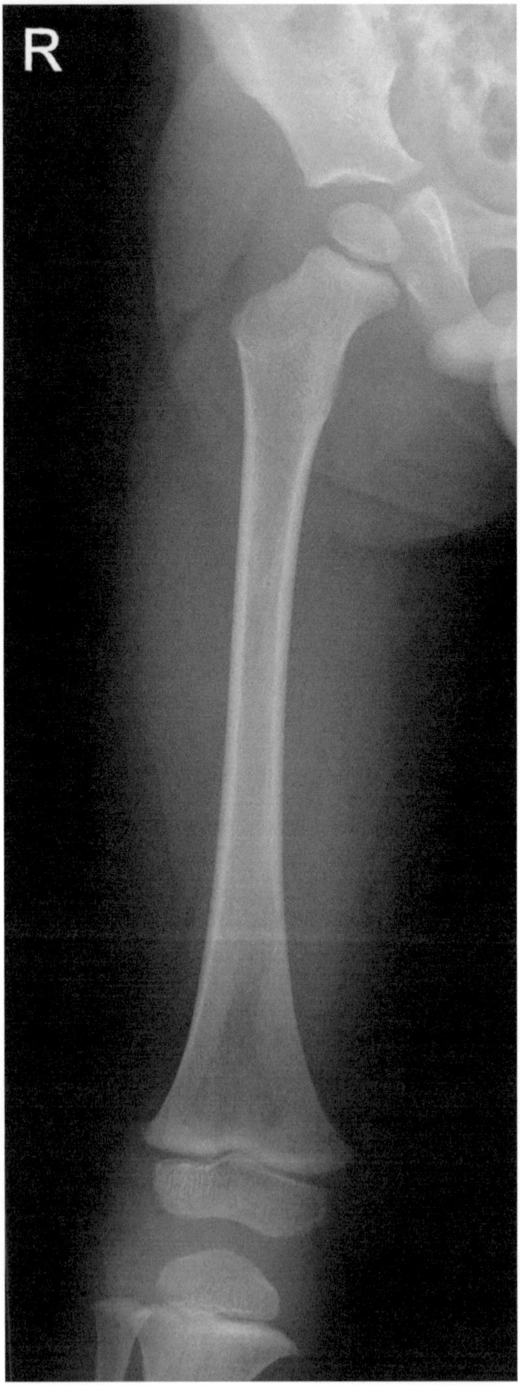

Image 8

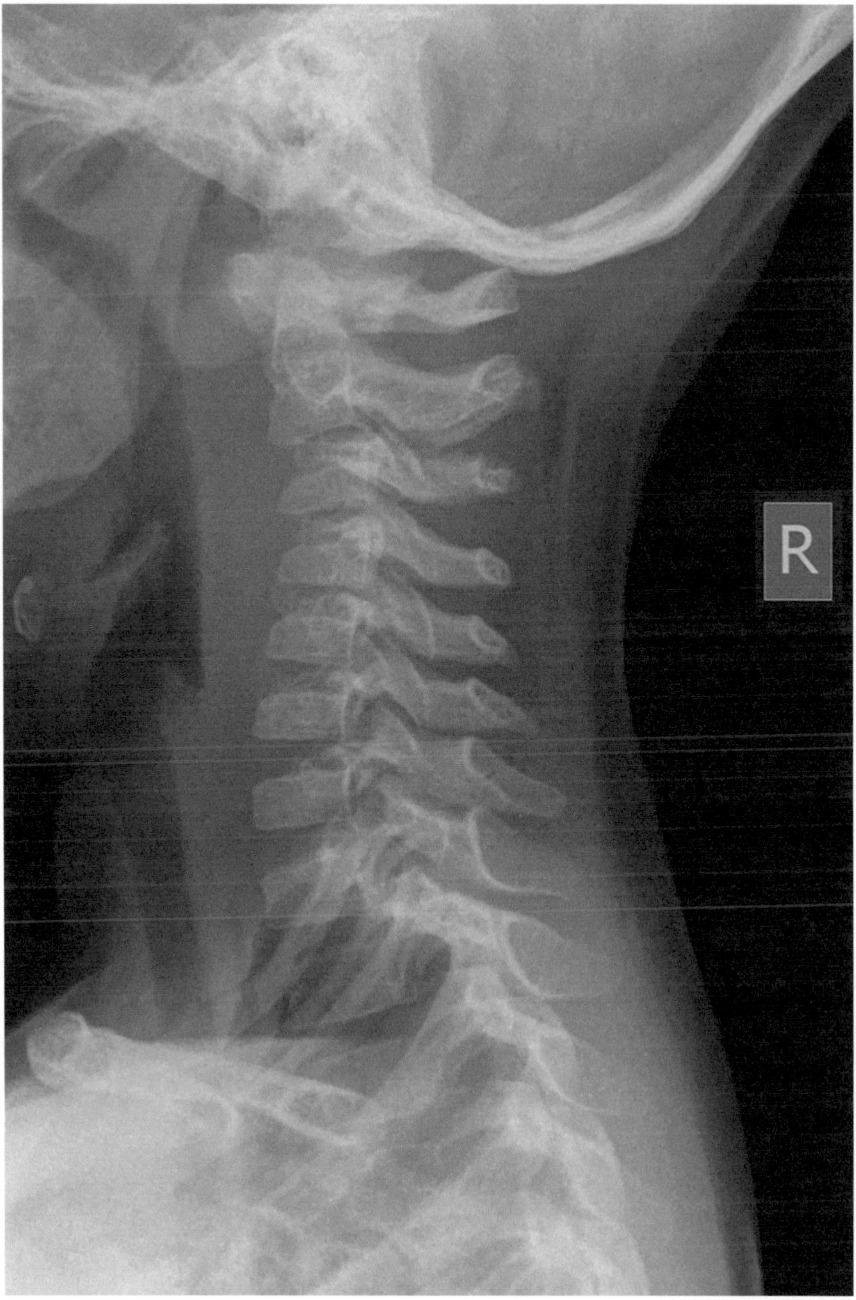

Image 9

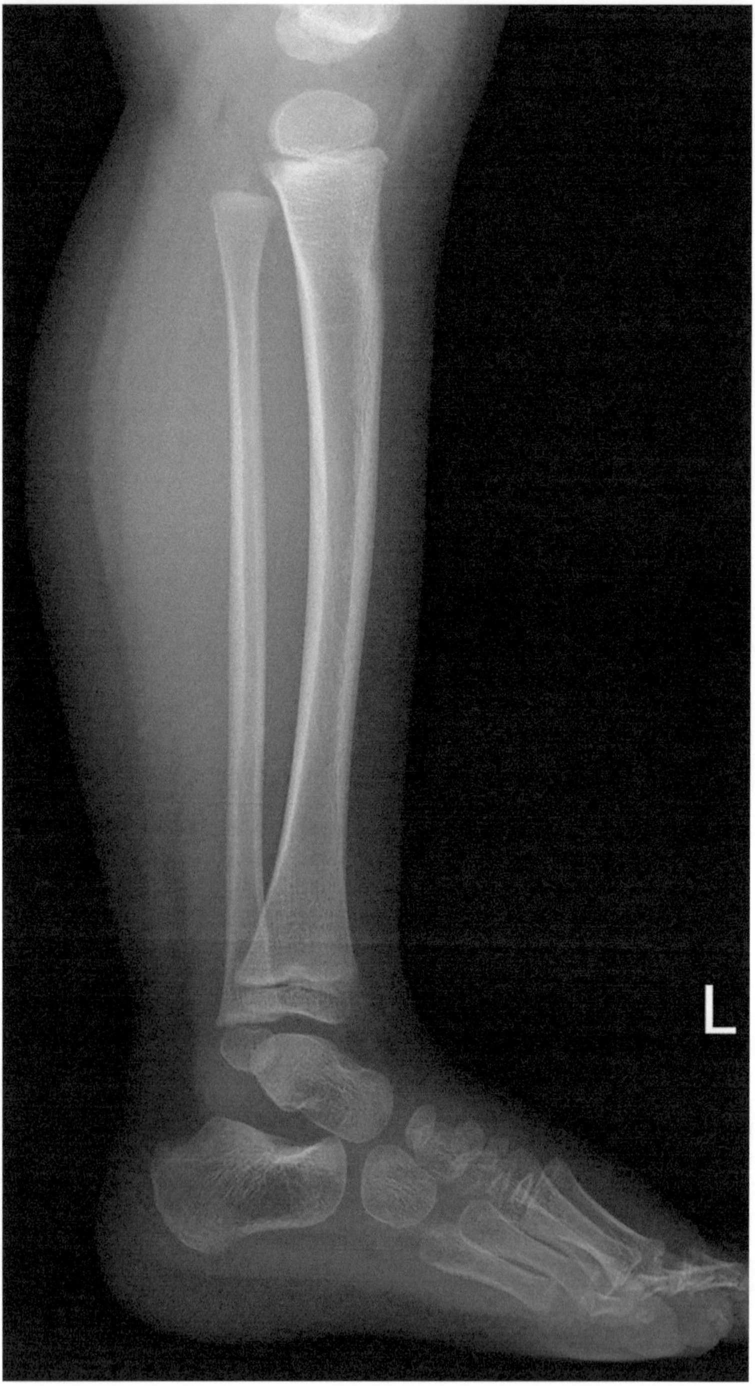

Image 10

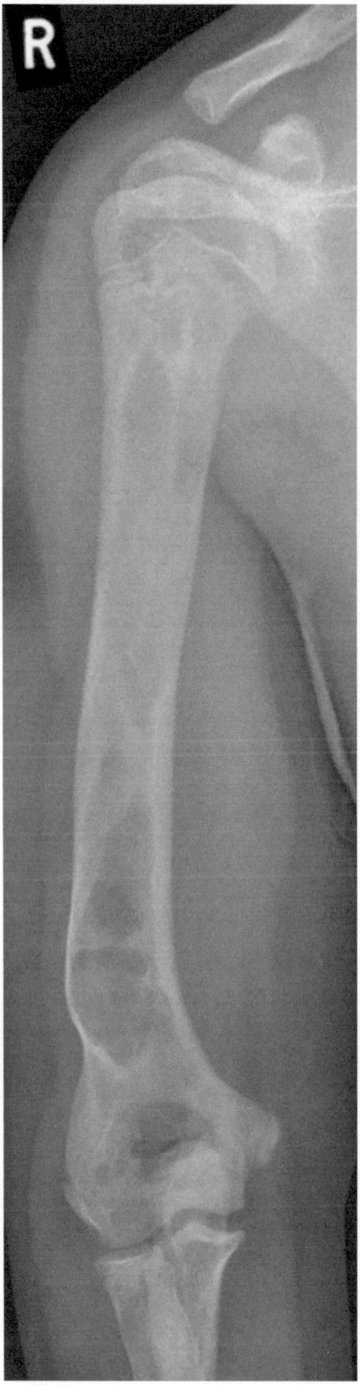

Image 11

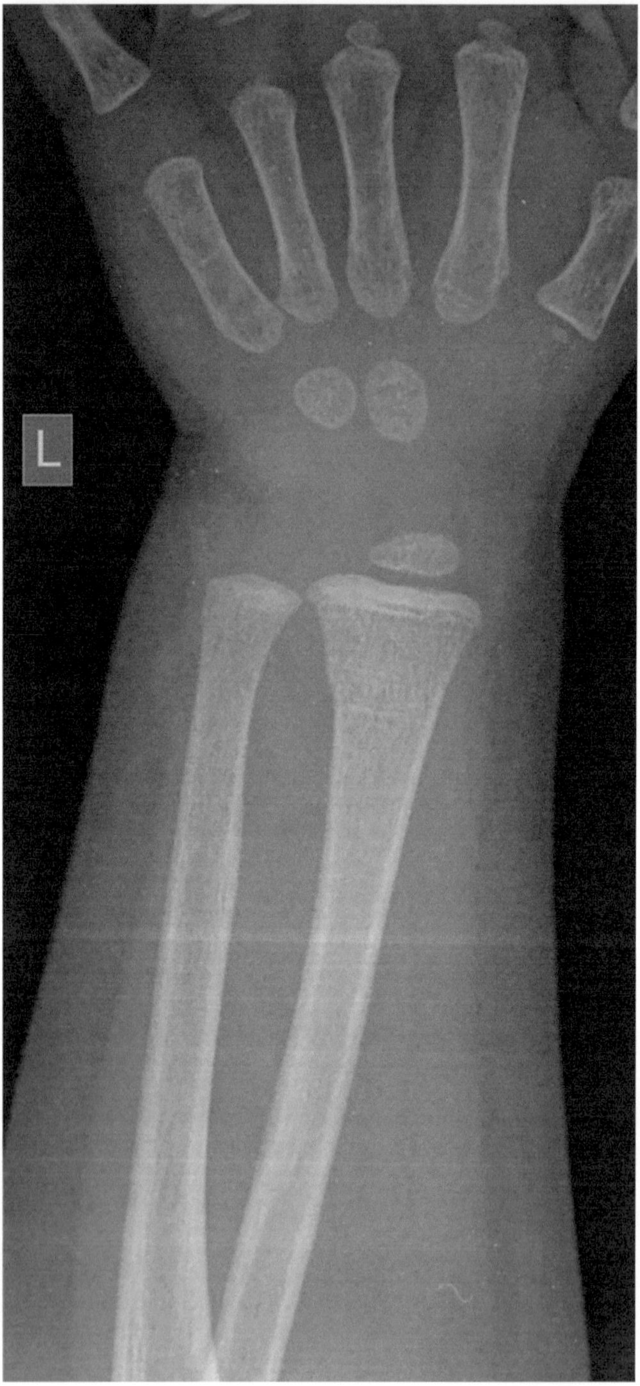

Image 12

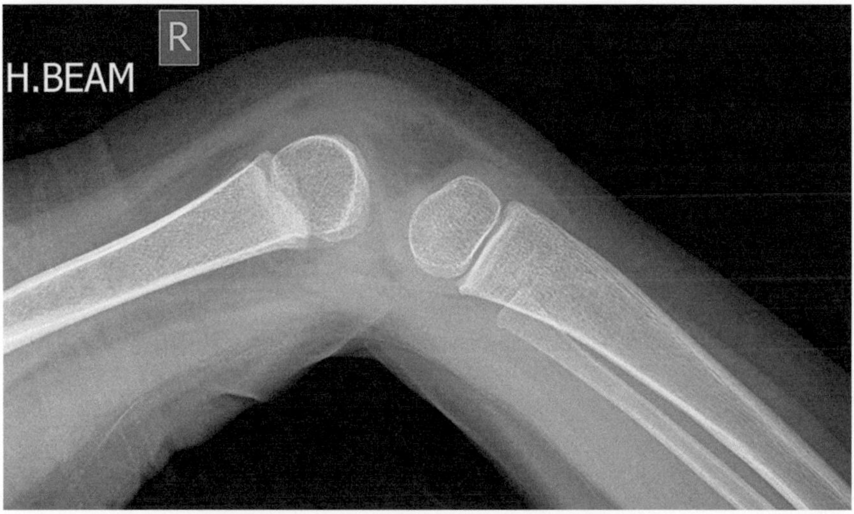

Image 13

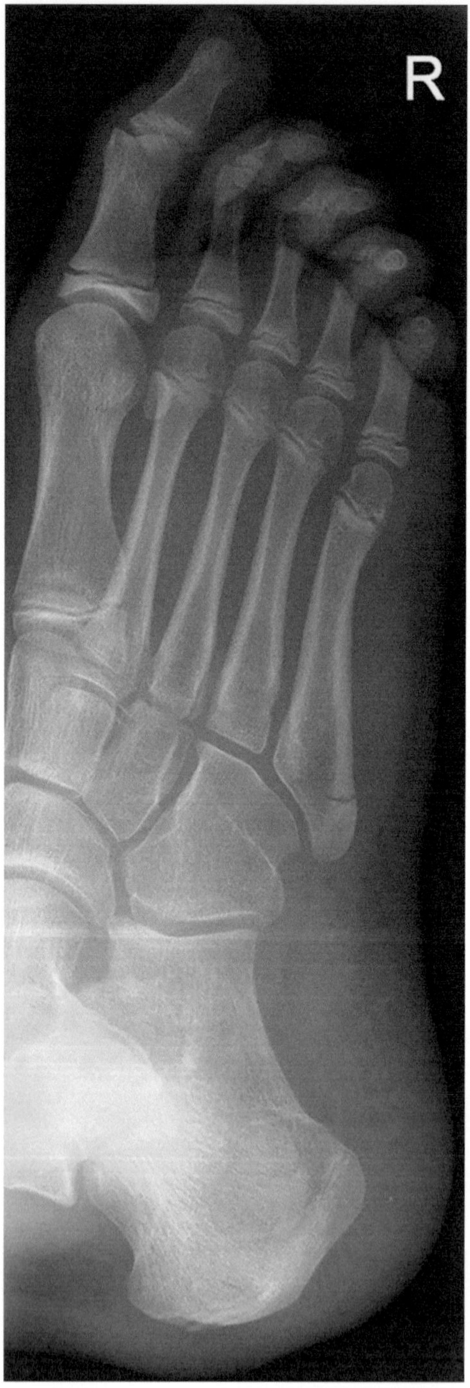

Image 14

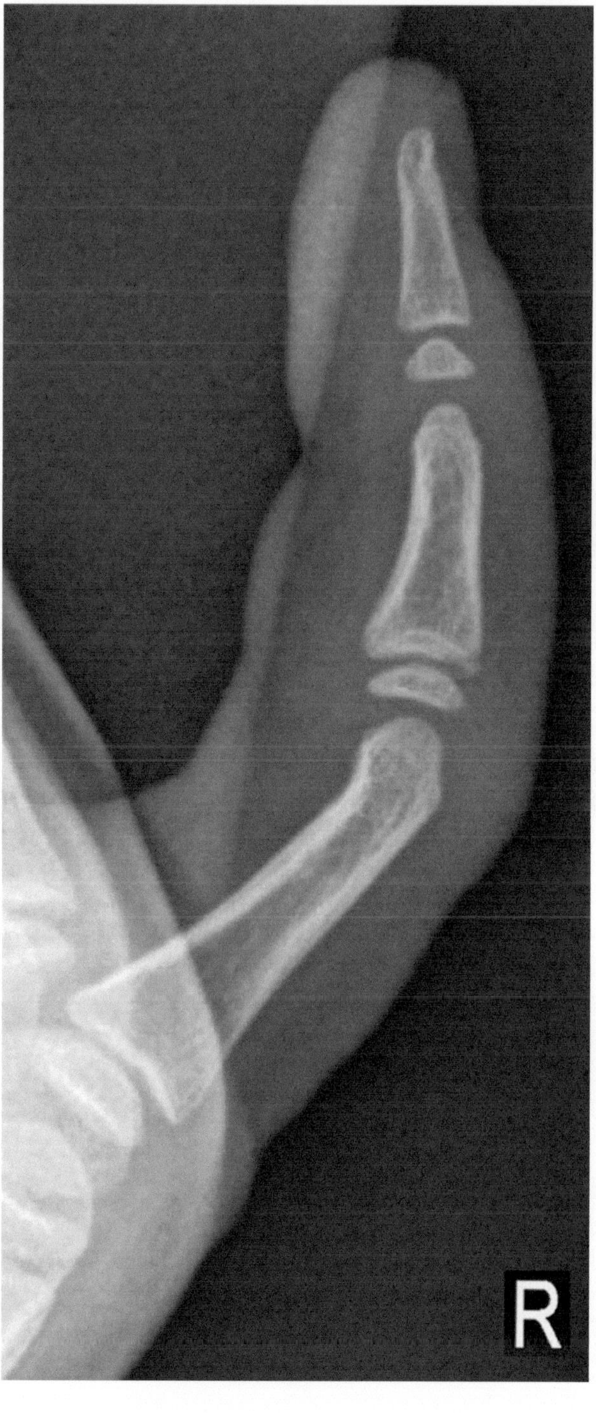

Image 15

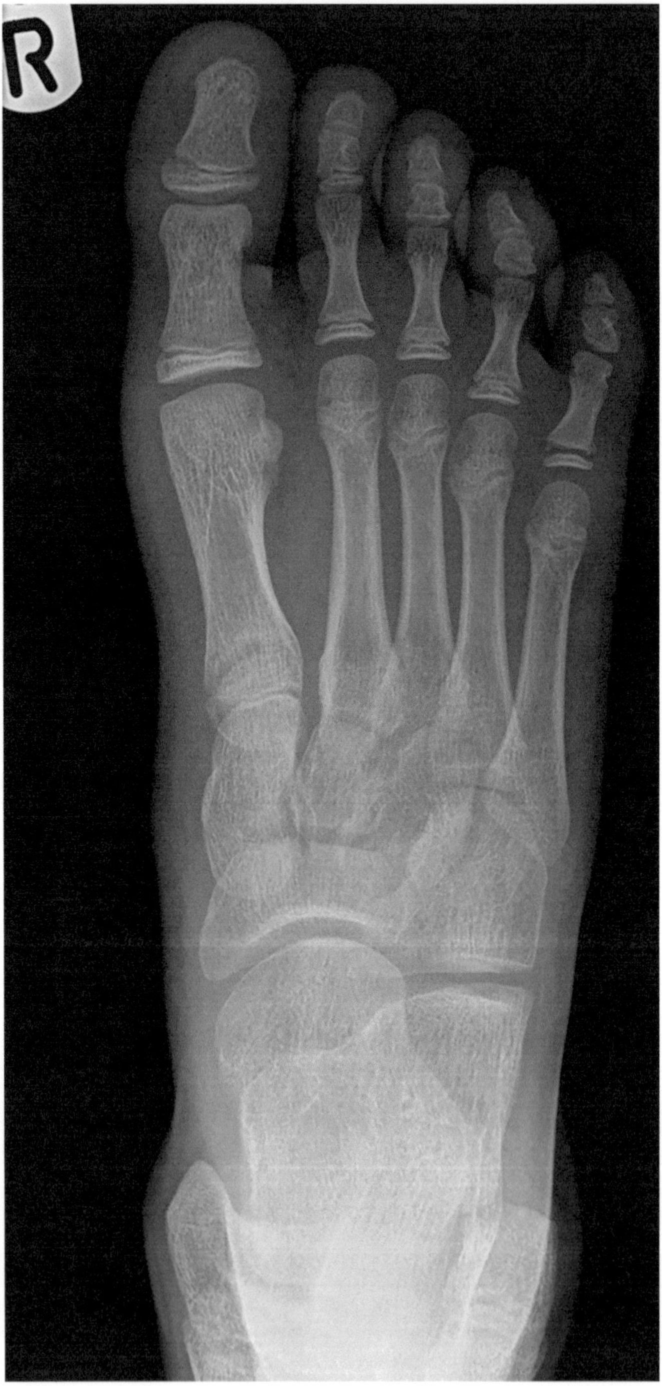

Image 16

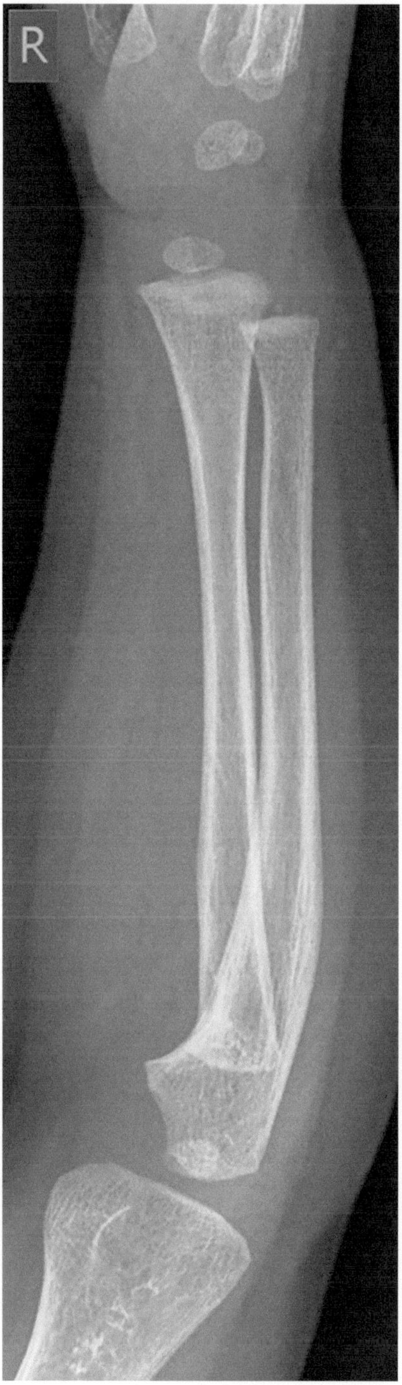

Image 17

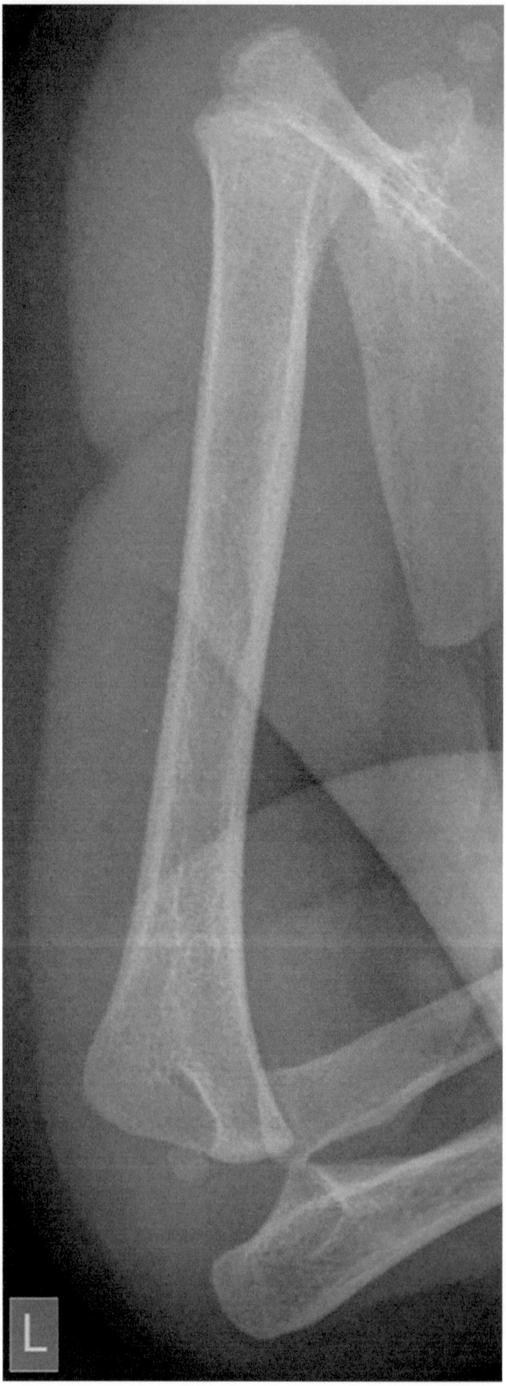

Image 18

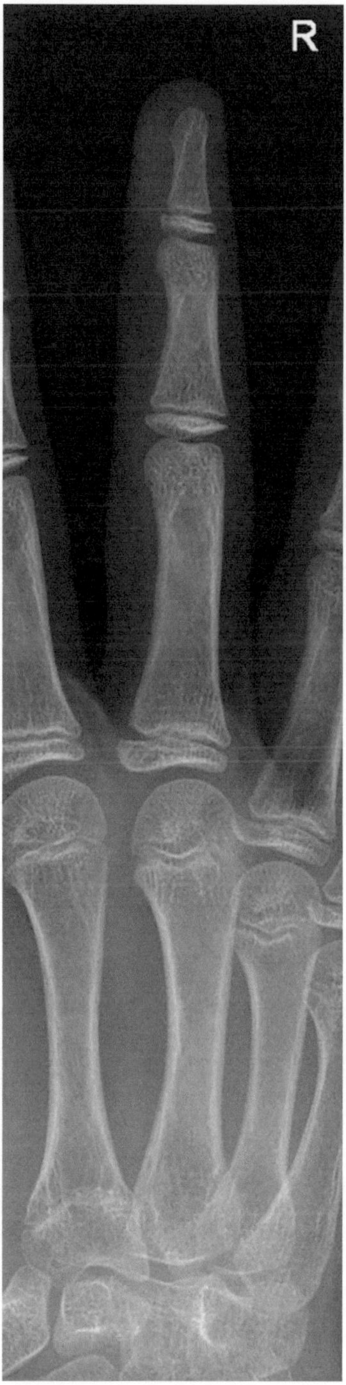

Image 19

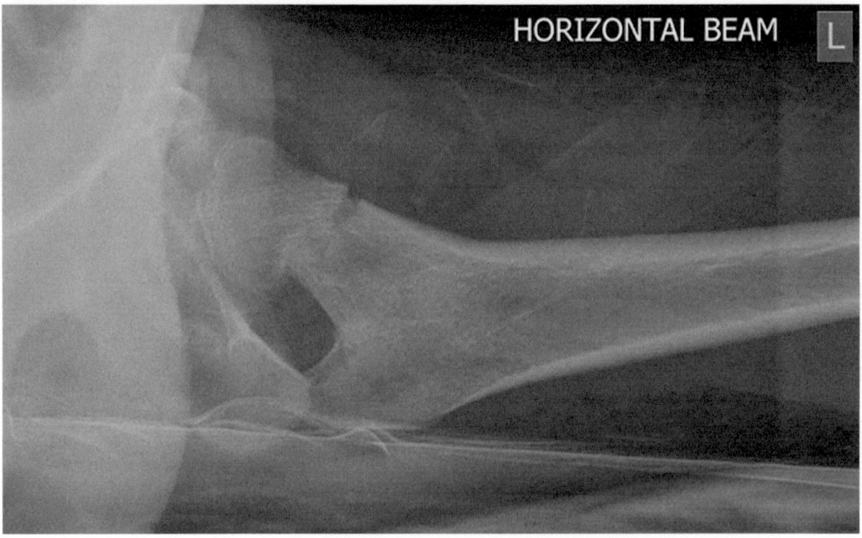

Image 20

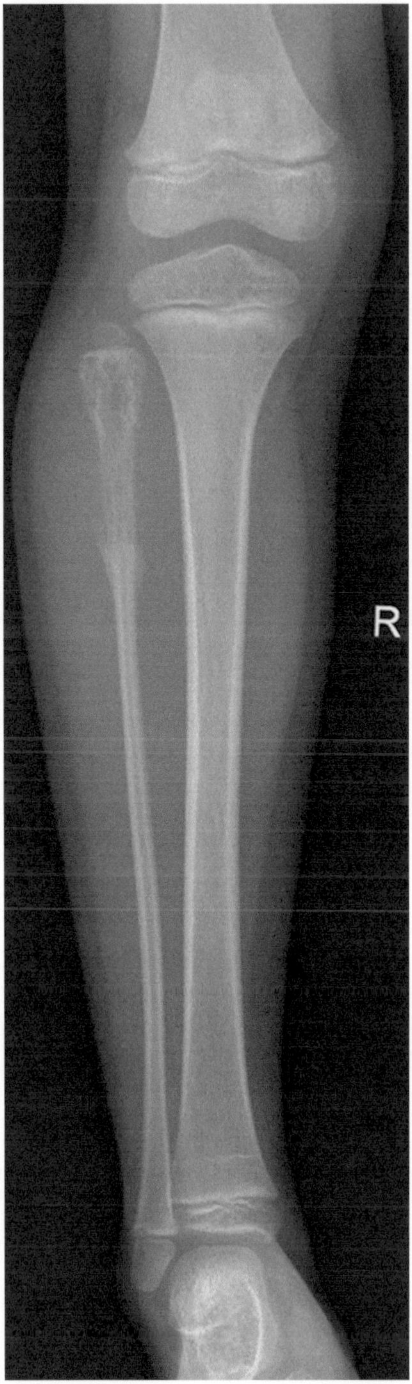

Image 21

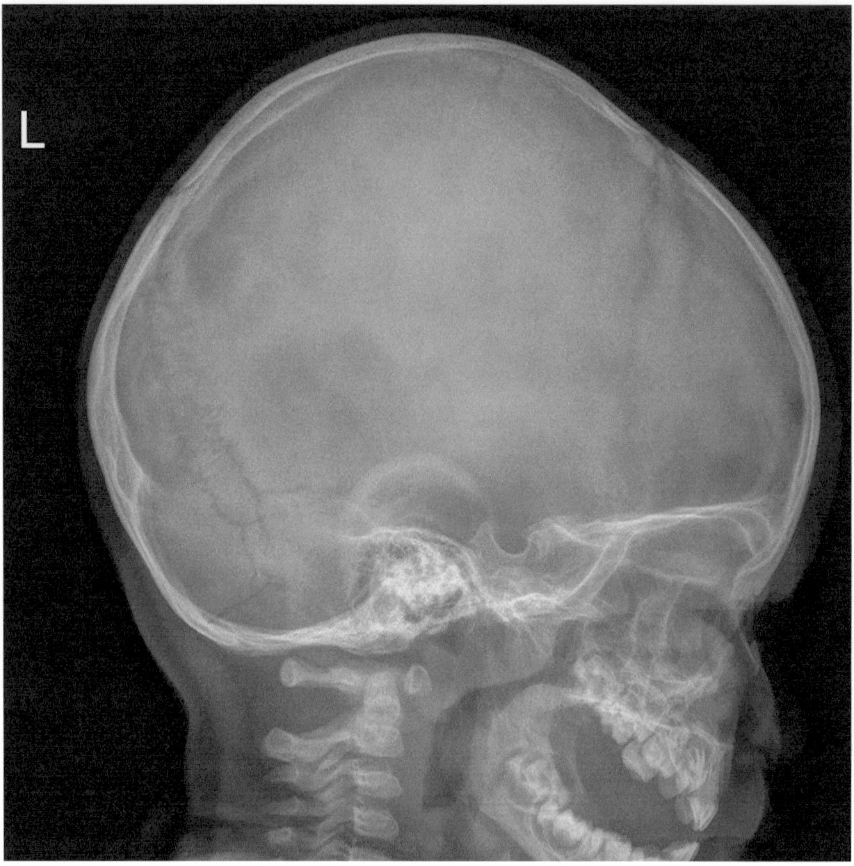

Image 22

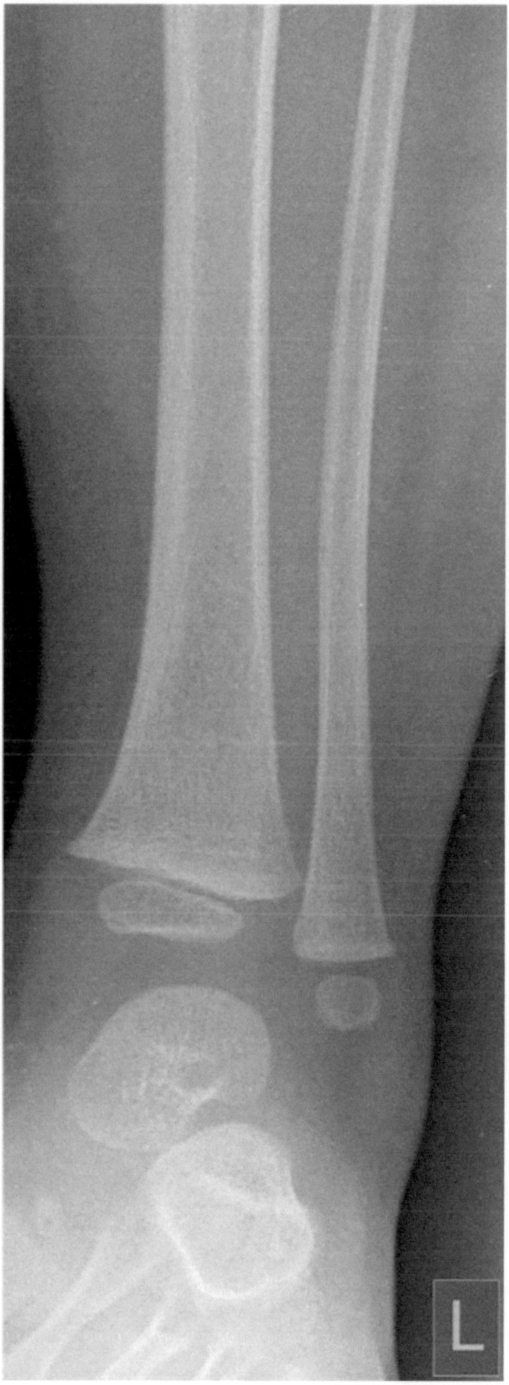

Image 23

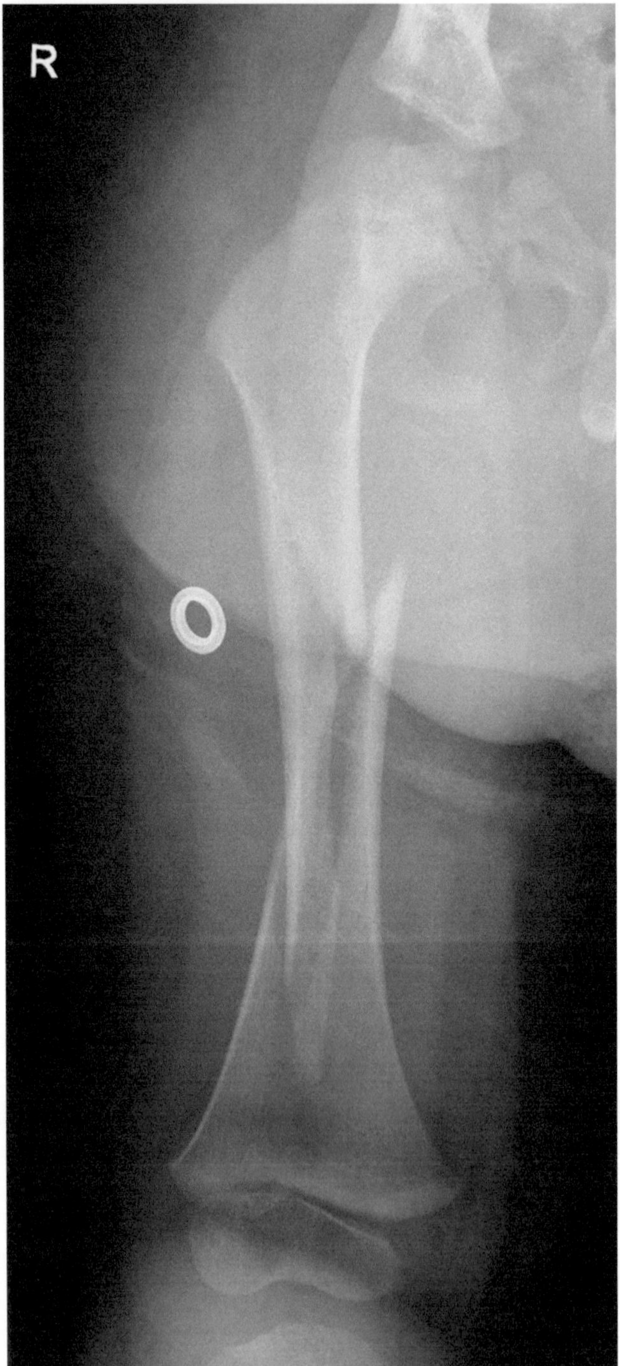

Image 24

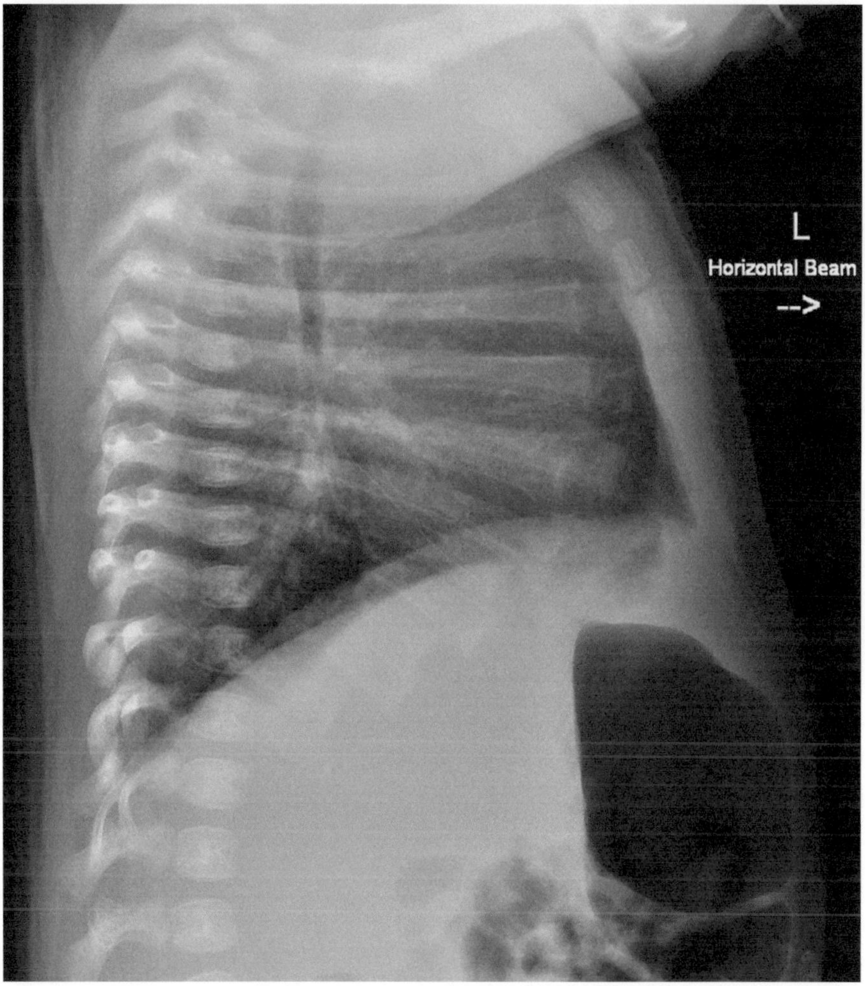

Image 25

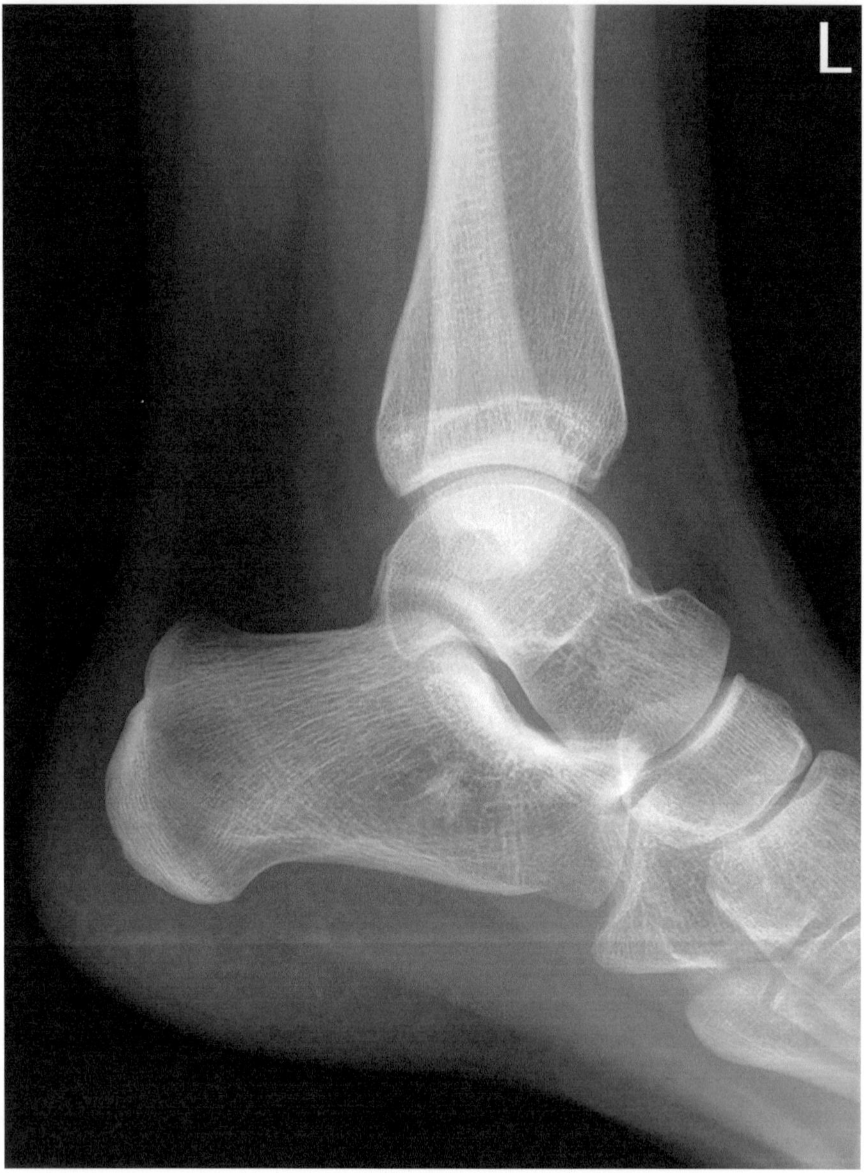

Image 26

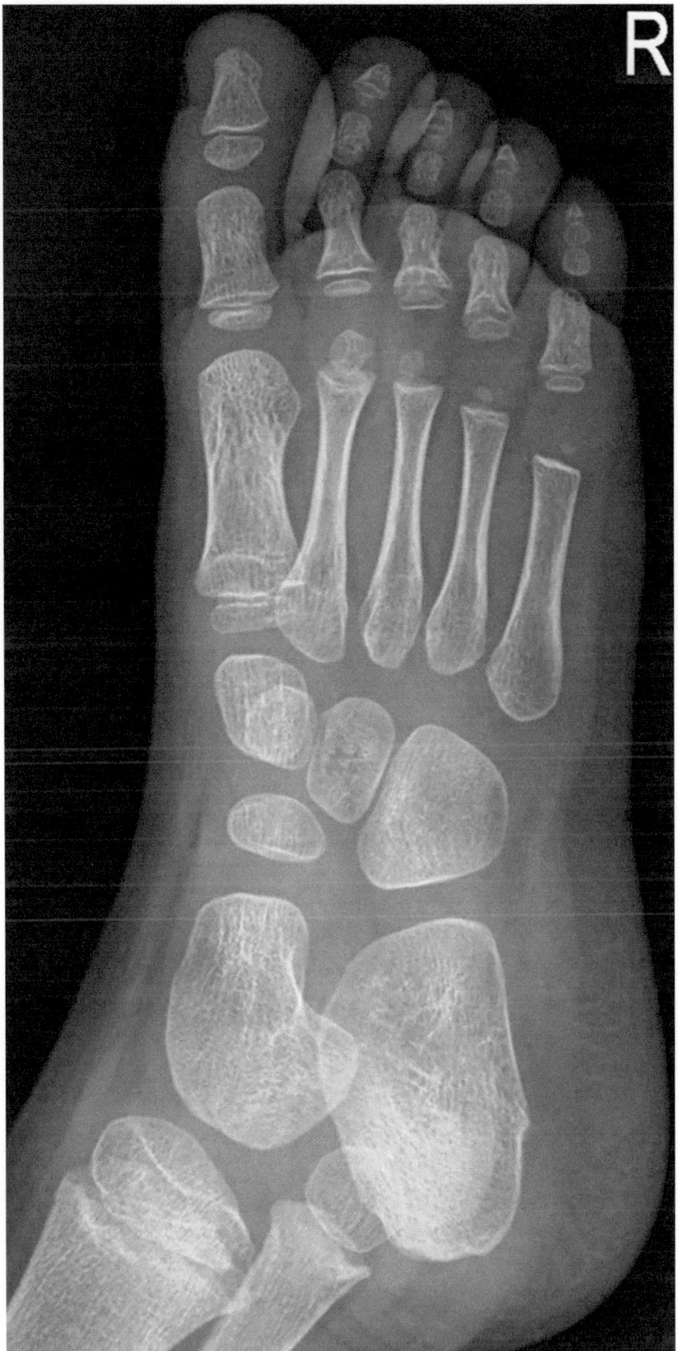

Image 27

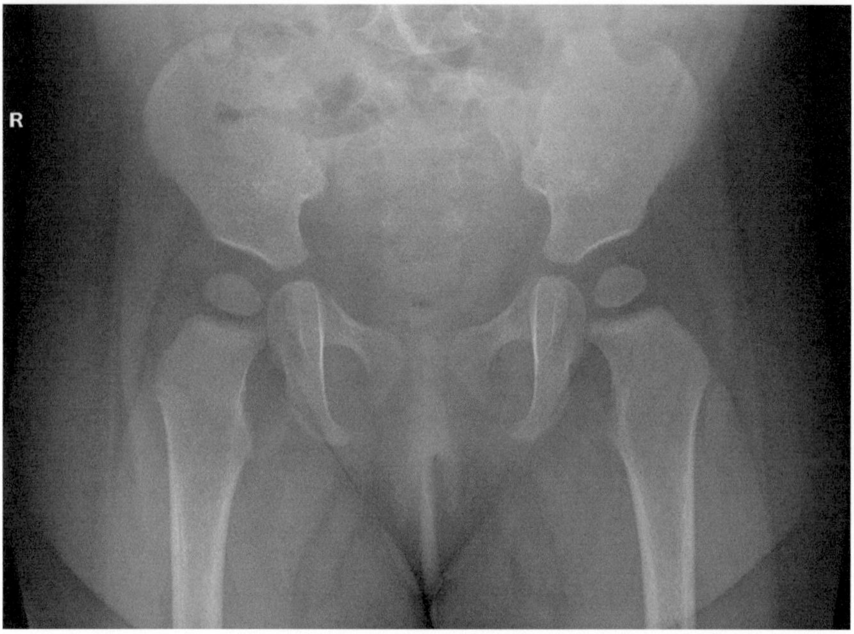

Image 28

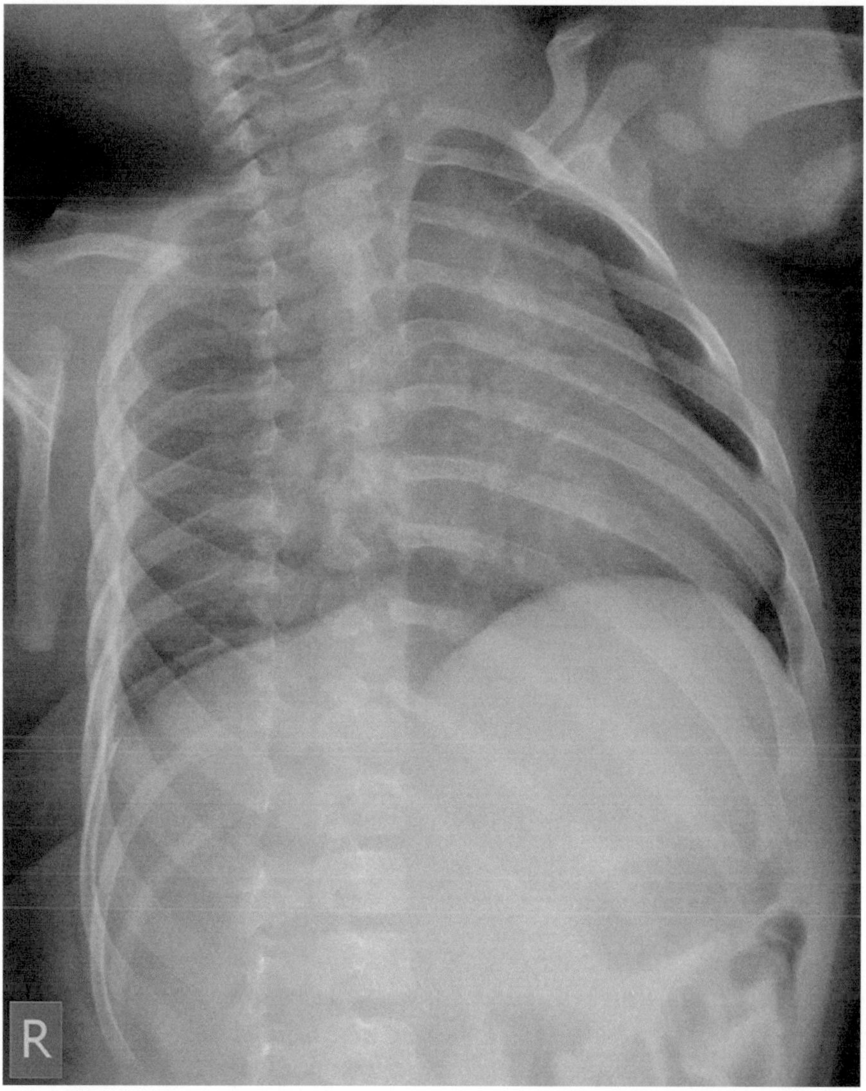

Image 29

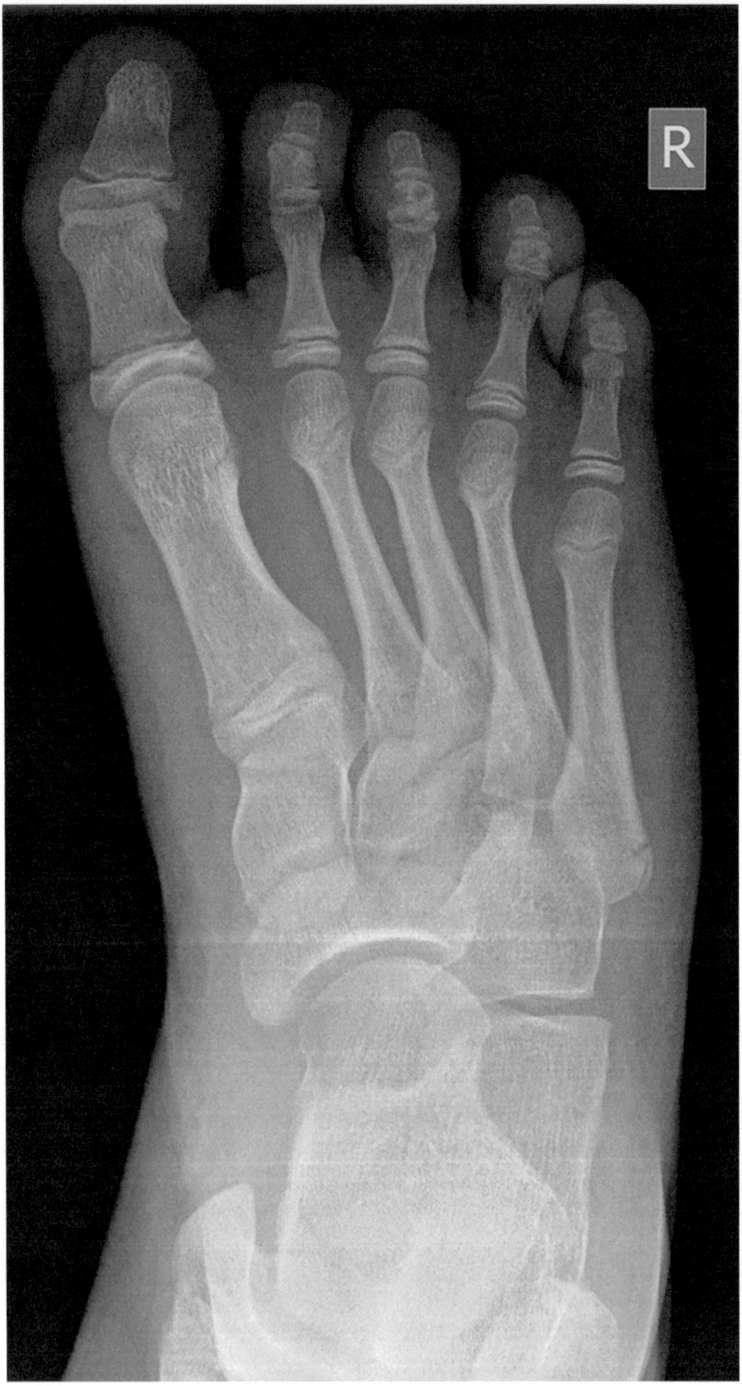

Image 30

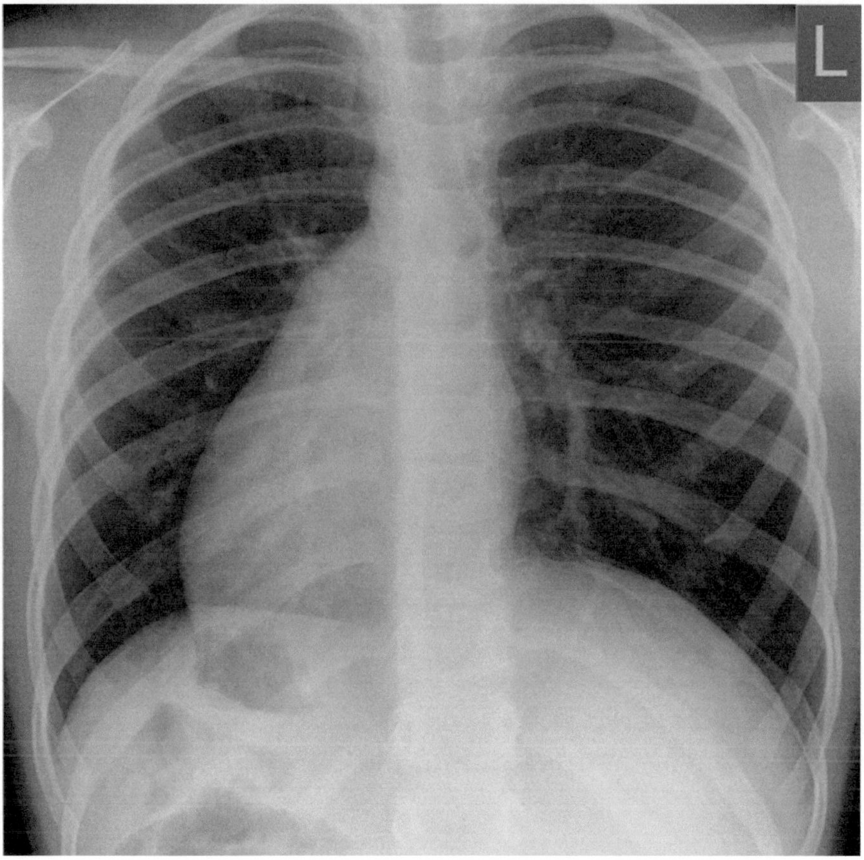

3.2 Answers

Image	Normal	Abnormal	Diagnosis/abnormality (only if abnormal)
1	✓		
2		✓	Metaphyseal # L distal fibula
3		✓	AVN L proximal femoral epiphysis
4	✓		
5		✓	# L supracondylar humerus
6		✓	R pulmonary nodules
7	✓		
8		✓	Prevertebral soft tissue thickening
9	✓		
10		✓	Fibrous dysplasia R humerus and proximal radius
11		✓	Buckle # L distal radius metaphysis
12	✓		
13		✓	# R fifth metatarsal base
14		✓	SH2 # dorsal aspect R little finger middle phalanx
15		✓	SH2 # R fifth toe proximal phalanx
16	✓		
17	✓		
18	✓		
19		✓	# L neck of femur
20		✓	Aggressive bone lesion R proximal fibula
21	✓		
22	✓		
23		✓	Spiral # R femoral diaphysis
24	✓		
25	✓		
26	✓		
27	✓		
28	✓		
29		✓	# R fifth metatarsal base
30		✓	Situs inversus

3.3 Explanations

2. **Metaphyseal # L distal fibula**
Metaphyseal fractures (also known as classic metaphyseal lesions, CMLs), along with posterior rib and complex skull fractures, are highly specific fractures for physical abuse in infants and young children. CMLs are rare in the 'normal handling' of an otherwise normal, healthy child (i.e., no underlying bone dysplasia or metabolic disease). They may have 'corner' or 'bucket handle' fracture configurations on tangential and angled radiographic projections, respectively. This illustrated case has a "corner fracture" appearance of the left distal fibula. Note the overlying soft tissue swelling with blurring of the adjacent muscle-fat planes, and the normal physiological periosteal reaction of the left tibial diaphysis.
Children under the age of 1 year, and in particular those less than 4 months, have the highest incidence of metaphyseal and abusive fractures. CMLs are less common in older children who are able to walk. The commonest locations for metaphyseal fractures include the distal femur, the proximal and distal tibia, and the proximal humerii. These fractures are reported to be the commonest long-bone fracture in fatally abused infants, specifically bilateral asymmetric tibial CMLs.
Physical child abuse is insidious, transcends racial and socio-economic groups, can present at any time, and may do so in an unrelated context. As clinical radiologists, we *must* remain vigilant to identify such highly specific radiographic findings for physical abuse so that child protection measures can be initiated promptly. Discuss the local pathways with your paediatric radiologists and safeguarding/child protection team.

3. **Avascular necrosis L proximal femoral epiphysis**
The crescentic subchondral lucency in the anteromedial aspect of the left proximal femoral epiphysis along with its reduced height and increased density (sclerosis) are radiographic features consistent with avascular necrosis (AVN). As previously discussed, idiopathic AVN of the proximal femoral epiphysis is known as Perthes disease. See the explanation for Image 1 of Test 1.

5. **# L supracondylar humerus**
There is a left supracondylar fracture and an associated elbow joint effusion, indicated by the elevated anterior and posterior fat pads, as a result of intra-articular extension of the fracture. Supracondylar fractures are usually better appreciated on lateral projections than anteroposterior (AP) projections, e.g. as seen in Image 15 of Test 1. The radiocapitellar and anterior humeral alignment are normal in this image and should be assessed on every elbow radiograph. See the explanations for Image 11 and 15 of Test 1.

6. **R pulmonary nodules**

There are two well-circumscribed nodules in the right lung: the first is projected over the right anterior second rib, the second over the right anterior seventh/posterolateral tenth rib. Sitting back and comparing the right and left hemithoraces increases the conspicuity of these nodules. The staging chest, abdomen and pelvis computed tomography (CT) demonstrated both of these pulmonary nodules along with a large soft tissue pelvic mass which was confirmed as rhabdomyosarcoma on subsequent biopsy. The pulmonary nodules were fluorodeoxyglucose (FDG) avid on positron emission tomography-computed tomography (PET-CT), consistent with metastases.

In children, pulmonary metastases may arise from the following non-exhaustive list of solid tumours (in order of frequency):

- Osteosarcoma.
- Ewing's sarcoma.
- Wilms' tumour.
- Hepatoblastoma.
- Neuroblastoma.
- Rhabdomyosarcoma.
- Well-differentiated thyroid cancer.
- Non-rhabdomyosarcoma soft tissue sarcoma (NRSTS).
- Adrenocortical carcinoma.

8. **Prevertebral soft tissue thickening**

There is increased prevertebral soft tissue anterior to the C2 to C5 vertebral bodies resulting in loss of the normal cervical lordosis and an almost kyphotic appearance from C2 to C4. Increased cervical prevertebral soft tissue can occur in the setting of infection (fluid and inflammation), trauma (haemorrhage) and neoplasia. Note also the:

- Pseudosubluxation of C2 on C3 which refers to the anterior displacement of the C2 vertebral body with respect to the C3 vertebral body. This is a common *normal* finding in children less than 7 years of age due to ligamentous immaturity resulting in laxity.
- Radiolucent horizontal line through the middle of the C2 vertebral body which represents the synchondrosis between the ossification of the dens and the anterior body of C2—this is *not* a fracture. Remember that the C2 vertebral body is formed by the fusion of *four* separate ossification centres which is usually complete (fully fused) by the age of 12 years.

Alignment of the upper cervical spine should be assessed on every lateral cervical spine radiograph. See the magnified and annotated normal image below in a different (older) paediatric patient:

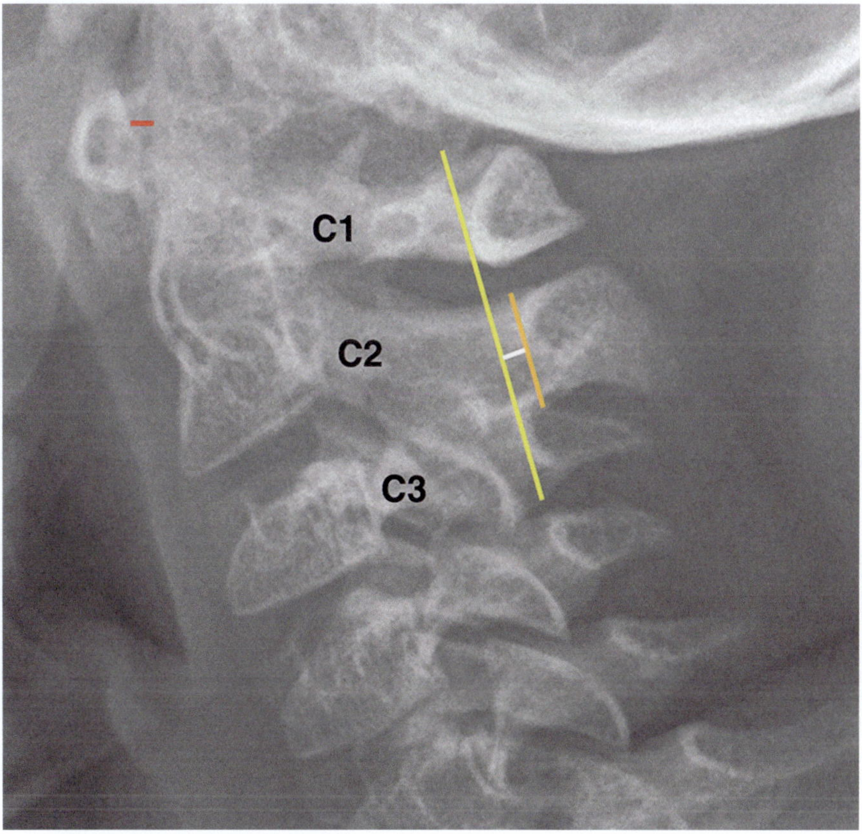

Yellow line—this is Swischuk's line which connects the anterior aspects of the posterior arches of C1 and C3.

Orange line—the anterior aspect of the posterior arch of C2.

White line—the *normal* distance between the yellow and orange lines should measure 1–2 mm, as on this radiograph. If there is:

- Deviation <2 mm, appearances would be consistent with a pseudosubluxation, as described above.
- Deviation >2 mm, a *true* subluxation is indicated.

Red line—this is the atlantodental interval, the horizontal distance between the posterior cortex of the anterior arch of C1 (the atlas) and the anterior cortex of the dens (or peg) of C2 (the axis). The *normal* distance should measure <5 mm in children, which is greater than the 3 mm limit in adults, secondary to ligamentous laxity in children. These lines and distances should be assessed on every paediatric lateral cervical spine radiograph, particularly in the context of trauma. One caveat is that normal upper cervical spine alignment is *insufficient* to exclude a 'Hangman's fracture', i.e. bilateral pars interarticularis fractures of C2 from a hyperextension-distraction injury resulting in anterior spondylolisthesis.

Assessment of cervical spine alignment can be difficult in children when a true lateral projection cannot be obtained due to movement/patient distress and the resultant obliquity limits evaluation. In the appropriate clinical context (i.e. traumatic injury), cervical spine CT may be indicated. Maintain close liaison with Emergency Department (ED) colleagues in an acute setting.

It is important to assess for the presence of gas whenever prevertebral soft tissue swelling is identified, which may indicate gas-forming organisms in the context of a retropharyngeal abscess. Up to three-quarters of retropharyngeal abscesses in children occur before the age of 5 years. Occasionally, retropharyngeal abscesses may result from foreign body ingestion, an important point to remember when discussing cases with clinical colleagues, as children may ingest all manner of objects without their parents or caregivers' knowledge! Contrast enhanced CT better evaluates the extent and nature of any abscess, confirms the retropharyngeal location, assesses for evidence of mediastinal extension/mediastinitis, and helps to differentiate from retropharyngeal oedema/cellulitis (i.e., without abscess). Compression or narrowing of the airway is also better assessed on CT, which is an important anaesthetic consideration prior to any planned surgical intervention, if indicated.

Tip for the viva:
Consider the following points:

- Infection: the abscess may lie in the prevertebral space, *not* the retropharyngeal space, and thus may extend into the epidural space, resulting in discitis/osteomyelitis/epidural abscess.
- Grisel syndrome: atlantoaxial subluxation from inflammatory ligamentous laxity secondary to a retropharyngeal abscess causing torticollis. Whilst this is an uncommon cause of torticollis in infants and young children, knowledge of this condition is imperative given that affected patients are often not able to verbalise their symptoms.
- Lemierre syndrome: internal jugular vein (IJV) thrombophlebitis and/or thrombosis in the setting of oropharyngeal infection, i.e. retropharyngeal abscess.

10. **Fibrous dysplasia R humerus and proximal radius**
There are well-circumscribed, mildly expansile lucent lesions throughout the humeral diaphysis *and* the proximal radial metadiaphysis which demonstrate internal ground-glass matrix. There is surrounding reactive sclerosis/cortical thickening known as the 'rind sign'. Note also the endosteal scalloping, i.e. thinning of the inner cortex. The findings are consistent with fibrous dysplasia affecting both sides of the joint, as is typical, and the involvement is polyostotic given that more than one bone is affected. There is also resultant bowing deformity of the lateral distal humeral diaphysis. This child has McCune-Albright syndrome, the triad of:
    - Polyostotic fibrous dysplasia.
    - Endocrinopathy (precocious puberty).
    - Characteristic *café au lait* cutaneous pigmentation in the shape of the coast of Maine.

    Tip for the viva:
    - If a lucent bone lesion has been identified, it is important to look for a pathological fracture (which may be subtle) in the context of pain.

11. **Buckle # L distal radius metaphysis**
See the explanation for Image 18 of Test 1.

12. *Normal right knee radiograph*
The relative density in the region of the patella relates to the cartilaginous as yet unossified patella ossification centre—this is a normal finding. The patella starts to ossify between the ages of 3 and 5 years, with eventual coalescence of its ossification centres; a multipartite patella results if this fails and is often an incidental finding. Remember that patella ossification, when present, can be variable at all ages and may appear fragmented. See the explanation for Image 8 of Test 2.

13. **# R fifth metatarsal base**
See the explanation for Image 7 of Test 1.

14. **Salter-Harris 2 # dorsal aspect R little finger middle phalanx**
See the explanation for Image 30 of Test 1.

15. **Salter-Harris 2 # R fifth toe proximal phalanx**
This fracture is better visualised in the magnified image below:

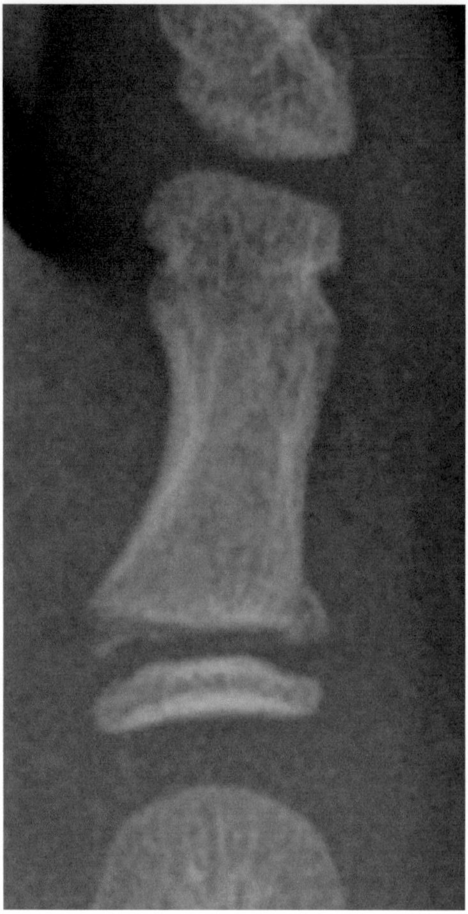

19. **# L neck of femur**

Neck of femur fractures in children are rare and account for less than 1% of all paediatric fractures. They typically result from a high energy impact such as a fall from a height or a road traffic accident (RTA). This 13-year-old girl presented to the Emergency Department (ED) with severe left hip pain and decreased range of movement after a fall on ice.

This portable projection was the only image that was able to be obtained in the ED on the patient's bed because of pain and immobility. As reflects real-life clinical practice, you should be able to offer an opinion on any imaging obtained, even if it is limited by patient factors and/or considered suboptimal (which may be more common with children). That being said, the complete subcapital/transcervical neck of femur fracture is clearly visualised in this image. It is mildly displaced, and the capital femoral epiphysis is at risk of AVN due to disrupted blood supply—early surgical reduction and fixation of the fracture is indicated.

20. **Aggressive bone lesion R proximal fibula**

There is a destructive, moth-eaten and permeative appearance of the right proximal fibular metaphysis and metadiaphysis with an associated soft tissue component (note the adjacent soft tissue swelling) but *without* an osteoid matrix (cf. the tumour matrix calcification seen with osteosarcoma, which may be ill-defined and 'cloud-like'). Note the associated Codman's triangle periosteal reaction in the proximal fibular diaphysis. The radiographic findings are consistent with Ewing's sarcoma which was subsequently diagnosed in this 5-year-old boy presenting with leg pain.

Ewing's sarcoma is the second most common primary malignant osseous tumour of childhood (following osteosarcoma) arising from the medullary cavity. It typically occurs between 10 and 20 years of age with a slight male predilection involving the:

- Long bones: it most commonly involves the lower extremities. The majority of cases (approximately 60%) affect the metadiaphysis followed by the mid-diaphysis, of the femur (most common), tibia, and humerus.
- Flat bones: the pelvis; scapula; and ribs. Regarding the latter two locations, consider Ewing's sarcoma of the chest wall: formally known as Askin tumour, these peripheral primitive neuroectodermal tumours (pPNET) belong to the Ewing's sarcoma family of tumours.

Systemic chemotherapy is the mainstay of treatment. Surgery and consideration of adjuvant radiotherapy depends on the location and size of the primary tumour. Imaging evaluation is similar to that for osteosarcoma and typically involves:

- Magnetic resonance imaging (MRI) of the affected limb/area to assess the primary tumour and "skip" lesions.
- CT staging to assess for metastases and lymphadenopathy. Prognosis is significantly impacted by the presence of distant metastases at the time of diagnosis, which can be pulmonary and/or bony (to the pelvis and extremities).
- Technetium-99m bone scintigraphy and PET-CT may also be employed (depending on patient age and clinical circumstances) to assess tumour extent and the presence of metastases.

21. *Normal lateral skull radiograph*
    It is worth noting that lateral skull radiographs are frequently oblique and hinder an accurate interpretation of (non-dedicated) cervical spine imaging (if included).

23. **Spiral # R femoral diaphysis**
    This pre-ambulant female infant was presented to the ED as being unsettled after "rolling off the bed" and landing on the floor; examination revealed right thigh swelling with crepitus. When considering femoral fractures in infants and young children, one must consider the age and developmental status of the child. Broadly speaking, infants can be divided into whether they are ambulant or pre-ambulant, and specifically whether they are able to pull themselves up, cruise, stand or toddle, unaided or with support. The spiral fracture is the commonest abusive femoral fracture and implies the application of significant torsional force. Any femoral fracture in a *pre-ambulant* infant without an appropriate history is suspicious.

28. *Normal sternal ossification centres*
    It is important that sternal ossification centres (also known as sternal segments or sternebrae) are *not* mistaken for healing rib fractures on oblique chest projections. Occasionally, these segments can line up perfectly along the ribs simulating callus from healing rib fractures but in fact represent *normal* sternal ossification. See the magnified image below—we have included an asterisk on each of the sternal ossification centres:

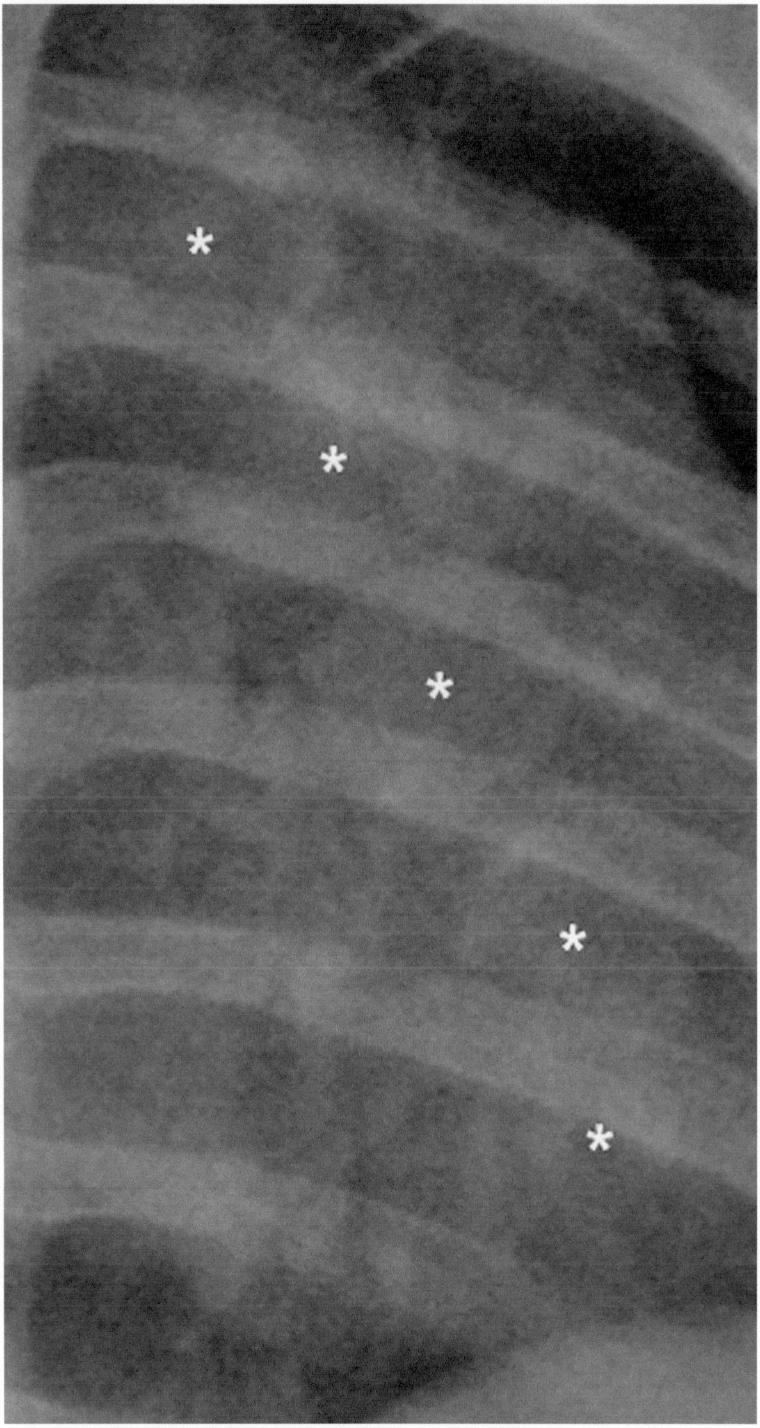

Overcalling these segments as healing fractures can have a significant impact on patient management, not only for the child but also the family unit. We have included this radiograph to emphasise the recognition of this *normal* finding. See Image 14 of Test 2 for a further example of the normal sternal segments projected over the ribs in a different patient.

Tip for the viva:

- Remember to look at the AP and contralateral oblique chest projections to confirm/exclude healing rib fractures.

29. **# R fifth metatarsal base**
See the explanation for Image 7 of Test 1.

30. **Situs inversus**
Note the side marker in the top right corner of the image which correctly indicates the left side of the patient. This is situs inversus and *not* dextrocardia given the positions of the cardiac apex, the aortic knuckle, the stomach bubble (which lies under the right hemidiaphragm) and the liver (which elevates the left hemidiaphragm). Dextrocardia exists in isolation, i.e. not in the context of situs inversus; in which case the stomach bubble lies under the left hemidiaphragm and the liver under the right (as expected).

Up to 20% of patients with situs inversus may have Kartagener syndrome, a primary ciliary dyskinesia which is inherited in an autosomal recessive fashion and is characterised by abnormal ciliary structure or function leading to impaired mucociliary clearance. It is comprised of the following triad:

- Situs inversus.
- Chronic sinusitis/nasal polyposis.
- Bronchiectasis.

Males with Kartagener syndrome may experience subfertility and females have an increased rate of ectopic pregnancy due to the underlying ciliopathy affecting the fallopian tubes.

Further Reading

Image 6

Davidoff AM, Heaton TE (2016) Surgical treatment of metastases in pediatric solid tumors. Semin Pediatr Surg 25(5):311–317

Image 8

Bell D et al (2022) Lemierre syndrome. https://radiopaedia.org/articles/lemierre-syndrome. Accessed Feb 2023

Bickle I et al (2018) Pseudosubluxation of the cervical spine. https://radiopaedia.org/articles/pseudosubluxation-of-the-cervical-spine. Accessed Feb 2023

Goergen S, Ditchfield M, Babl F et al (2015) Paediatric cervical spine trauma. Education Modules for Appropriate Imaging Referrals: Royal Australian and New Zealand College of Radiologists. https://www.ranzcr.com/our-work/quality-standards/education-modules. Accessed Feb 2023

Hoang JK, Branstetter BF 4th, Eastwood JD et al (2011) Multiplanar CT and MRI of collections in the retropharyngeal space: is it an abscess? AJR Am J Roentgenol 196(4):W426–W432

Knipe H et al (2016) Grisel syndrome. https://radiopaedia.org/articles/grisel-syndrome-2. Accessed Feb 2023

National Institute for Health and Care Excellence (2014, updated 2019) 'Head injury', NICE clinical guideline 176. National Clinical Guideline Centre, London. https://www.nice.org.uk/guidance/cg176. Algorithm 4: selection of children from imaging of the cervical spine. https://www.nice.org.uk/guidance/cg176/resources/imaging-algorithm-pdf-498950893. Accessed Feb 2023

O'Brien TW Sr, Shen P, Lee P (2015) The dens: normal development, developmental variants and anomalies, and traumatic injuries. J Clin Imaging Sci 30(5):38

Swischuk LE (1977) Anterior displacement of C2 in children: physiologic or pathologic. Radiology 122(3):759–763

Yousaf M et al (2023) Hangman fracture. https://radiopaedia.org/articles/hangman-fracture. Accessed Feb 2023

Image 10

Iqbal S et al (2022) McCune-Albright syndrome. https://radiopaedia.org/articles/mccune-albright-syndrome. Accessed Feb 2023

Shah JN, Cohen HL, Choudhri AF et al (2017) Pediatric benign bone tumors: what does the radiologist need to know? Radiographics 37(3):1001–1002

Yongjing G, Huawei L, Zilai P et al (2001) McCune-Albright syndrome: radiological and MR findings. JBR-BTR 84(6):250–252

Image 12

El-Feky M et al (2022) Multipartite patella. https://radiopaedia.org/articles/multipartite-patella. Accessed July 2023

Image 19

Al Khatib N, Younis MH, Hegazy A et al (2019) Early versus late treatment of paediatric femoral neck fractures: a systematic review and meta-analysis. Int Orthop 43(3):677–685

Image 20

Kaste SC (2011) Imaging pediatric bone sarcomas. Radiol Clin North Am 49(4):749–765

Lustosa L et al (2022) Codman triangle periosteal reaction. https://radiopaedia.org/articles/codman-triangle-periosteal-reaction. Accessed Feb 2023

Saber M et al (2021) Askin tumour. https://radiopaedia.org/articles/askin-tumour-1. Accessed Feb 2023

Yap J et al (2022) Ewing sarcoma. https://radiopaedia.org/articles/ewing-sarcoma. Accessed Feb 2023

Image 23

Hui C, Joughin E, Goldstein S et al (2008) Femoral fractures in children younger than three years: the role of nonaccidental injury. J Pediatr Orthop 28:297–302

Kemp AM, Dunstan F, Harrison S et al (2008) Patterns of skeletal fractures in child abuse: systematic review. BMJ 337:a1518

Paddock M, Sprigg A, Offiah AC (2017) Re: Imaging and reporting considerations for suspected physical abuse (non-accidental injury) in infants and young children. Part 1: initial considerations and appendicular skeleton. A reply. Clin Radiol 72(5):422

Image 28

McAloon J, O'Neill C (2011) Ossification centres, not rib fractures. Arch Dis Child 96(3):284

Image 30

Baba Y et al (2020) Kartagener syndrome. https://radiopaedia.org/articles/kartagener-syndrome-1. Accessed Feb 2023

Berdon WE, Willi U (2004) Situs inversus, bronchiectasis, and sinusitis and its relation to immotile cilia: history of the diseases and their discoverers-Manes Kartagener and Bjorn Afzelius. Pediatr Radiol 34(1):38–42

Test 4

4

M. Paddock et al., *Paediatric Radiology Rapid Reporting*,
https://doi.org/10.1007/978-3-031-48255-7_4

4.1 Images

Image 1

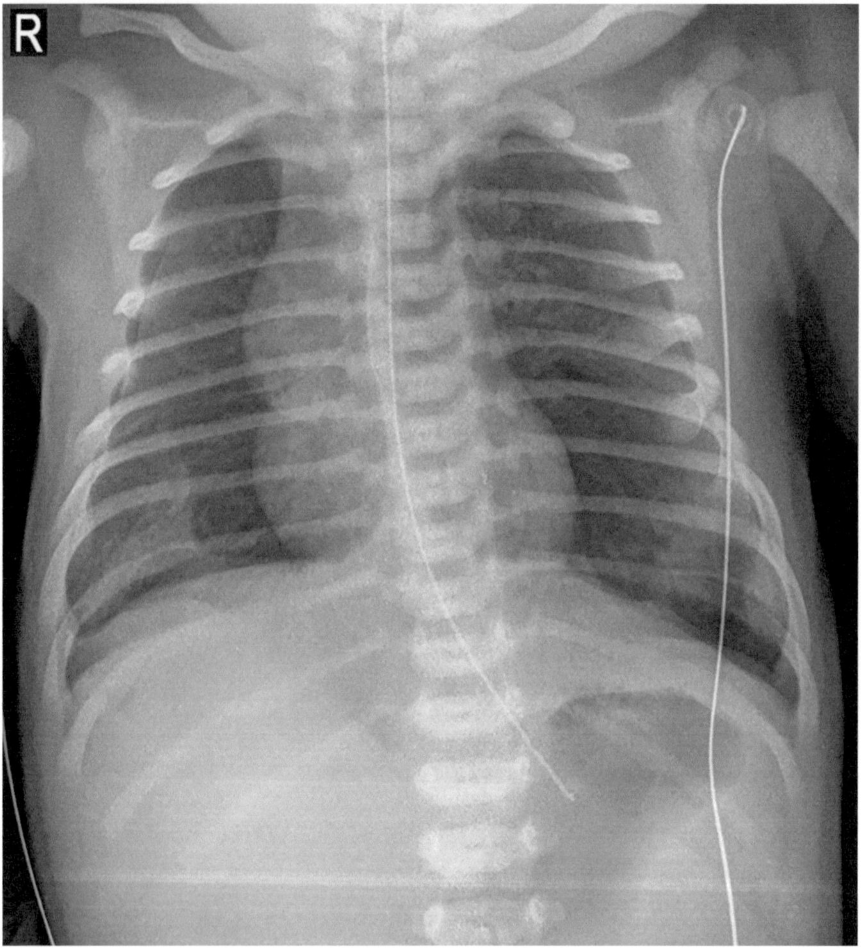

Image 2

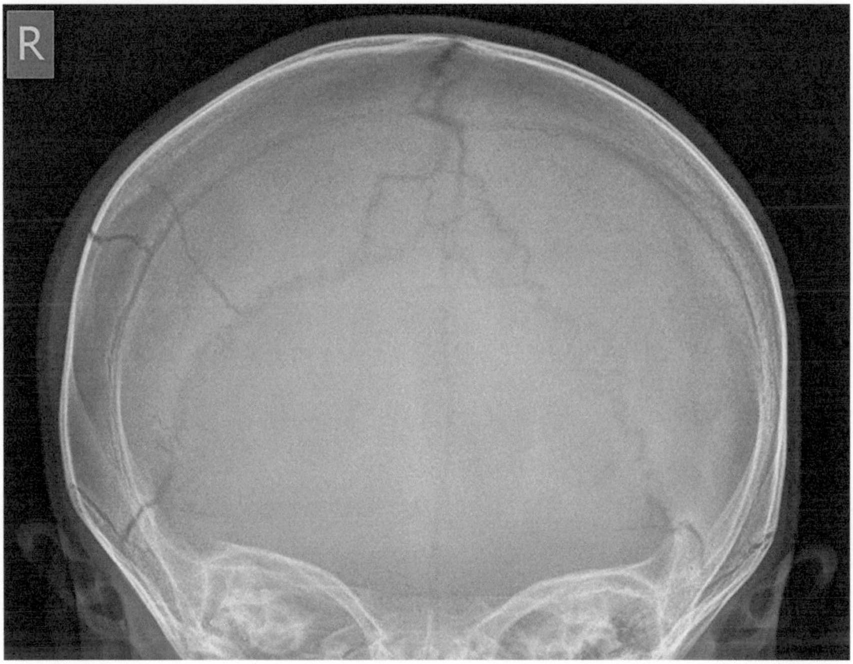

Image 3

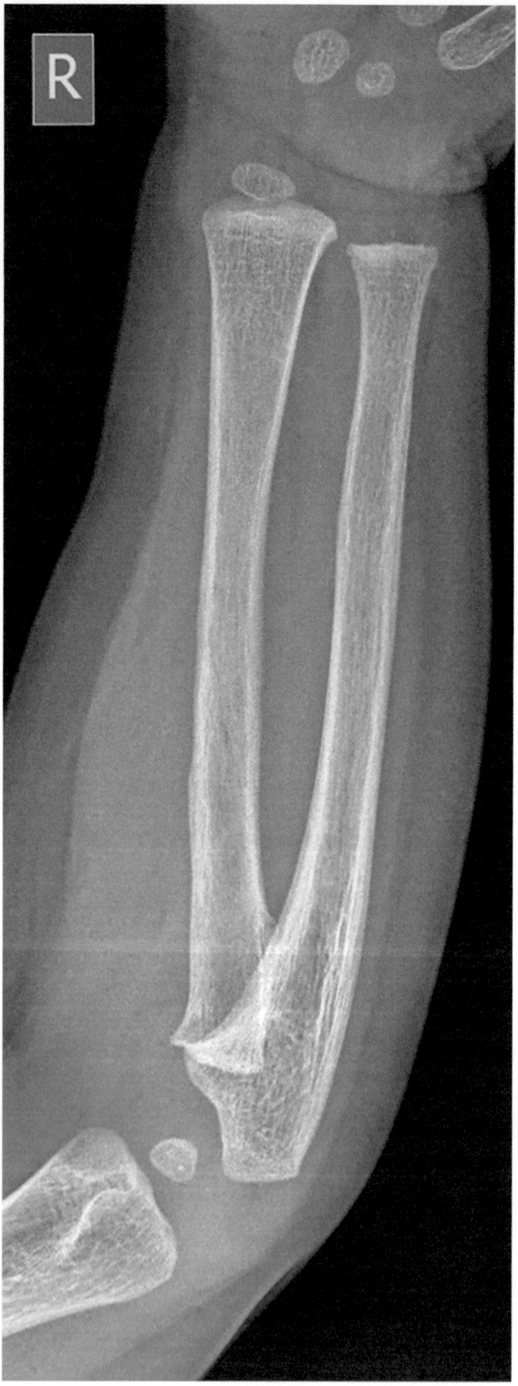

Image 4

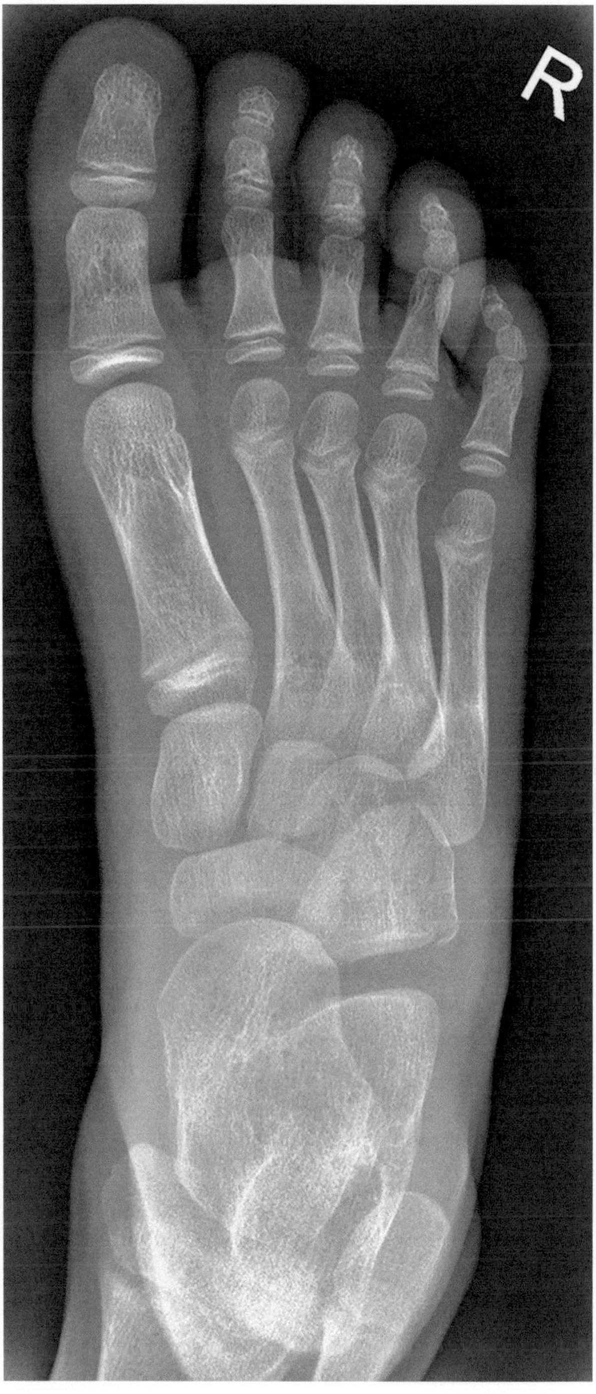

Image 5

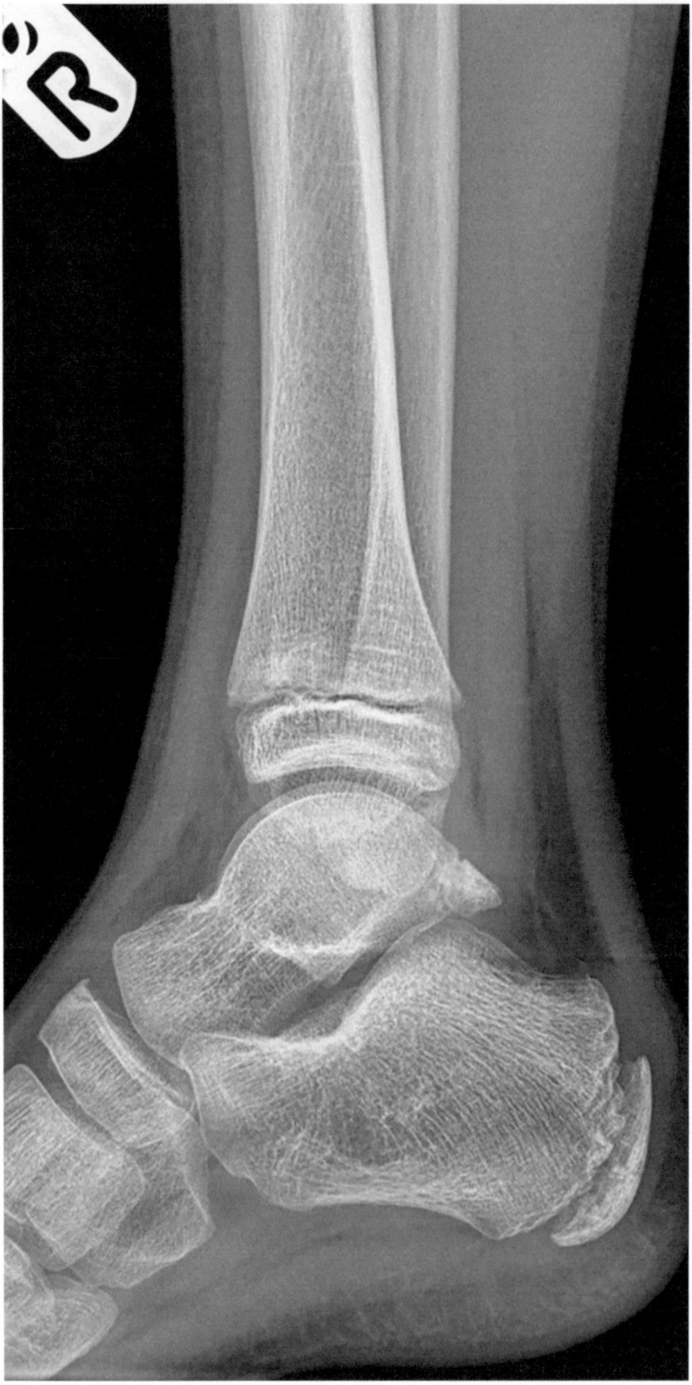

Image 6

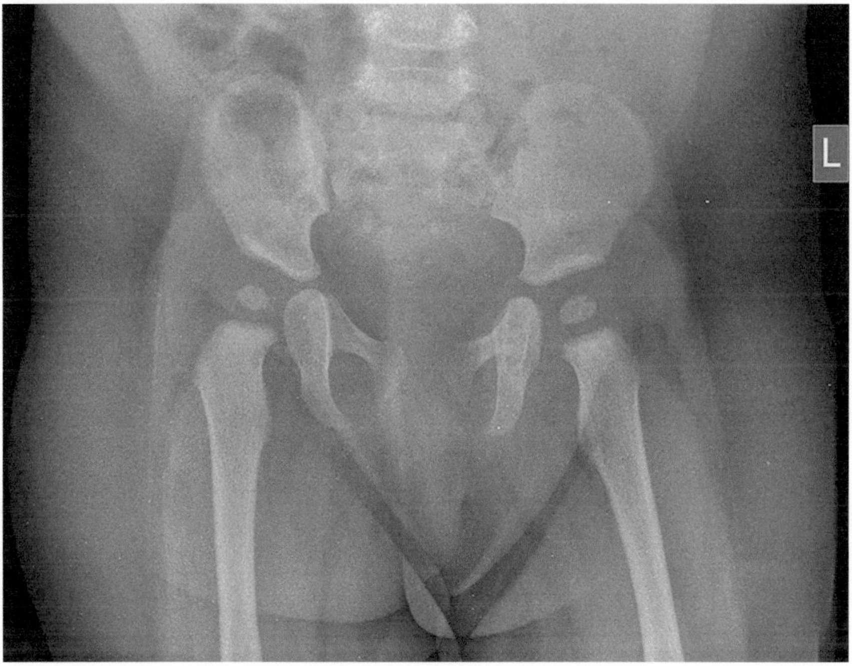

Image 7

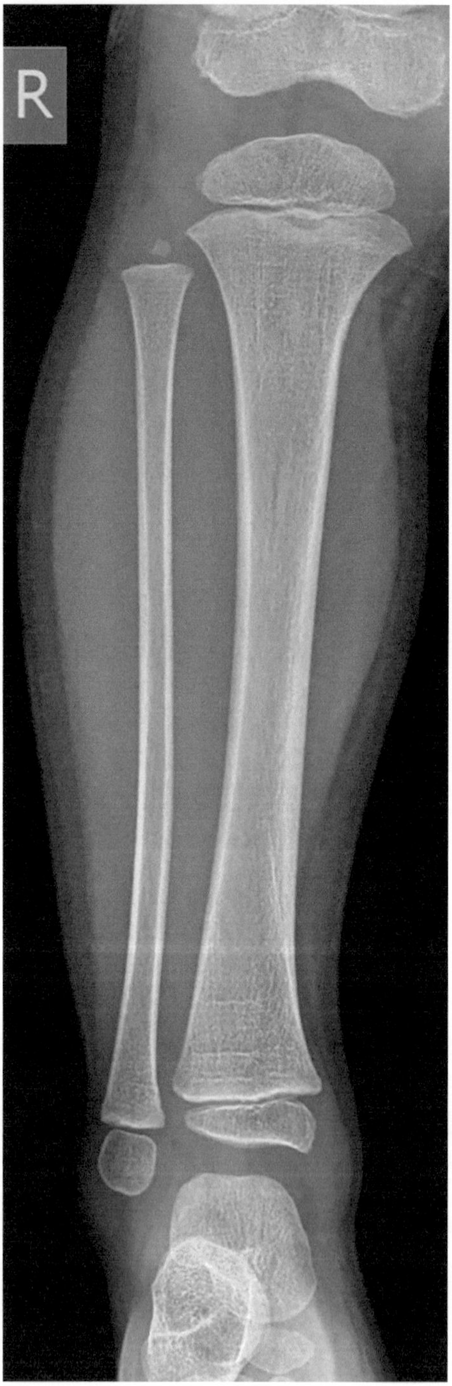

Image 8

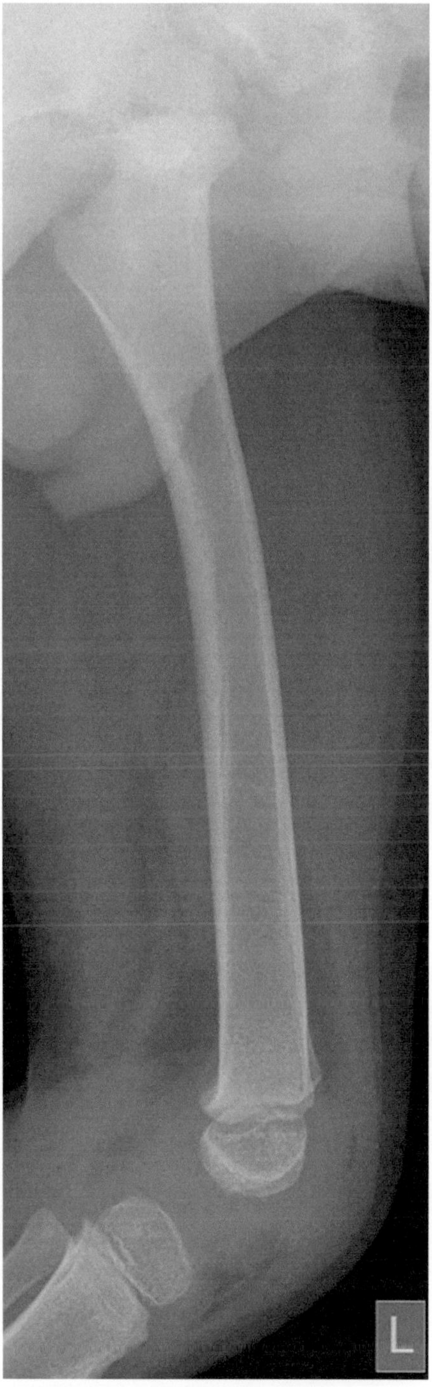

Image 9

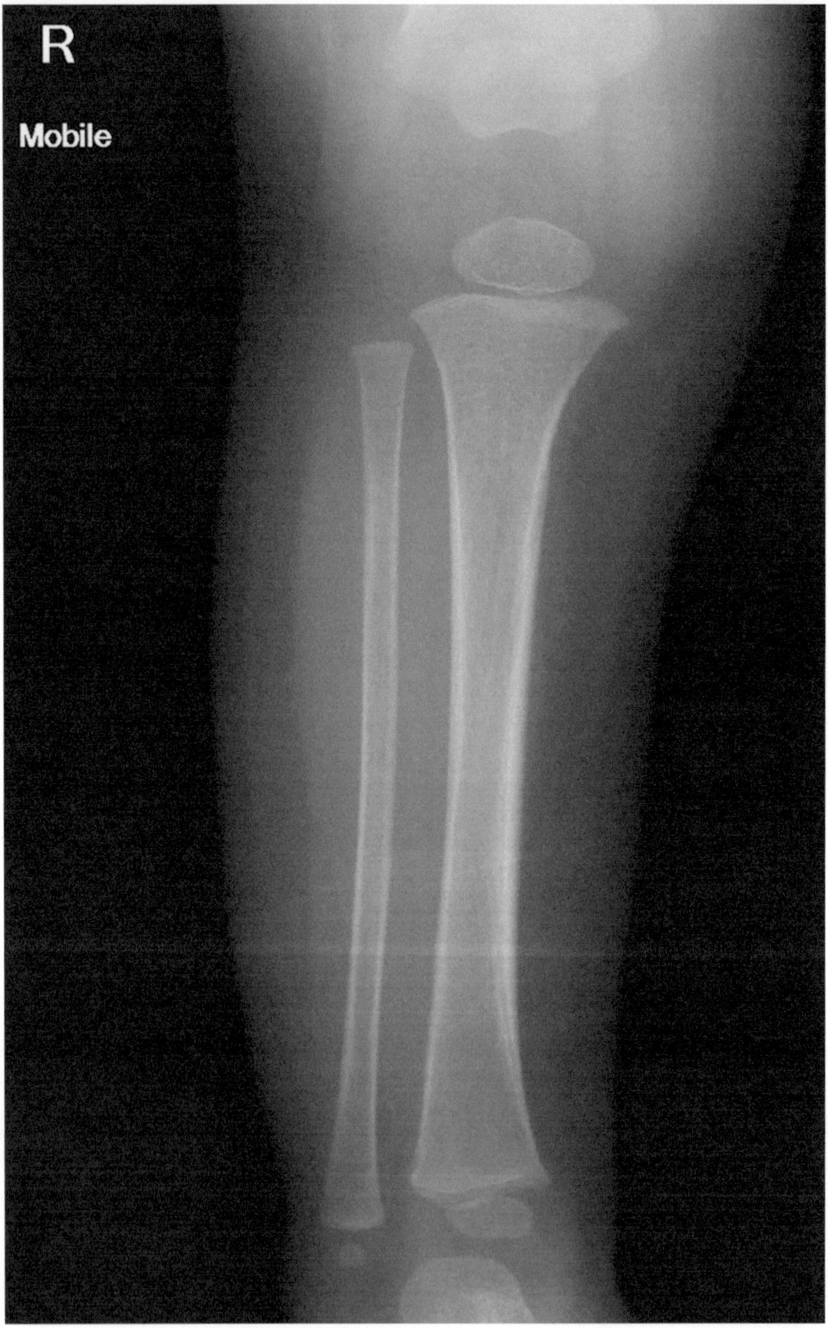

Image 10

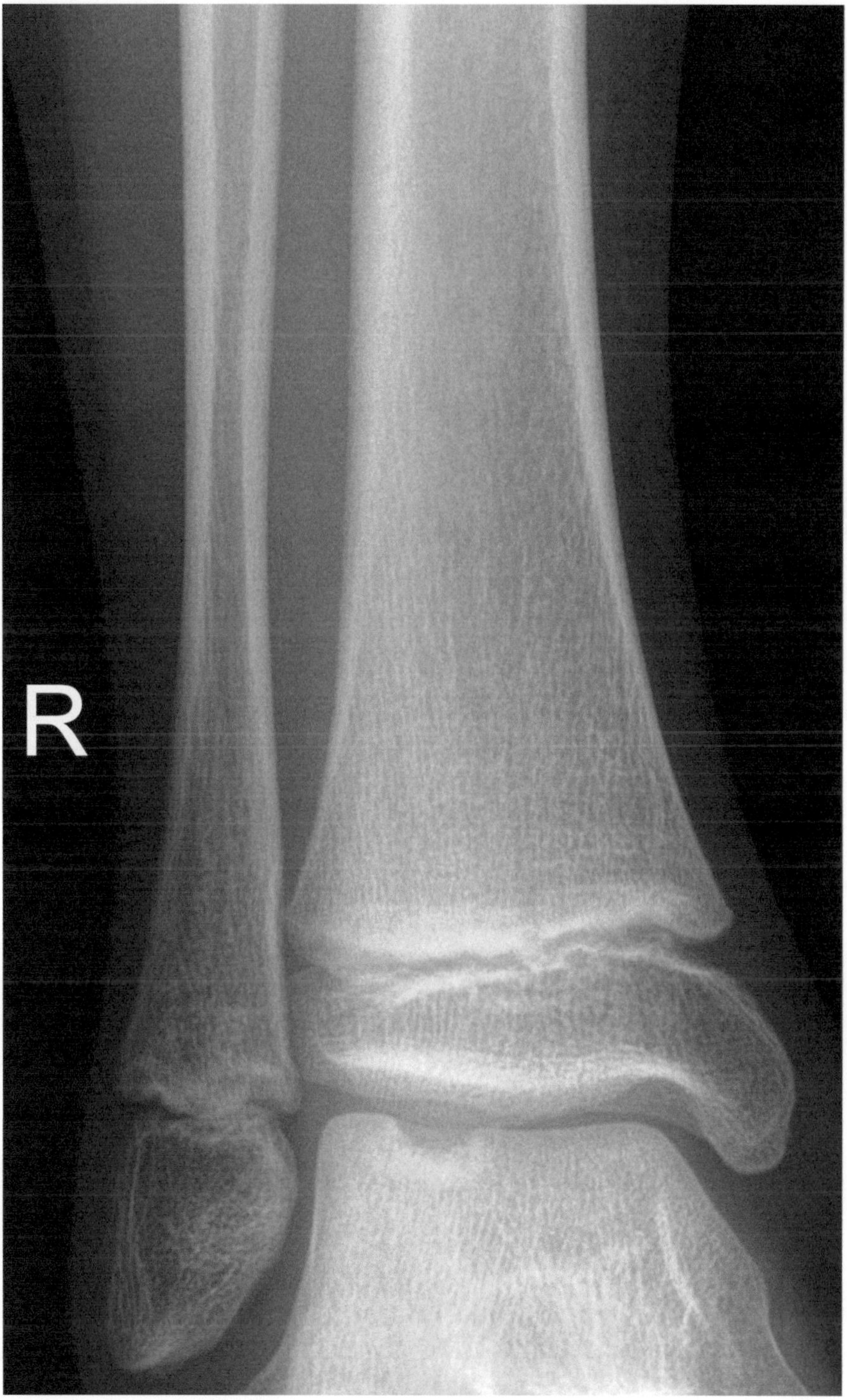

Image 11

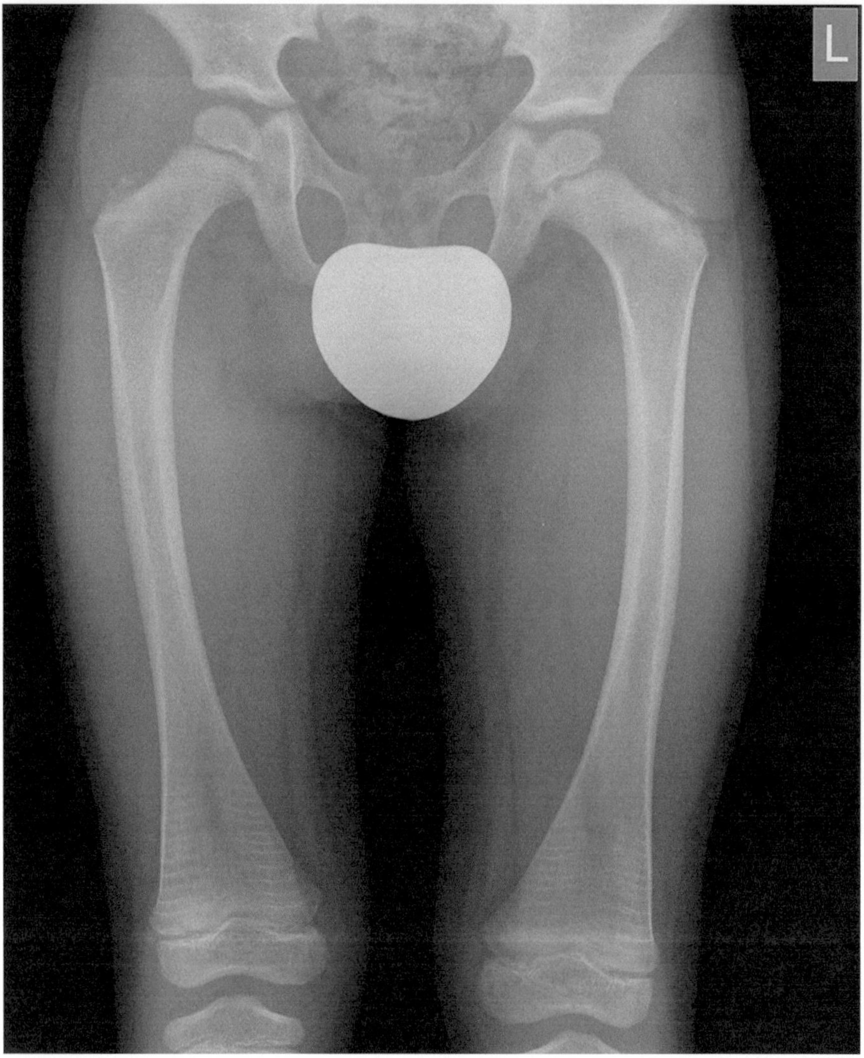

Image 12

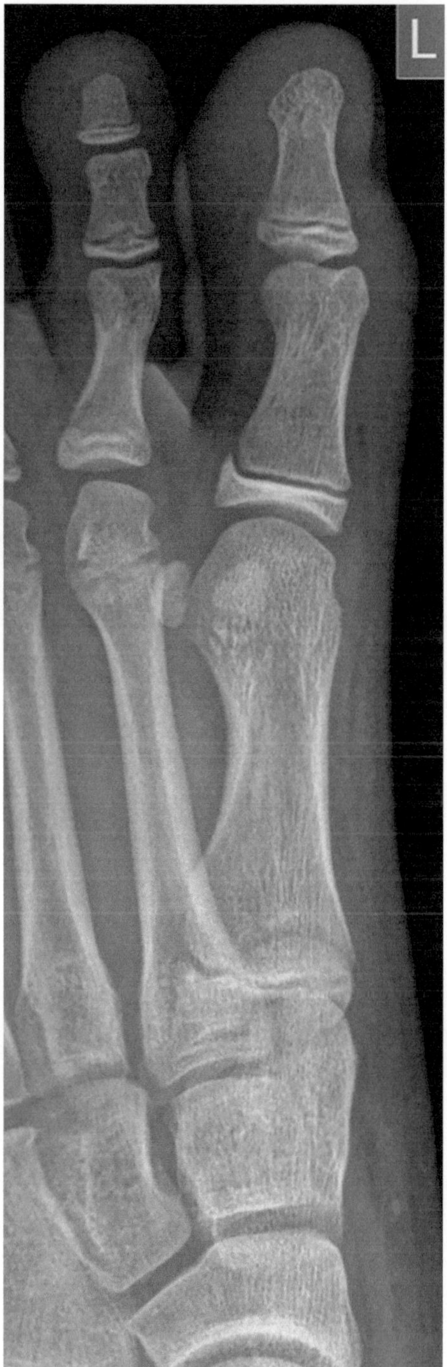

Image 13

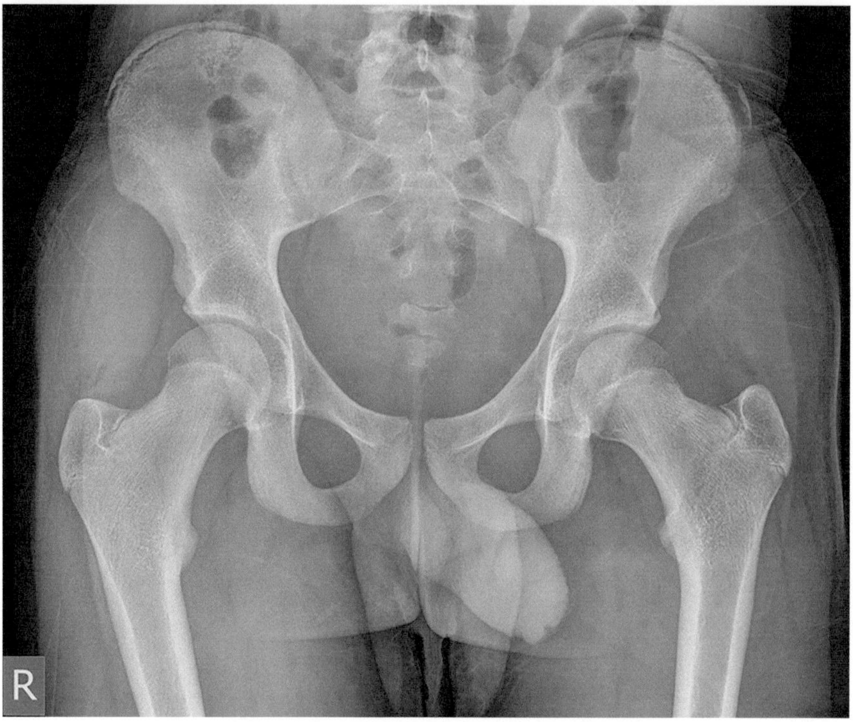

Image 14

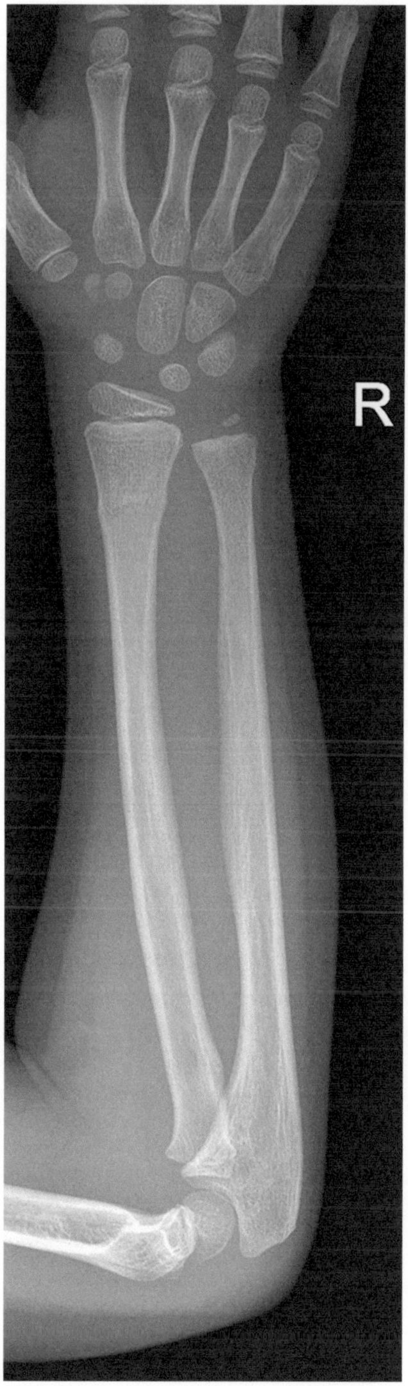

Image 15

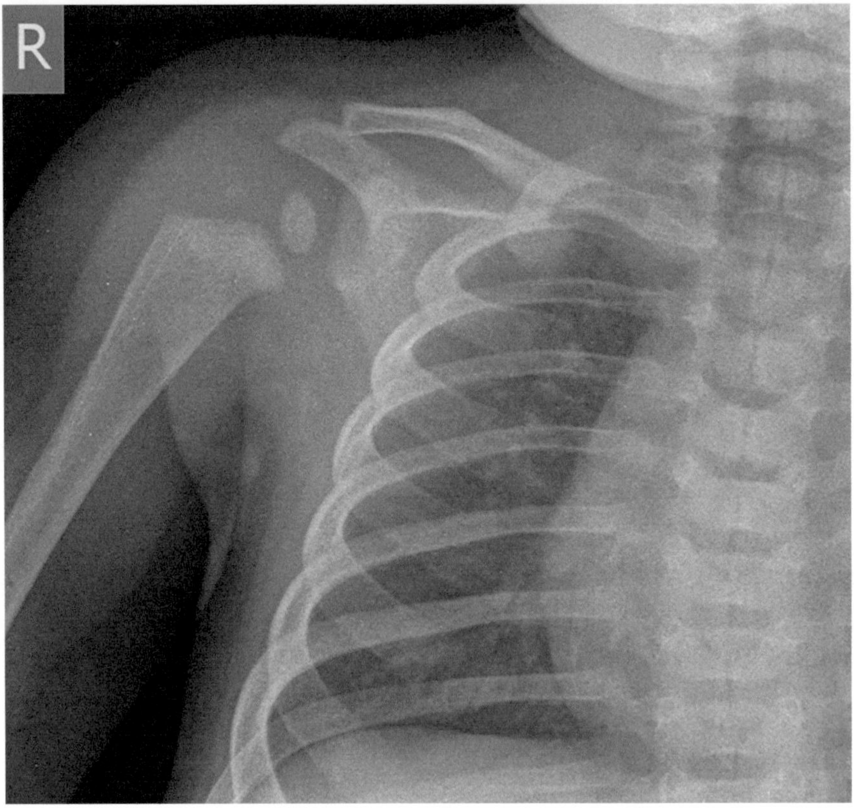

Image 16

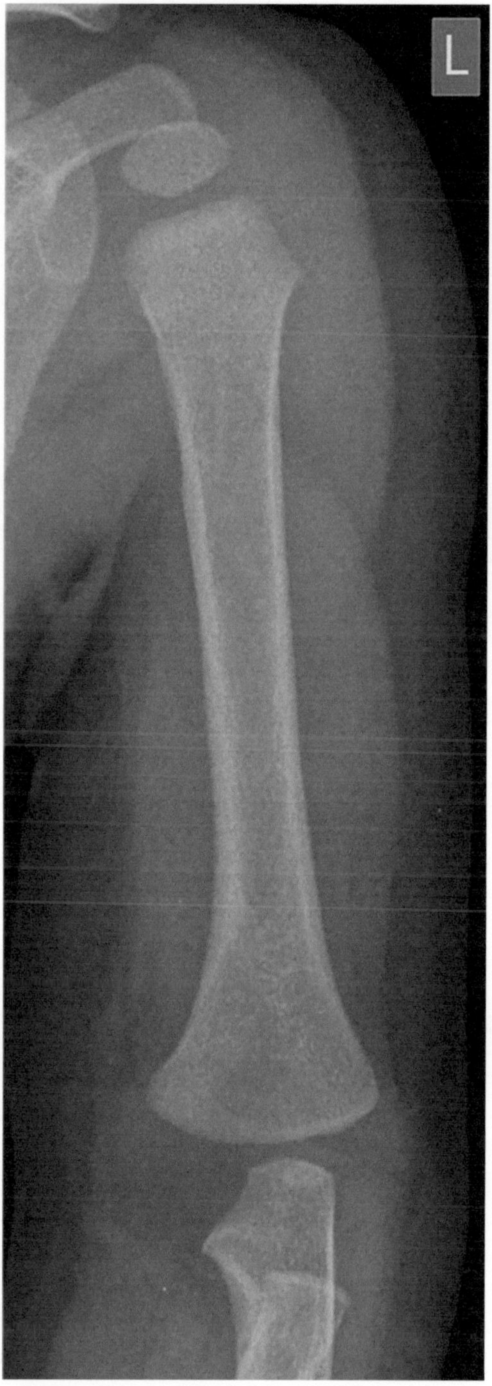

Image 17

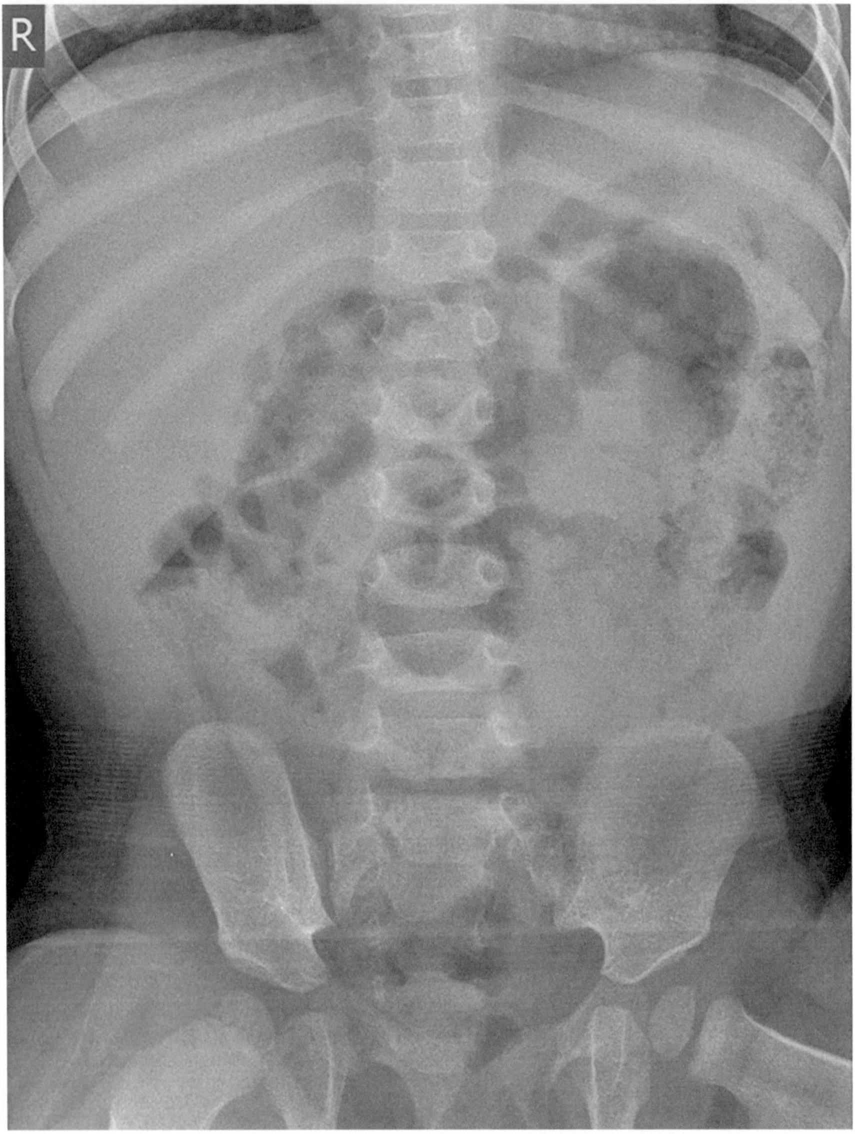

Image 18

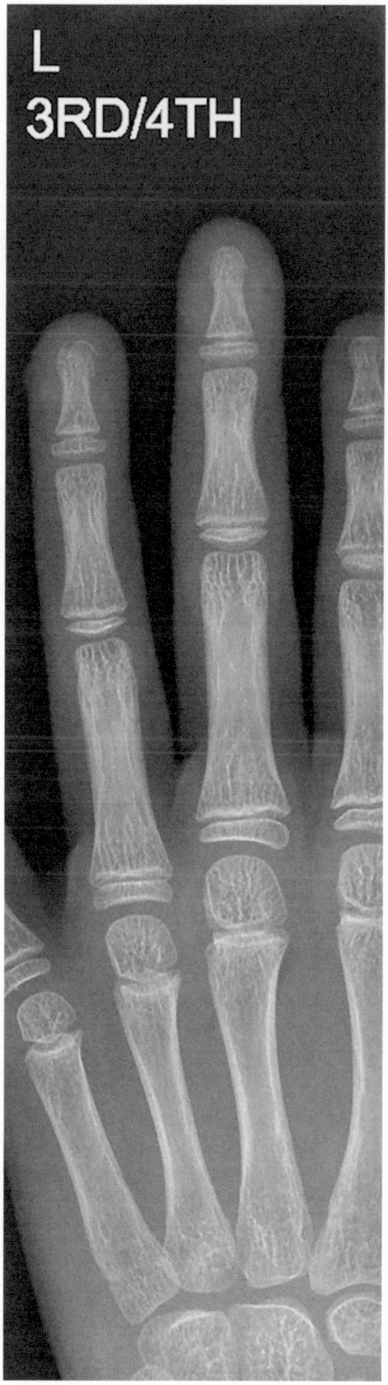

Image 19

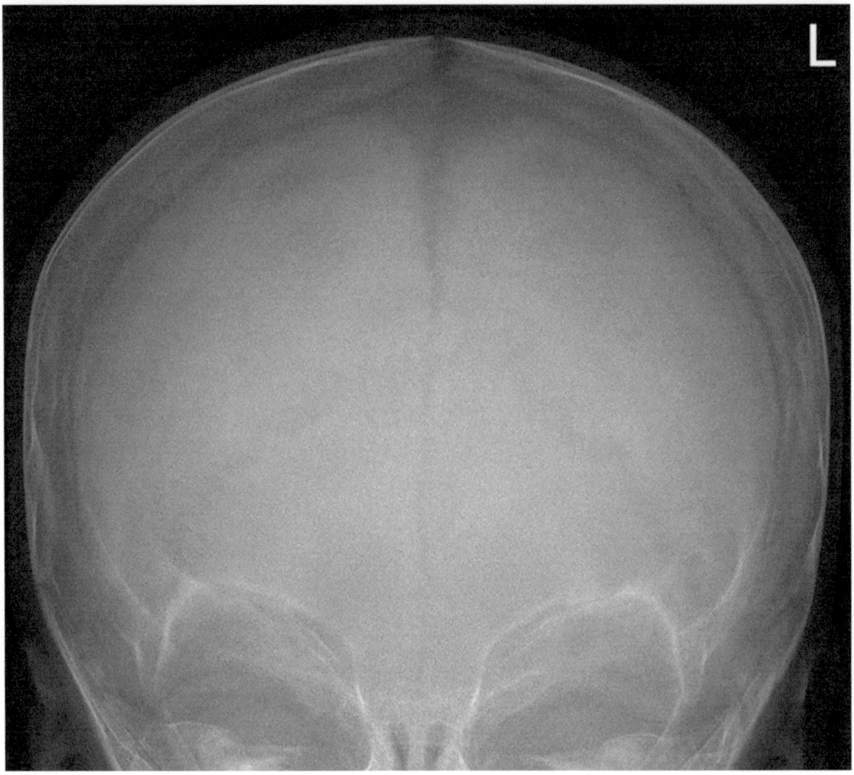

Image 20

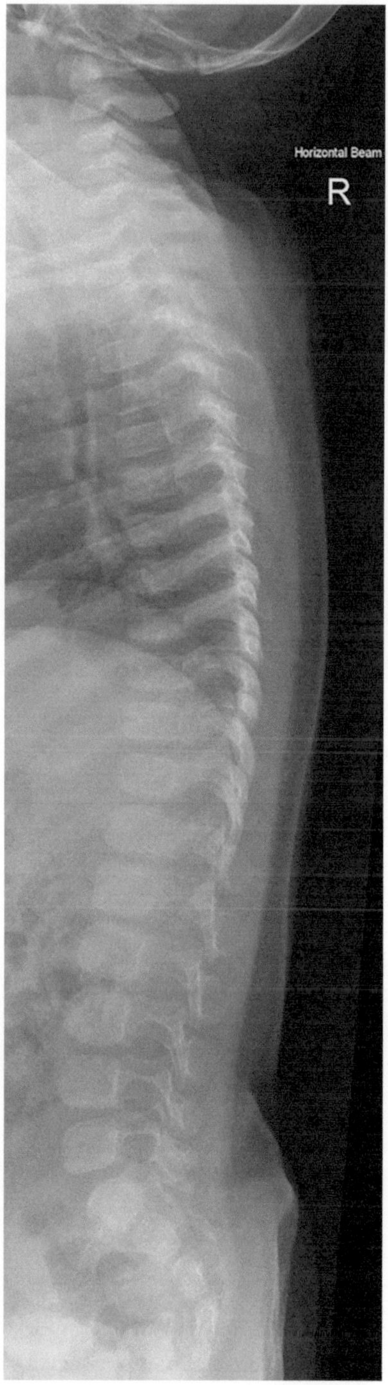

Image 21

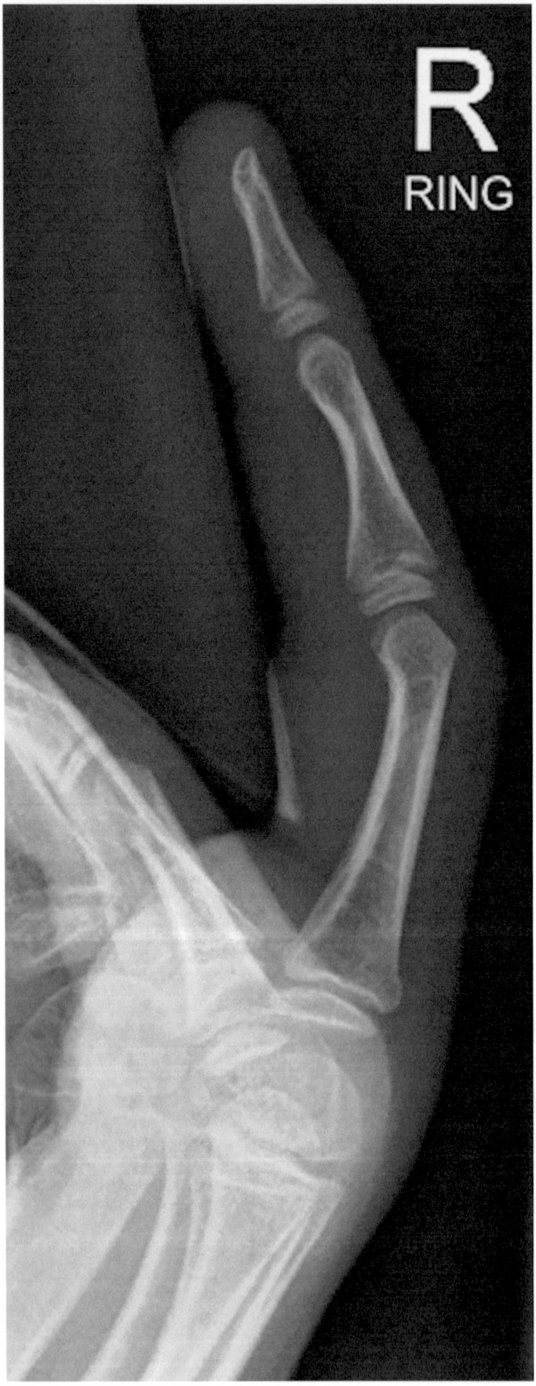

Image 22

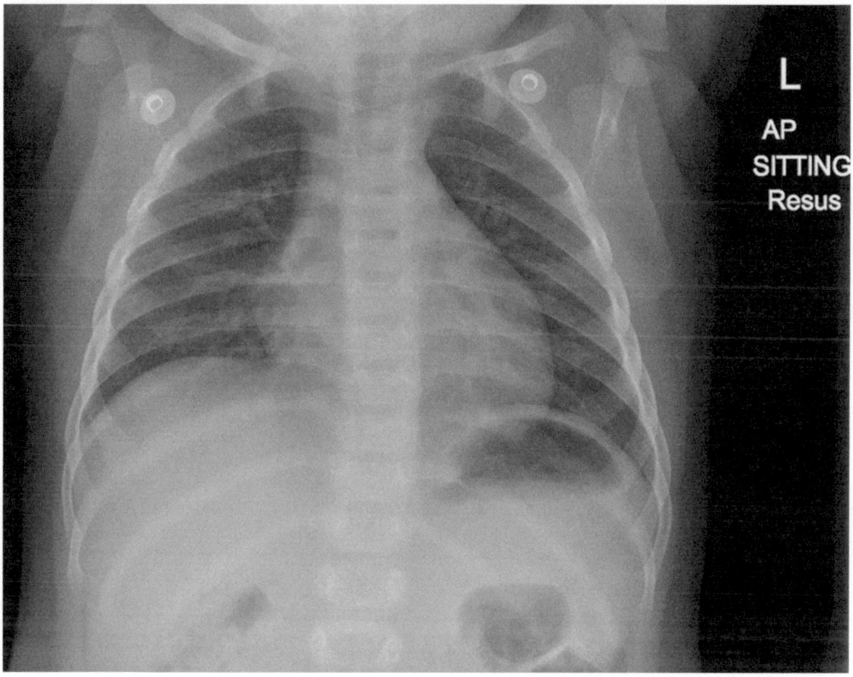

Image 23

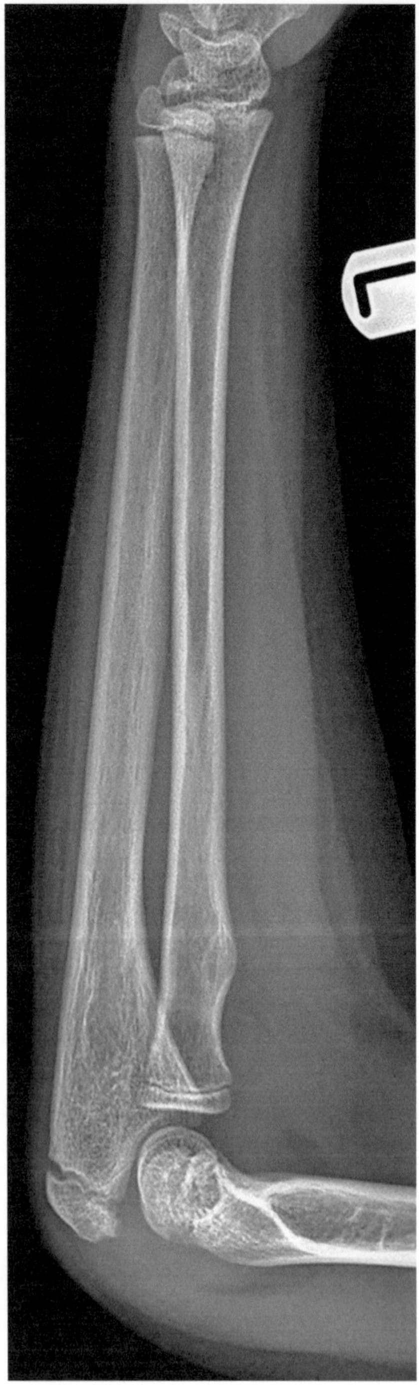

Image 24

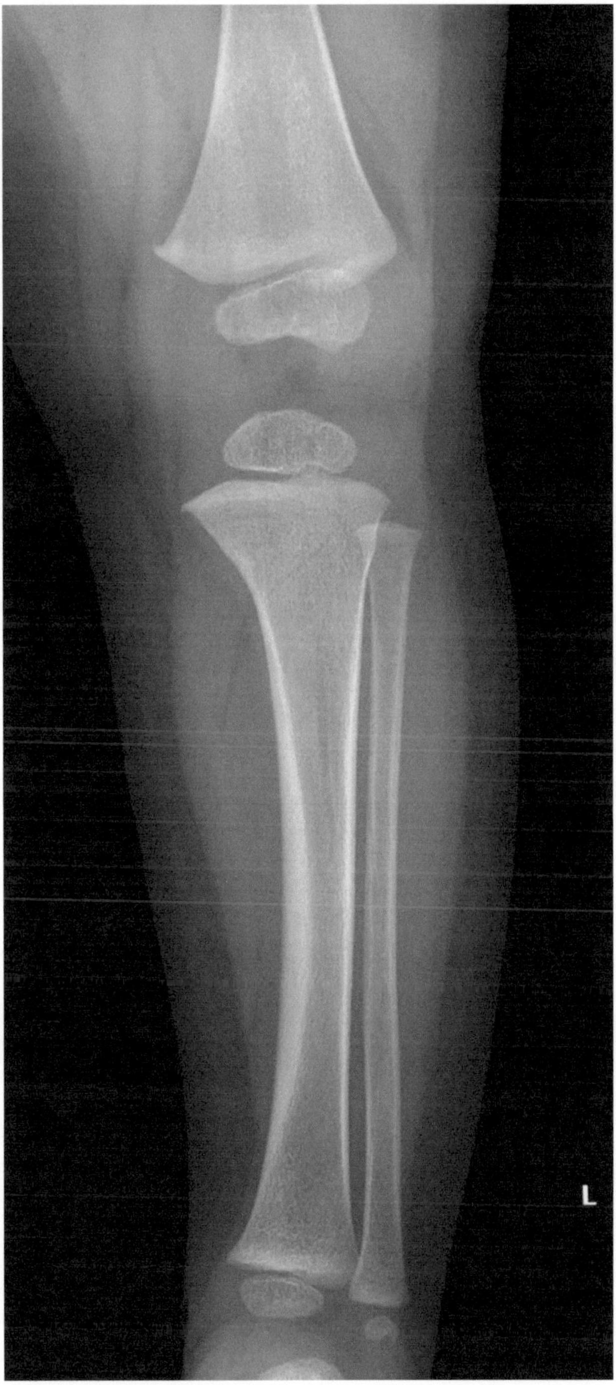

Image 25

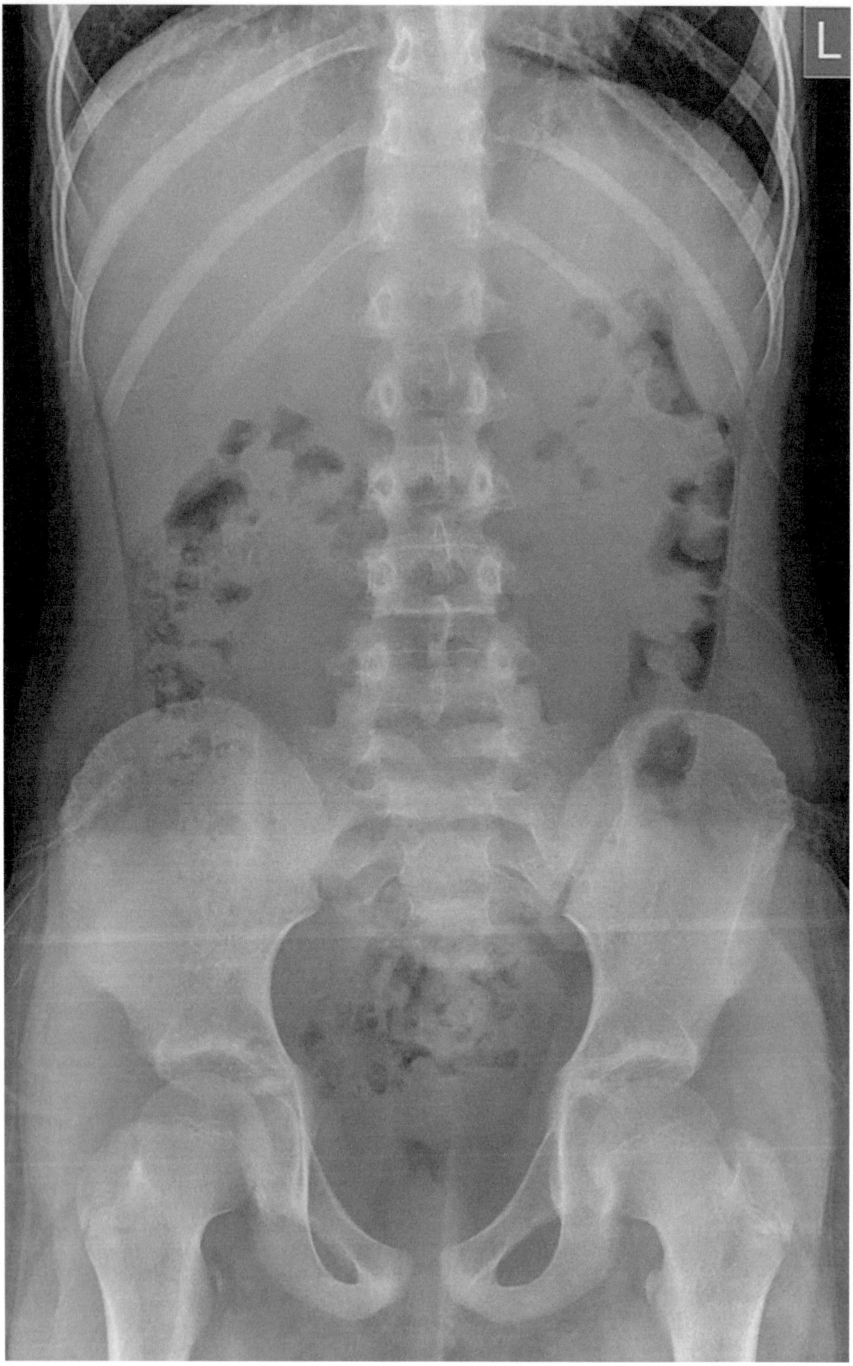

Image 26

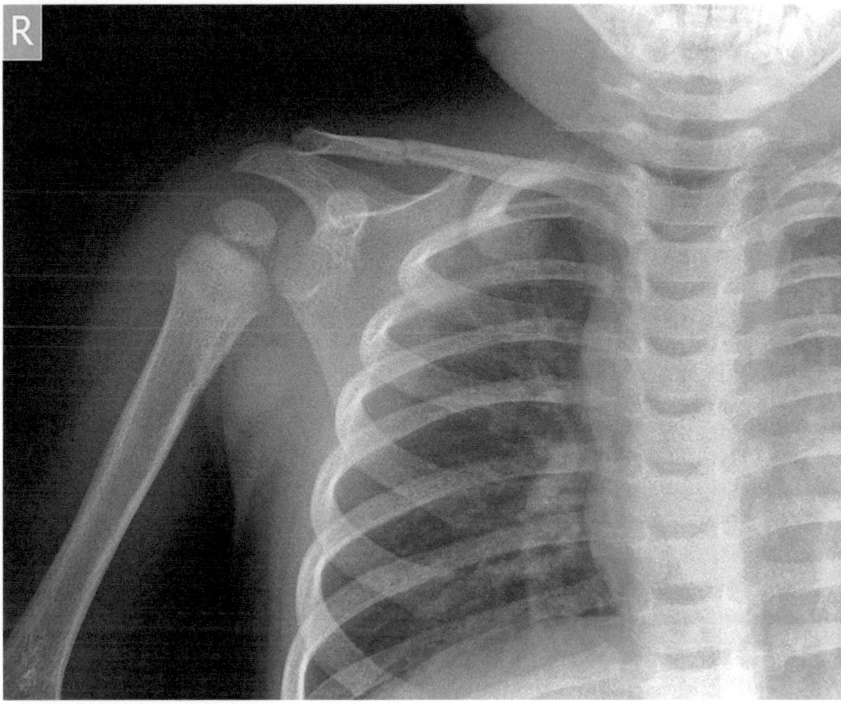

Image 27

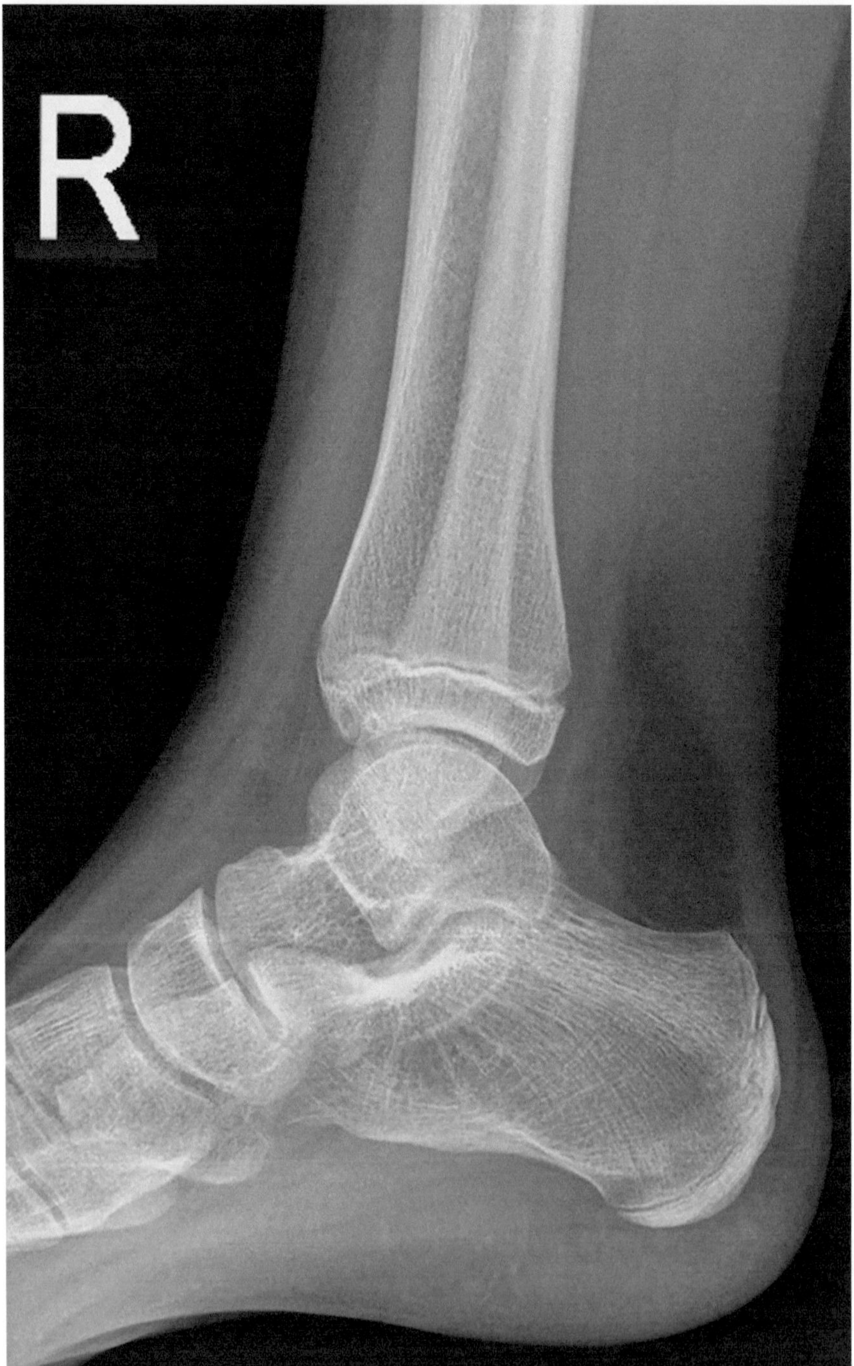

Image 28

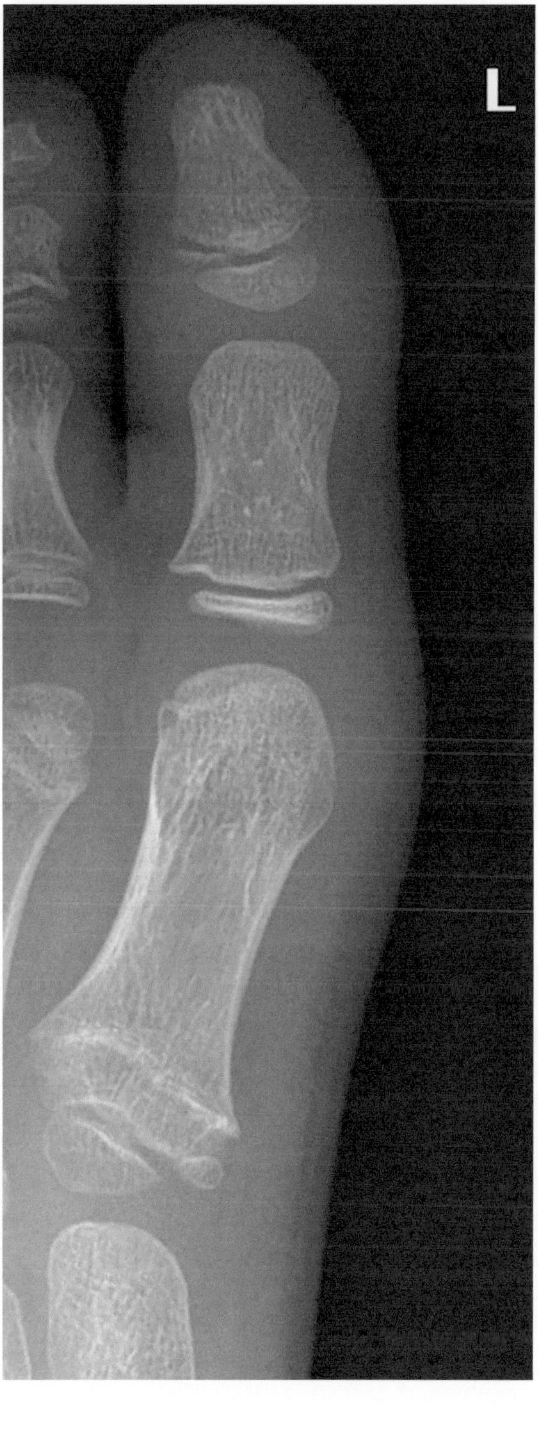

Image 29

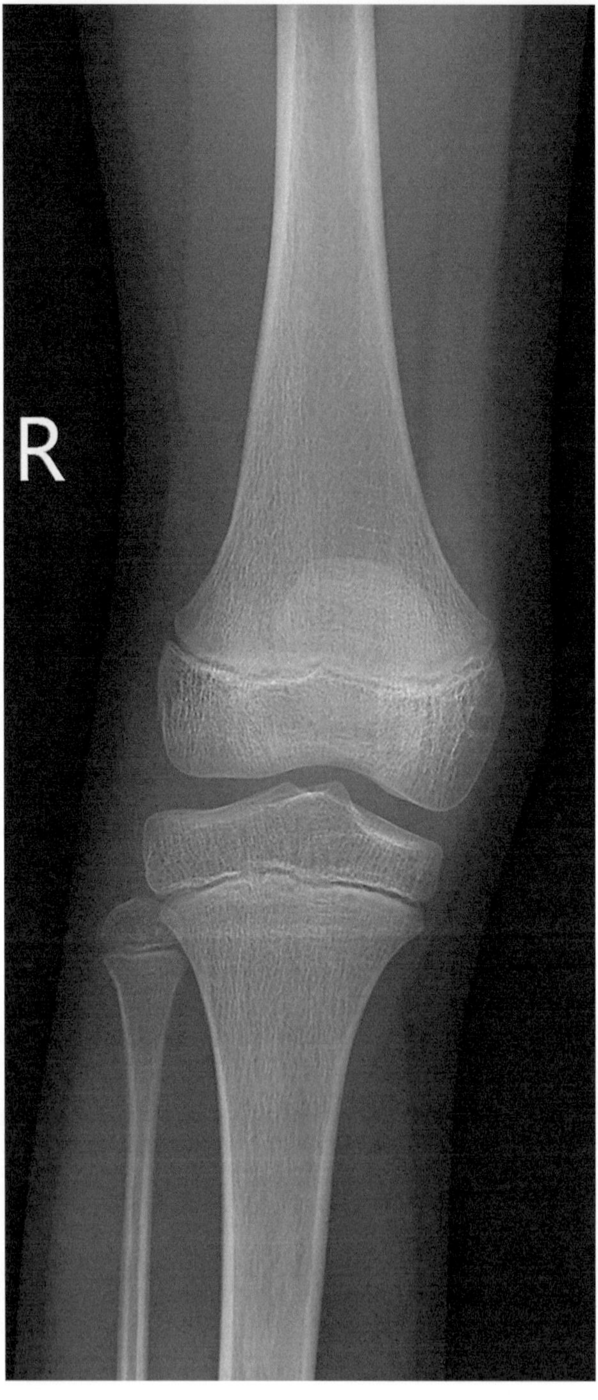

Image 30

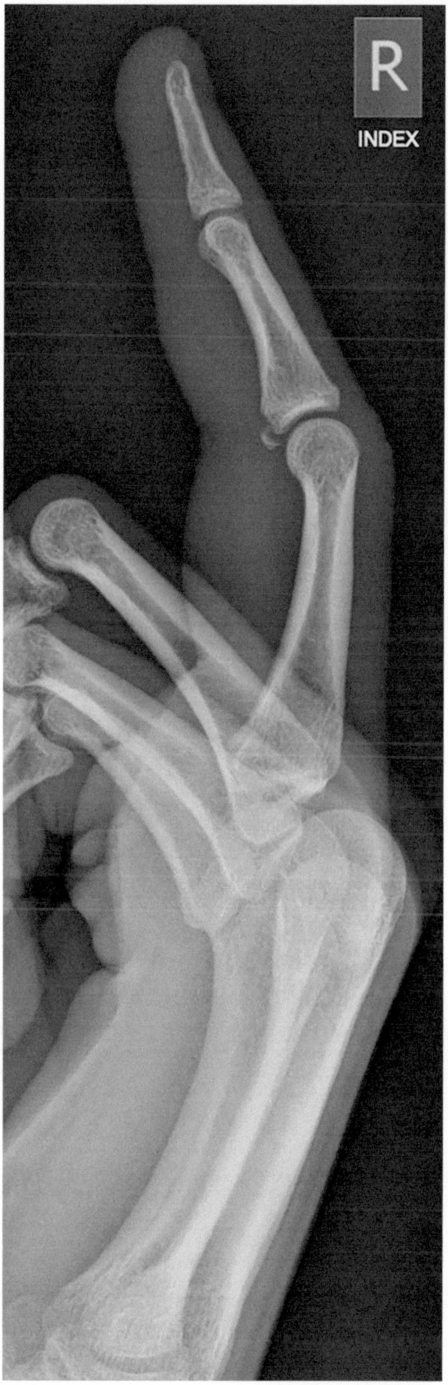

4.2 Answers

Image	Normal	Abnormal	Diagnosis/abnormality (only if abnormal)
1		✓	Bilateral pneumothoraces
2		✓	# R parietal bone
3	✓		
4		✓	# R cuboid
5	✓		
6		✓	R DDH
7	✓		
8	✓		
9	✓		
10		✓	OCD R talus
11		✓	Alternating dense/lucent lines both distal femora
12	✓		
13		✓	Avulsion # L iliac crest apophysis
14		✓	Buckle #s R distal radius and ulna
15	✓		
16	✓		
17	✓		
18		✓	# L ring finger distal phalanx terminal tuft
19	✓		
20	✓		
21		✓	Buckle # dorsal aspect R ring finger proximal phalanx
22	✓		
23		✓	L elbow joint effusion
24		✓	Buckle fracture L proximal tibial metaphysis
25	✓		
26		✓	# distal 1/3 R clavicle
27	✓		
28		✓	SH2 # L hallux distal phalanx
29	✓		
30		✓	Volar plate # R index finger intermediate phalanx

4.3 Explanations

1. **Bilateral pneumothoraces**

   There are bilateral pneumothoraces as evidenced by the increased lucency along the lateral aspects of both hemithoraces in between the lung and thoracic bony cage, enabling visualisation of the lungs edges, deepening of both costophrenic angles (the deep sulcus sign), more so on the right, along with crisp mediastinal and diaphragmatic margins. See the explanation for Image 10 of Test 1.

   Note the right-sided prominence of the superior mediastinum, which is consistent with the thymus and is a normal appearance in this age group (neonate).

2. **# R parietal bone**

   Linear skull fractures of the parietal bone are the most common skull fractures and result from both accidental and inflicted head injuries. Multiple, complex, diastatic, and depressed skull fractures suggest high-energy trauma and may be more suspicious for inflicted injury (physical abuse) depending on the patient age, the presenting clinical context, and the developmental ability of the child, i.e. if present in pre-ambulant (usually less than 12 months of age) or non-mobile infants. See the references for Image 14 of Test 2 for a more detailed discussion regarding the imaging findings of suspected physical abuse (SPA) in infants and young children.

4. **# R cuboid**

   Whilst cuboid fractures are rare in the paediatric population, they can disrupt the normal mechanics of the foot, resulting in deformity and disability. Children may be presented to the Emergency Department (ED) with a limp, pain, swelling, and the inability to bear weight on the lateral aspect of their foot. In this image, the fracture is visualised along the inferolateral margin of the right cuboid. Given their rarity, cuboid fractures may be missed on radiographic evaluation, which reinforces the importance of tracing the outline of every imaged bone. Most commonly, they are isolated avulsion fractures but occasionally may be associated with other midfoot fractures, dislocations, or Lis-Franc joint injuries.

   The 'nutcracker' fracture refers to a cuboid fracture associated with an avulsion fracture of the navicular—this results from compression between the calcaneus and the bases of the fourth and fifth metatarsals during traumatic abduction of the forefoot.

5. *Normal right ankle radiograph*

   There are two incidental accessory ossicles present in this image which are *not* the result of acute fractures:

   - The *os trigonum*, which lies posterior to the talus and represents a failure of fusion of the lateral tubercle of the posterior talar process.
   - The *os supranaviculare*, which lies at the proximal aspect of the dorsal navicular or talonavicular joint and is found in approximately 1% of the population.

Whilst ossicles may have variable appearances at all ages, they are usually well-corticated and appear in expected anatomic locations. However, if there is a history of trauma, focal pain, associated overlying soft tissue swelling, and/or joint effusion, an acute bony injury such as an avulsion fracture should be considered.

6. **Developmental dysplasia of the right hip**
In this radiograph, the right acetabular roof appears shallow when compared to the left, and the right proximal femoral ossific nucleus is smaller and appears 'off centre'. The lateral margin of the right ossific nucleus is aligned with the lateral most aspect of the acetabular roof, indicating a degree of lateral subluxation. This is more formally assessed by drawing a horizontal line along the inferior aspects of both triradiate cartilages, known as the Hilgenreiner line. The Perkin line can then be drawn perpendicular to the Hilgenreiner line (which is used for reference) along the lateral most aspect of the acetabular roof. The proximal femoral ossific nucleus on each side should lie inferomedial to the intersection of these two lines, i.e. medial to the Perkin line and inferior to the Hilgenreiner line, or the inner lower quadrant produced by the intersection of these two lines.
The Hilgenreiner line is also used as a reference line to calculate the acetabular angle, which is the angle between the Hilgenreiner line and a further line drawn tangential to the acetabular roof. As the normal hip joints mature, they become progressively shallower. In developmental dysplasia of the hip (DDH), and in neuromuscular disorders such as cerebral palsy and some skeletal dysplasias, the acetabular angle will be increased. There are excellent illustrations of these lines and angles in the references provided.
This radiograph is a subtler example of DDH when compared to the image from Image 17 of Test 2—see this explanation for a detailed discussion of DDH. These findings must be reported to enable prompt orthopaedic referral and early initiation of treatment to improve patient outcomes.

10. **Osteochondral defect R talus**
Osteochondral defects (OCDs), or lesions, are focal areas of damage to the articular cartilage with injury to the adjacent subchondral bone, which may occur secondary to: repeated microtrauma; an impaction injury; avascular necrosis (AVN); or a subchondral insufficiency fracture (i.e. articular collapse). The commonest sites for osteochondral defects are:
    - Femoral condyle (most common): typically the **L**ateral **A**spect of the **M**edial (**E**pi)condyle (mnemonic, **LAME**).
    - Capitellum (of the humerus): anterolateral or central aspect.
    - Talus: posteromedial.
    - Humeral head.

    Magnetic resonance imaging (MRI) is the test of choice and is essential in determining management. High T2 signal separating the fragment from the bone (known as the 'rim sign') indicates an unstable lesion that requires surgical fixation. However, an important caveat is that focal oedema can mimic this appearance resulting in a false positive. Be sure to look for any high signal subchondral cystic change and other intra-articular loose bodies.

Note that the term *osteochondritis dissecans* is the end result of aseptic separation of an osteochondral fragment which results in an *osteochondral defect*; the two are closely related.

11. **Alternating dense/lucent lines both distal femora**
There are sclerotic lines alternating with less dense (relatively more radiolucent) native bone in the distal femoral metaphyses resulting in a horizontal striped appearance. The underlying condition in this case is osteogenesis imperfecta (OI), a group of congenital disorders of collagen type 1 production which affect the bones and connective tissues. The treatment involves repeated episodes of cyclical bisphosphonate therapy which work by inhibiting osteoclast function: the resultant new bone formation is represented by the linear sclerosis (dense lines). Thus, this appearance may be termed 'bisphosphonate lines' if there is a history of bisphosphonate treatment, or 'zebra lines'. Importantly, excessive doses may lead to iatrogenic osteopetrosis. If you are considering a diagnosis of OI, look for the associated features such as acute and/or healing fractures with associated bony remodelling, osteopenia, Wormian bones (see below), and platybasia.
There are several causes for alternating dense/lucent metaphyseal lines which include:
- Growth arrest/resumption lines (also known as Harris or Park lines): seen after periods of 'metabolic stress', i.e. an acute illness where growth is arrested and then resumes when the acute stressor has resolved. They may be distinguished from bisphosphonate lines in that growth arrest lines rarely cross from one cortex to the other.
- Bisphosphonate therapy (as in this case).
- Rickets: particularly those on prolonged treatment in cases of vitamin D dependent rickets.
- Osteopetrosis.
- Chemotherapy.
- Chronic anaemia: seen in haemoglobinopathies such as sickle cell disease and thalassemia.
- Treated leukaemia.

Tips for the viva:
- Small bones may be visualised in the cranial sutures, most commonly the lambdoid sutures, i.e. intrasutural bones, which are also known as Wormian bones. They are considered a normal variant when present but raise the possibility of pathology when ten or more Wormian bones have been identified. The differential diagnosis for multiple Wormian bones can be remembered using the mnemonic **PORKCHOPS**:
  - **P**yknodysostosis.
  - **O**steogenesis imperfecta.
  - **R**ickets.
  - **K**inky hair syndrome (also known as Menkes disease).
  - **C**leidocranial dysplasia/dysostosis.
  - **H**ypothyroidism; **H**ypophosphatasia.

- **O**topalatodigital syndrome.
- **P**rimary acro-osteolysis (also known as Hajdu-Cheney); **P**achydermo-periostosis.
- **S**yndrome of Down's (Trisomy 21).

- In this case, note the flaring of the distal femoral metaphyses, reminiscent of the Erlenmeyer flask deformity seen in several conditions which can be remembered using the mnemonic **LORA CHONG**:
  - **L**ead poisoning; **L**eukaemia.
  - **O**steopetrosis: the infantile subtype is autosomal recessive (remember that it is re**C**essive in **C**hildren) whereas the benign a**D**ult subtype is autosomal **D**ominant. Also look for diffuse bony sclerosis and sclerotic vertebral end-plates (known as sandwich vertebrae); **O**steochondromatosis.
  - **R**ickets; **R**heumatoid arthritis.
  - **A**chondroplasia: the most common skeletal dysplasia which results from a mutation in fibroblast growth factor gene 3 (*FGFR3*). The dominant feature is rhizomelic (from the Greek *rhizo* meaning 'root' and *melia* meaning 'limb') dwarfism where there is proximal (i.e. humeral and femoral, the 'root') limb shortening.
  - **C**raniometaphyseal dysplasias: these are rare autosomal dominant skeletal dysplasias characterised by thickening of the skull, abnormal facies, cranial nerve dysfunction and metaphyseal irregularities.
  - **H**aemoglobinopathies: sickle cell disease; thalassaemia.
  - **O**ther dysplasias: fibrous dysplasia; Pyle disease, a rare autosomal recessive metaphyseal dysplasia characterised by flared metaphyses (Erlenmeyer flask) which appear relatively lucent because of the relative constriction and sclerosis of the diaphyses. When there is cranial involvement, it is termed craniometaphyseal dysplasia (above).
  - **N**iemann-Pick disease: a collection of autosomal recessive lysosomal storage disorders characterised by the underlying metabolic deficiency (acid sphingomyelinase deficiency or impaired intracellular cholesterol trafficking).
  - **G**aucher disease: an autosomal recessive lysosomal storage disorder resulting from a deficiency of glucocerebrosidase. See the explanation for Image 1 of Test 1.

13. **Avulsion # L iliac crest apophysis**

Careful inspection reveals an avulsion fracture of the left iliac crest apophysis. Apophyseal avulsion injuries may be found on pelvic/hip radiographs performed for pain in sporty/active children. In the paediatric population, the tendons are stronger than the apophyses on to which they attach such that a strong muscular contraction results in an avulsion of the apophysis rather than a sprain or tear of the tendon.

Bony structure—Tendinous attachment (from proximal to distal):

- Iliac crest—Abdominal muscles (external and internal obliques, transversus abdominis).

- Anterior superior iliac spine (A**SIS**)—**S**artorius and ten**s**or fa**s**cia latae.
- Anterior inferior iliac spine (A**IIS**)—Rectus femor**is**.
- **G**reater trochanter—**G**luteus medius and minimus.
- Lesser trochanter—Iliopsoas.
- Pubic symphysis—Adductors.
- Ischial tuberosity—Hamstrings.

Tip for the viva:

This is common examination fodder and can appear in any component of the 2B examination: *the above pairings should be learnt rote.*

14. **Buckle #s R distal radius and ulna**

Did you also spot the right distal ulna fracture? Note the subtle undulation of the cortical margins of the right distal ulna consistent with a buckle fracture. Remember that radius and ulna fractures commonly occur *together*—see the explanation for Image 18 of Test 1 and the Introduction section. Both fractures are better visualised in the magnified image below:

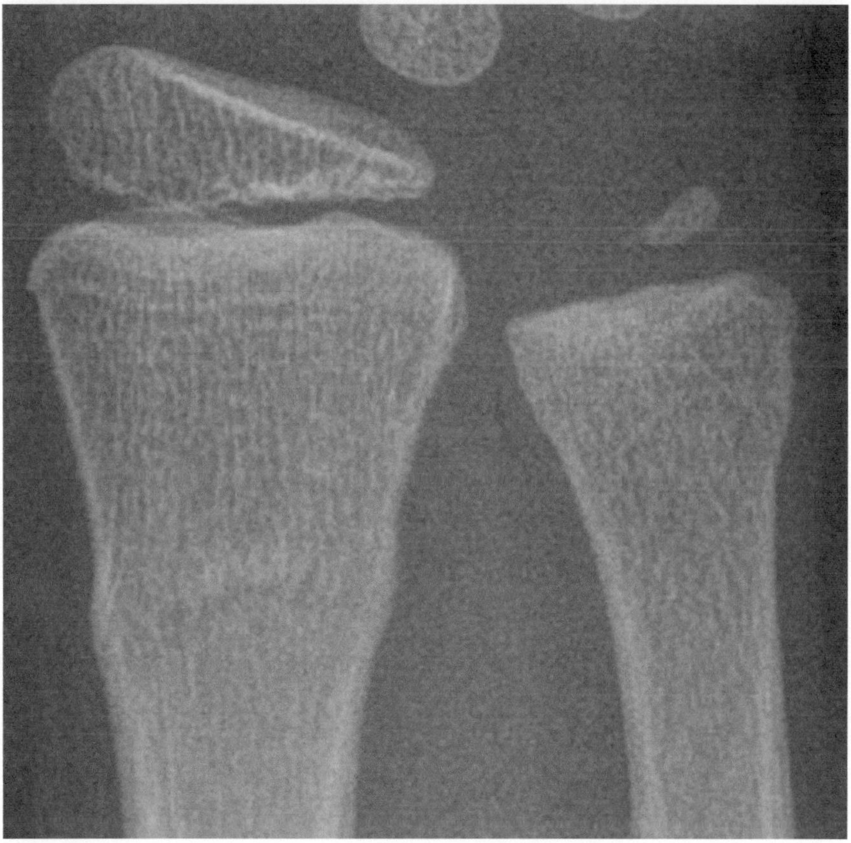

18. **# L ring finger distal phalanx terminal tuft**
There is a minimally displaced fracture through the terminal tuft of the left ring finger distal phalanx. These fractures usually result from a crush injury, often with an overlying injury to nail matrix or pulp.

21. **Buckle # dorsal aspect R ring finger proximal phalanx**
This child was presented to the ED with finger pain and reduced range of movement following a basketball injury. Whilst this finding is subtle, it is real: tracing the outline of every bone reveals a 'bump' in the dorsal cortex of the base of the right finger proximal phalanx consistent with a buckle fracture. See the explanation for Image 18 of Test 1.

23. **L elbow joint effusion**
Note the elevated anterior and posterior fat pads at the bottom of this left forearm radiograph consistent with a large left elbow joint effusion; however, no acute bony injury is identified. See the explanation for Image 11 of Test 1.

24. **Buckle fracture L proximal tibial metaphysis**
Buckle or transverse fractures of the proximal tibial metaphysis are commonly known as 'trampoline fractures'. These typically occur in children aged 2–5 years of age and are thought to result when a second, usually older/heavier child causes the trampoline surface to recoil upwards to meet the 'descending' child who is usually younger/lighter. The 'excessive load' is thought to result in this characteristic fracture pattern seen in the magnified image below (the subtle bulge in the cortices of the proximal tibia, more so of the lateral cortex):

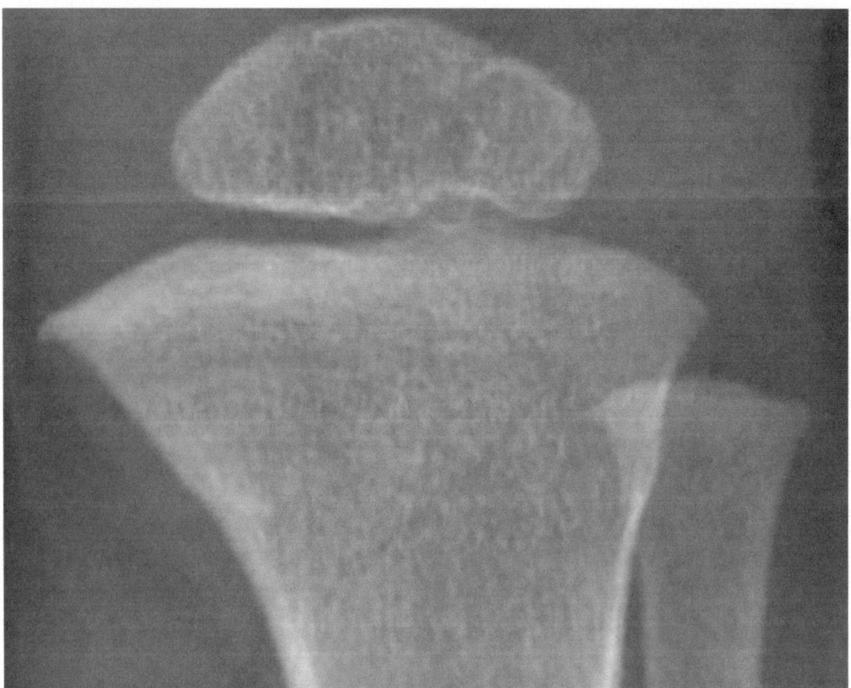

There is a documented propensity for these fractures to develop a late valgus angulation deformity, known as Cozen's phenomenon, named for the orthopaedic surgeon who first described this deformity. This is usually self-limiting and resolves in 1–2 years following the acute injury. Whilst better remodelling potential may be expected in younger children, corrective hemi-epiphysiodesis may be required. Early recognition of this complication is important so that an early orthopaedic assessment and appropriate management can be instigated, if required.

26. **# distal 1/3 R clavicle**
Clavicle fractures account for 15% of all upper extremity injuries in children with half of all clavicle fractures occurring below the age of 7 years. They may result from a fall onto an outstretched hand (FOOSH), direct trauma to the lateral aspect of the shoulder, or birth injury following a difficult delivery. Toddlers may be presented to the ED with arm neglect, i.e. 'not using their arm', if the trauma/fall has not been witnessed.
The Allman classification can be used and categorises the injury depending upon which portion of the bone has been affected:
    - Type 1: the middle third or midshaft (most common, approximately 80%); may be associated with shortening, comminution and angulation (typically apex cranial).
    - Type 2: the lateral (or distal) third, at the level of, or distal to the coracoclavicular ligament. They have higher rates of non-union (failure of fracture healing which may require intervention); approximately 15%.
    - Type 3: the medial (or proximal) third which can be associated with sternoclavicular dislocation; approximately 5%.

    However, in clinical practice, the fracture is usually just described, e.g. there is a minimally displaced fracture at the junction of the middle and distal thirds of the right clavicle, as in this case.

28. **Salter-Harris 2 # L hallux distal phalanx**
This Salter-Harris 2 fracture resulted from a plant pot falling on the left hallux. Interphalangeal joint alignment is preserved. Non-displaced phalangeal fractures of the foot (toes 2 to 5) often only require neighbour strapping/buddy taping with closed fractures rarely requiring reduction. Surgical fixation is typically reserved for significantly displaced or angulated fractures, open fractures and intra-articular fractures of the hallux.

30. **Volar plate # R index finger intermediate phalanx**
Intra-articular avulsion fractures of the proximal interphalangeal joint volar plate result from hyperextension injuries. Fractures which involve a significant portion of the articular surface can result in joint instability given that a greater portion of the stabilising collateral ligaments are attached to the avulsed fracture fragment. These injuries may require surgical fixation.

Further Reading

Image 4

Angoules AG, Angoules NA, Georgoudis M et al (2019) Update on diagnosis and management of cuboid fractures. World J Orthop 10(2):71–80

Weerakkody Y et al (2021) Nutcracker fracture of the cuboid. https://radiopaedia.org/articles/nutcracker-fracture-of-the-cuboid. Accessed July 2023

Image 5

Kasáč Z et al (2023) Os trigonum. https://radiopaedia.org/articles/os-trigonum. Accessed Feb 2023

Niknejad M et al (2022) Os supranaviculare. https://radiopaedia.org/articles/os-trigonum. Accessed July 2023

Image 6

Gaillard F et al (2008) Hilgenreiner's and Perkin's line (diagram). https://radiopaedia.org/cases/hilgenreiners-and-perkins-line-diagram. Accessed Feb 2023

Knipe H et al (2022) Acetabular angle. https://radiopaedia.org/articles/acetabular-angle. Accessed Feb 2023

Murphy A et al (2022) Hilgenreiner line. https://radiopaedia.org/articles/hilgenreiner-line. Accessed Feb 2023

Weerakkody Y et al (2022) Perkin line. https://radiopaedia.org/articles/perkin-line. Accessed Feb 2023

Image 9

Please see the references for Image 14 of Test 2 regarding the imaging of suspected physical abuse in infants and young children.

Image 10

Jadeja R et al (2023) Osteochondritis dissecans. https://radiopaedia.org/articles/osteochondritis-dissecans. Accessed Feb 2023

Skalski M et al (2023) Osteochondral defect. https://radiopaedia.org/articles/osteochondral-defect. Accessed Feb 2023

Thapa MM, Chaturvedi A, Iyer RS et al (2012) MRI of pediatric patients: part 2, normal variants and abnormalities of the knee. AJR Am J Roentgenol 198(5):W456–W465

Image 11

Al Muderis M, Azzopardi T, Cundy P (2007) Zebra lines of pamidronate therapy in children. J Bone Joint Surg Am 89(7):1511–1516

Baba Y et al (2023) Metaphyseal dysplasia. https://radiopaedia.org/articles/metaphyseal-dysplasia. Accessed July 2023

Bandegi P et al (2023) Erlenmeyer flask deformity mnemonic. https://radiopaedia.org/articles/erlenmeyer-flask-deformity-mnemonic. Accessed July 2023

Bell DJ et al (2018) Growth arrest lines. https://radiopaedia.org/articles/growth-arrest-lines. Accessed Mar 2023

Bell DJ et al (2020) Niemann Pick disease. https://radiopaedia.org/articles/niemann-pick-disease. Accessed July 2023

Niknejad M et al (2022) Alternating radiolucent and radiodense metaphyseal lines. https://radiopaedia.org/articles/alternating-radiolucent-and-radiodense-metaphyseal-lines Accessed March 2023

Worsley C et al (2022) Erlenmeyer flask deformity. https://radiopaedia.org/articles/erlenmeyer-flask-deformity-1. Accessed July 2023

Yap J et al (2023) Achondroplasia. https://radiopaedia.org/articles/achondroplasia. Accessed July 2023

Image 13

Bomer J, Holscher H (2015) Hip pathology in children: imaging findings. https://radiologyassistant.nl/pediatrics/hip/hip-pathology-in-children. Accessed Mar 2023

Shaath K, Andras L (2021) Pelvis fractures—pediatric. https://www.orthobullets.com/pediatrics/3000/pelvis-fractures%2D%2Dpediatric. Accessed Mar 2023

Sheikh Y et al (2022) Apophyseal avulsion fractures of the pelvis and hip. https://radiopaedia.org/articles/apophyseal-avulsion-fractures-of-the-pelvis-and-hip. Accessed Mar 2023

Stevens MA, El-Khoury GY, Kathol MH et al (1999) Imaging features of avulsion injuries. Radiographics 19(3):655–672

Image 24

El-Feky M et al (2023) Trampoline fracture. https://radiopaedia.org/articles/trampoline-fracture. Accessed Aug 2023

Jeong C, Lee SU, Kim HG et al (2021) Trampoline-related fractures of the proximal tibia in children. J Orthop Surg Res 16(1):551

Luijkx T et al (2018) Cozen fracture. https://radiopaedia.org/articles/cozen-fracture-1. Accessed Aug 2023

Macknet D, Swarup I, Sink E (2021) Proximal tibia metaphyseal fractures—pediatric. https://www.orthobullets.com/pediatrics/4025/proximal-tibia-metaphyseal-fractures%2D%2Dpediatric. Accessed Aug 2023

Yang BW, Shore BJ, Rademacher E et al (2019) Prevalence of Cozen's phenomenon of the proximal tibia. J Pediatr Orthop 39(6):e417–e421

Image 26

Andras L, Shirley E, Skaggs DL (2023) Clavicle shaft fracture—pediatric. https://www.orthobullets.com/pediatrics/322128/clavicle-shaft-fracture%2D%2Dpediatric. Accessed July 2023

El-Feky M et al (2022) Fracture non-union. https://radiopaedia.org/articles/fracture-non-union-1. Accessed July 2023

The Royal Children's Hospital Melbourne (2023) Clavicle fractures—Emergency Department. https://www.rch.org.au/clinicalguide/guideline_index/fractures/clavicle_fractures_emergency_department/. Accessed July 2023

Vargas-Vila MA, Mehlman CT, Pennock AT (2019) The community orthopaedic surgeon taking trauma call: pediatric midshaft clavicle fracture pearls and pitfalls. J Orthop Trauma 33(Suppl 8):S1–S5

Image 28

Smit K (2023) Foot fractures—phalanx. https://posna.org/physician-education/study-guide/foot-fractures-phalanx. Accessed July 2023

Image 30

Knipe H et al (2022) Volar plate avulsion injury. https://radiopaedia.org/articles/volar-plate-avulsion-injury. Accessed Mar 2023

Test 5

5

M. Paddock et al., *Paediatric Radiology Rapid Reporting*,
https://doi.org/10.1007/978-3-031-48255-7_5

5.1 Images

Image 1

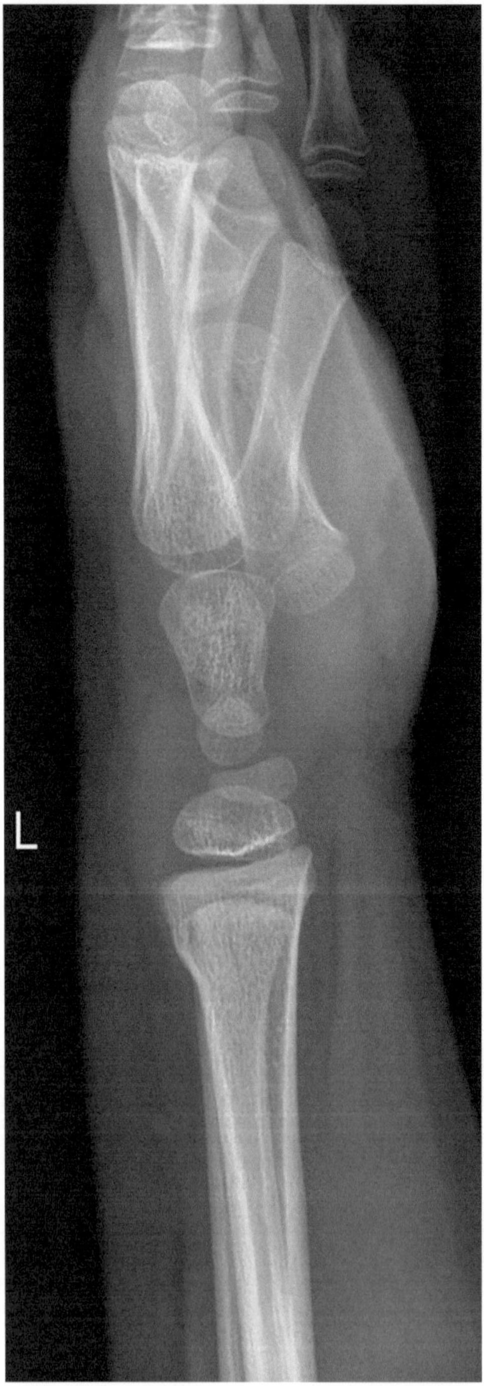

Image 2

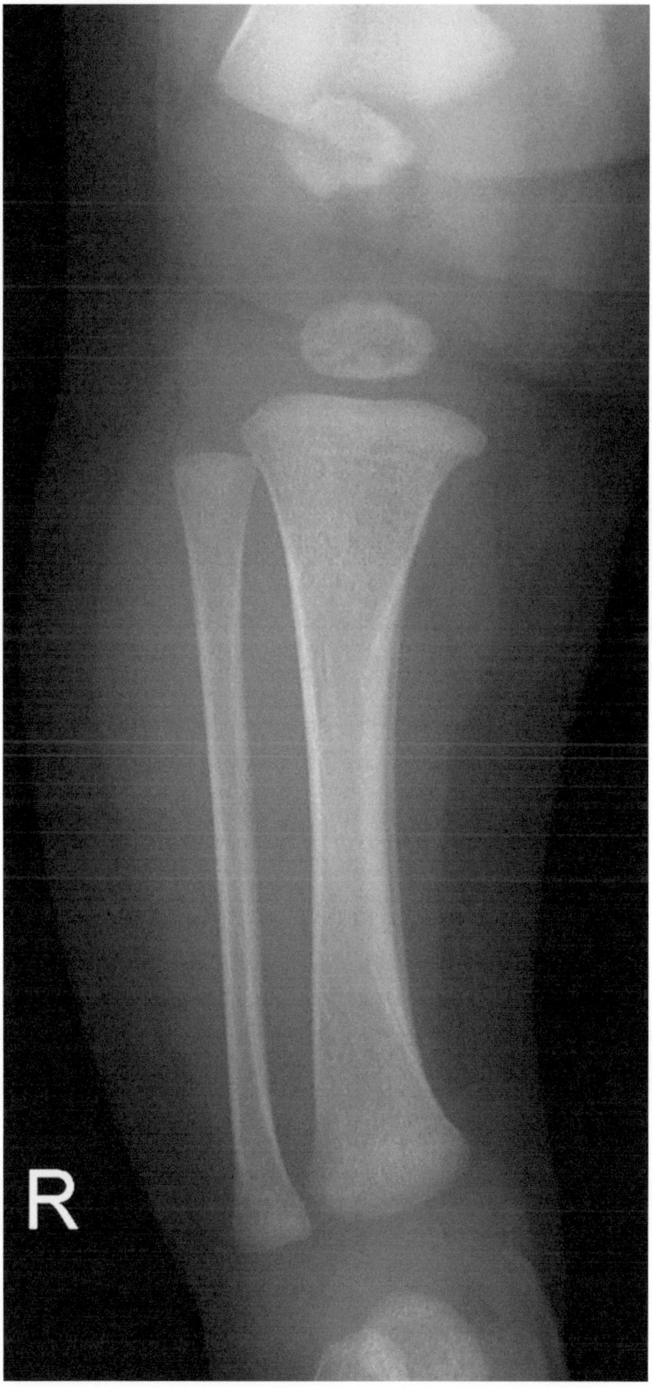

Image 3

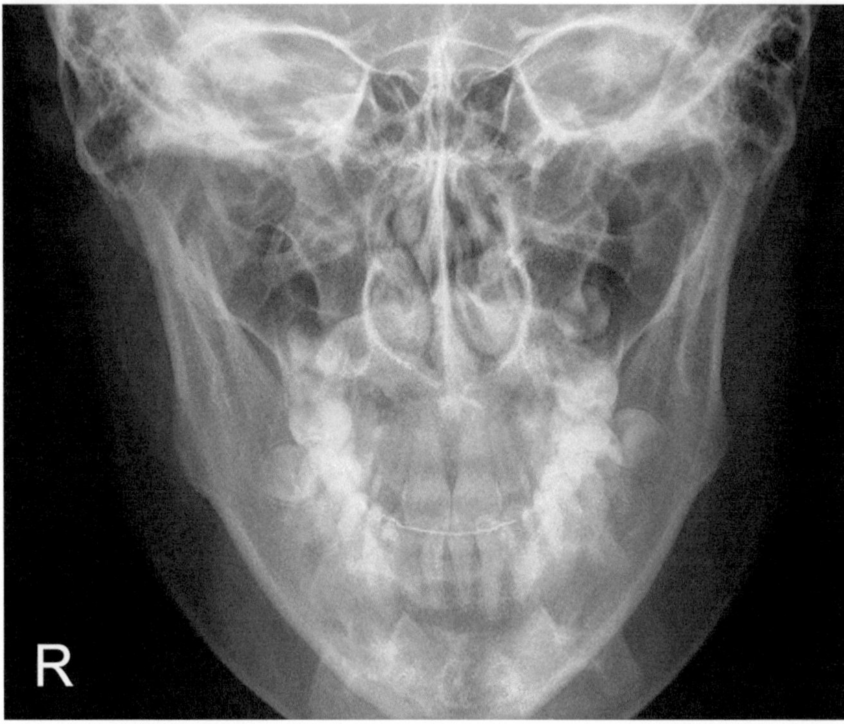

Image 4

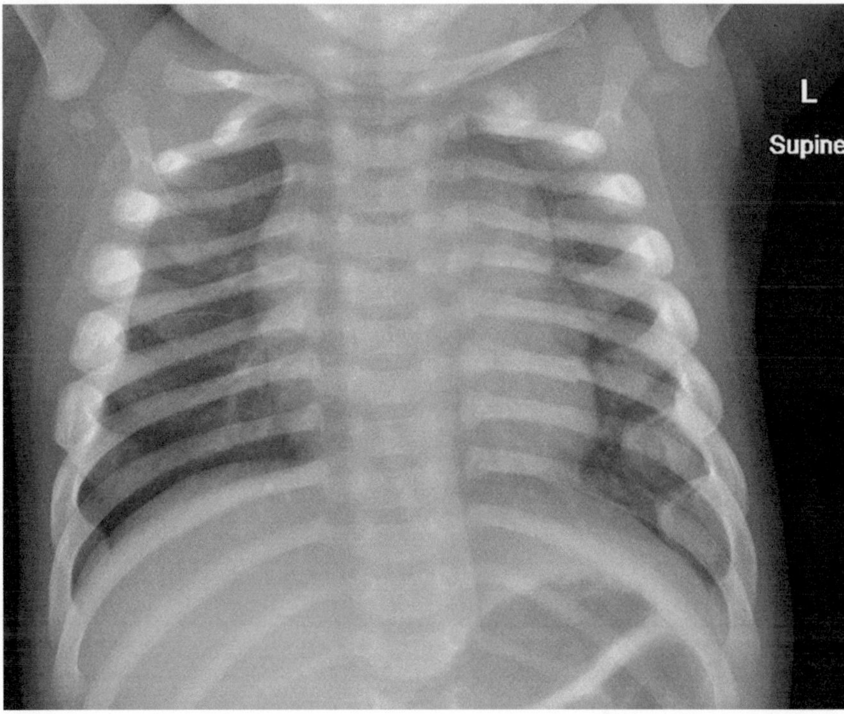

Image 5

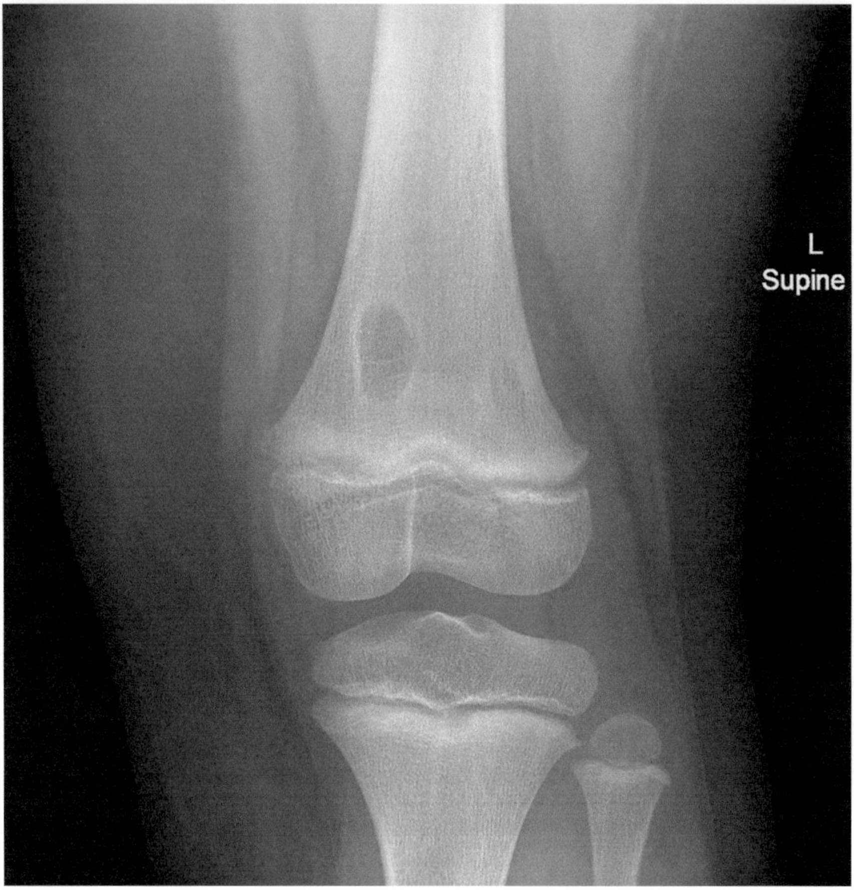

Image 6

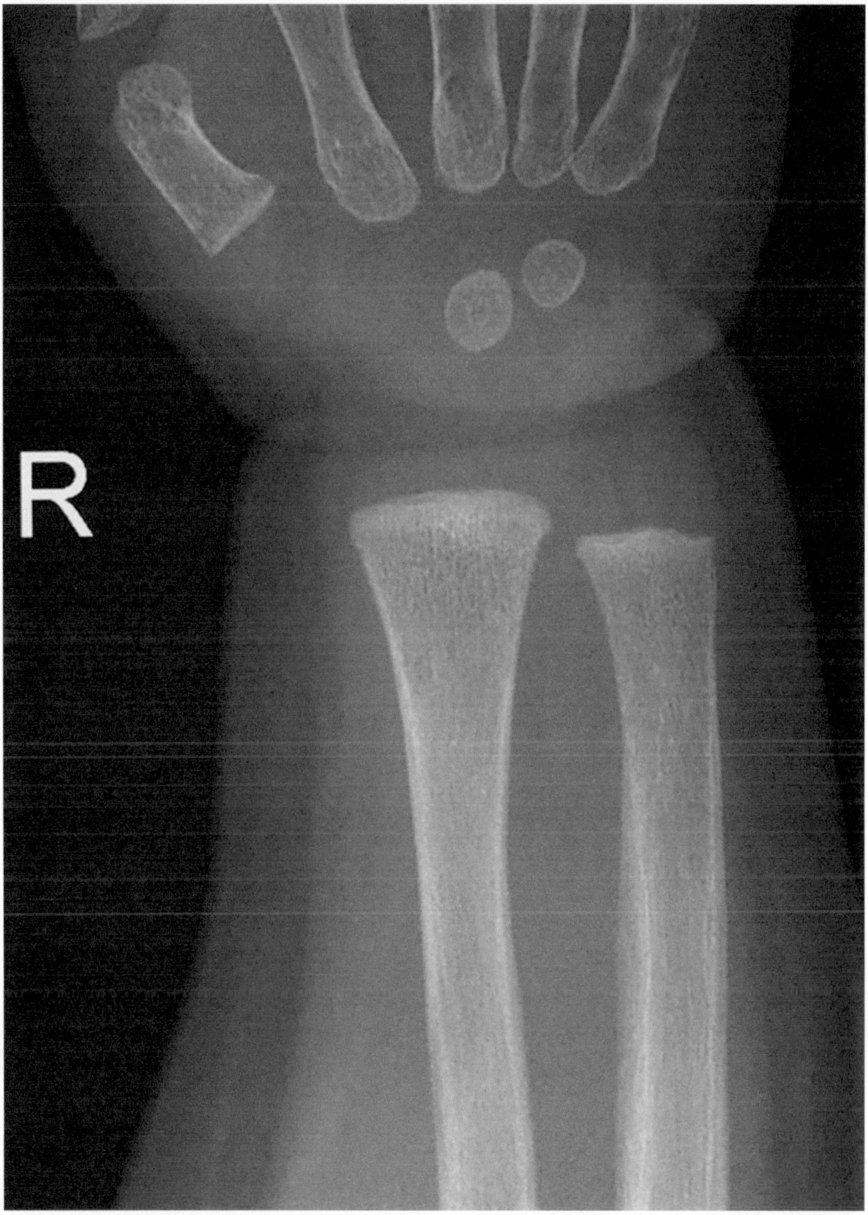

Image 7

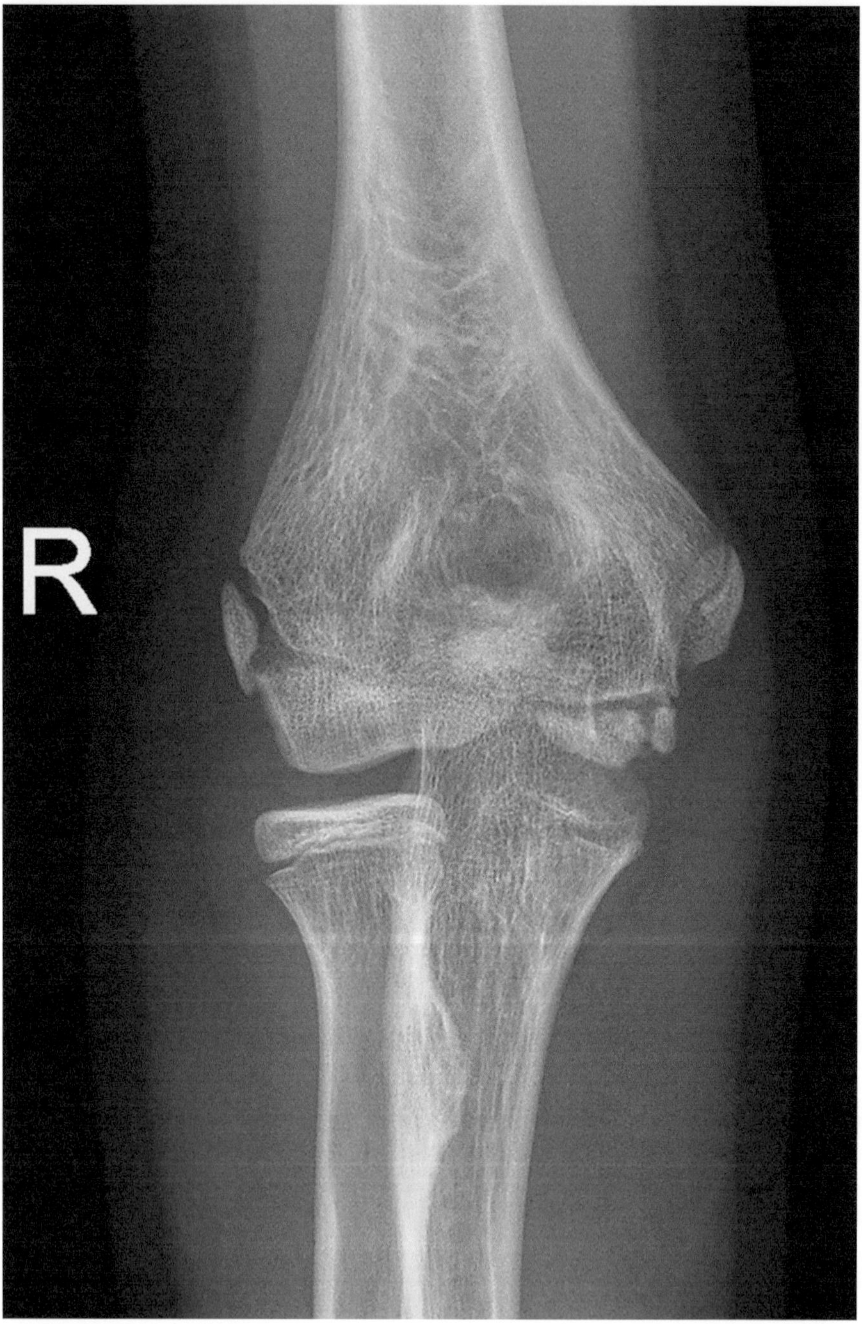

Image 8

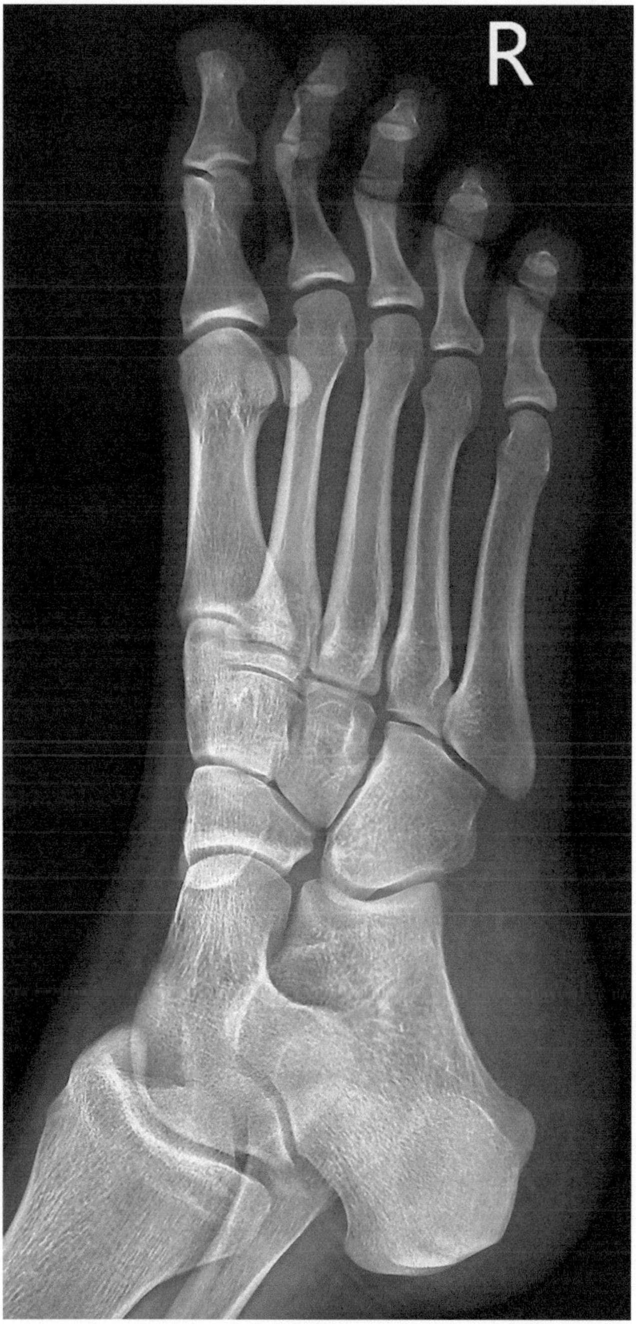

Image 9

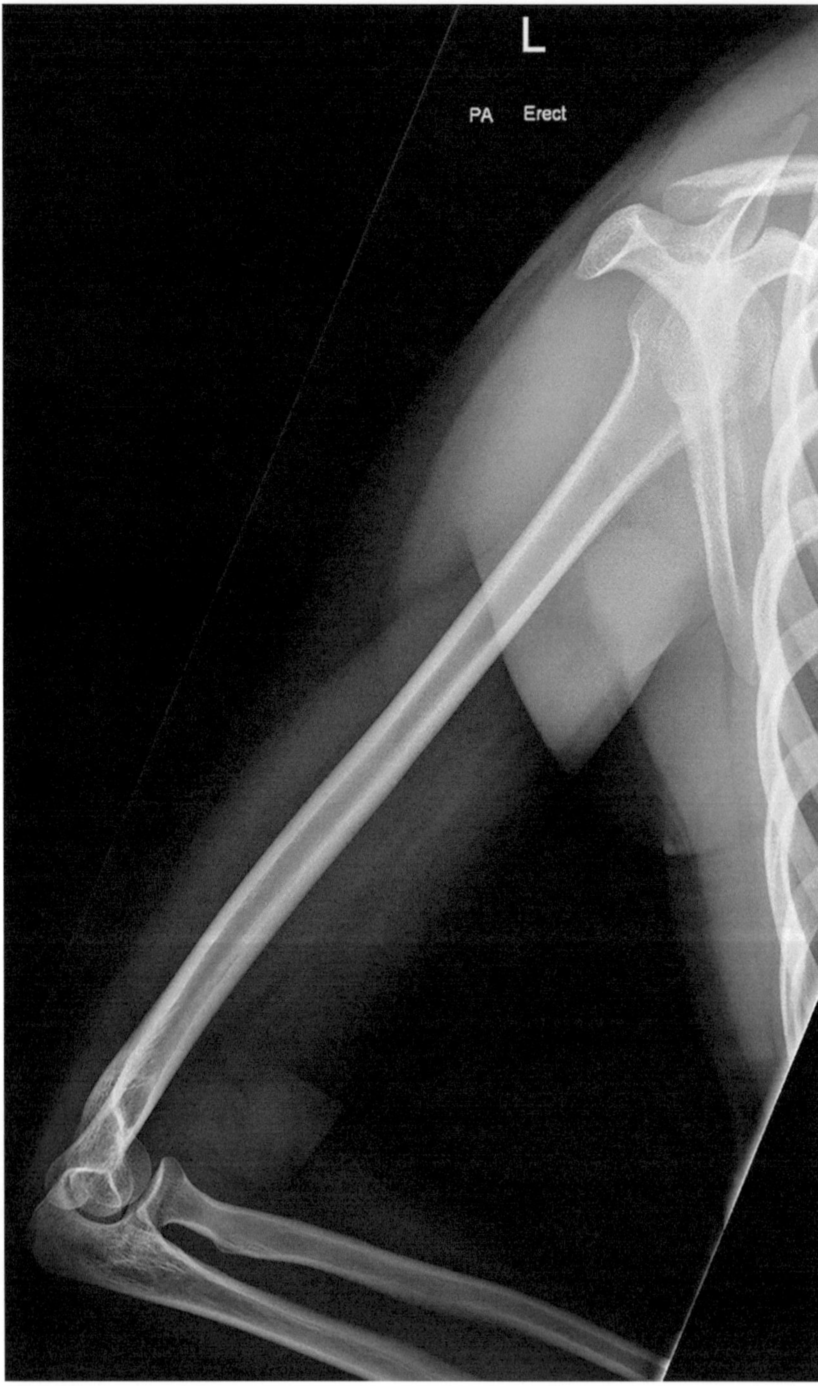

Image 10

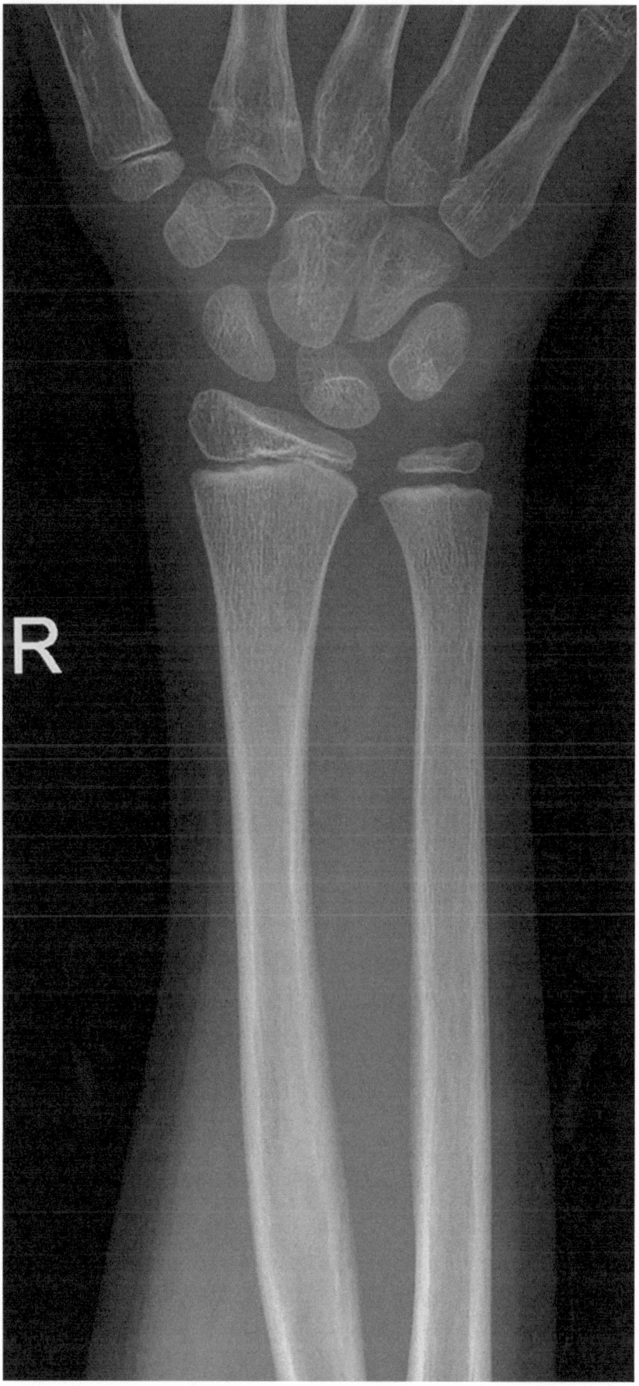

Image 11

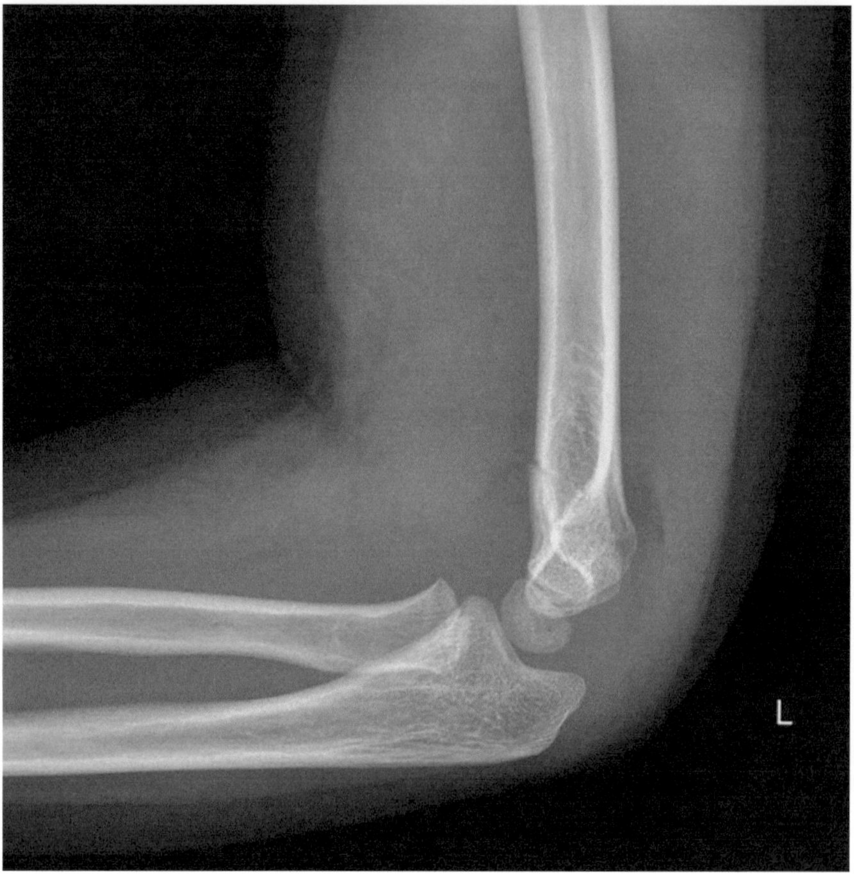

Image 12

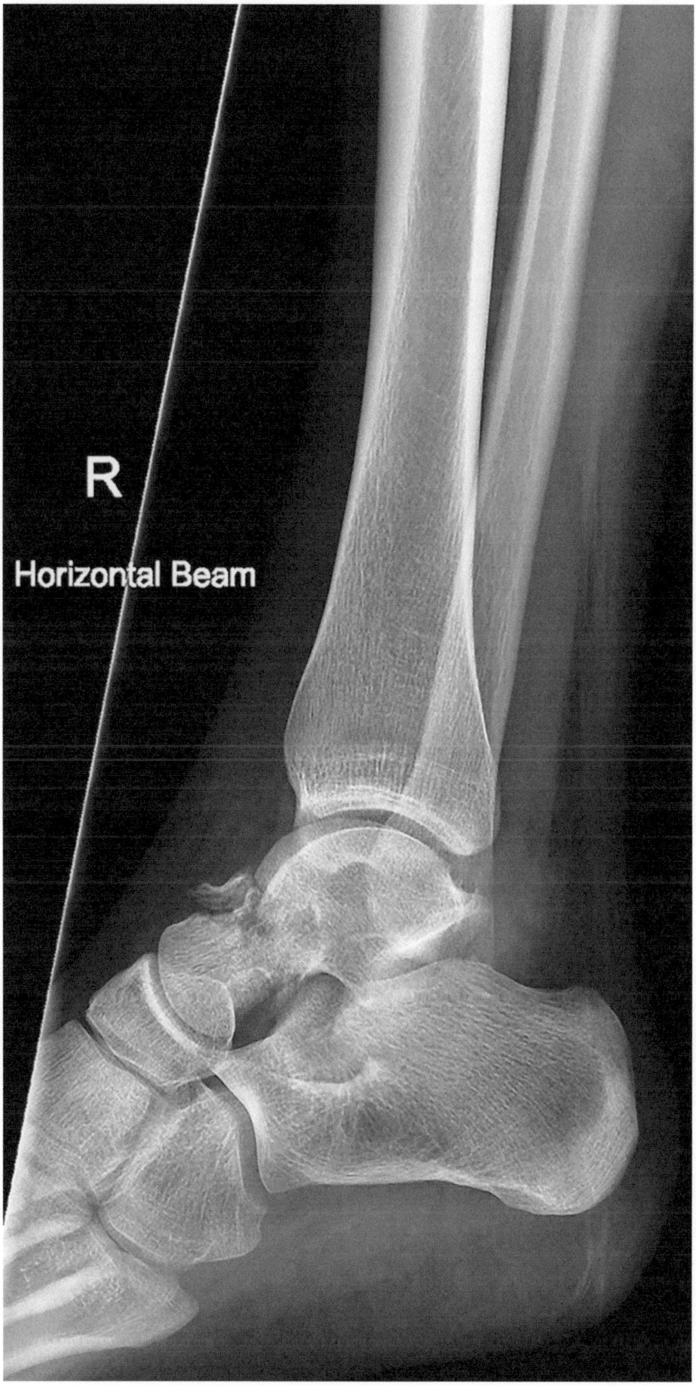

Image 13

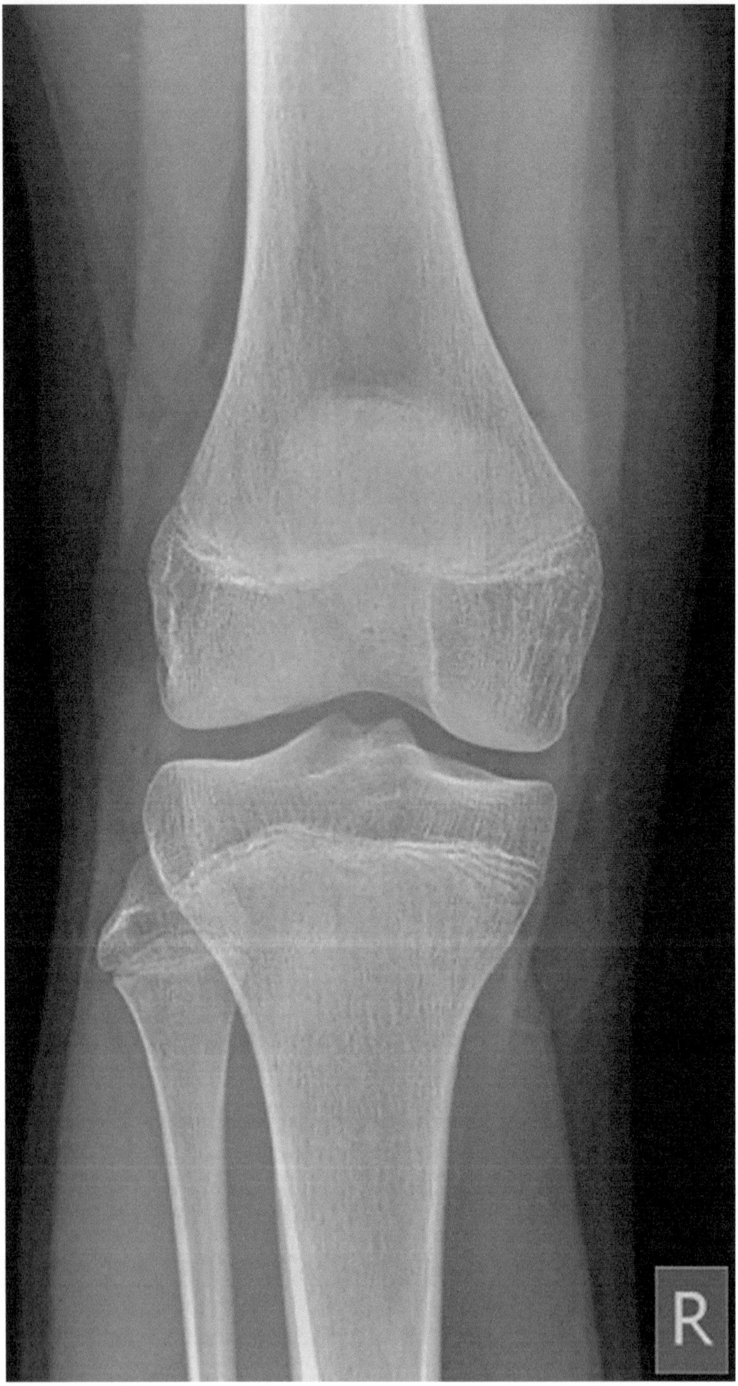

Image 14

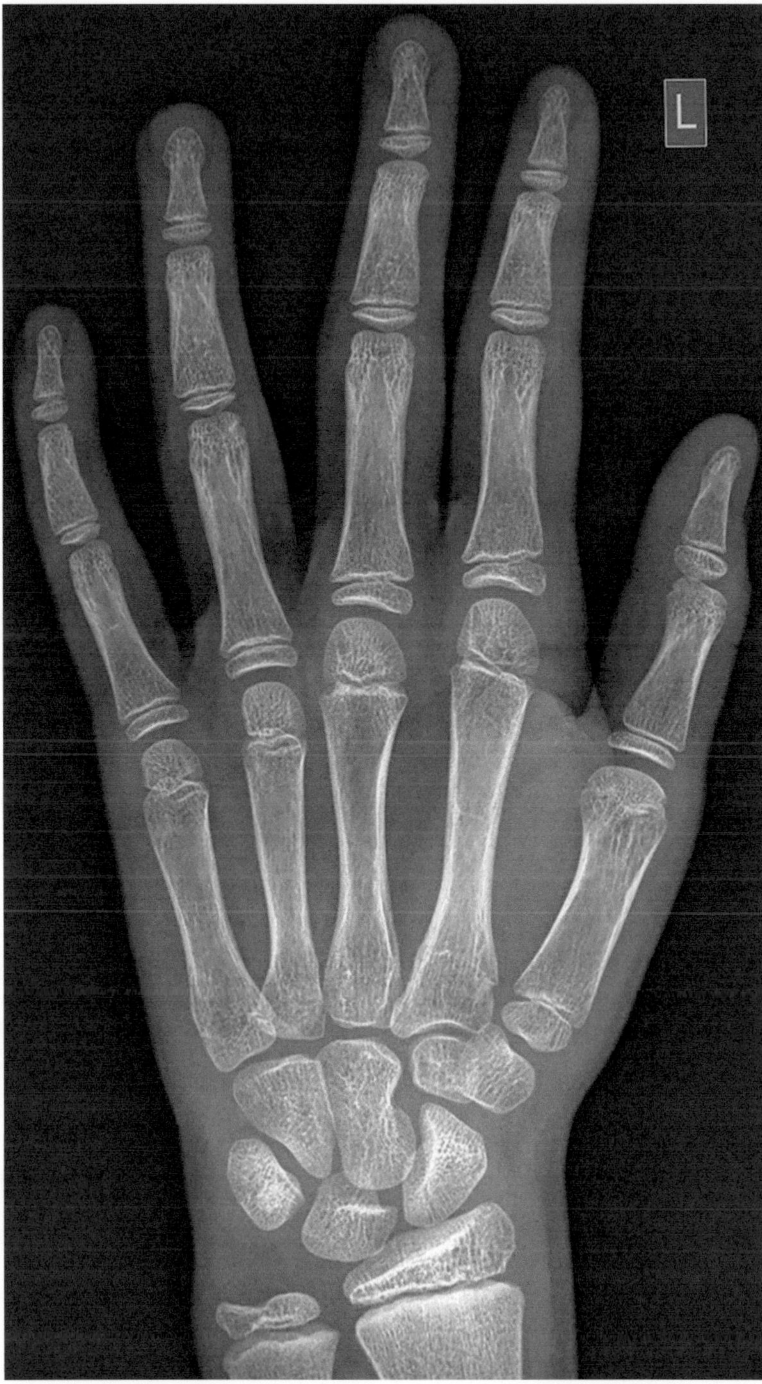

Image 15

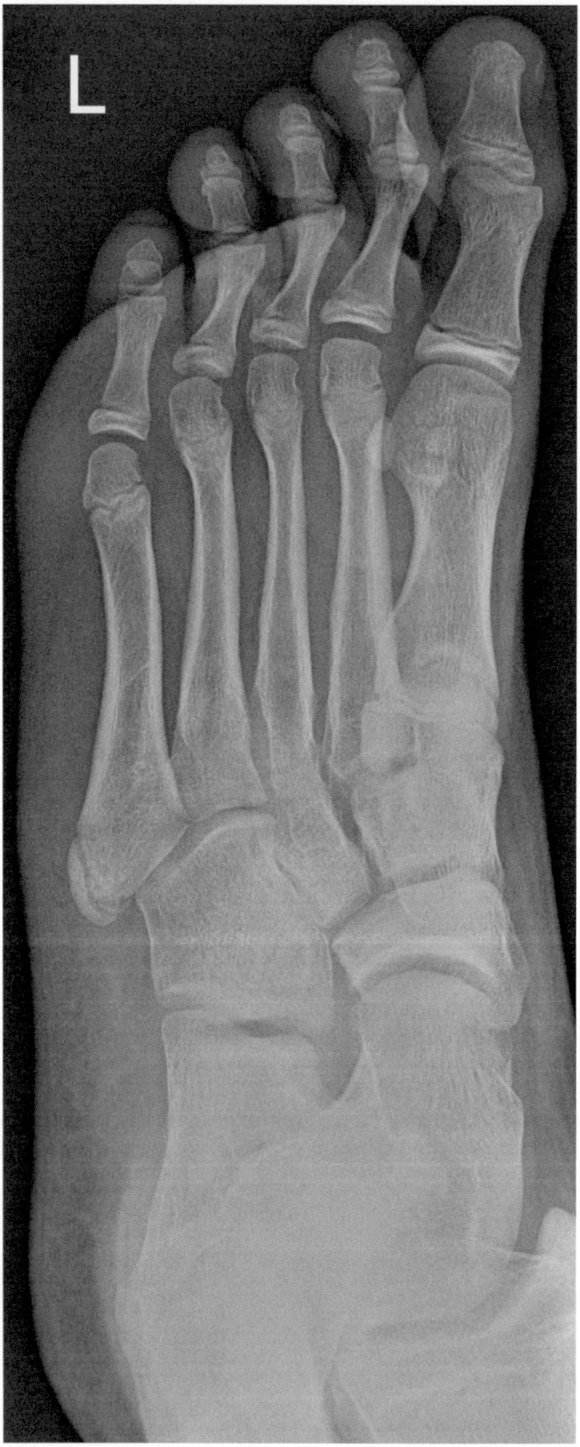

Image 16

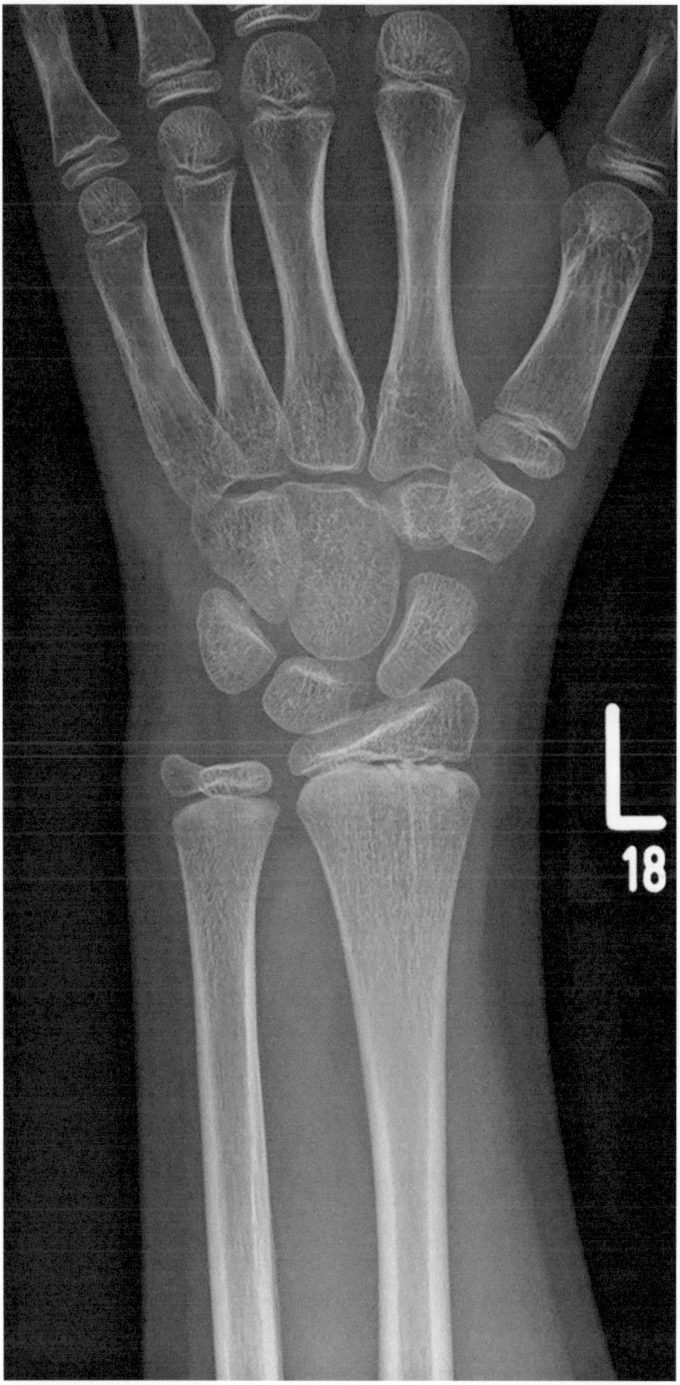

Image 17

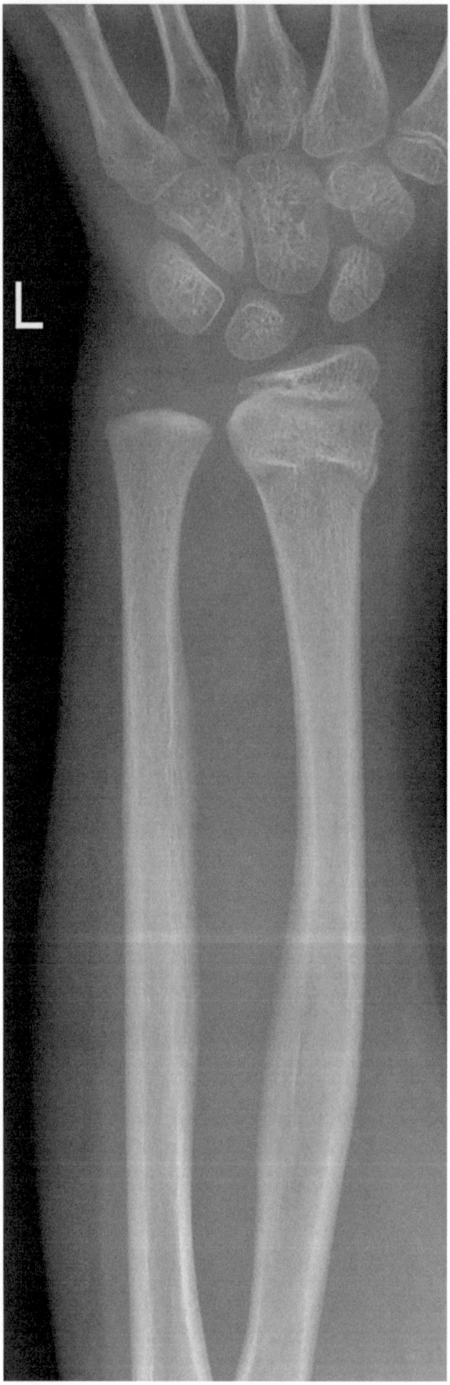

Image 18

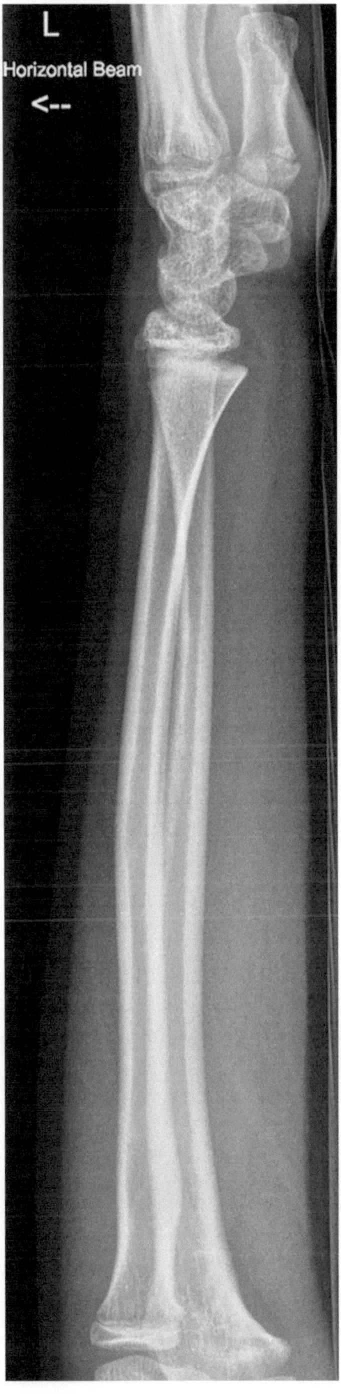

Image 19

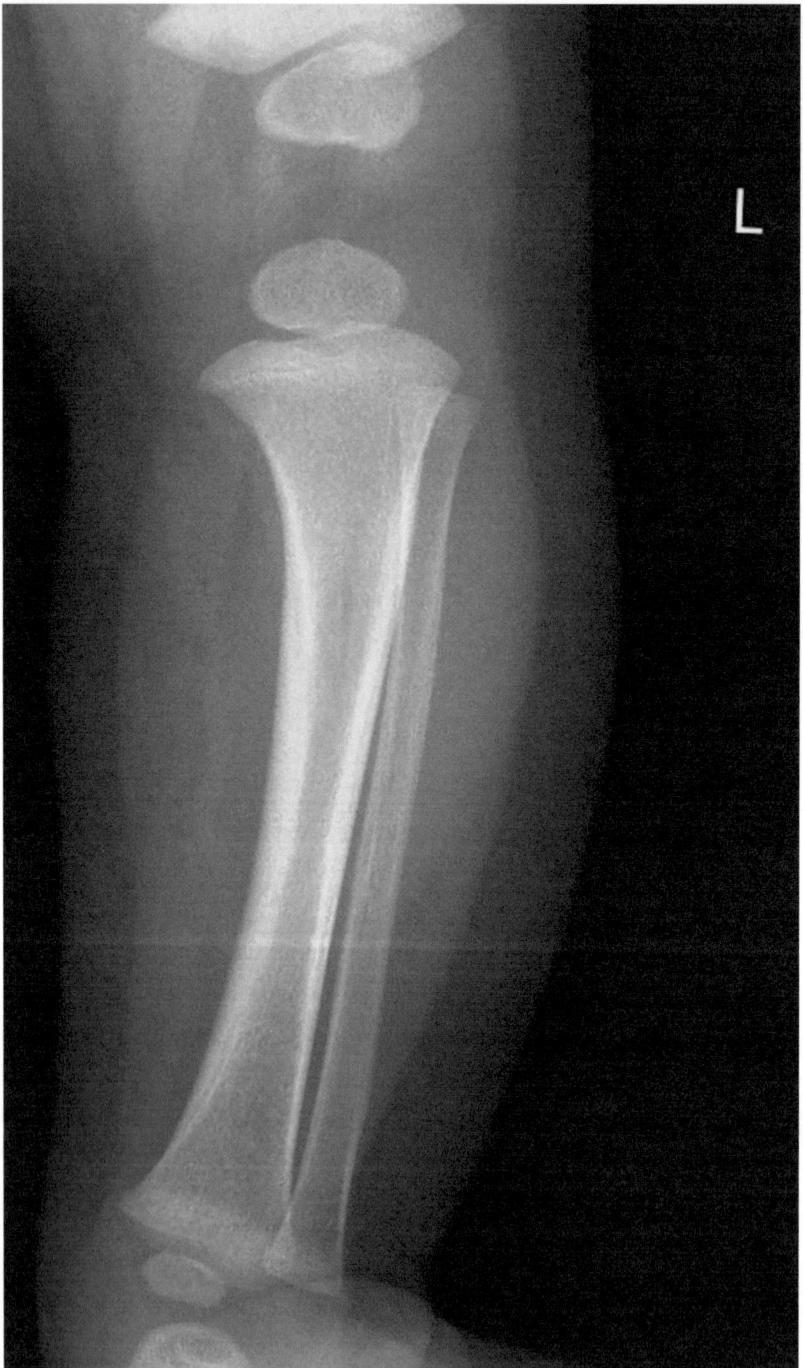

Image 20

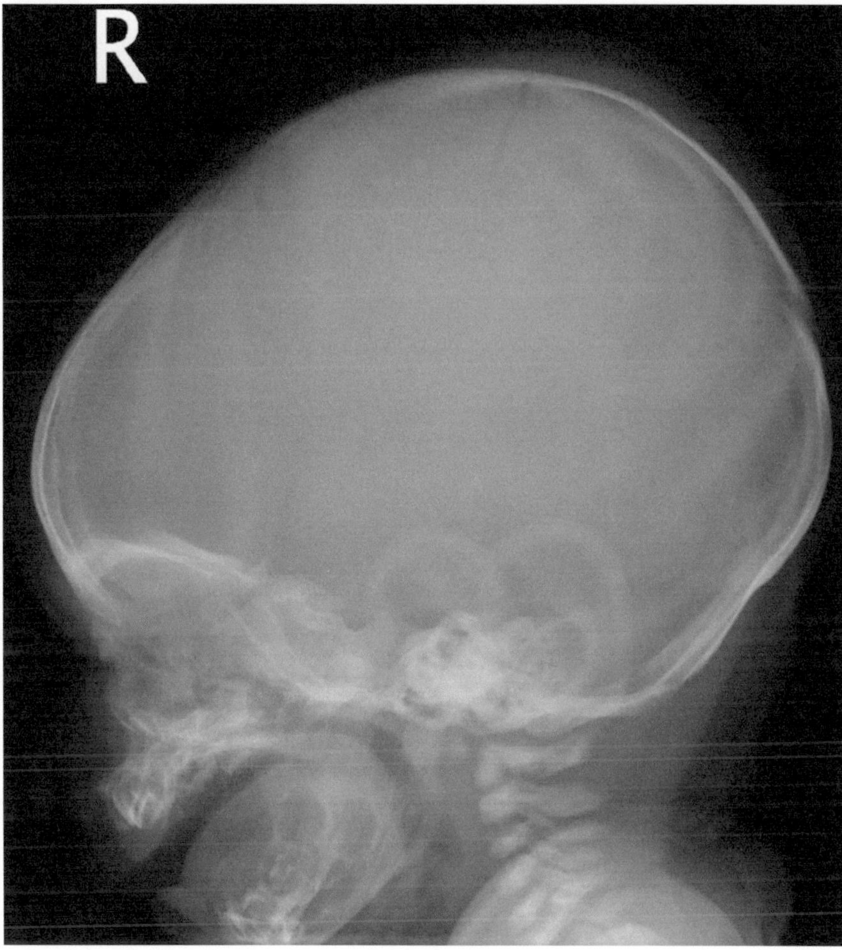

Image 21

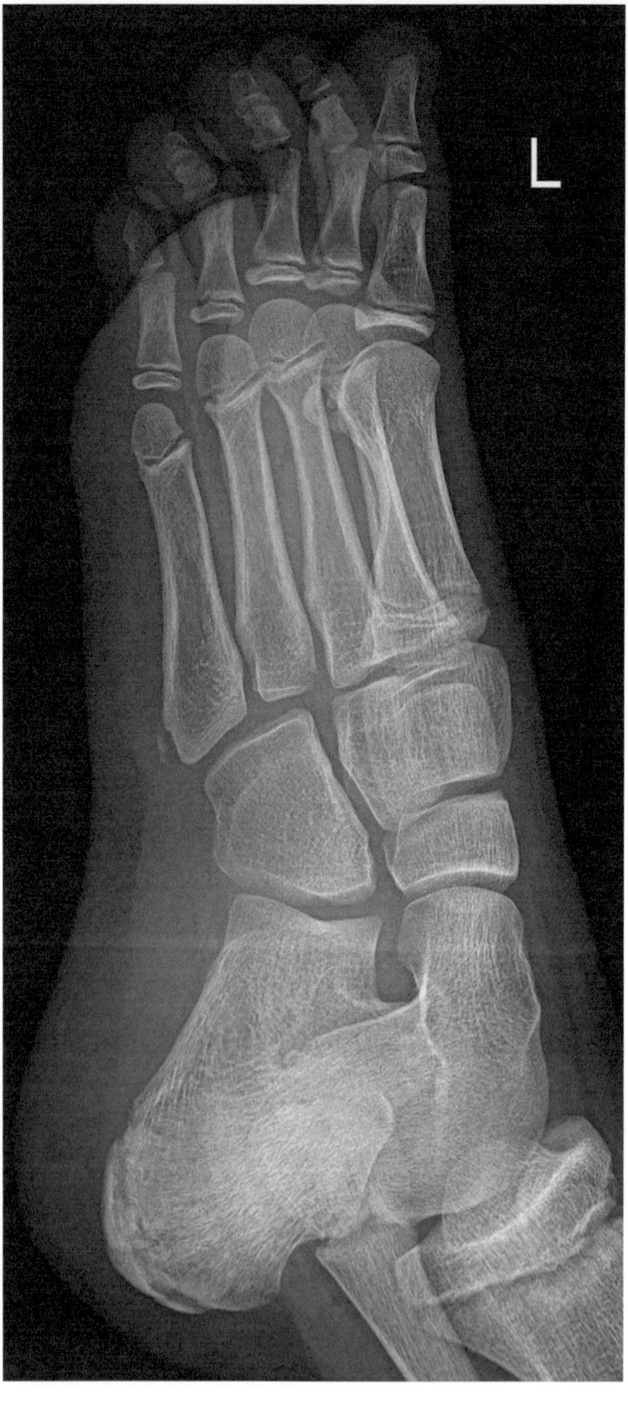

Image 22

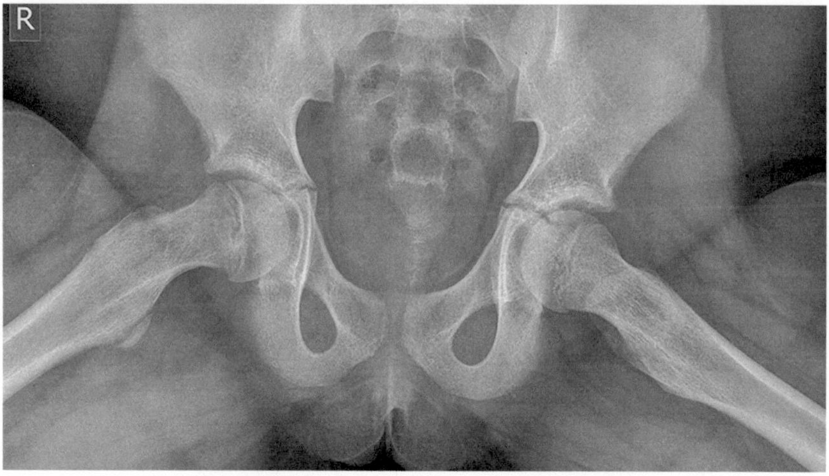

Image 23

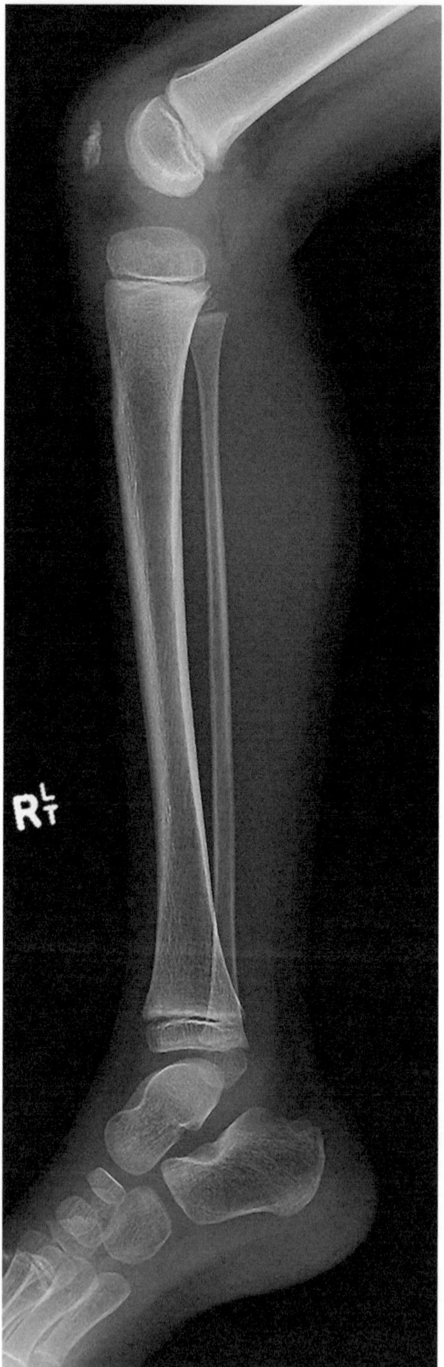

Image 24

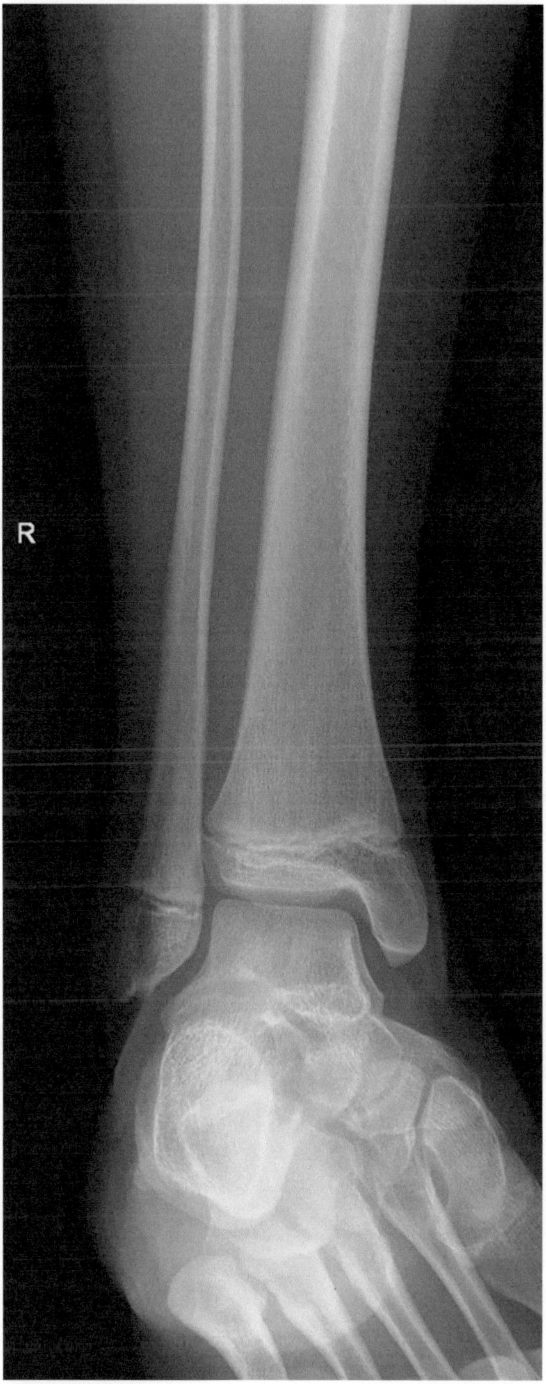

Image 25

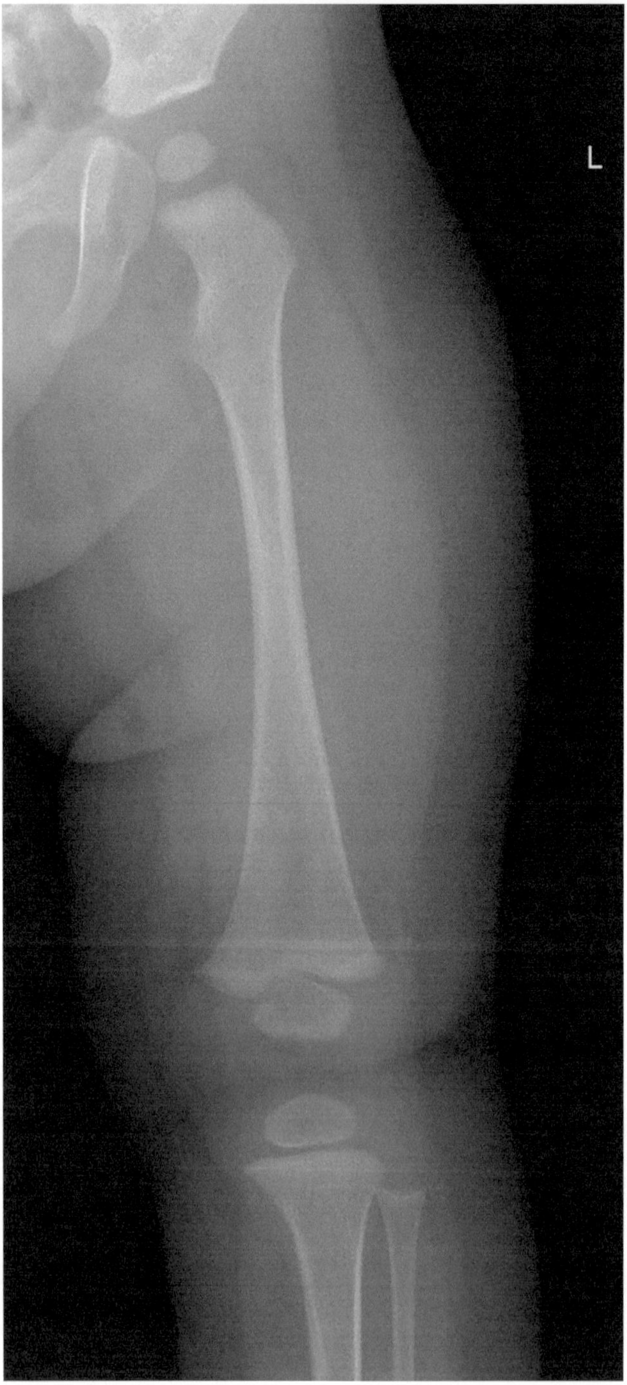

Image 26

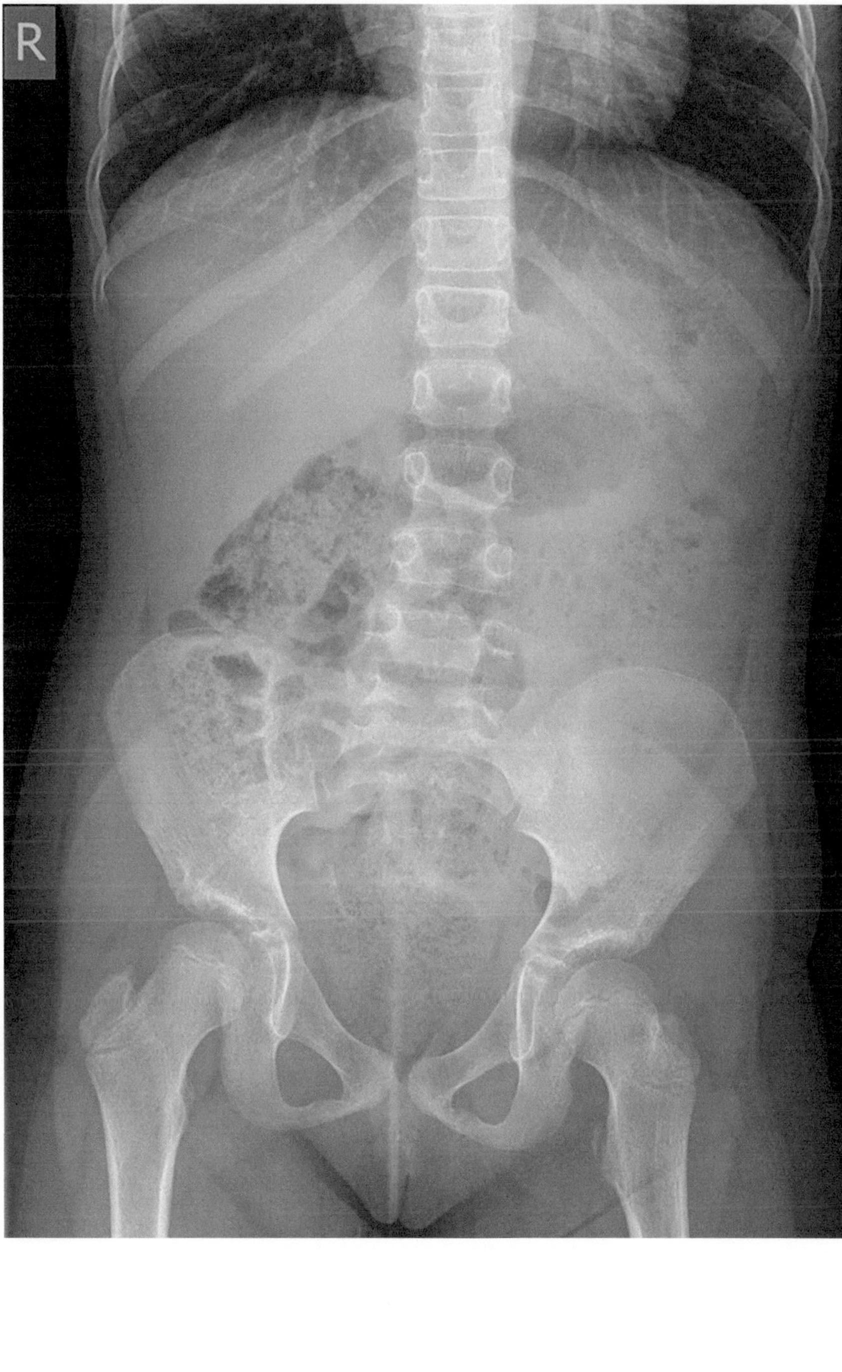

Image 27

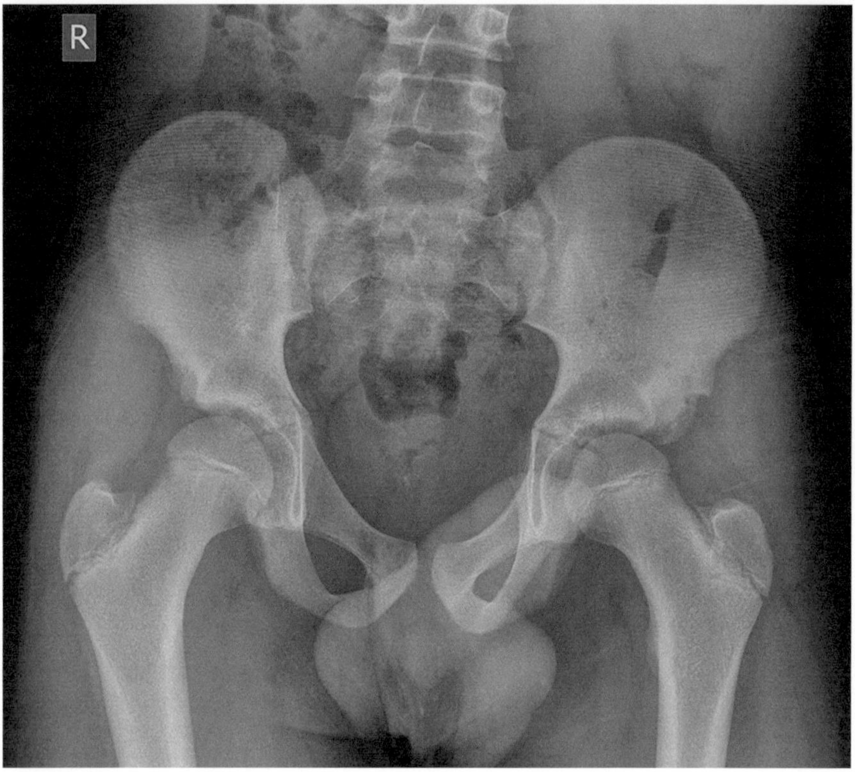

Image 28

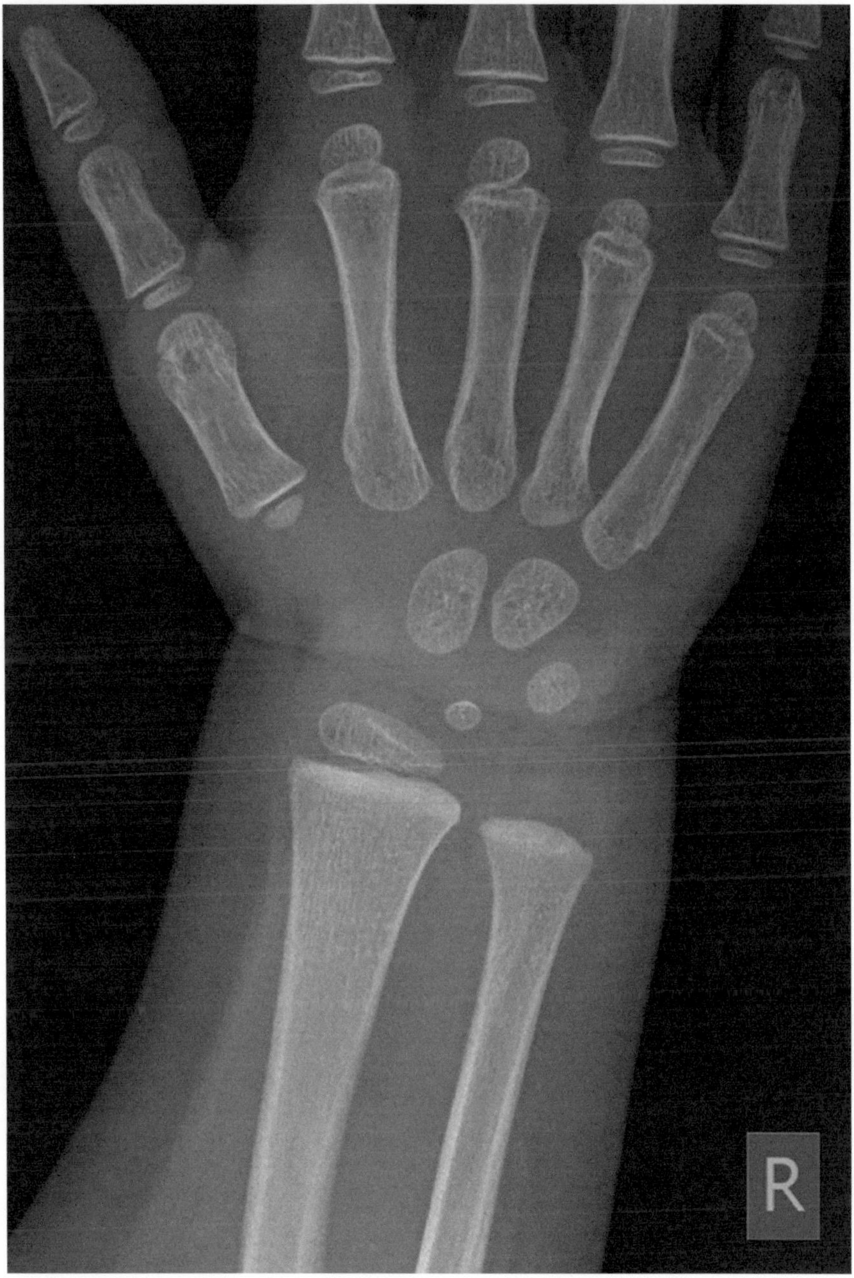

Image 29

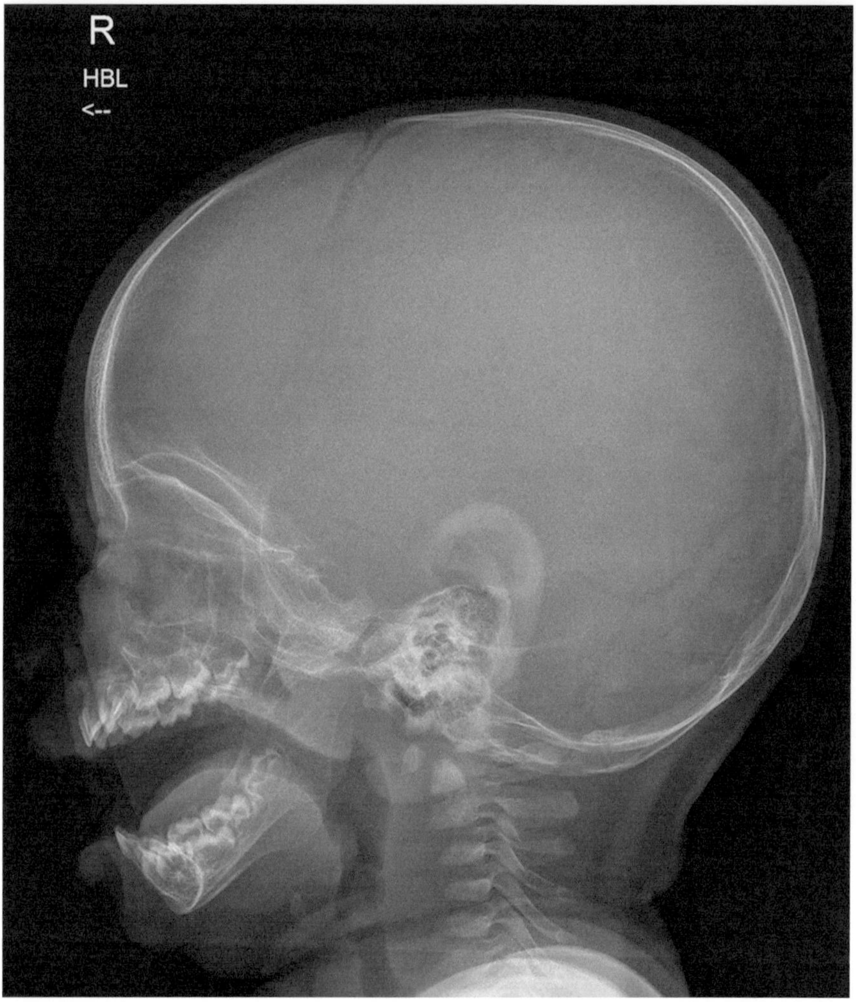

Image 30

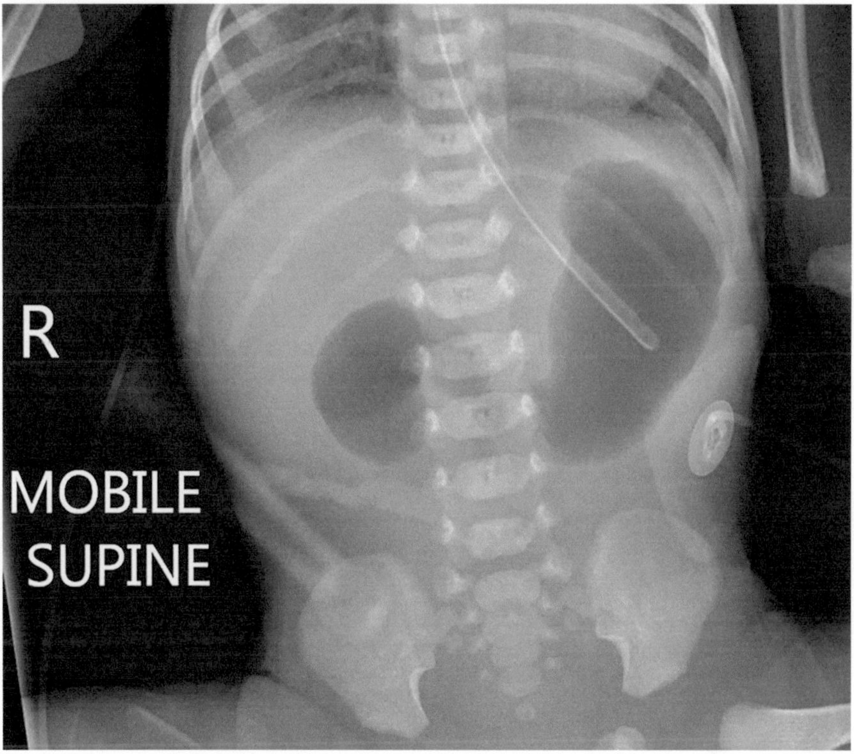

5.2 Answers

Image	Normal	Abnormal	Diagnosis/abnormality (only if abnormal)
1		✓	Buckle # L distal radius metaphysis
2	✓		
3	✓		
4		✓	Multiple acute and healing rib #s
5		✓	Fibrous cortical defect L medial distal femoral metaphysis
6	✓		
7	✓		
8		✓	# R little toe proximal phalanx
9	✓		
10	✓		
11		✓	# L supracondylar humerus
12		✓	# R talar neck
13	✓		
14	✓		
15		✓	# L fifth metatarsal base
16	✓		
17		✓	Transverse # L distal radial metaphysis
18		✓	SH1 # L distal radius
19	✓		
20		✓	# parietal bone
21	✓		
22		✓	R SUFE
23	✓		
24	✓		
25	✓		
26		✓	Multiple R distal ureteric calculi (Steinstrasse)
27		✓	Healing avulsion # L AIIS
28	✓		
29	✓		
30		✓	Double bubble sign

5.3 Explanations

1. **Buckle # L distal radius metaphysis**
   There is a buckle fracture of the dorsal cortex of the left distal radial metaphysis. There is no fracture line extending to the distal radial physis and so this is not a Salter-Harris injury. The distal ulna is intact, which is an important negative to note given that distal radius and ulnar fractures commonly occur together. See the explanation for Image 18 of Test 1.

2. *Normal physiological periosteal reaction*
   Normal physiological periosteal reaction ("of the newborn") is a common radiographic finding which can be seen in up to one-third of infants, usually between the ages of 1 and 4 months. The radiographic findings are typified by a 'benign' pattern of symmetrical periosteal reaction along the diaphyses which does *not* extend to the metaphyses. The long bones are involved, i.e. the femora, tibiae, and humerii, and less commonly, the radii and ulnae. This radiograph demonstrates the typical smooth, solid, and unilamellated periosteal reaction along the medial cortex of the right tibia which is a normal finding in this 3-month-old girl. See Image 2 of Test 3 for a further example of physiological periosteal reaction involving the tibia.
   Periosteal reaction can range from benign to aggressive:
   Solid/unilamellated < multilamellated/'onion skin' < spiculated/'hair-on-end'/'sunburst' < Codman's triangle.
   There is a differential diagnosis when periosteal reaction has been identified which depends on the patient age and the clinical context in which it is identified:
   - Prostaglandin E therapy: in infants who have a duct-dependent lesion, i.e. a congenital cardiac disorder or lesion which requires the ductus arteriosus (DA) to remain patent for survival, prostaglandin therapy is used to maintain DA patency, usually until definitive surgical correction. The periosteal reaction associated with prostaglandin E therapy may be diffuse. There is usually a history of extended prostaglandin use and admission to a neonatal intensive care unit (NICU)/special care baby unit (SCBU) to support this radiographic finding.
   - **TORCH** infections: these infections are acquired either transplacentally or at birth. The mnemonic stands for:
     - **T**oxoplasmosis.
     - **O**thers (human immunodeficiency virus [HIV], syphilis): A pathognomonic radiographic sign of congenital syphilis is the 'Wimberger sign' which refers to focal bilateral metaphyseal destruction of the medial aspect of the proximal tibiae. However, this must not be confused with the 'Wimberger *ring* sign' which refers to dense sclerosis/calcification around an epiphysis with relatively central radiolucency in the context of scurvy (hypovitaminosis C).
     - **R**ubella.
     - **C**ytomegalovirus (CMV).
     - **He**rpes simplex.

An important finding which may be seen in congenital rubella, syphilis, and CMV is irregularity, fraying, and longitudinally aligned linear bands of metaphyseal sclerosis termed ‘celery stalk metaphysis’.

- Suspected physical abuse (SPA)/inflicted injury.
- Caffey disease: A disorder characterised by periostitis and soft tissue inflammation which is usually self-limiting. It is also known as infantile cortical hyperostosis which helpfully describes the pathology and what is visualised radiographically. Infants can present within the first few months of life with systemic features such as fever, irritability, erythema, and tender soft tissue swelling. The flat bones are typically affected with the mandible constituting the majority of cases (75–80%). When long bones are involved, the ulnae are most commonly affected. The radiographic findings are typified by dense subperiosteal new bone formation/subperiosteal cortical hyperostosis, sclerosis, and associated soft tissue swelling. If it is not self-limiting, the long-term sequelae include remodelling, asymmetry, or synostosis of adjacent bones.
- Metastases.

4. **Multiple acute and healing rib #s**
This 5-month-old boy was presented to the Emergency Department (ED) with grunting after “falling off a couch onto a plug adaptor on a tiled floor”. He had bruising over his anterolateral ribs and flanks.

This radiograph demonstrates multiple bilateral healing rib fractures (of the left anterolateral first and third to seventh ribs and the right lateral third to sixth ribs) as evidenced by the florid callus formation. Additionally, there are several acute minimally displaced rib fractures (the posterior left third, fourth and seventh ribs). There may also be acute undisplaced fractures of the posterior left fifth and sixth ribs: these are difficult to assess on this image but were confirmed on the contemporaneous computed tomography (CT) thorax. Given the time constraints in the examination, it would be sufficient to write ‘multiple acute and healing rib #s’.

These fractures are better appreciated on the left and right lateral oblique projections below, which are taken from the subsequent skeletal survey:

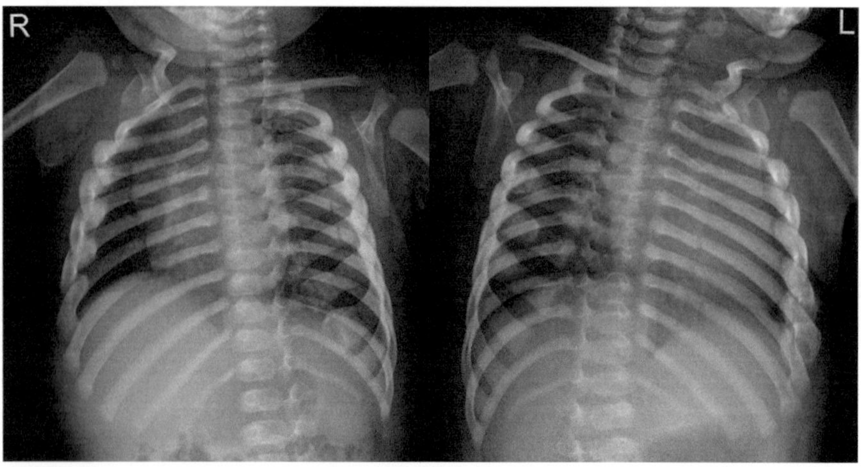

These projections image the ribs in profile which improves rib fracture detection, as well as having a higher sensitivity for identifying posterior rib fractures which are highly specific injuries for abuse.

SPA is investigated by a *two-part* radiographic examination: an initial skeletal survey and a follow-up skeletal survey performed 11–14 days after the initial examination. Acute rib fractures may be missed on (initial skeletal survey) chest radiographs because such fractures are often incomplete, minimally displaced, may be difficult to differentiate from bronchial and vascular markings, and may be obscured by overlapping structures. Rib fractures are more readily identified on follow-up radiographs due to their increased conspicuity as healing callus develops (as demonstrated in this radiograph). Mechanisms should be in place for those children who are not returned to the imaging department for their follow-up skeletal survey to complete their imaging examination.

Multiple rib fractures in different locations at different stages of healing imply several applications of force to the thorax at different times, i.e. repeated episodes of abuse, as in this case. Fractures of the first rib are highly suspicious as they require considerable application of force/energy to result in fracture, e.g. they may be seen following road traffic accidents (RTAs).

Physical abuse in infants and young children is insidious and may present at any time which is why radiologists must remain vigilant to any suspicious radiographic appearances. Acute and/or healing fractures may be detected on radiographs performed for another/unrelated indication, and as such, the radiologist may be the first person to raise the suspicion of abusive/inflicted injury. We emphasise that every rib (and indeed, every osseous structure) must be scrutinised on every paediatric chest radiograph, not only in the examination but also in clinical practice.

5. **Fibrous cortical defect L medial distal femoral metaphysis**
Fibrous cortical defects (FCDs) are common benign 'do not touch' lesions with a male predilection. These lucent lesions are confined to the cortex with no involvement of the underlying medullary cavity. They often have a thin rim of sclerosis with no associated periosteal reaction. They are typically oval with their long axis parallel to the long axis of the bone and are most commonly found in the metaphyses, often around the knee joint. Given their ubiquity and benignity, further imaging is not required (and discouraged). They tend to 'fill in' with time, i.e. sclerose/mineralise.

Tip for the viva:

- Non-ossifying fibromas (NOFs) are histologically identical to FCDs but by definition measure greater than 3 cm. FCDs measure less than 3 cm.

6. *Normal right wrist radiograph*
This radiograph is normal. The rectangular appearance at the distal radial and ulnar metaphyses represents the subperiosteal bone collar which is commonly visualised at the ends of long bones. This is a normal finding and does *not* represent a buckle fracture. See Image 8 of Test 1 and Image 2 of Test 2 for further examples of subperiosteal bone collars of the distal radius and ulna, and distal tibia and fibula, respectively.

7. *Normal right elbow radiograph*
The fragmented appearances of the trochlear ossification centre are normal and can continue to appear fragmented until fully ossified. The appearances of the capitellum, radial head and internal and external epicondyle ossification centres are also normal and the ossification centres are in their expected anatomic locations. The olecranon ossification is not well visualised on the anteroposterior (AP) projection but is better visualised on the lateral projection. The surrounding fat-muscle planes are preserved indicating that there is no soft tissue swelling to suggest an acute avulsion injury. The cortical irregularity and lucency of the right radial tuberosity is normal and represents the insertion site of the right biceps brachii tendon.

You must be familiar with the appearances of the elbow secondary ossification centres at different ages including when they first appear on radiographs, i.e. start to ossify. Familiarity with these appearances will help you differentiate between age-appropriate normal/developmental appearances and acute bony/avulsion injuries. This is particularly important because an avulsed ossification centre may mimic another normal ossification centre if significantly displaced. The order and age of appearance of the normal elbow secondary ossification centres is predictable and can be best remembered using the mnemonic **CRITOE** (or **CRITOL**):

- **C**apitellum: 1–2 years.
- **R**adial head: 2–4 years.
- **I**nternal (or medial) epicondyle: 4–6 years.
- **T**rochlea: 8–11 years.
- **O**lecranon: 9–11 years.
- **E**xternal (or **L**ateral) epicondyle: 10–11 years.

Any ossification centre which appears out of order or is apparently missing should be viewed with suspicion and the radiographs should be scrutinised for injury. Importantly, the age and order at which these ossification centres completely ossify, i.e. fuse to the distal humerus is independent of the age at which they begin to ossify. Note that the elbow ossification centres generally appear earlier in girls than in boys. See the references for relevant illustrations which reinforce the above information.

8. **# R little toe proximal phalanx**
Careful inspection reveals the minimally displaced oblique fracture of the right little toe proximal phalanx.

11. **# L supracondylar humerus**
    See the explanations for Images 11 and 15 of Test 1.

12. **# R talar neck**
    Talar neck fractures are the most common fractures of the talus. They result from high-energy injuries, usually due to axial loading to the hindfoot in forced dorsiflexion. Common complications include avascular necrosis (AVN), post-traumatic subtalar arthritis and varus malunion.

15. **# L fifth metatarsal base**
    There is an acute transversely oriented fracture fragment through the base of the left fifth metatarsal with adjacent minor soft tissue swelling. The normal base of fifth metatarsal apophysis is aligned to the vertical (longitudinal) plane of the metatarsals and is not fractured. We have included this image to help you differentiate the appearance of the normal left fifth metatarsal apophysis from an acute fracture. The acute fracture fragment is better visualised and distinguished from the adjacent normal apophysis in the magnified image below:

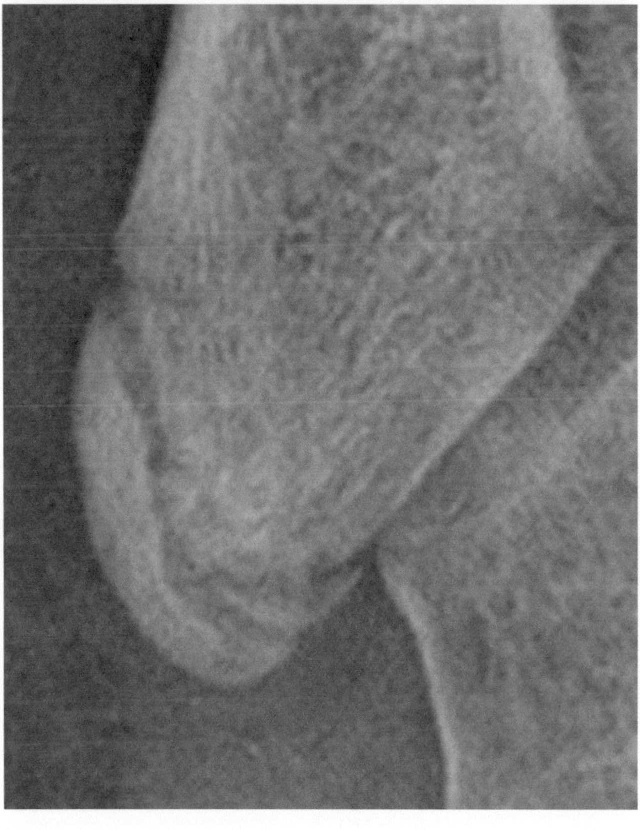

See the explanation for Image 7 of Test 1 for a further example of an acute base of fifth metatarsal fracture.

16. *Normal left wrist radiograph*
    The tiny focus of ossification projected over the joint space between the left triquetrum and the left hamate represents the ossification centre for the left pisiform bone.

17. **Transverse # L distal radial metaphysis**
    There is a complete transverse fracture of the left distal radial metaphysis. There is no concomitant fracture of the left distal ulna.

18. **Salter-Harris 1 # L distal radius**
    Note the widening of the left distal radial physis with associated dorsal slip of the epiphysis about the physis consistent with a Salter-Harris 1 injury. These fractures must not be overlooked. Often the key findings in these injuries are disproportionate overlying soft tissue swelling and a widened physis. See the explanation for Image 30 of Test 1.

20. **# parietal bone**
    There is a lucent line in the parietal bone with overlying soft tissue swelling/scalp haematoma consistent with an acute fracture. Whilst the sagittal suture is not visualised on this lateral image, the coronal (which can be visualised arising from the anterior fontanelle) and lambdoid sutures (which can be visualised arising from the posterior fontanelle) can be distinguished from the acute fracture. On the basis of this image, it cannot be determined if the left or right parietal bone is fractured.

    Given its superior diagnostic accuracy, head CT with multiplanar reconstructions (MPR) and volume rendered (VR) imaging supersedes the role of radiographs in the diagnosis of skull fracture (any indication). However, you may still be presented with a skull fracture in any component of the examination. As such, it is important that you are able to differentiate normal suture lines from acute fractures.

    Tip for the viva:
    - The simple linear parietal skull fracture is the commonest skull fracture in both accidental and inflicted injury. It is the presenting clinical context and history (or lack thereof) which discriminates between the two.

22. **R slipped upper femoral epiphysis**
    See the explanation for Image 12 of Test 2.

26. **Multiple R distal ureteric calculi (Steinstrasse)**
    The abnormality in this radiograph is subtle but again reinforces that you must adopt a systematic approach to radiographic interpretation. Once you have identified the asymmetry between both sides of the pelvis, it cannot be ignored. The abnormality is better appreciated in the magnified image below:

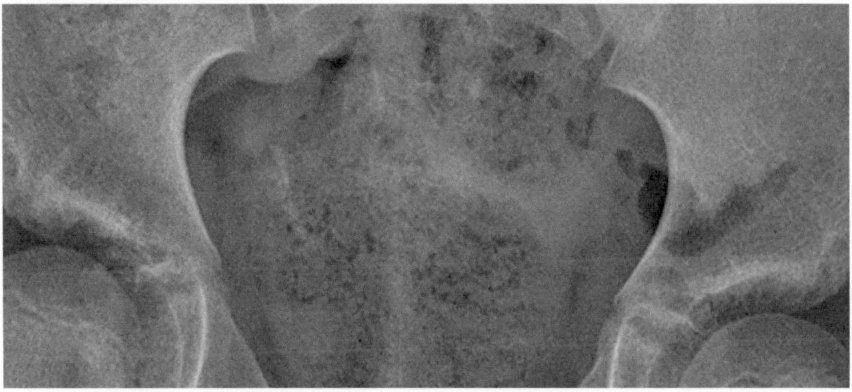

The term 'Steinstrasse', from the German meaning 'stone street', describes a column of impacted calculi in the ureter; however, the term is generally used in the context of distal ureteric obstruction as a complication of extracorporeal shock wave lithotripsy (ESWL). ESWL can be safely performed in children but post-procedure acute kidney injury may ensue.

27. **Healing avulsion # L anterior inferior iliac spine**
There is irregularity of the left anterior inferior iliac spine (AIIS) consistent with a healing injury. The AIIS is the insertion for the rectus femoris tendon. See the explanation for Image 13 of Test 4.

29. *Normal skull radiograph*
This radiograph is normal with normal appearances of both coronal and lambdoid sutures. There is no skull fracture or scalp swelling. Compare this normal image with the radiograph from Image 20 of this test which demonstrates an acute parietal bone fracture.

30. **Double bubble sign**
This radiograph shows the classic 'double bubble sign' of duodenal atresia. There is gas within the stomach and within the first part of the duodenum causing distension. There is an absence of distal gas indicating a complete atresia, i.e. a blind ending duodenum. This is thought to result from failure of recanalisation of the bowel lumen around the end of the first trimester. The bowel is a solid tube in fetal life before this time. Affected patients present with vomiting and abdominal distension secondary to the duodenal obstruction. The type of vomiting will depend upon the location of the atretic segment: if it is distal to the ampulla of Vater, it will be bilious; and non-bilious, if proximal to the ampulla.

Note that a complete or severely obstructing duodenal web (which often occurs in the second part of the duodenum) can also give a 'double bubble' appearance on radiography. However, if the web is partially or incompletely obstructing the duodenal lumen, there will usually be some distal gas. A 'triple bubble sign' may be seen with jejunal atresia which can occur anywhere from the ligament of Treitz, i.e. the duodenojejunal (DJ) flexure, to the jejunoileal junction. Additionally, there may be more than one atretic jejunal segment.

Duodenal atresia is associated with other conditions:

- **VACTERL** syndrome: comprises the following constellation of congenital abnormalities:
  - **V**ertebral anomalies: these include hemivertebrae, butterfly vertebrae, or block vertebrae; caudal regression; and/or spina bifida.
  - **A**norectal anomalies; **A**nal atresia; other gut **A**tresias:

    Jejunal atresia: described above.

    Ileal atresia.

    Anal atresia: this can range from a membranous separation to complete congenital absence. Following clinical evaluation by surgical colleagues, a lower GI contrast examination may be required to delineate the anatomy and assess for the presence of a fistula, e.g. recto-vesical or recto-vaginal.
  - **C**ardiac anomalies: clinical examination and echocardiography are indicated to exclude a structural defect.
  - **T**racheo-o**E**sophageal fistula (TEF in the USA; TOF in the UK) ± oesophageal atresia (OA): the history is typically that of antenatal polyhydramnios and failure to successfully pass a nasogastric tube (NGT) into the stomach at birth. Radiographs will show that the distal portion of the NGT coils in the proximal oesophageal pouch. The NGT is usually replaced with a Replogle tube (a double lumen tube which in contrast to an NGT has a number of side holes). The Replogle tube rests in the proximal oesophageal pouch to simultaneously irrigate and aspirate secretions/debris. There are five types of TOF with which you should be familiar. The most common type (type A, 85%) comprises proximal OA with a distal TOF. The presence of gas in the stomach and bowel on radiography indicates that a TOF must be present. If there was an isolated OA with no fistula, there would be no way for gas to enter the gastrointestinal tract and, therefore, this would not be seen radiographically.
  - **R**enal anomalies: these include the spectrum of:

    Cystic renal disease: autosomal recessive polycystic kidney disease (ARPKD); multicystic dysplastic kidney (MCDK)

    Pre-tumorous renal conditions: nephroblastomatosis

    Tumorous renal conditions: mesoblastic nephroma; multilocular cystic nephroma

    Obstructive renal disease: congenital pelviureteric junction obstruction (PUJO)

Positional abnormalities: crossed fused renal ectopia
Renal dysgenesis and agenesis

- **R**adial ray anomalies: these are characterised by unilateral or bilateral absence (aplasia/hypoplasia) of varying portions of the radius and thumb. Whilst these anomalies are rare, their presence necessitates exclusion of other associated anomalies.
- **L**imb anomalies: usually polydactyly.

- Down syndrome (Trisomy 21): approximately 30% of infants with duodenal atresia have Down syndrome; conversely approximately 3% of those with Down syndrome have duodenal atresia.
- Annular pancreas: this is a developmental/embryonic abnormality in which the pancreas may encase the duodenum and result in duodenal obstruction.

Tip for the viva:

- Note the appropriately positioned NGT tip projected over the stomach in this case. You may be presented with a radiograph in which a Replogle tube has already been placed so you should be familiar with its appearance as it is distinct from an NGT.
- Most paediatric surgical centres will have a pathway for evaluating infants with suspected VACTERL syndrome which you should discuss with your local paediatric radiologists and surgeons.

Further Reading

Image 2

Bell DJ et al (2017) Celery stalk metaphysis. https://radiopaedia.org/articles/celery-stalk-metaphysis. Accessed July 2023

Kwon DS, Spevak MR, Flecther K, Kleinman PK (2002) Physiologic subperiosteal new bone formation: prevalence, distribution and thickness in neonates and infants. AJR Am J Roentgenol 179(4):985–988

O'Shea P et al (2022) Wimberger sign. https://radiopaedia.org/articles/wimberger-sign-1. Accessed July 2023

Qureshi PAAA et al (2020) Wimberger ring sign. https://radiopaedia.org/articles/wimberger-ring-sign-1. Accessed July 2023

University of Washington (2018) Periosteal reaction. https://rad.washington.edu/about-us/academic-sections/musculoskeletal-radiology/teaching-materials/online-musculoskeletal-radiology-book/periosteal-reaction/. Accessed July 2023

van der Woude JH, Smithuis R (2010) Bone tumor—systemic approach and differential diagnosis. http://www.radiologyassistant.nl/en/p494e15cbf0d8d/bone-tumor-systematic-approach-and-differential-diagnosis.html#i4b331f308764e. Accessed July 2023

Image 5

Blaz M, Palczewski P, Swiatkowski J, Golebiowski M (2011) Cortical fibrous defects and nonossifying fibromas in children and young adults: the analysis of radiological features in 28 cases and a review of literature. Pol J Radiol 76(4):32–39

Foo M et al (2023) Fibrous cortical defect. https://radiopaedia.org/articles/fibrous-cortical-defect. Accessed July 2023

Hacking C et al (2023) Non-ossifying fibroma. https://radiopaedia.org/articles/non-ossifying-fibroma-1. Accessed July 2023

Image 7

Lustosa L et al (2023) Ossification centres of the elbow. https://radiopaedia.org/articles/ossification-centres-of-the-elbow. Accessed July 2023

Lustosa L et al (2023) Elbow ossification mnemonic. https://radiopaedia.org/articles/elbow-ossification-mnemonic. Accessed July 2023

Patel B, Reed M, Patel S et al (2009) Gender-specific pattern differences of the ossification centers in the pediatric elbow. Pediatr Radiol 39:226–231

Image 12

Weatherford B (2023) Talar neck fractures. https://www.orthobullets.com/trauma/1048/talar-neck-fractures. Accessed Sept 2023

Image 26

Akin Y, Yucel S (2014) Long-term effects of pediatric extracorporeal shockwave lithotripsy on renal function. Res Rep Urol 28(6):21–25

Knipe H et al (2023) Steinstrasse. https://radiopaedia.org/articles/steinstrasse. Accessed July 2023

Image 29

Marti B, Sirinelli D, Maurin L, Carpentier E (2013) Wormian bones in a general paediatric population. Diagn Interv Imaging 94(4):428–432

Yap J et al (2023) Wormian bones (mnemonic). https://radiopaedia.org/articles/wormian-bones-mnemonic. Accessed July 2023

Image 30

Bickle I et al (2023) Congenital tracheo-oesophageal fistula. https://radiopaedia.org/articles/congenital-tracheo-oesophageal-fistula. Accessed July 2023

El-Feky M et al (2023) Double bubble sign (duodenum). https://radiopaedia.org/articles/double-bubble-sign-duodenum. Accessed July 2023

Jones J et al (2023) Anal atresia. https://radiopaedia.org/articles/anal-atresia. Accessed July 2023

Khalid S, Faizan M, Alam MM et al (2013) Congenital longitudinal radial deficiency in infants: spectrum of isolated cases to VACTERL syndrome. J Clin Neonatol 2(4):193–195

Sharma R et al (2023) Triple bubble sign. https://radiopaedia.org/articles/triple-bubble-sign. Accessed July 2023

Vadera S et al (2023) Annular pancreas. https://radiopaedia.org/articles/annular-pancreas. Accessed July 2023

Yap J et al (2022) VACTERL association. https://radiopaedia.org/articles/vacterl-association-1. Accessed July 2023

Yap J et al (2023) Duodenal atresia. https://radiopaedia.org/articles/duodenal-atresia. Accessed July 2023

Test 6

6

M. Paddock et al., *Paediatric Radiology Rapid Reporting*,
https://doi.org/10.1007/978-3-031-48255-7_6

6.1 Images

Image 1

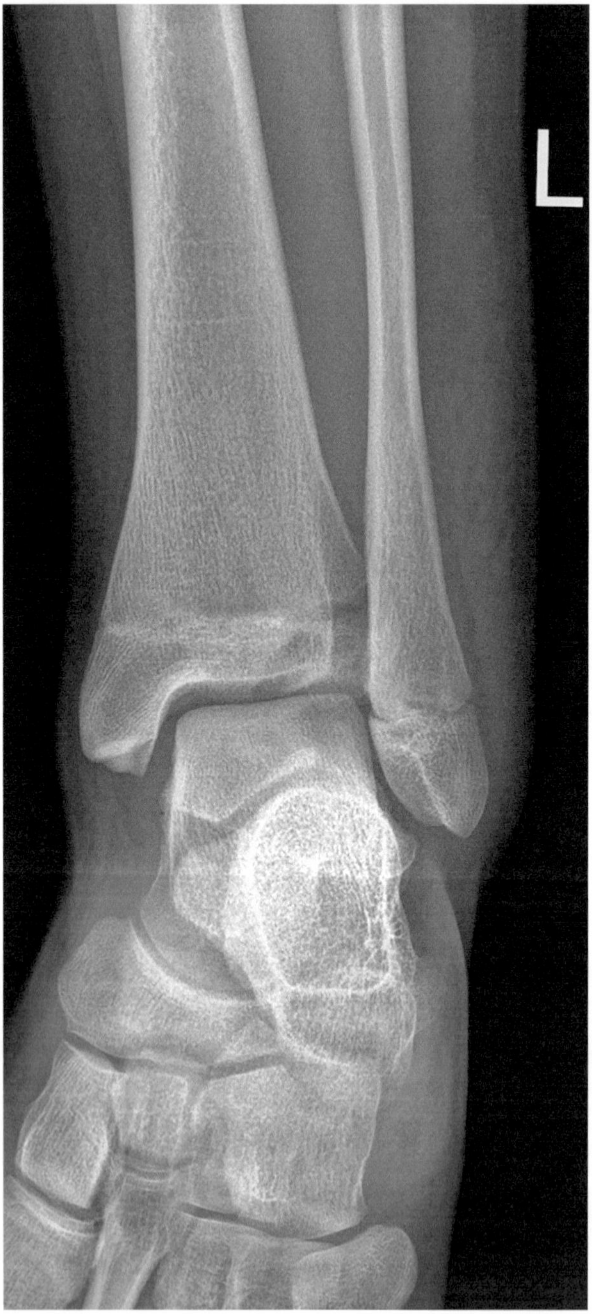

Image 2

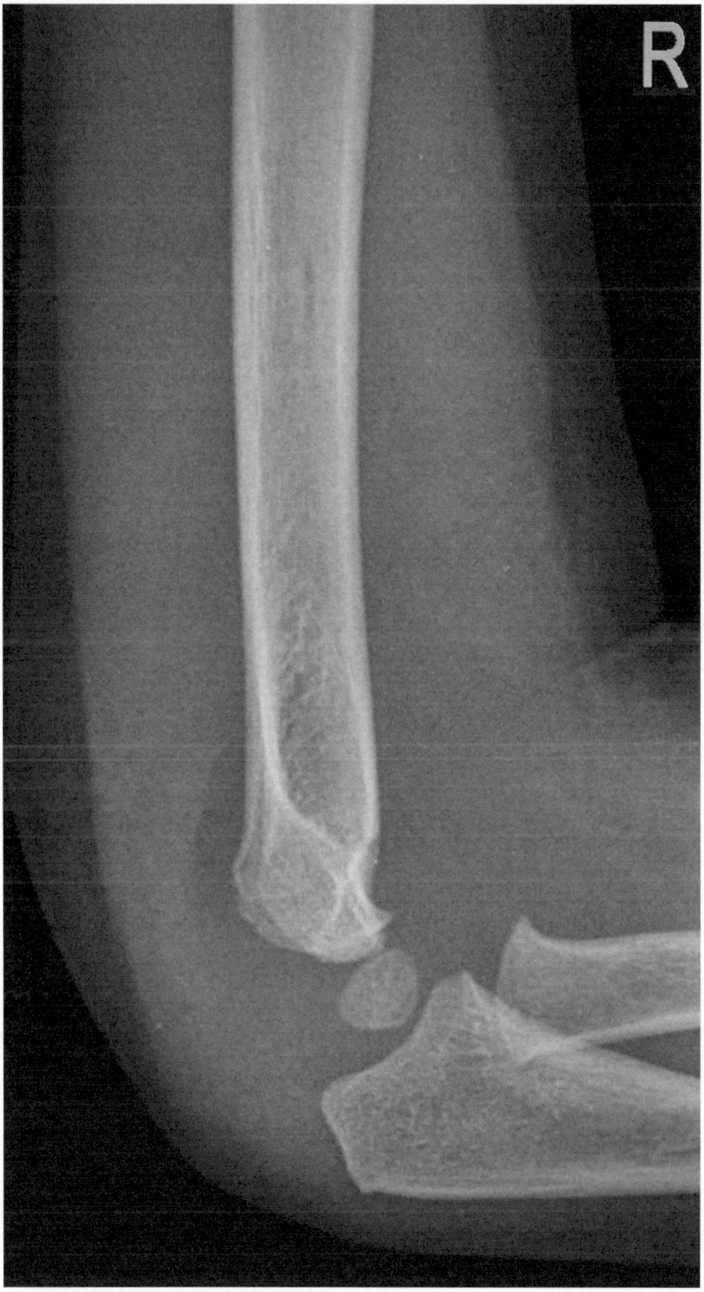

Image 3

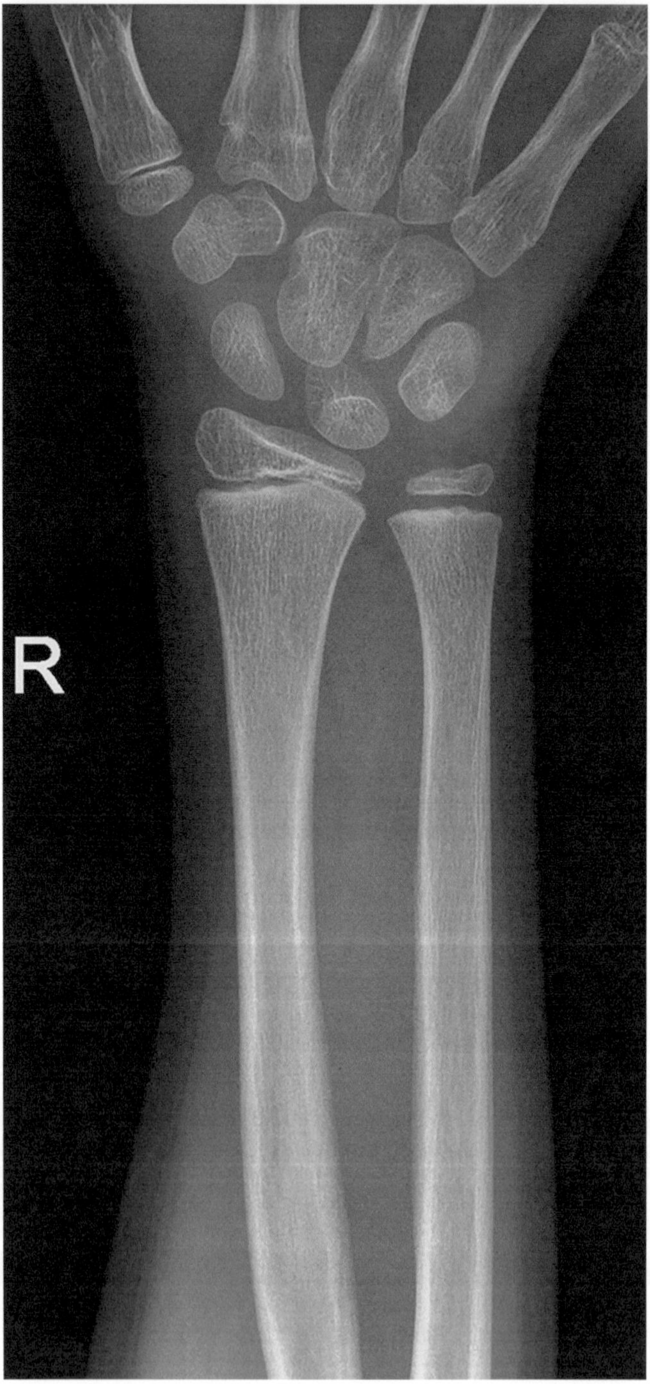

Image 4

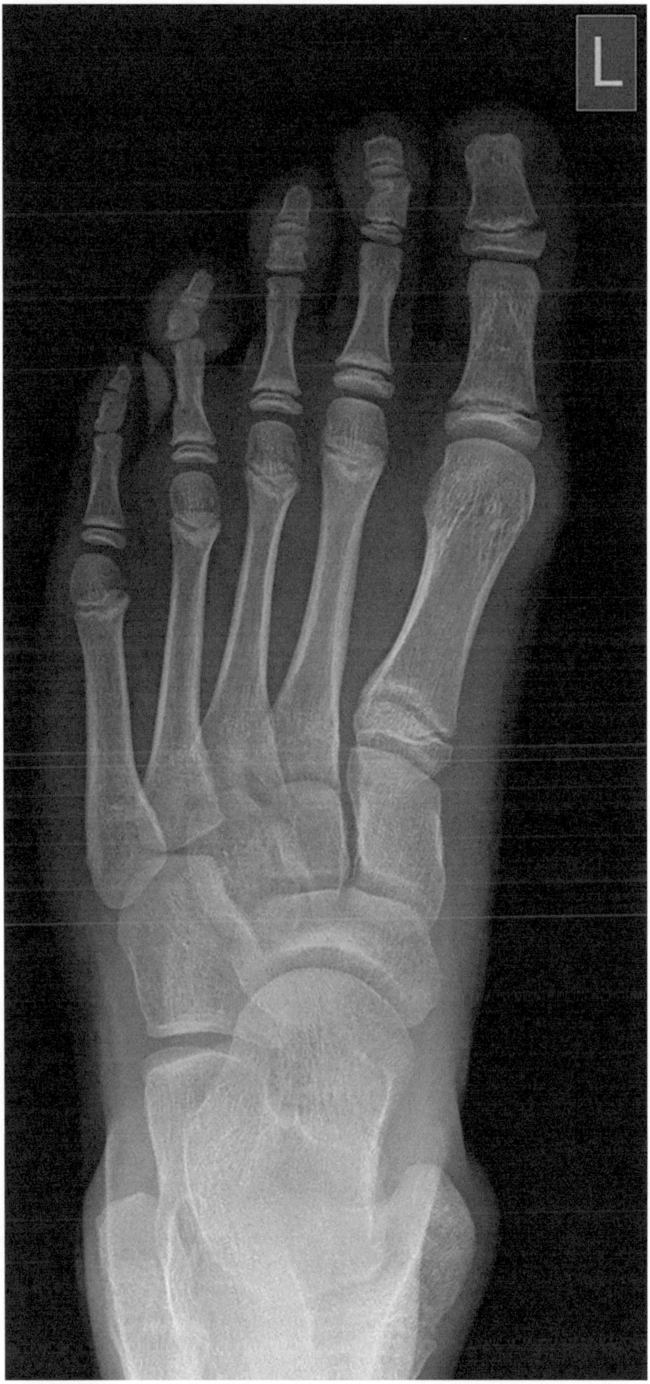

Image 5

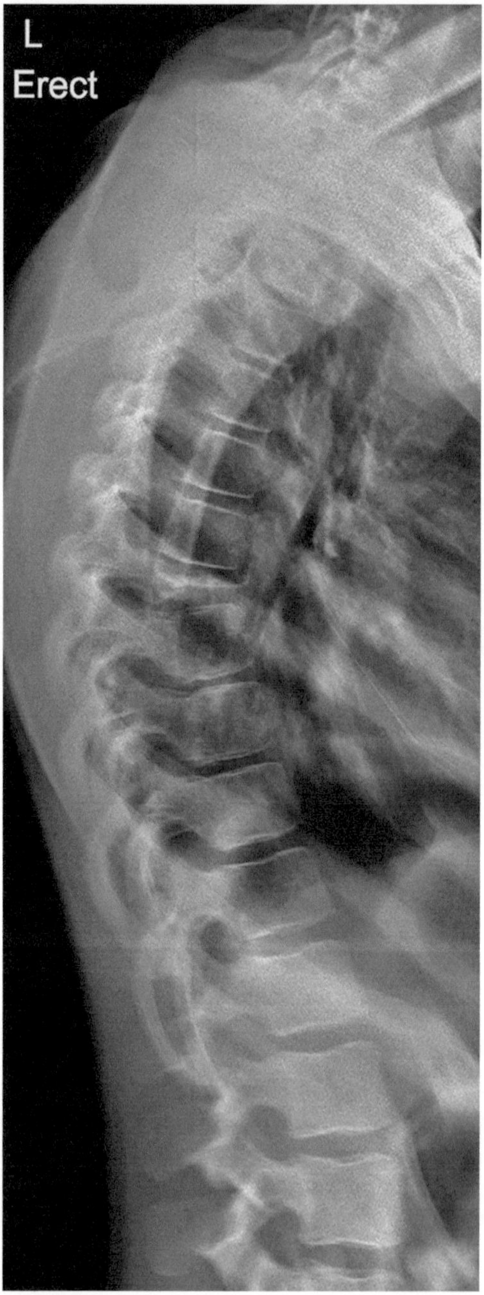

Image 6

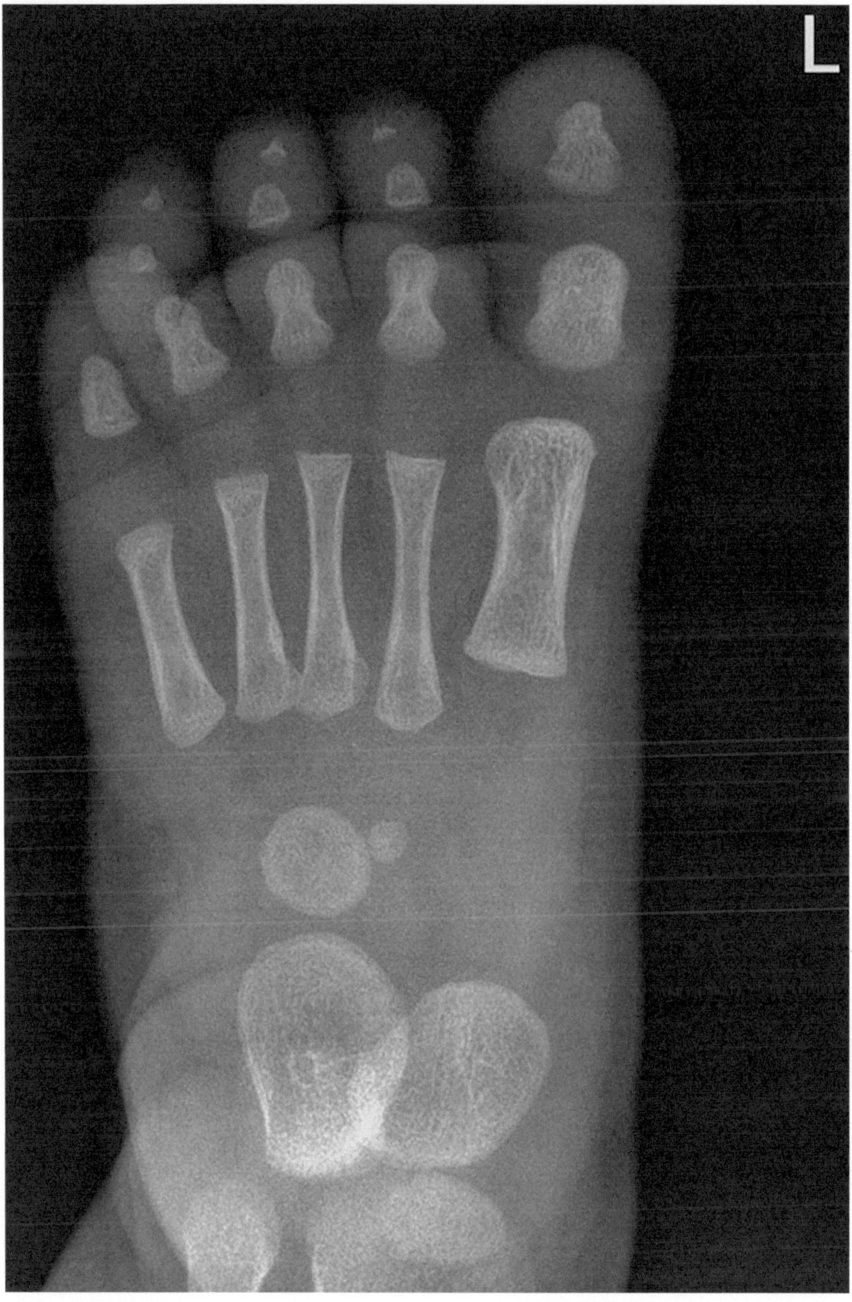

Image 7

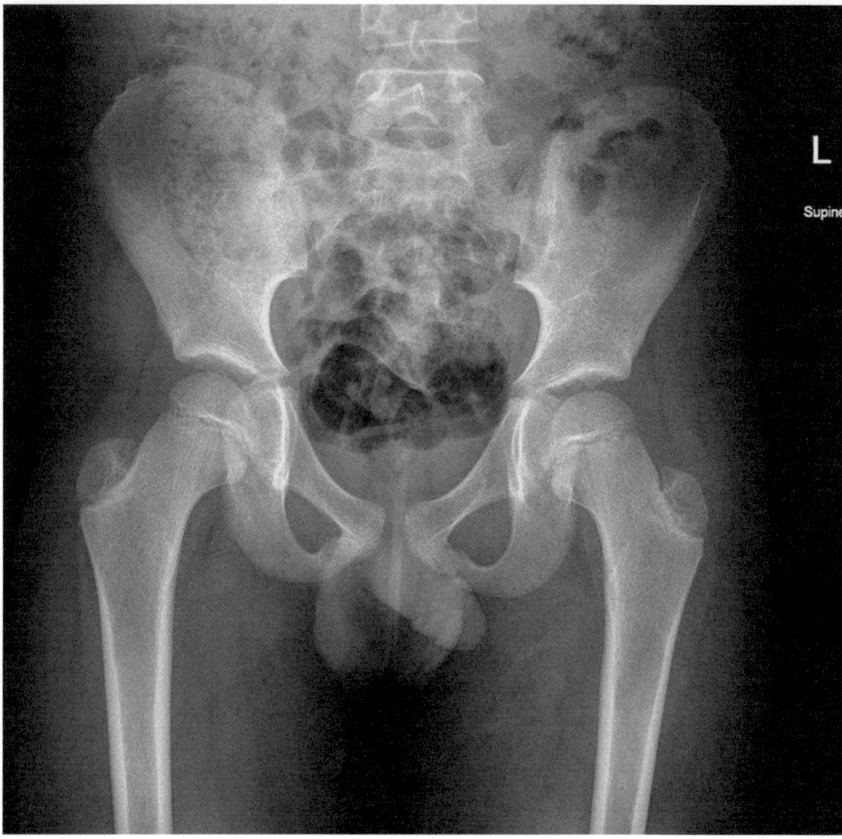

Image 8

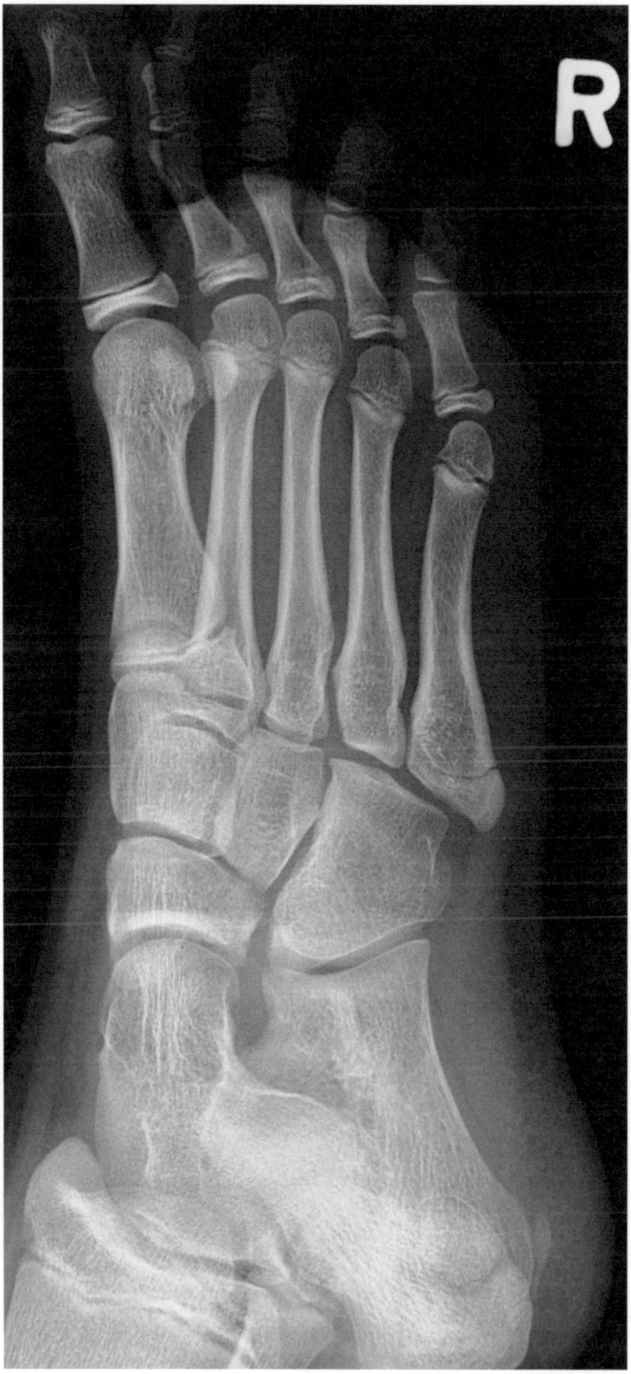

Image 9

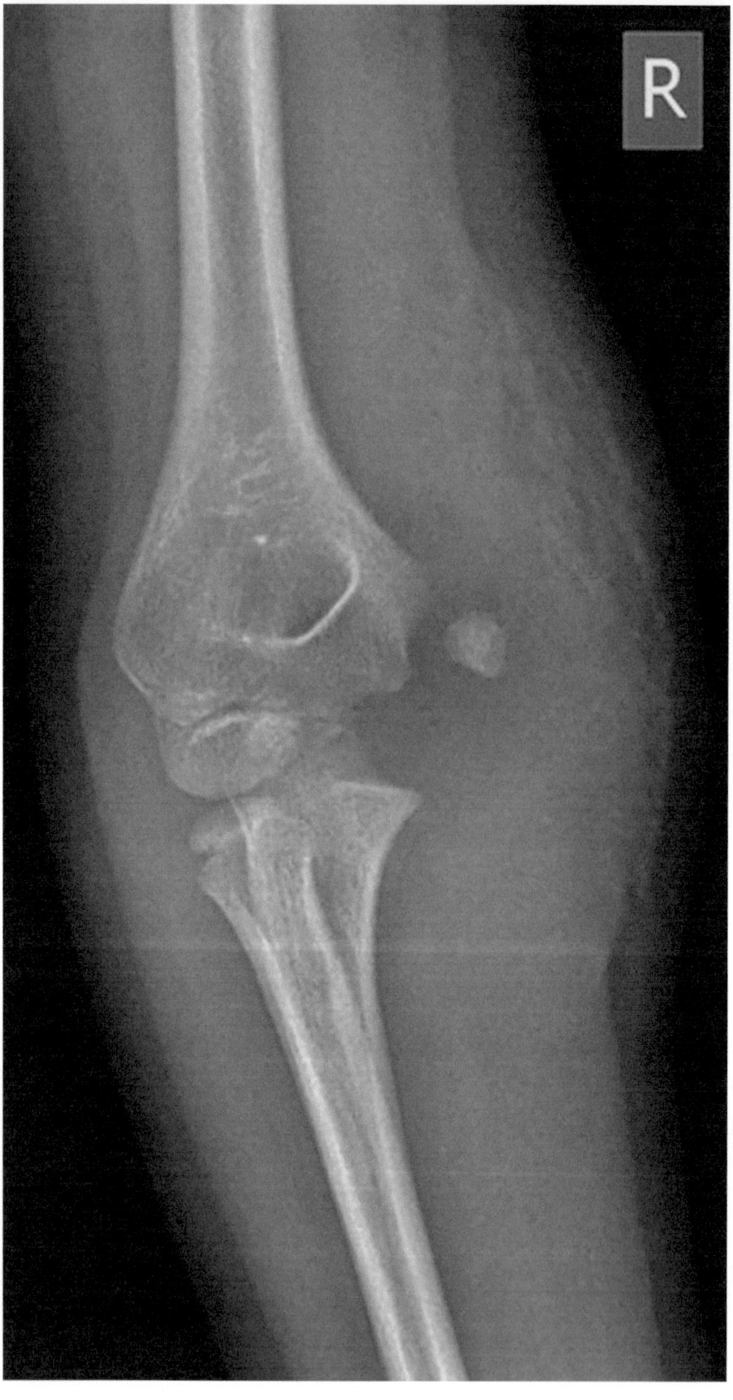

Image 10

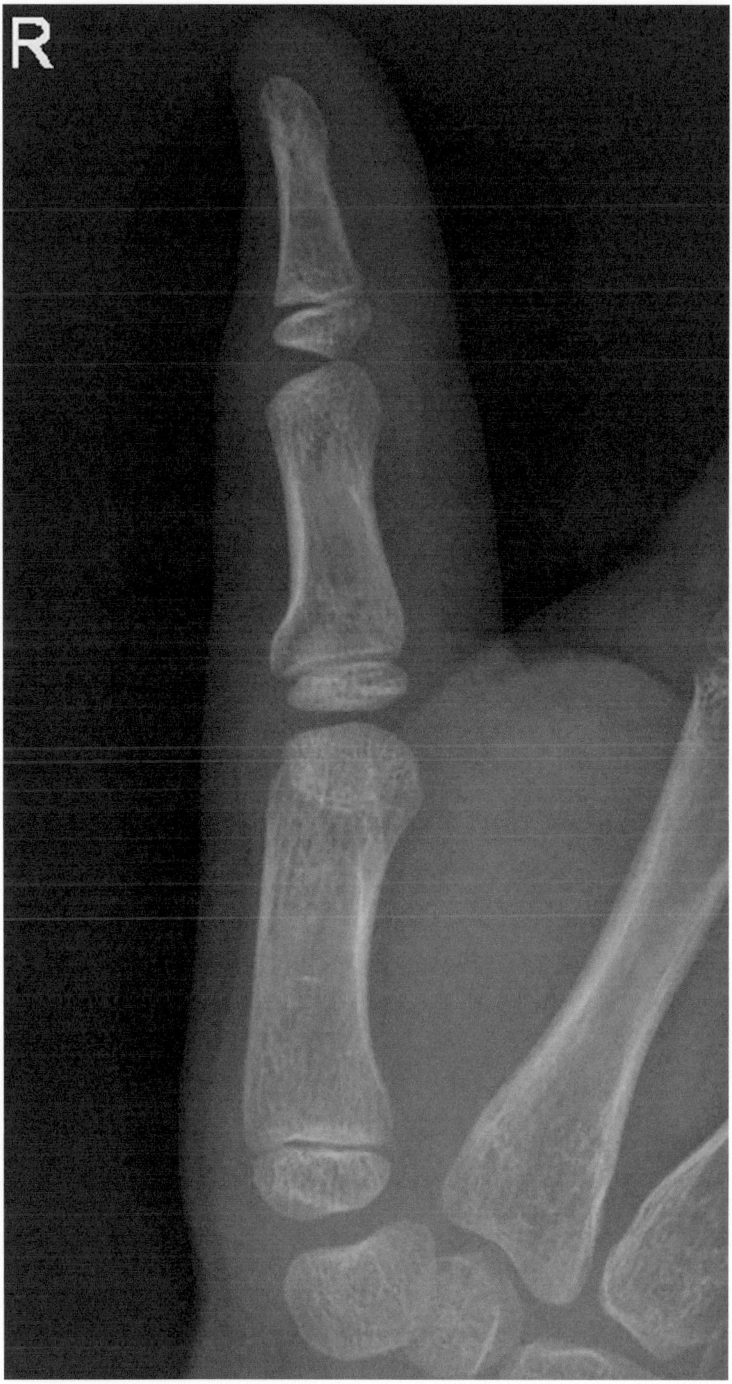

Image 11

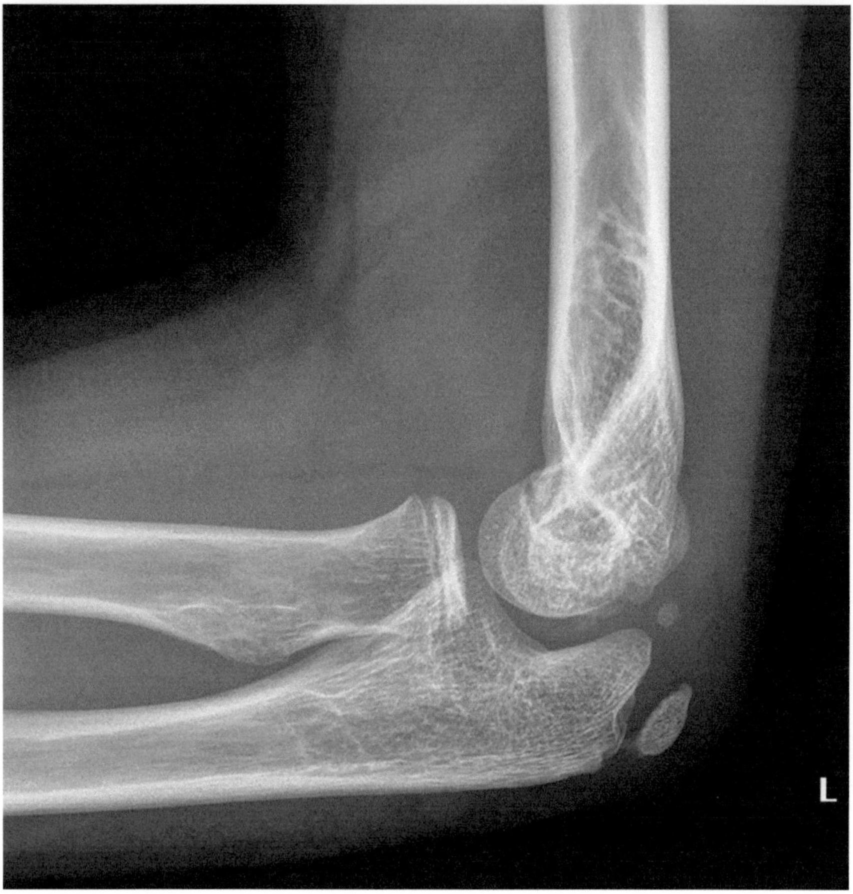

Image 12

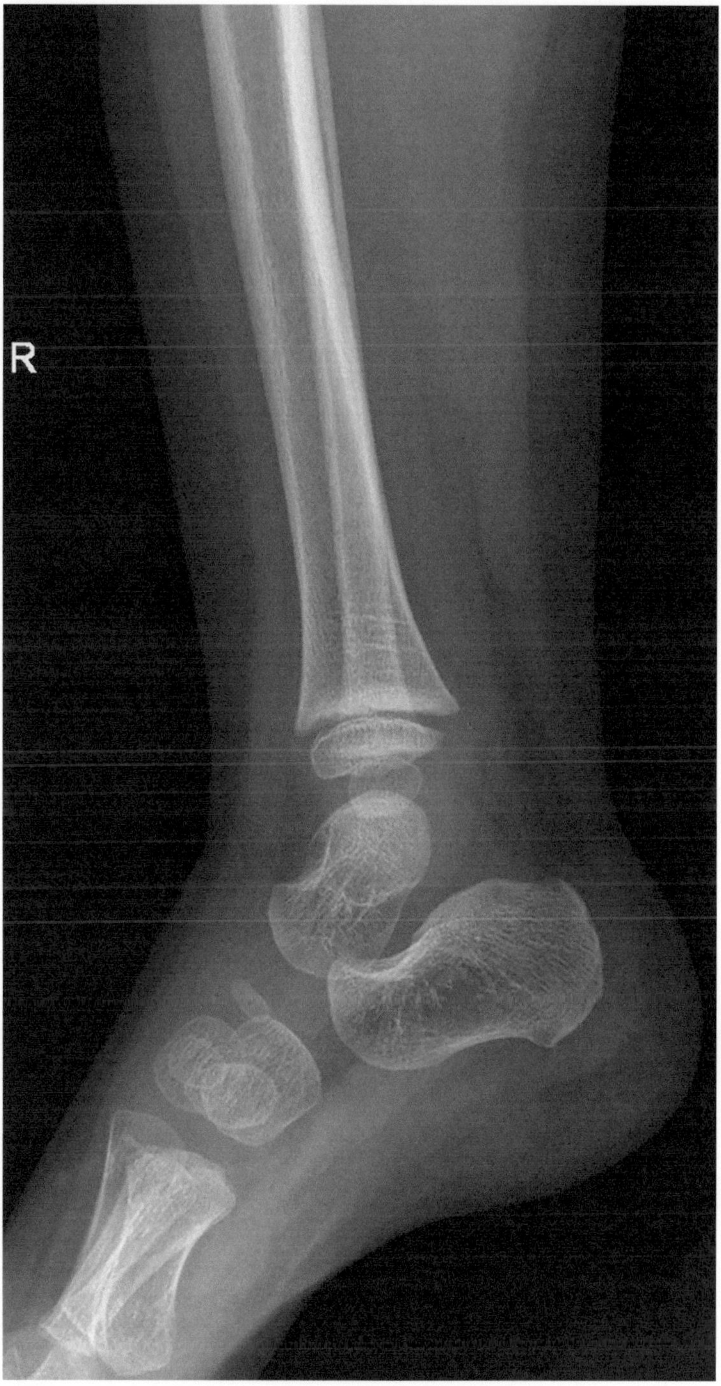

Image 13

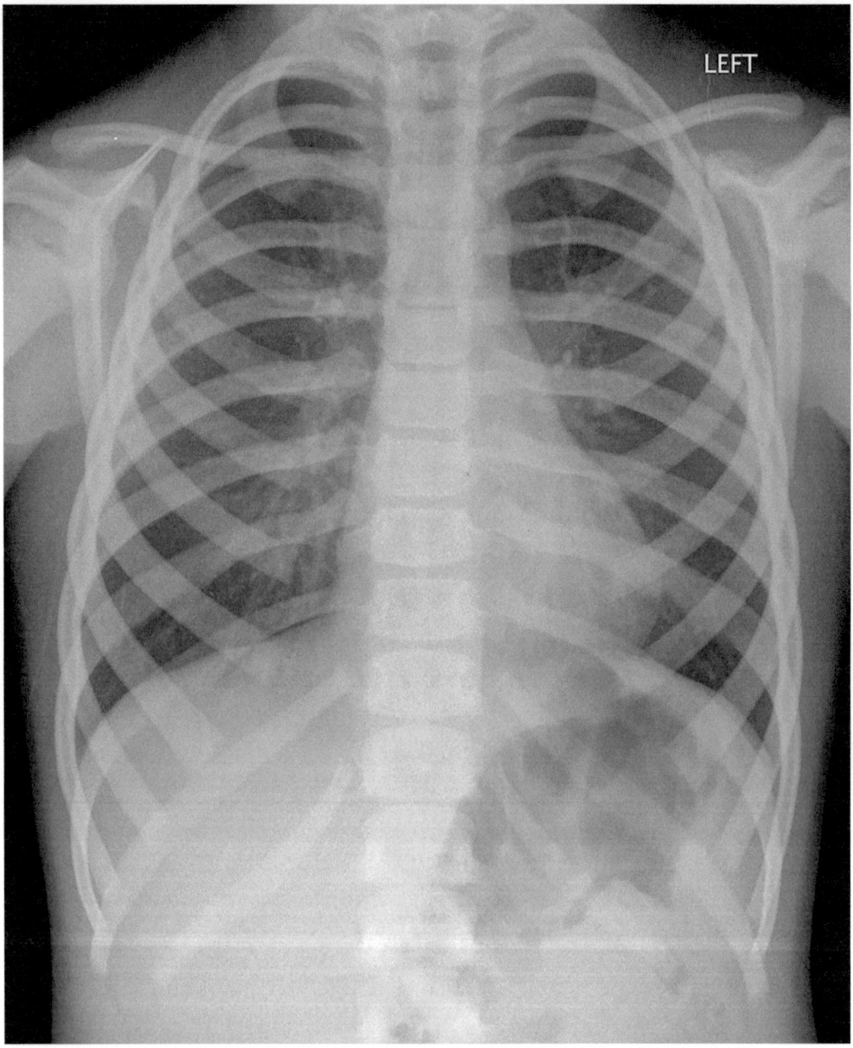

Image 14

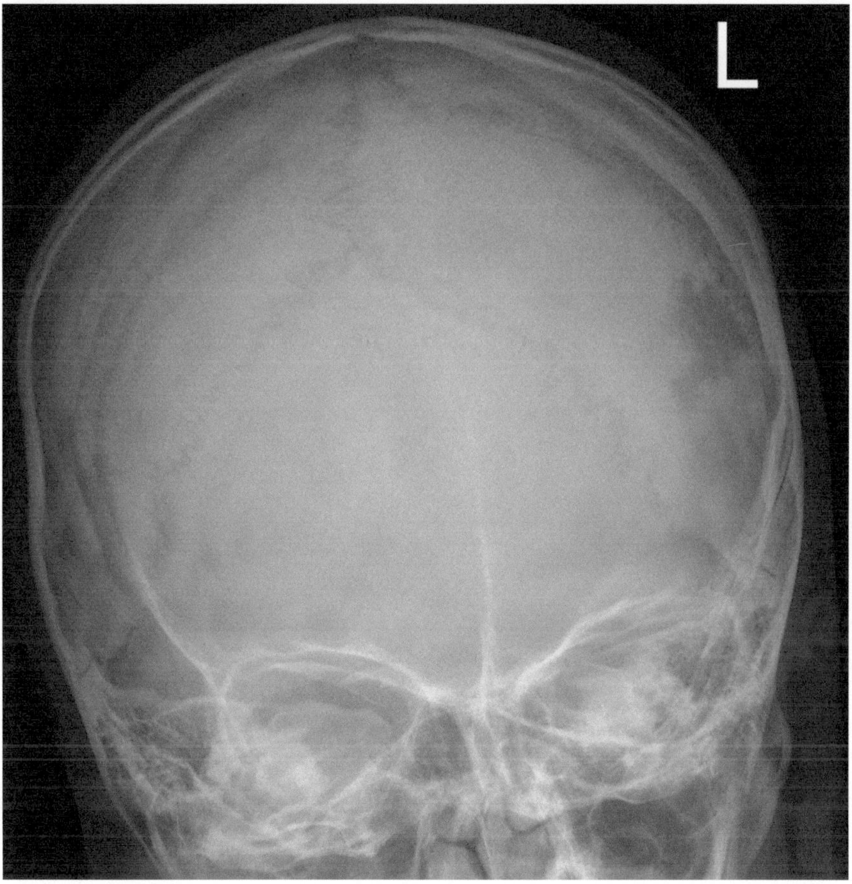

Image 15

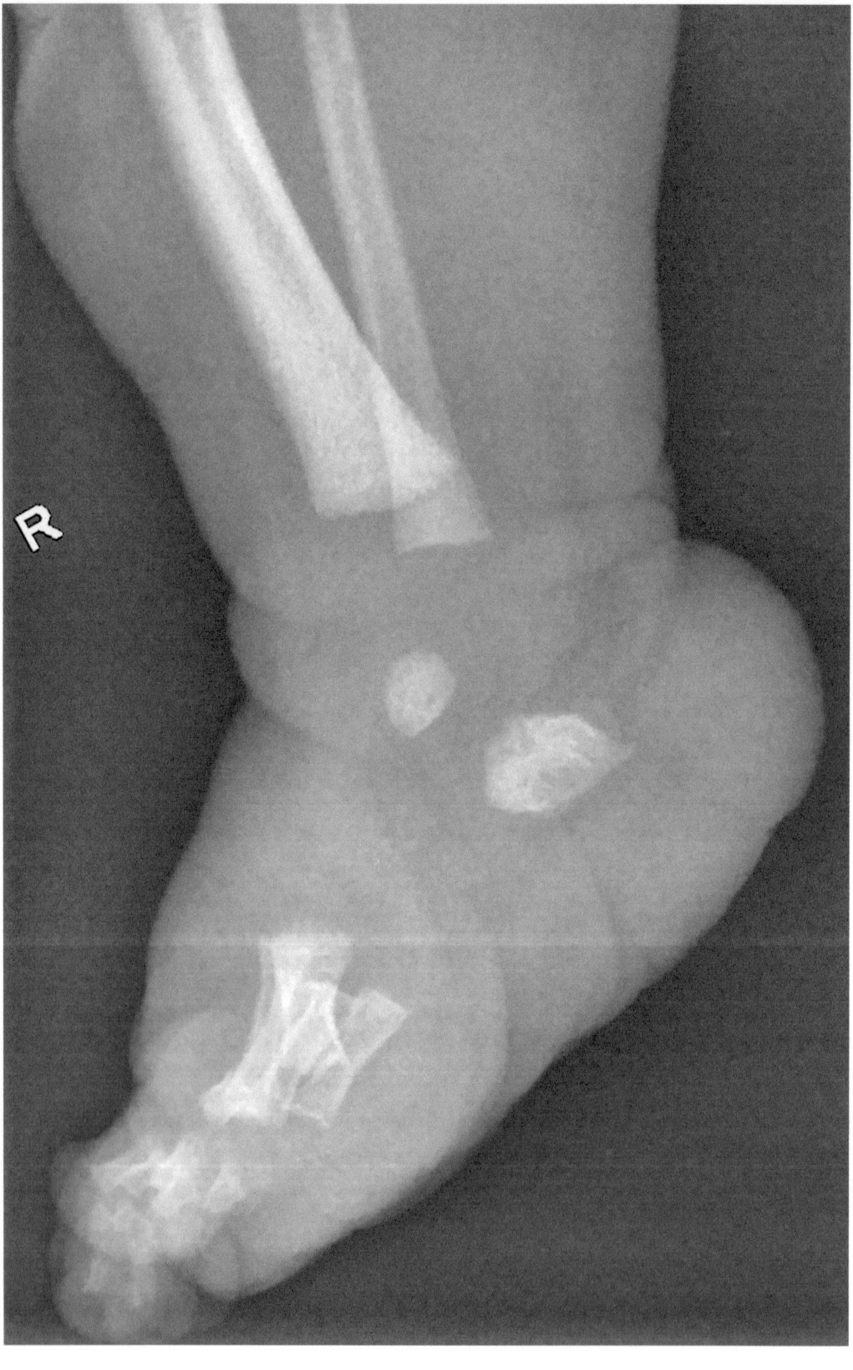

Image 16

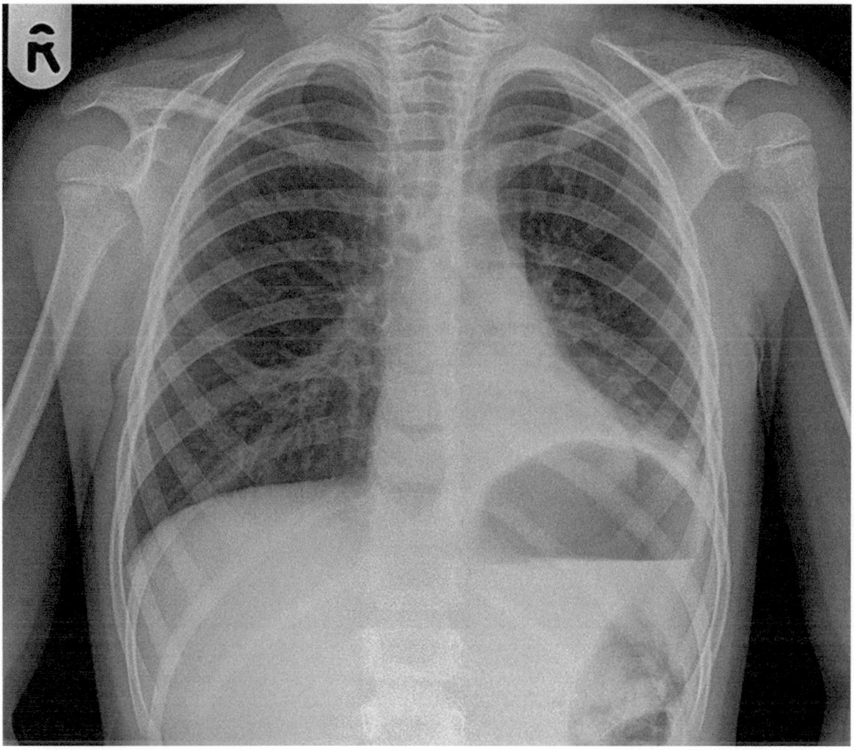

Image 17

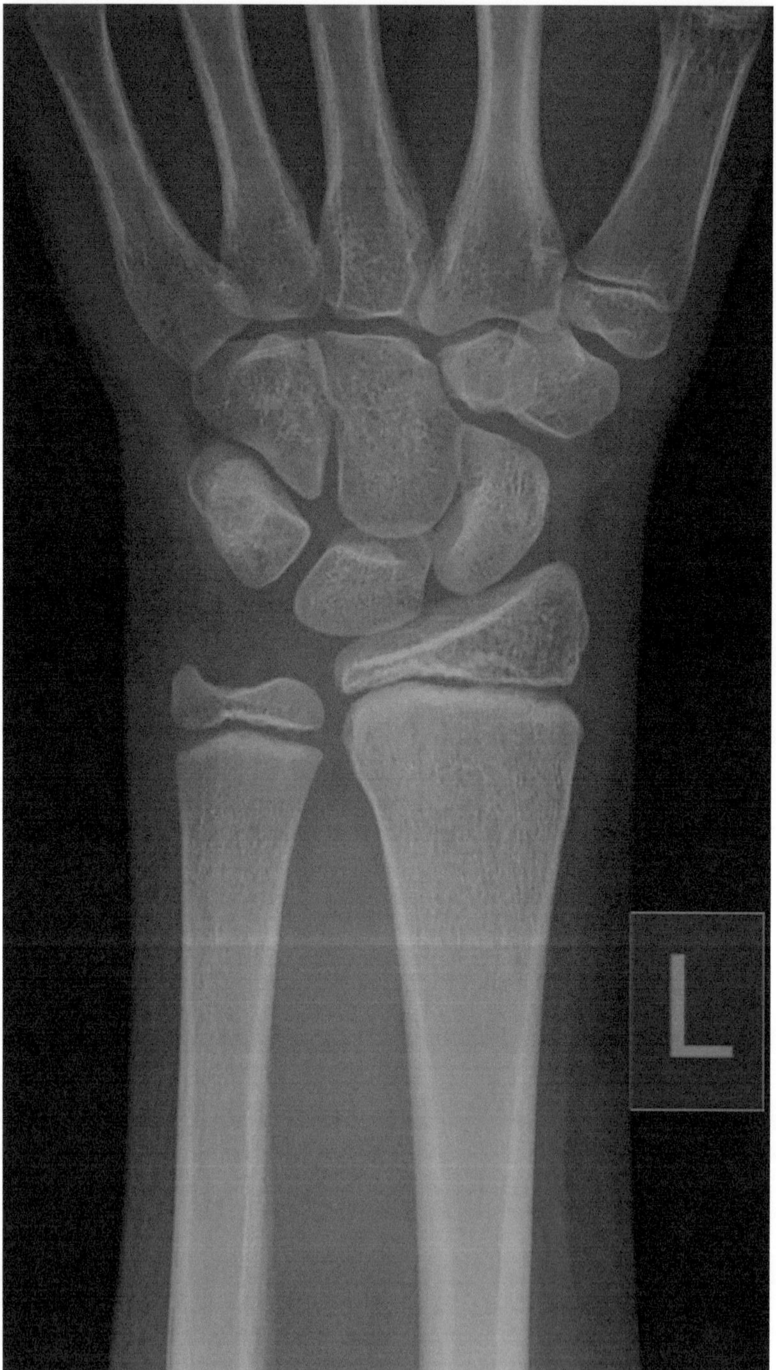

Image 18

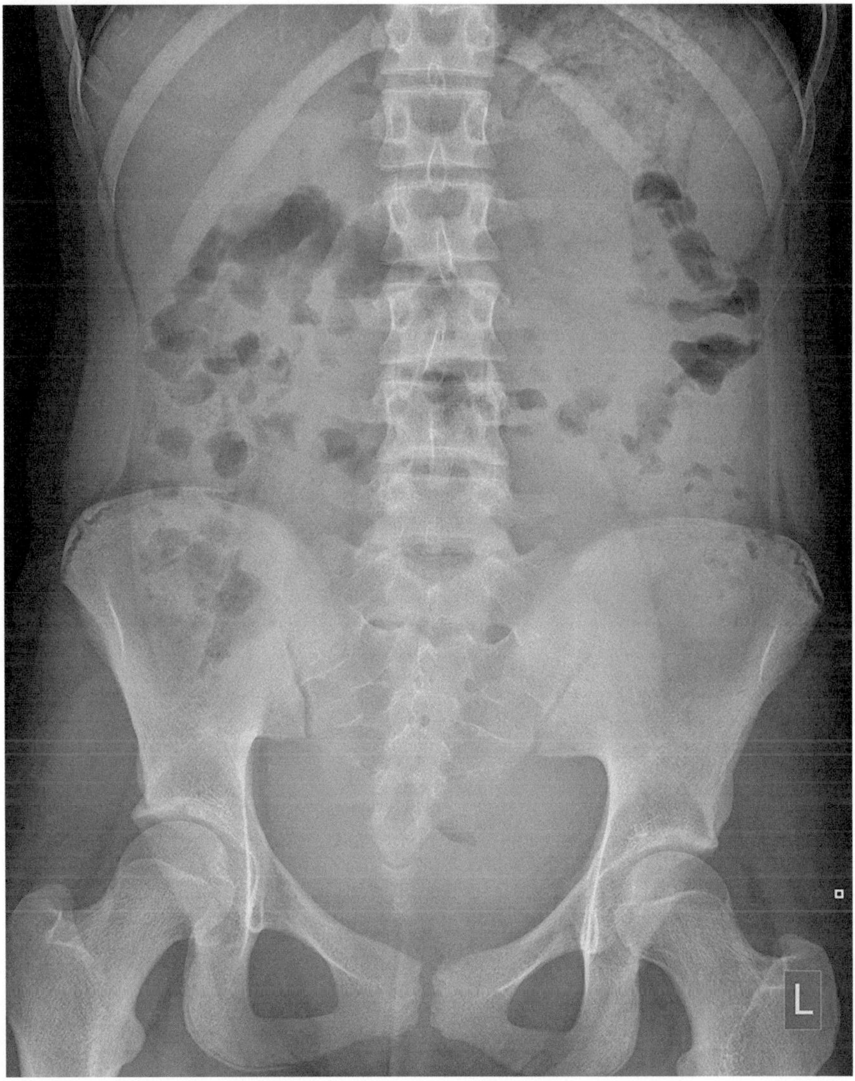

Image 19

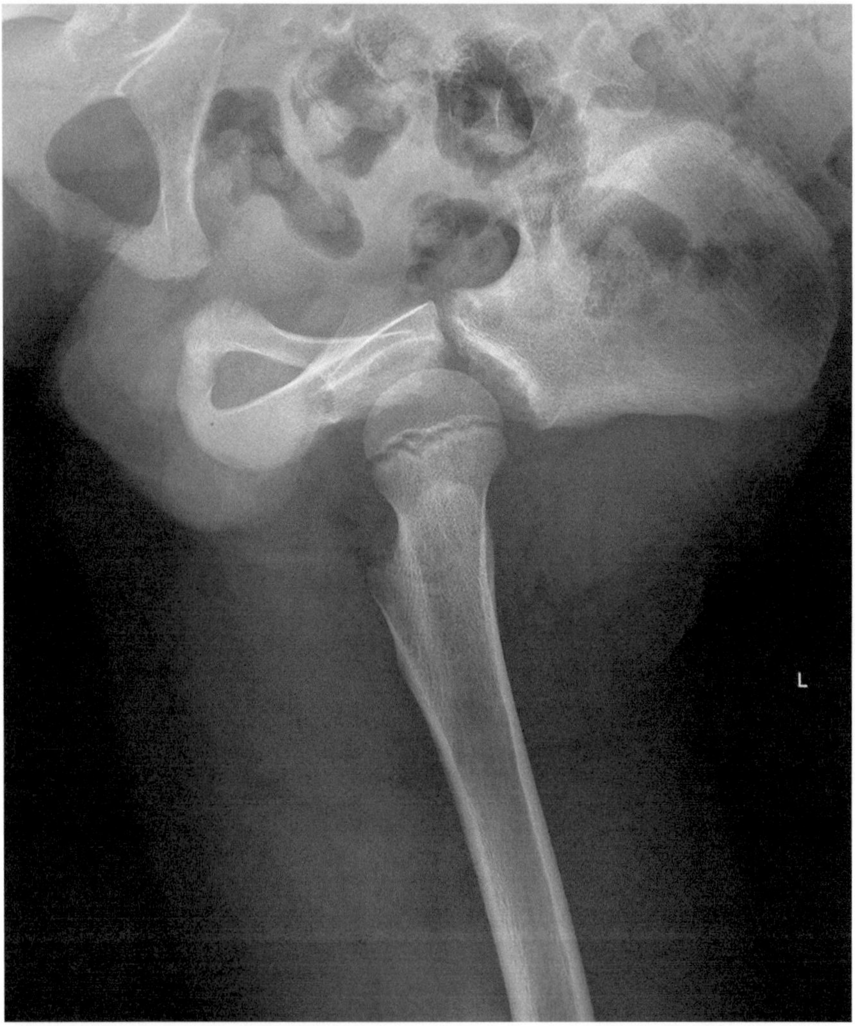

Image 20

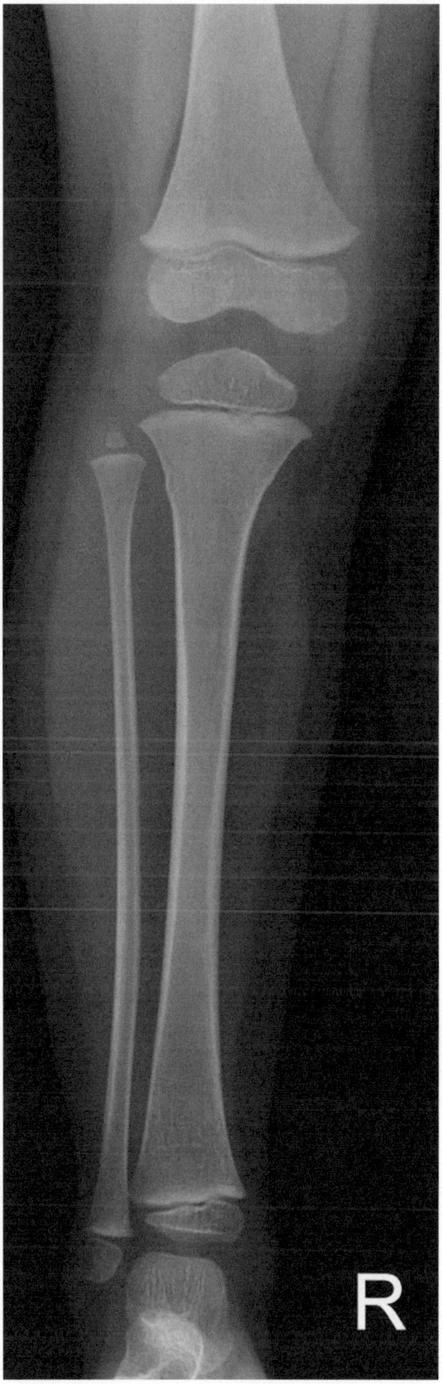

Image 21

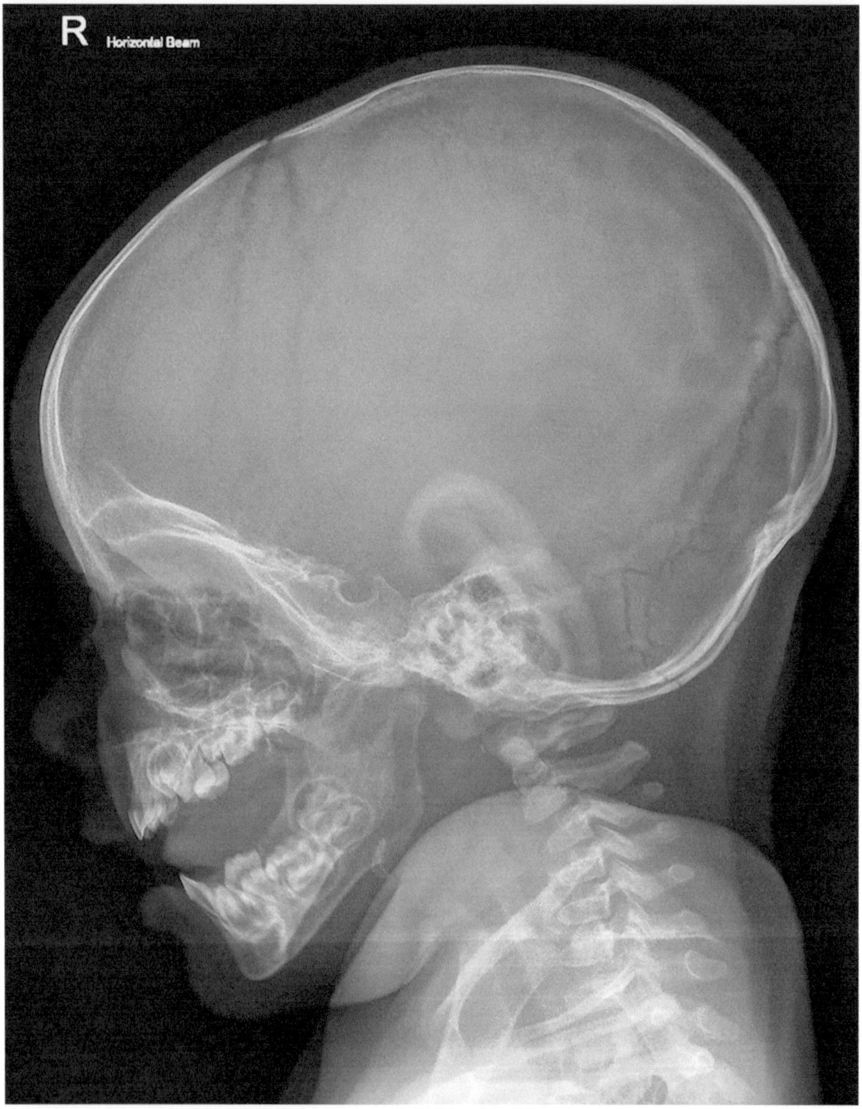

Image 22

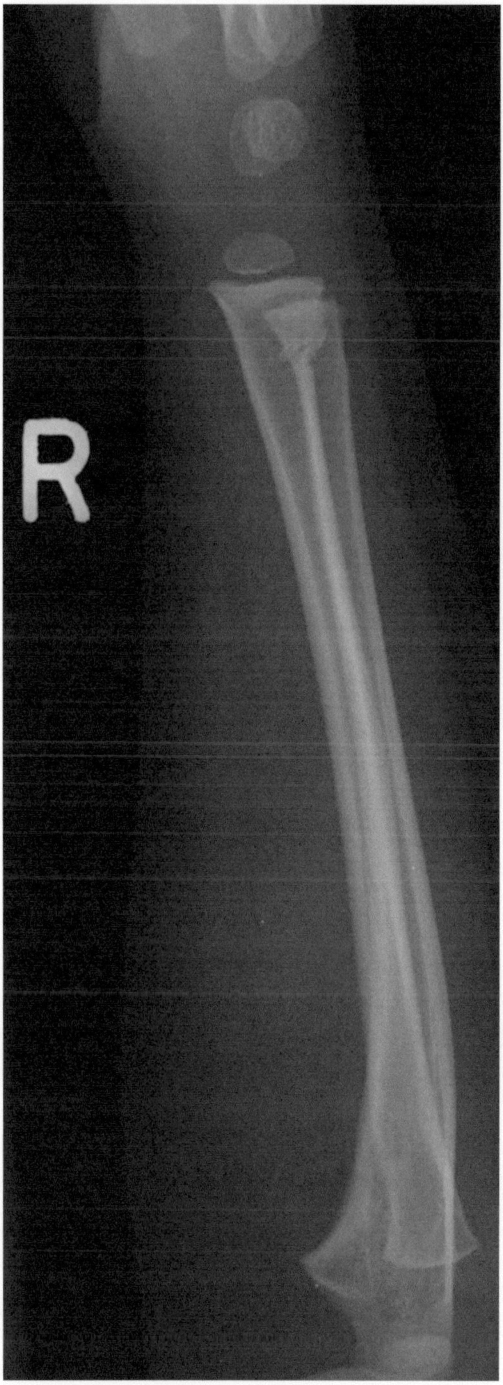

Image 23

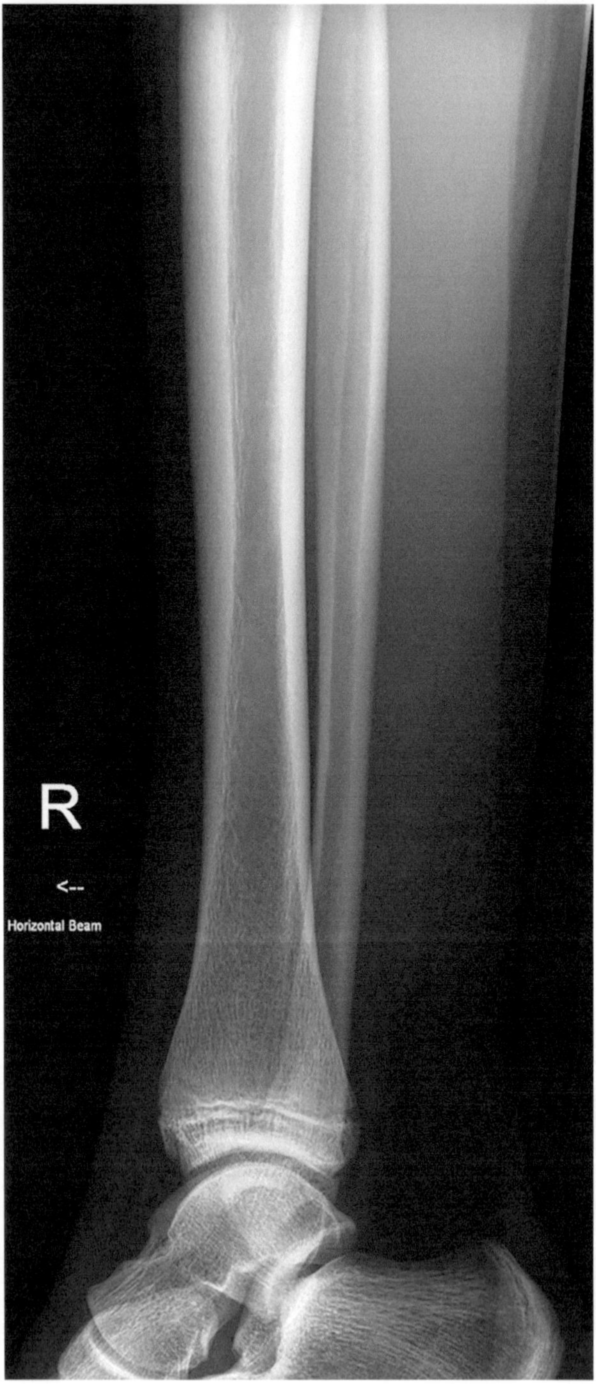

Image 24

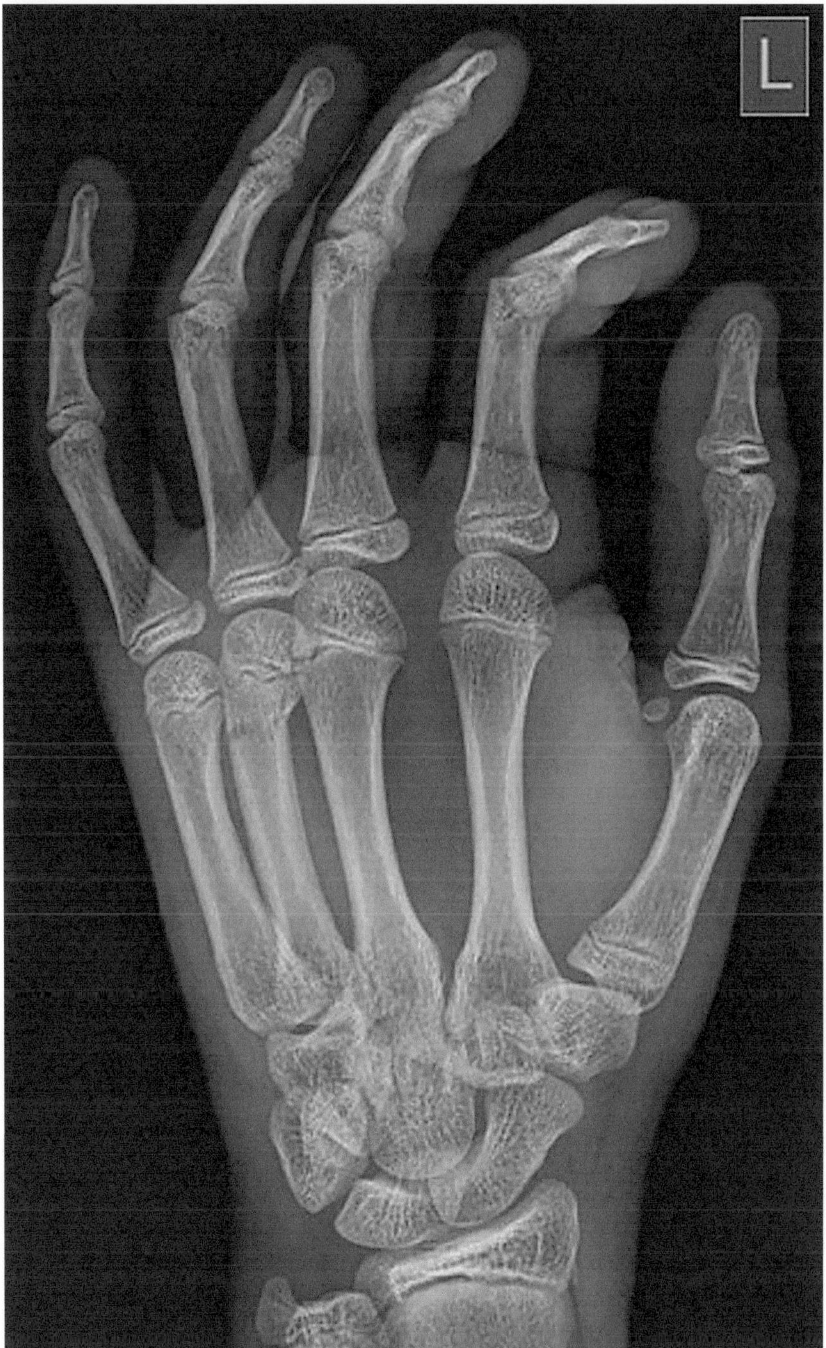

Image 25

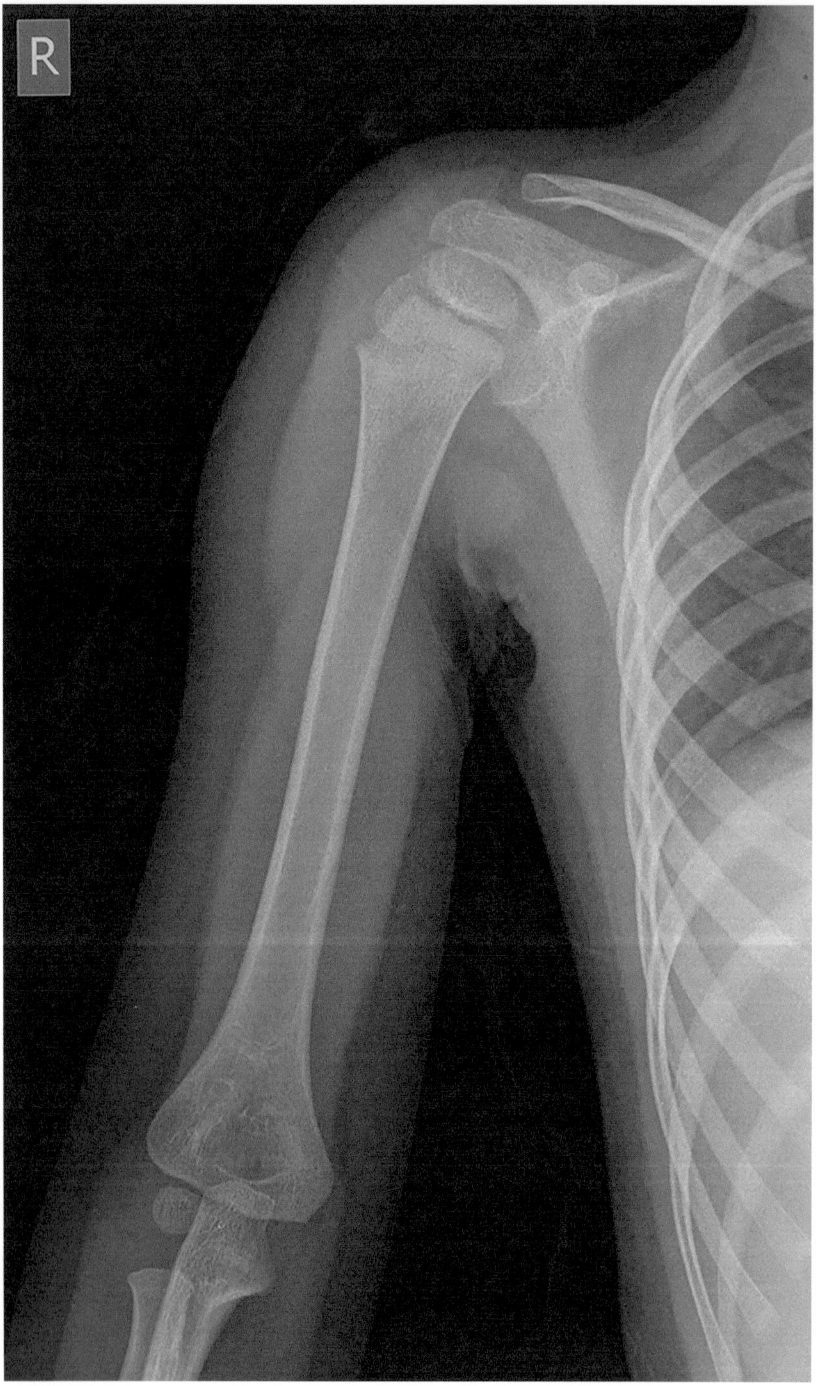

Image 26

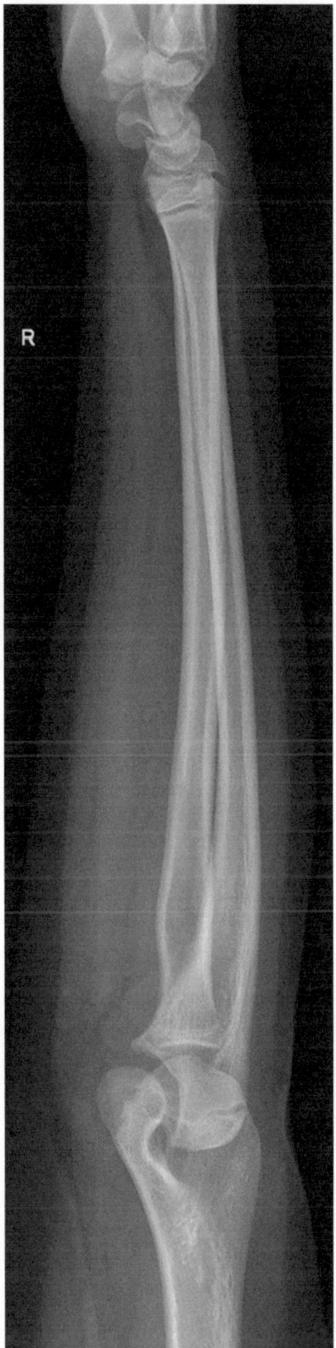

Image 27

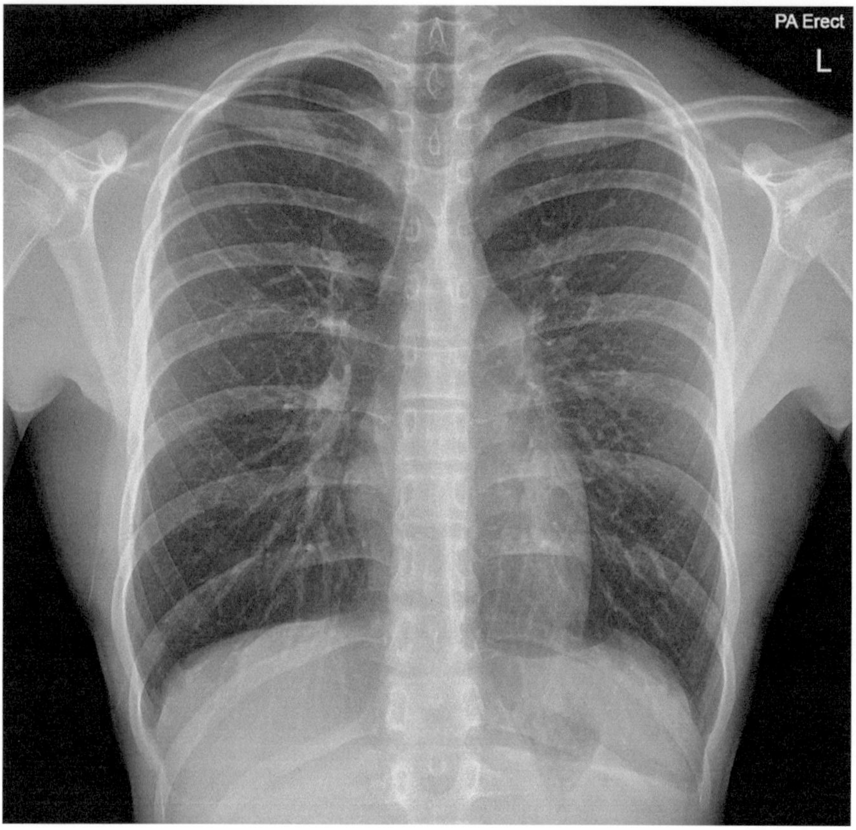

Image 28

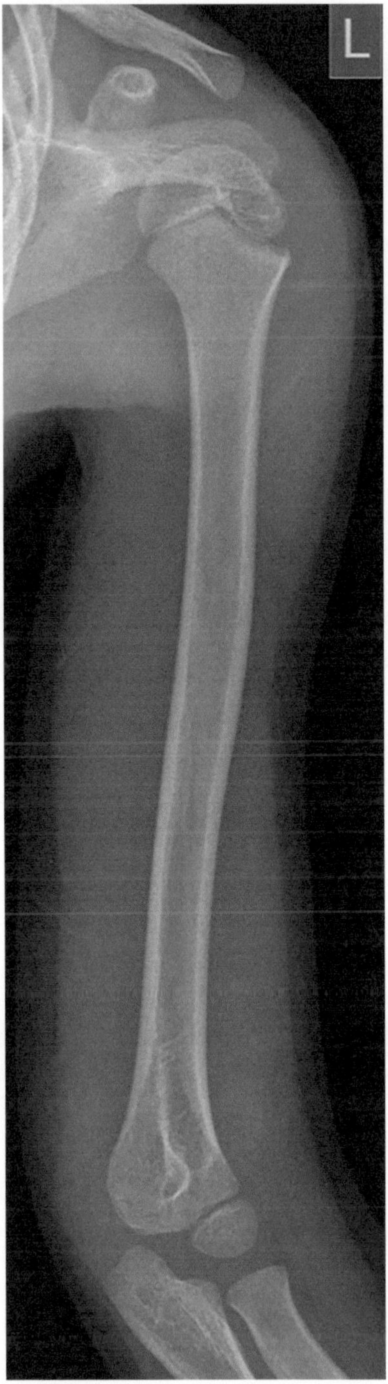

Image 29

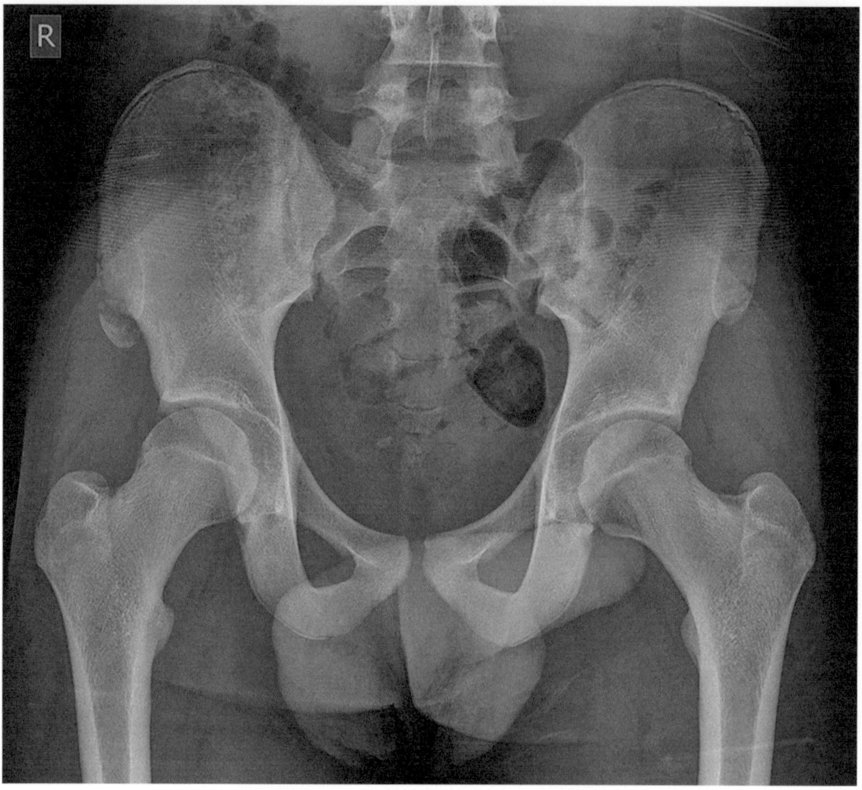

Image 30

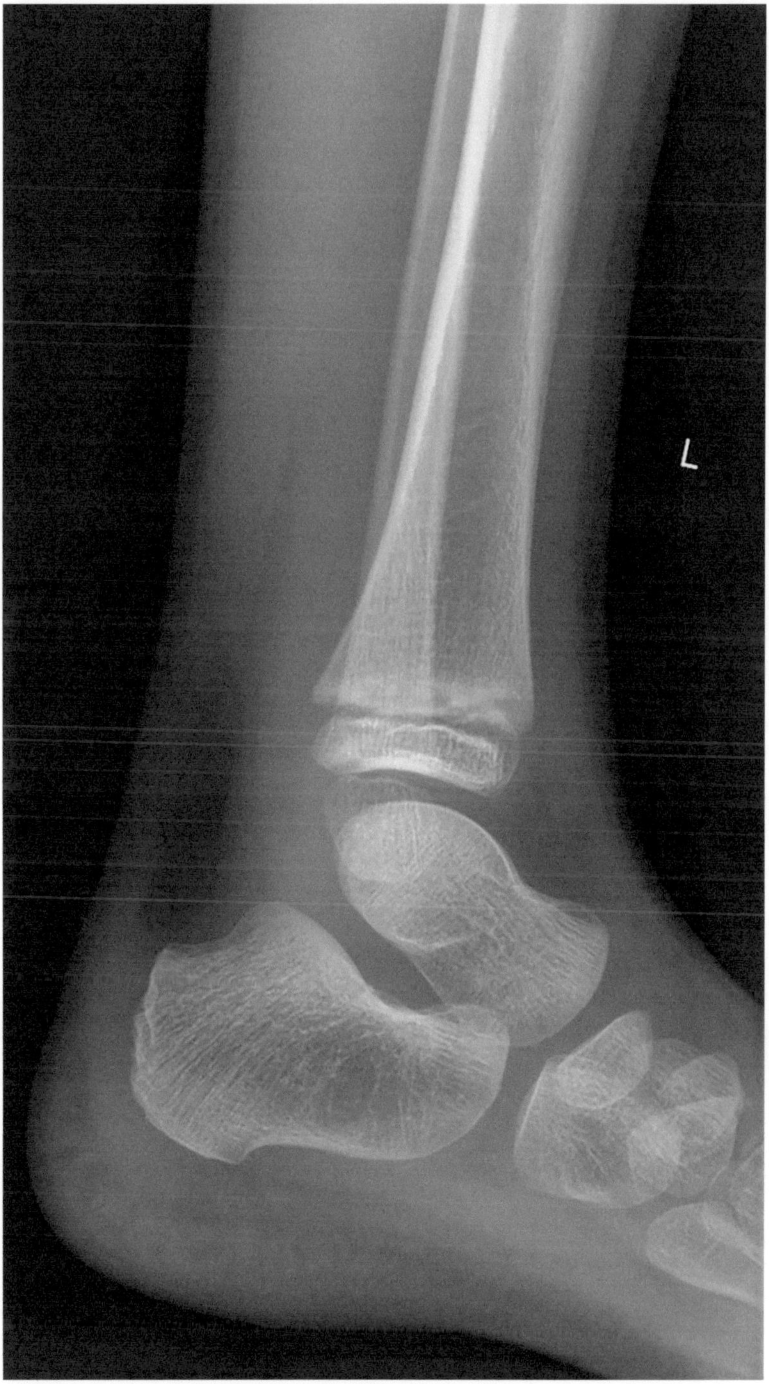

6.2 Answers

Image	Normal	Abnormal	Diagnosis/abnormality (only if abnormal)
1		✓	L Tillaux #
2		✓	# R supracondylar humerus
3	✓		
4		✓	# L fourth toe proximal phalanx
5		✓	Vertebra plana T8
6	✓		
7	✓		
8		✓	# R fifth metatarsal base
9		✓	Avulsion # R medial epicondyle
10		✓	Buckle # dorsal aspect R thumb proximal phalanx base
11	✓		
12	✓		
13		✓	Diffuse bony sclerosis
14		✓	Lucent lesion L skull
15	✓		
16		✓	L lower lobe collapse
17		✓	Buckle # L distal radial metaphysis
18		✓	Pelvic mass/paucity of pelvic bowel gas
19	✓		
20		✓	Buckle # R proximal tibial metaphysis
21	✓		
22		✓	Buckle #s R distal radial and ulnar metaphyses
23	✓		
24		✓	Transverse # L fourth metacarpal neck
25	✓		
26	✓		
27	✓		
28	✓		
29		✓	Avulsion # R ASIS
30	✓		

6.3 Explanations

1. **L Tillaux #**
   A Salter-Harris 3 fracture through the *lateral* aspect of the distal tibial epiphysis is known as a Tillaux fracture (after the French surgeon and anatomist). This fracture is associated with an avulsion of the anterior tibiofibular ligament following an abduction-external rotation mechanism of injury. These injuries occur more often in older children and adolescents, at which age the medial aspect of the distal tibial physis has usually fused. Remember that the distal tibial physis fuses from *medial to lateral*, i.e. the medial aspect of the distal tibial physis fuses before the lateral aspect, with the latter fusing at around 12–15 years of age.
   See the explanation for Image 30 of Test 1 for a discussion regarding the Salter-Harris classification.

2. **# R supracondylar humerus**
   See the explanations for Images 11 and 15 of Test 1.

4. **# L fourth toe proximal phalanx**
   Close inspection reveals the minimally displaced transverse fracture of the left fourth toe proximal phalanx reinforcing that scrutiny of every bony structure is required. The fracture is magnified below:

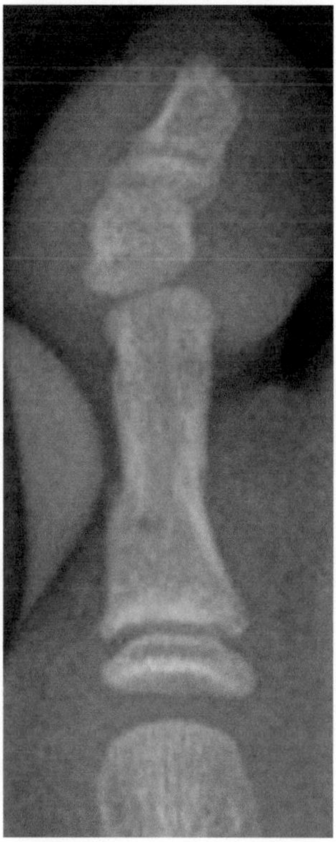

5. **Vertebra plana T8**

Vertebra plana describes the advanced collapse of a vertebral body which has lost almost all of its anterior, middle, and posterior height. Compare this to the wedging of a vertebral body in which only the anterior vertebral height is lost. Vertebral body height loss can occur due to:

- Failure of the anterior column secondary to trauma or decreased mineral bone density
- Platyspondyly, which refers to multiple flattened vertebral bodies, usually in the context of a skeletal dysplasia

Compare the advanced collapse of the T8 vertebral body to the adjacent normal height vertebral bodies in the magnified image below:

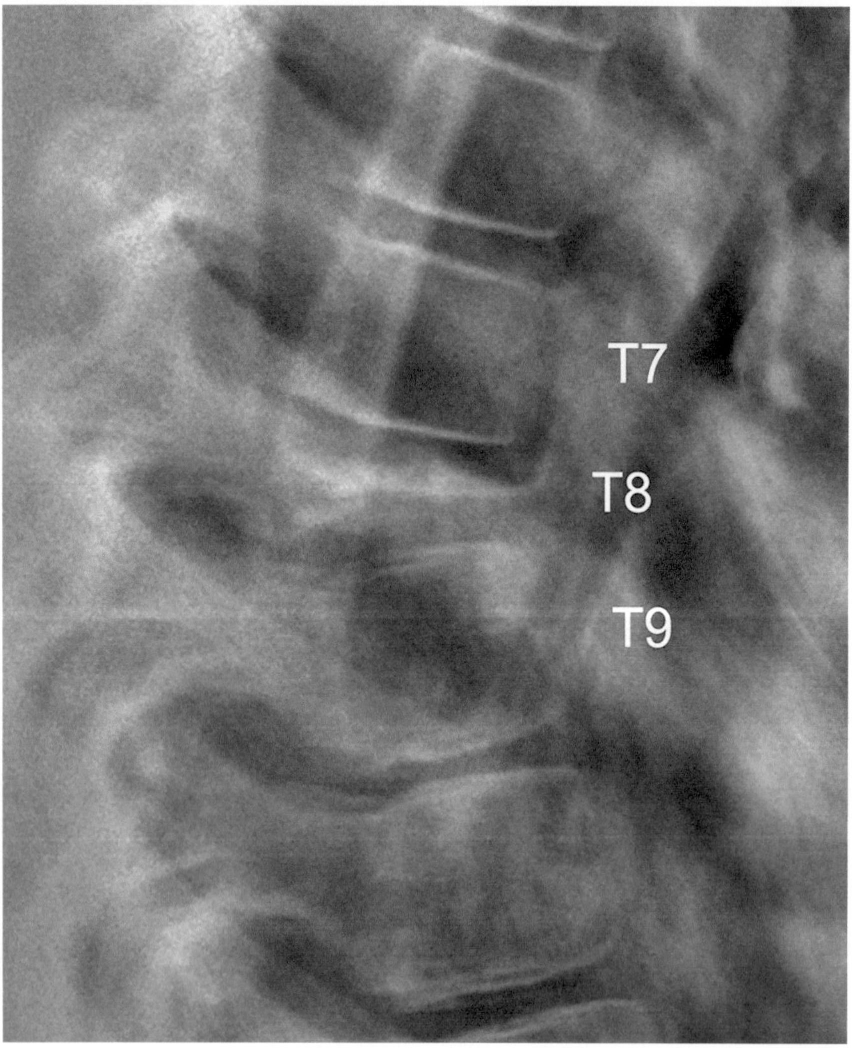

In this case, the T8 vertebral body can be identified by first identifying the T12 vertebral body by its articulation with the lowest pair of ribs and then counting up. When the whole spine has been imaged, it is best practice to identify the C2 vertebral body and then count down. This is not a perfect method because it assumes that vertebral body segmentation is normal (7 cervical, 12 thoracic, 5 lumbar and 5 [fused] sacral vertebrae) and that there are 12 pairs of ribs, which may not be the case in every child. However, if only a portion of the spine is available for review, it would generally be safe to assume that the lowermost pair of ribs articulates with the T12 vertebral body. You could note this in your report for the long case component and mention it should it come up in your viva. For the purposes of the examination, you are unlikely to be penalised if you report this as 'vertebra plana lower thoracic vertebral body'.

The differential diagnosis of a *single level* vertebra plana in *children* includes:

- Langerhans' cell histiocytosis (LCH): the most common cause (and the cause in this case).
- Ewing's sarcoma.
- Osteomyelitis: look for associated disc destruction (loss of disc height) along with vertebral endplate destruction in bacterial infection. When the disc heights are relatively preserved in the context of vertebral bony destruction, consider tuberculous spondylitis and look for an associated paraspinal abscess if cross-sectional imaging has been performed. A rare cause of vertebra plana in children is chronic recurrent multifocal osteomyelitis (CRMO).
- Aneurysmal bone cyst (ABC).

The differential diagnosis of *multilevel* vertebra plana in *children* includes:

- Gaucher's disease (see the explanation for Image 1 of Test 1).
- Leukaemia: the most common primary malignancy in children.
- Lymphoma.
- Metastatic disease.
- Trauma.

7. *Normal pelvic radiograph*

   Note the slight asymmetry of the ischiopubic synchondroses which is commonly visualised on paediatric pelvic radiographs and represents normal development/ossification.

8. **# R fifth metatarsal base**

   See the explanation for Image 7 for Test 1.

9. **Avulsion # R medial epicondyle**

   This radiograph demonstrates a displaced avulsion fracture of the medial epicondyle ossification centre with significant overlying soft tissue swelling. Medial epicondyle avulsion fractures are the most common avulsion injuries of the paediatric elbow. Whilst the findings are fairly obvious on this radiograph, often the disproportionate soft tissue swelling may be the only sign of injury, particularly in those below 7 years of age, as the medial apophysis has not yet begun to ossify. Also look for any subtle widening of the physis (which may indicate a Salter-Harris 1 injury) and displacement and/or angulation of the apophysis.

The medial epicondyle ossification centre is classed as an *apophysis* as it does not contribute to the longitudinal growth of the humerus or to the formation of the elbow joint. Remember that apophyses are sites of ligamentous or tendinous attachment.

Avulsion of the medial epicondyle ossification centre results from an extreme valgus force when a child falls onto an outstretched arm (FOOSH). This force can also temporarily open the joint space into which the avulsed medical epicondyle ossification centre can be displaced. On radiographs, this may simulate the trochlear ossification centre where a displaced avulsed medical epicondyle ossification centre can be overlooked. This is a significant injury that should *not* be missed: retention of an avulsion fragment in the joint space can lead to severe articular damage and early secondary osteoarthritis. See the explanation for Image 7 of Test 5 for a discussion of the normal ossification pattern of the paediatric elbow.

10. **Buckle # dorsal aspect R thumb proximal phalanx base**
    There is abnormal undulation of the dorsal metaphyseal cortex of the right thumb proximal phalanx base consistent with a buckle fracture. Compare with the dorsal cortices of the right thumb distal phalanx and metacarpal, which are normal in appearance with a 'smooth' contour.

11. *Normal left elbow radiograph*
    There is no fracture or effusion, radiocapitellar alignment is normal and there is no associated soft tissue swelling to indicate an acute injury. See the explanation for Image 11 of Test 1 for a discussion regarding elbow joint alignment.

13. **Diffuse bony sclerosis**
    The differential diagnosis for diffuse bony sclerosis in children can be divided into broad categories and is best remembered using the mnemonic, **PPIMS:**
    - **P**oisoning:
      - Lead.
      - Fluorosis.
      - Hypervitaminosis D.
      - Chronic hypervitaminosis A.
    - **P**hysiological neonatal sclerosis.
    - **I**diopathic:
      - Caffey disease: see the explanation for Image 2 of Test 5.
      - Idiopathic hypercalcaemia of infancy.
    - **M**etabolic:
      - Renal osteodystrophy.

- Skeletal dysplasia:
  - Osteopetrosis: see the explanation for Image 11 of Test 4.
  - Pyknodysostosis: a rare autosomal recessive skeletal dysplasia characterised by osteosclerosis and short stature, as was the cause in this case.

14. **Lucent lesion L skull**

The differential diagnosis for a lucent skull lesion in a *child* is wide and includes:

- Eosinophilic granuloma/LCH (the cause in this case).
- Metastases from:
  - Neuroblastoma.
  - Medulloblastoma.
  - Leukaemia.
- Osteomyelitis.
- Dermoid/epidermoid cyst.
- Fibrous dysplasia.
- Haemangioma.
- Leptomeningeal cyst: this term is a misnomer as the abnormality is not a cyst but thought to result from herniation of the leptomeninges and/or cerebral parenchyma through a dural tear following a skull fracture. Over time, cerebrospinal fluid (CSF) pulsations of the herniated contents result in fracture expansion and eventual non-union. As such, they may also be referred to as 'growing' skull fractures and may complicate approximately 1% of skull fractures. When present, they may be seen a few months after the initial trauma adjacent to areas of post-traumatic encephalomalacia and typically present as an enlarging scalp mass in children less than 3 years of age.
- Surgical defect: e.g. previous burr hole.
- Meningocele.
- Normal variant: arachnoid granulation; emissary vein; venous lake.

It cannot be confidently determined in which bone the lucent lesion lies on the basis of this solitary anteroposterior (AP) projection. The orthogonal lateral projection confirmed this lesion to lie in the left frontal bone. Note the appearance of the normal cranial sutures.

16. **L lower lobe collapse**

This radiograph demonstrates the distinctive features of left lower lobe collapse, including:

- Increased retrocardiac/posteromedial left lung opacification.
- Volume loss in the left hemithorax, resulting in:
  - Mediastinal deviation to the left.
  - Elevation of the left hemidiaphragm: in this example, there is gastric distention and an air-fluid level. In the absence of gastric distension, the border of the left hemidiaphragm would usually be obscured/obliterated.
- Edge of the collapsed left lower lobe creates a 'double cardiac contour'.

In the setting of asthma or airways inflammation/infection a common cause of lobar collapse in children is mucous plugging. Foreign body inhalation/aspiration is also an important cause which should *always* be considered in young children. Remember that non-radiopaque foreign bodies will not be visualised on radiographs.

17. **Buckle # left distal radial metaphysis**
Paediatric bones have decreased density and increased porosity when compared to mature adult bones. This permits a greater absorption of energy and restriction of fracture propagation which explains the spectrum of bony injuries seen in children (i.e. plastic deformation, greenstick fractures, buckle/torus fractures, transverse undisplaced and displaced oblique fractures, and spiral fractures) when compared to adults. The subtle buckling of the left distal radial metaphysis is best appreciated by 'standing back' from the image to visualise the mild cortical bulging/undulation.
Whilst there is no associated ulnar buckle fracture in this case, it is important that one does not suffer 'satisfaction of search'. When the distal radial injury has been identified, the ulna must also be scrutinised for injury in every case. See the explanation for Image 18 of Test 1.

18. **Pelvic mass/paucity of pelvic bowel gas**
The paucity of bowel gas in the pelvis is noticeable once you know to look for it. 'Standing back' to evaluate the radiograph, one's eye is drawn to the pelvic area where there is increased opacification with commensurate paucity of bowel gas. Furthermore, the gas-filled bowel loop in the central abdomen is displaced superiorly.
This 14-year-old female presented with abdominal pain. Following this radiograph, a transabdominal ultrasound was performed, which revealed a large, distended fluid-filled structure with internal echoes. The anatomy was difficult to delineate given its size. Subsequent magnetic resonance imaging (MRI) revealed haematometrocolpos, a blood-filled distended uterus and vagina. An imperforate hymen is the most common cause, preventing evacuation of menstrual blood. Occasionally, the distension can be so great as to cause ureteric obstruction and dilation of the proximal renal tracts. There may also be an associated Müllerian duct anomaly/malformation, such as:
- Müllerian agenesis.
- Obstructing vaginal septum.
- Unicornuate uterus.
- Bicornuate uterus.
- Uterus didelphys.
- Septate uterus.

The kidneys should be thoroughly assessed in the context of a Müllerian duct anomaly for any of the frequently associated renal anomalies such as renal agenesis, duplex kidney, and cross fused renal ectopia. Remember that the

Müllerian ducts, also known as the paramesonephric ducts, are of embryologic mesodermal origin and track parallel to the urogenital ridge and terminate as the primitive urogenital sinus.

The differential diagnosis for the radiographic appearance in this case would also include: bladder outflow obstruction/urinary retention; megaureter; or another pelvic mass such as a rhabdomyosarcoma, large adnexal mass/cyst, or hydrosalpinx. A gravid uterus (and indeed, ectopic pregnancy) should also be considered in *any* young female of child-bearing age presenting with abdominal pain.

20. **Buckle # R proximal tibial metaphysis**
    See the explanation for Image 24 of Test 4.

22. **Buckle #s R distal radius and ulnar metaphyses**
    See the explanation for Image 18 of Test 1.

24. **Transverse # L fourth metacarpal neck**
    There is a transverse fracture through the left fourth metacarpal neck with a minor degree of volar angulation. This type of fracture usually results from direct trauma (punch injury with a clenched fist) or axial loading.

29. **Avulsion # R anterior superior iliac spine**
    Comparing the right hemipelvis to the left, there is an avulsion fracture of the right anterior superior iliac spine (ASIS) which is the insertion for the sartorius and tensor fascia latae tendons. See the explanation for Image 13 of Test 4.

Further Reading

Image 1

Murphy A et al (2023) Tillaux fracture. https://radiopaedia.org/articles/tillaux-fracture. Accessed Aug 2023

Smithius R (2018) Special cases of ankle fracture. Detection of 'not so obvious' fractures. https://radiologyassistant.nl/musculoskeletal/ankle/special-fracture-cases. Accessed Aug 2023

Image 5

El-Feky M et al (2023) Vertebra plana. https://radiopaedia.org/articles/vertebra-plana. Accessed Aug 2023

Wheeless CR (2012) Eosinophilic granuloma of the spine. https://www.wheelessonline.com/bones/spine/eosinophilic-granuloma-of-the-spine/. Accessed Aug 2023

Image 9

Lustosa L et al (2022) Medial epicondyle fracture. https://radiopaedia.org/articles/medial-epicondyle-fracture-1. Accessed Aug 2023

Qadeer A, Paddock M (2019) Intra-articular displacement of an avulsed medial (internal) epicondyle ossification centre in the paediatric elbow: a radiographic finding not to be missed. BMJ Case Rep 12(11):e231635

Smithuis R (2008) Elbow fractures in children. https://radiologyassistant.nl/pediatrics/hip/fractures-in-children-1. Accessed Aug 2023

Image 11

El-Feky M et al (2022) Anterior humeral line. https://radiopaedia.org/articles/anterior-humeral-line. Accessed Aug 2023

Image 13

Bell D et al (2022) Generalised increased bone density in children. https://radiopaedia.org/articles/generalised-increased-bone-density-in-children. Accessed Aug 2023

Boulet C, Madani H, Lenchik L et al (2016) Sclerosing bone dysplasias: genetic, clinical and radiology update of hereditary and non-hereditary disorders. Br J Radiol 89(1062):20150349

Vadera S et al (2022) Pyknodysostosis. https://radiopaedia.org/articles/pyknodysostosis. Accessed Aug 2023

Image 14

Anan RA et al (2022) Solitary lucent skull lesion. https://radiopaedia.org/articles/solitary-lucent-skull-lesion. Accessed Aug 2023

Ibrahim D et al (2022) Leptomeningeal cyst. https://radiopaedia.org/articles/leptomeningeal-cyst. Accessed Aug 2023

Image 16

Hacking C et al (2018) Left lower lobe collapse. https://radiopaedia.org/articles/left-lower-lobe-collapse. Accessed Aug 2023

Image 18

Ibrahim AY et al (2023) Haematometrocolpos. https://radiopaedia.org/articles/haematometrocolpos. Accessed May 2018

Test 7

7

M. Paddock et al., *Paediatric Radiology Rapid Reporting*,
https://doi.org/10.1007/978-3-031-48255-7_7

7.1 Images

Image 1

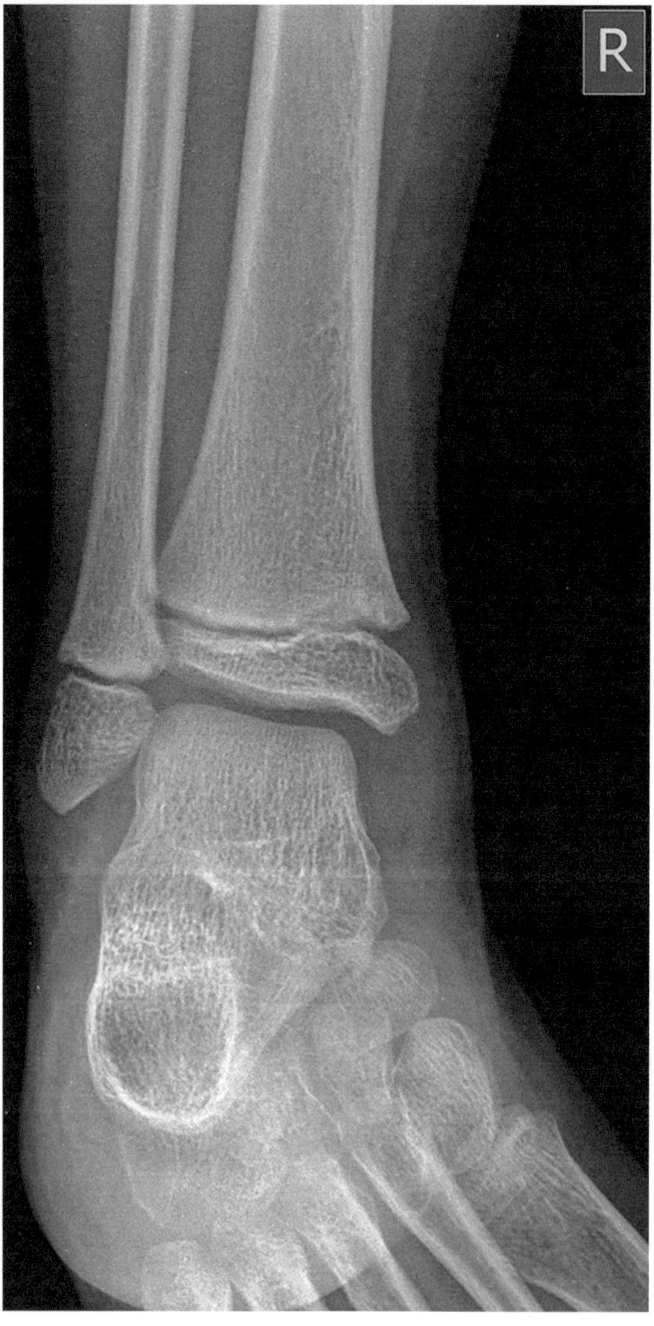

Image 2

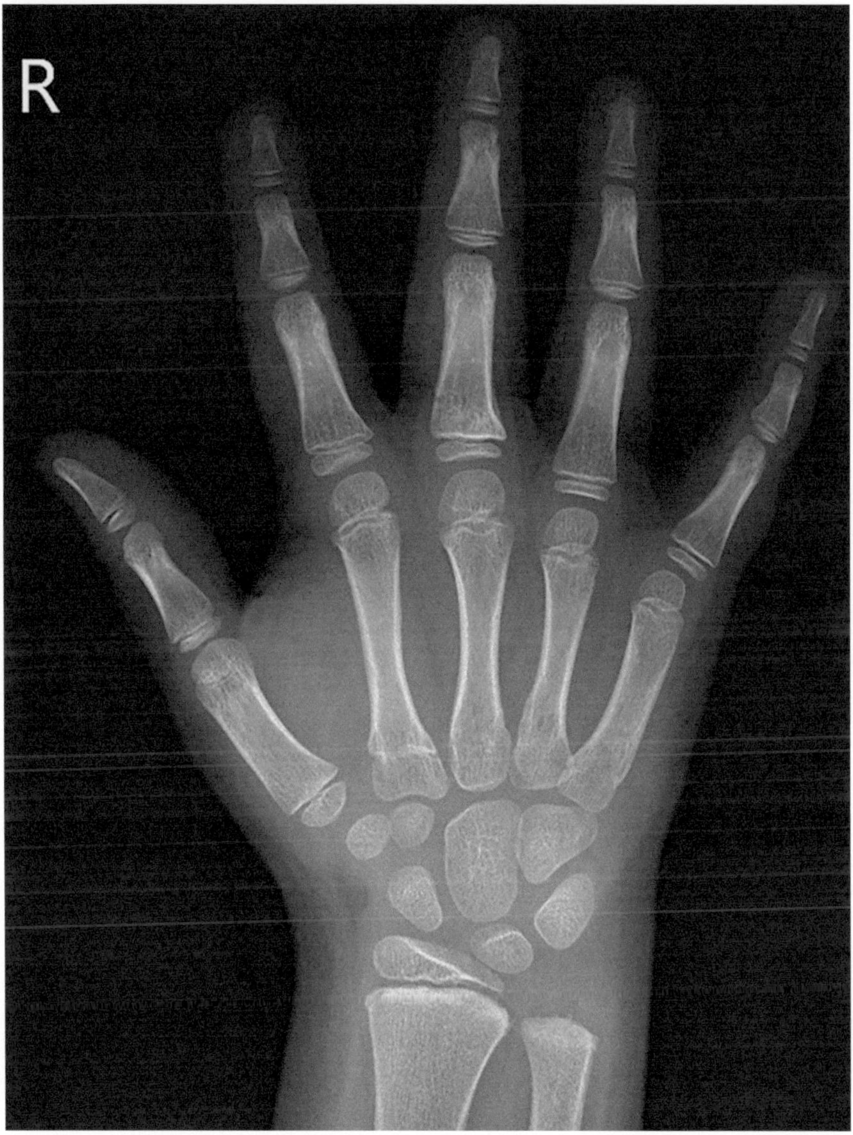

Image 3

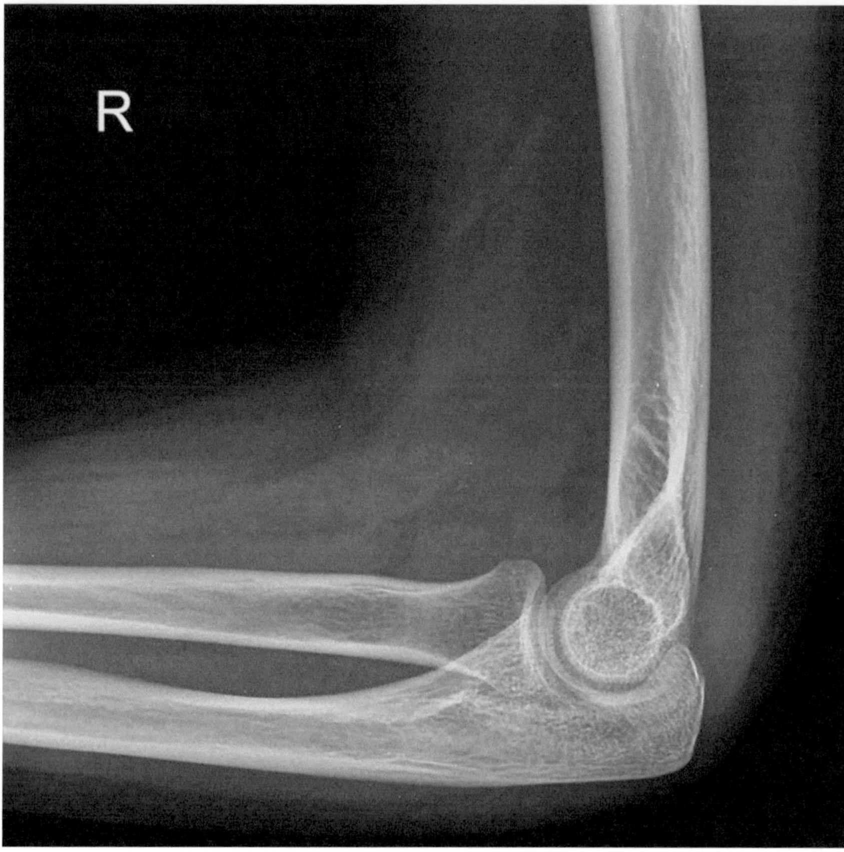

Image 4

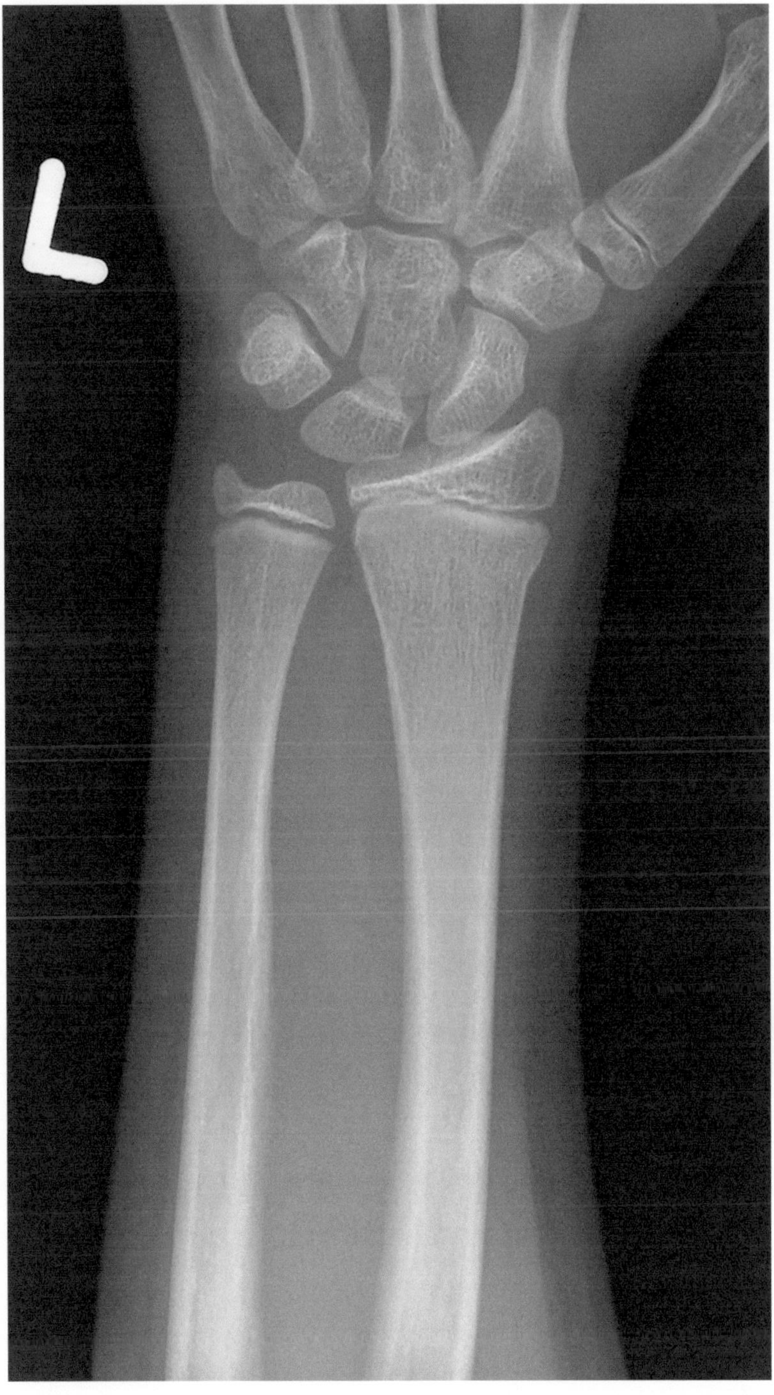

Image 5

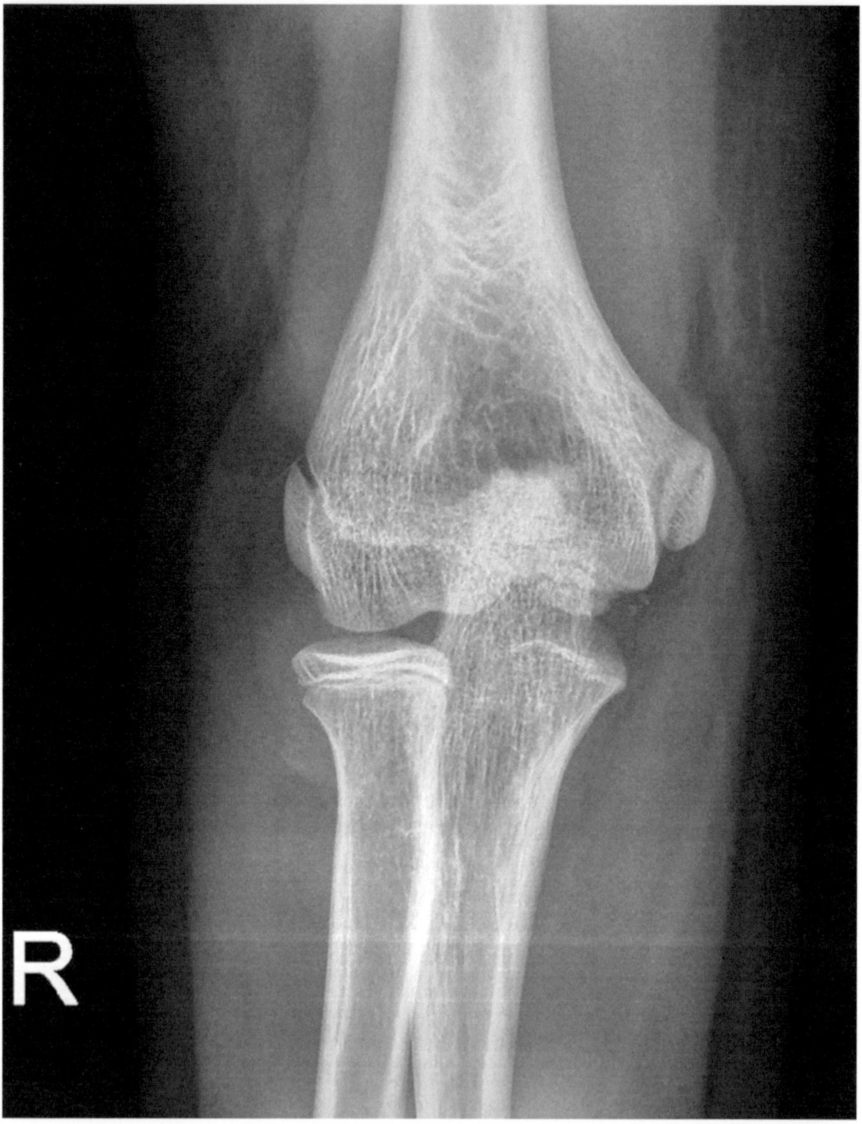

Image 6

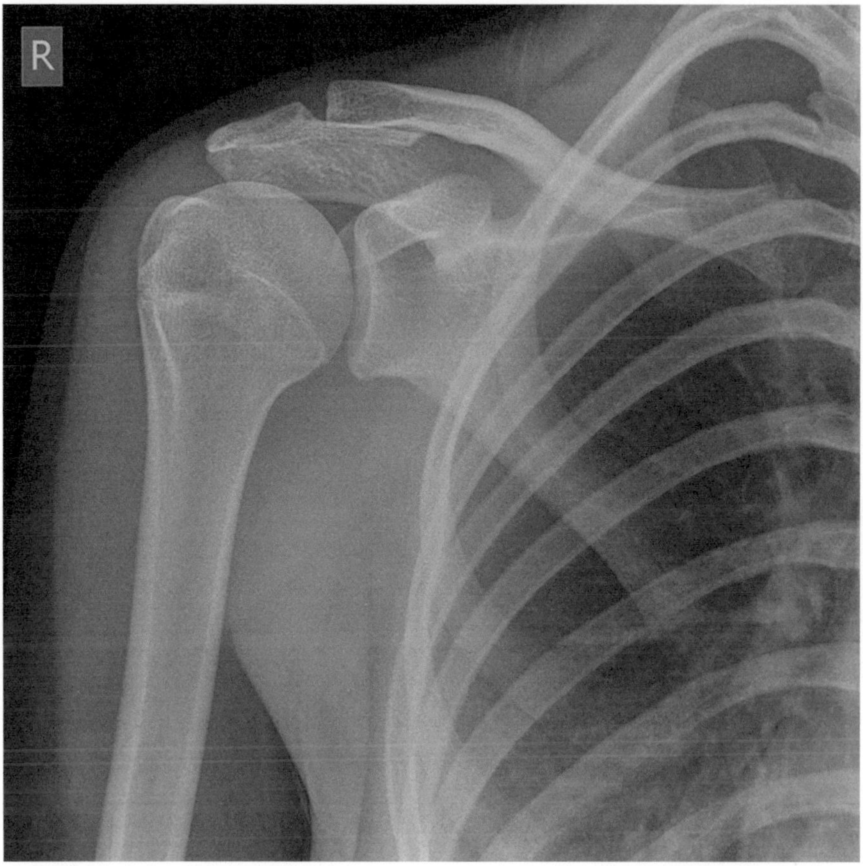

Image 7

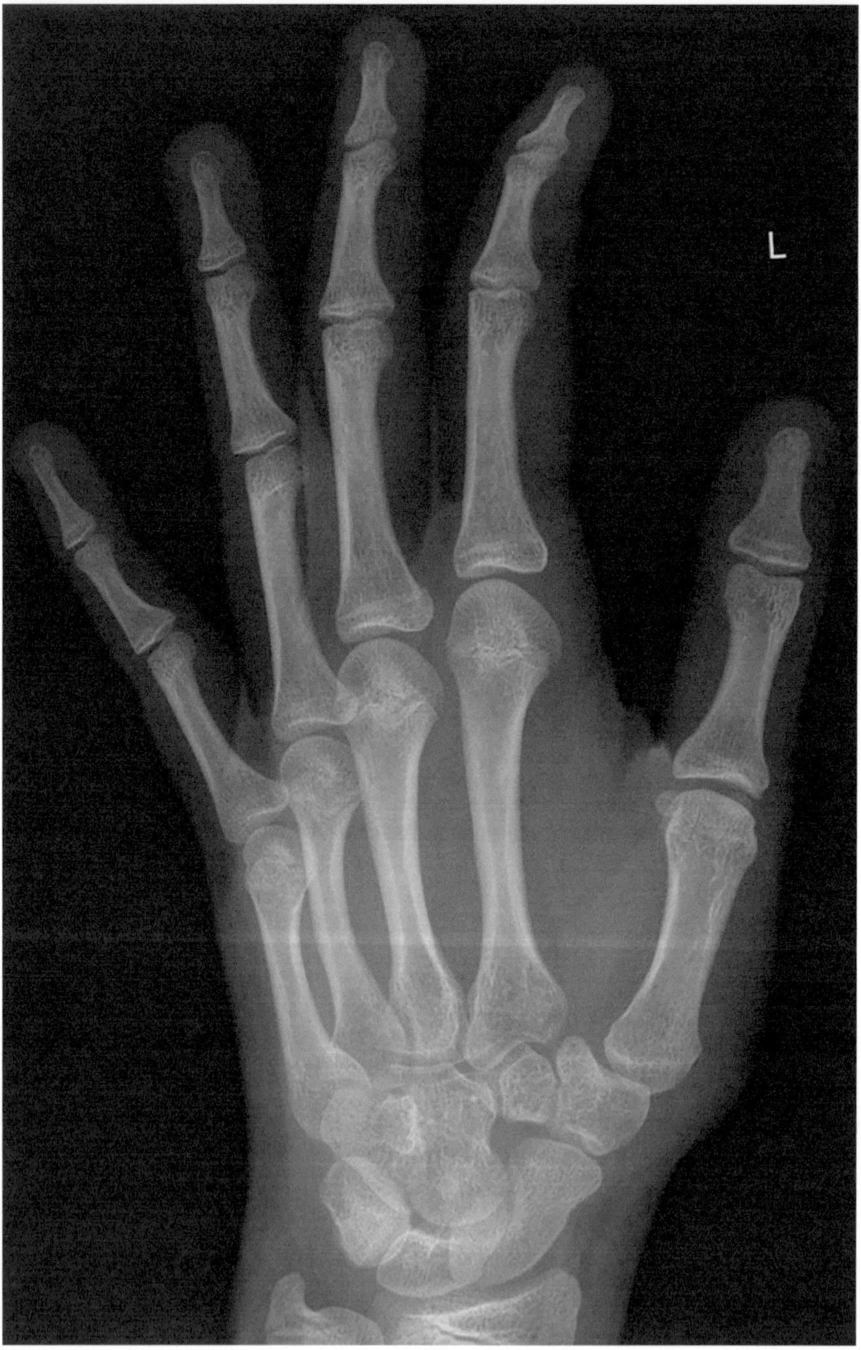

Image 8

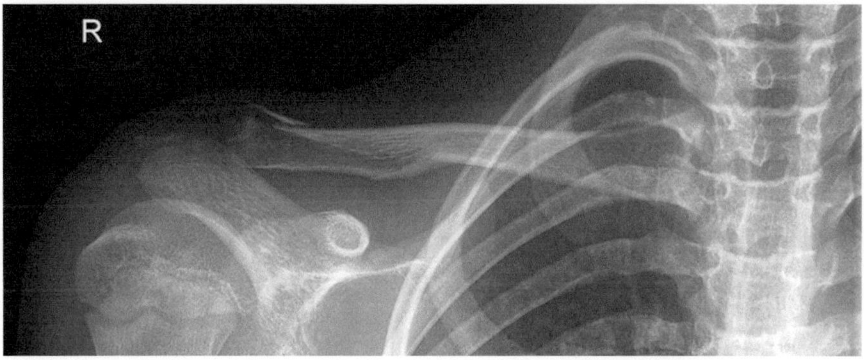

Image 9

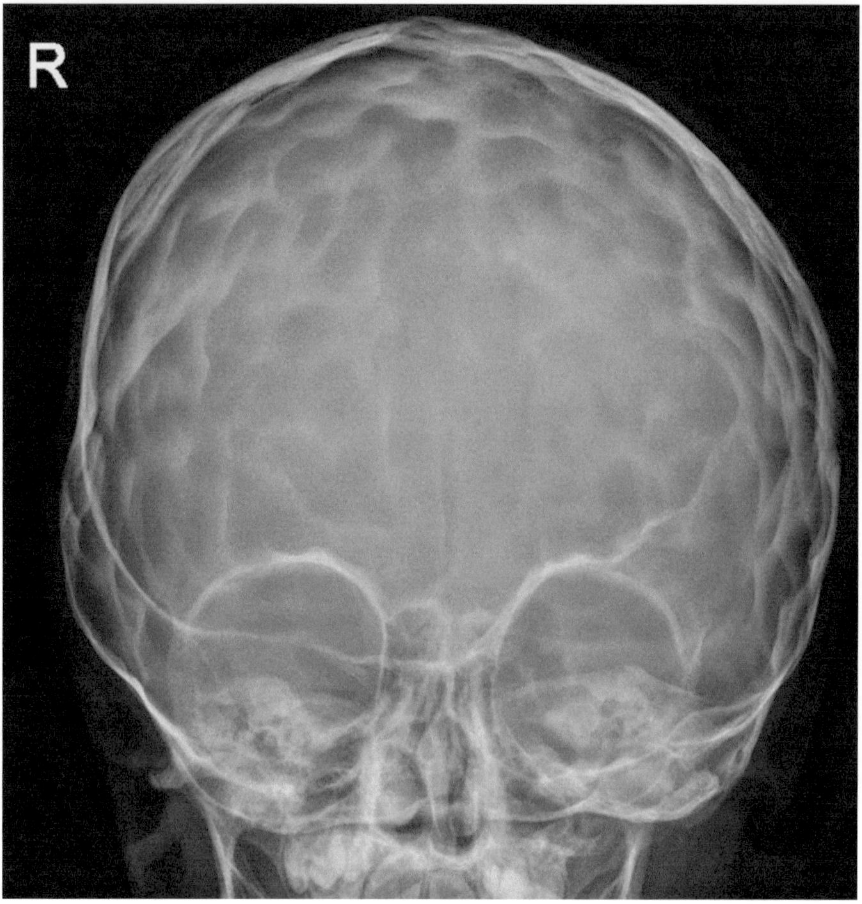

Image 10

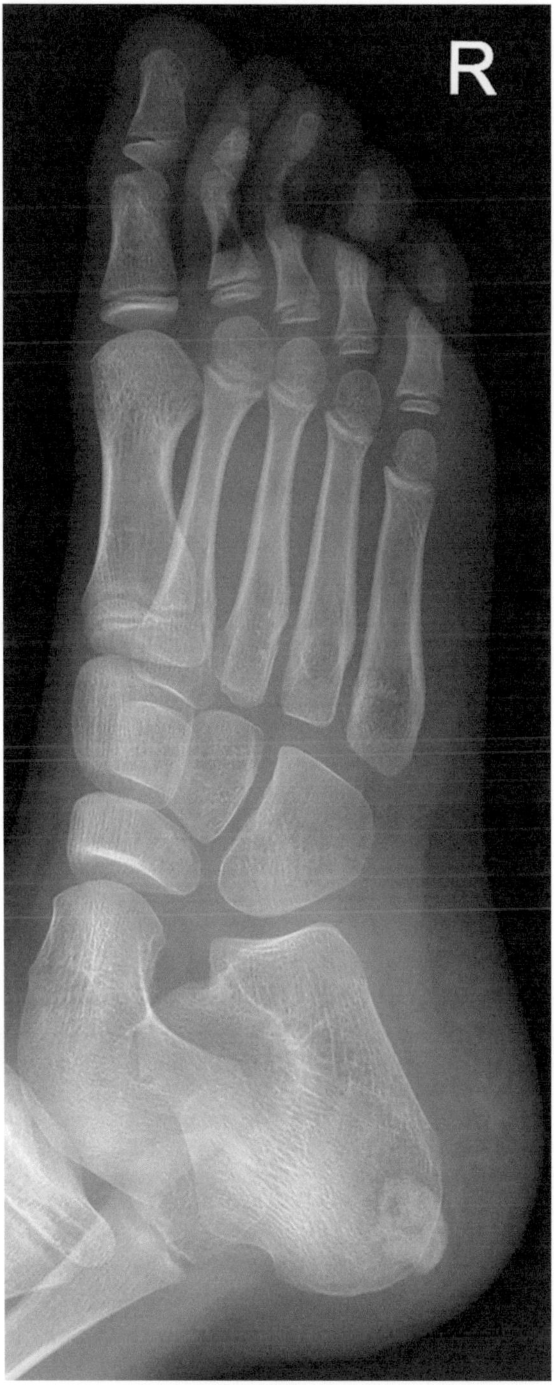

Image 11

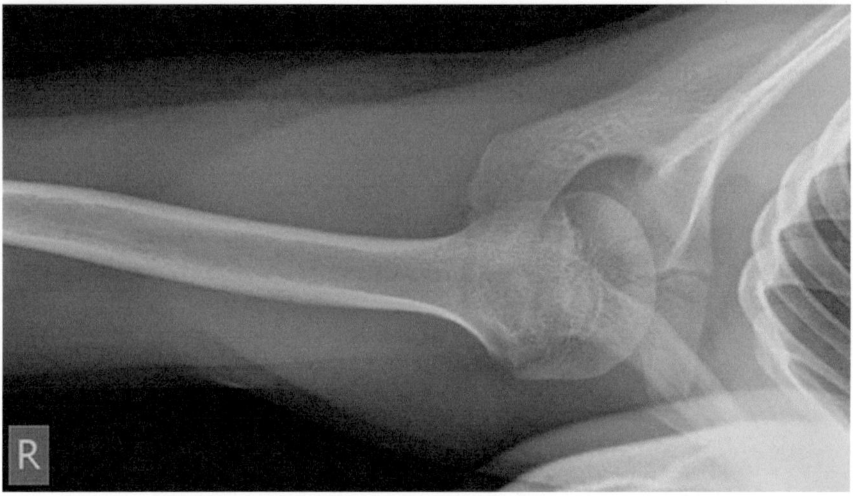

Image 12

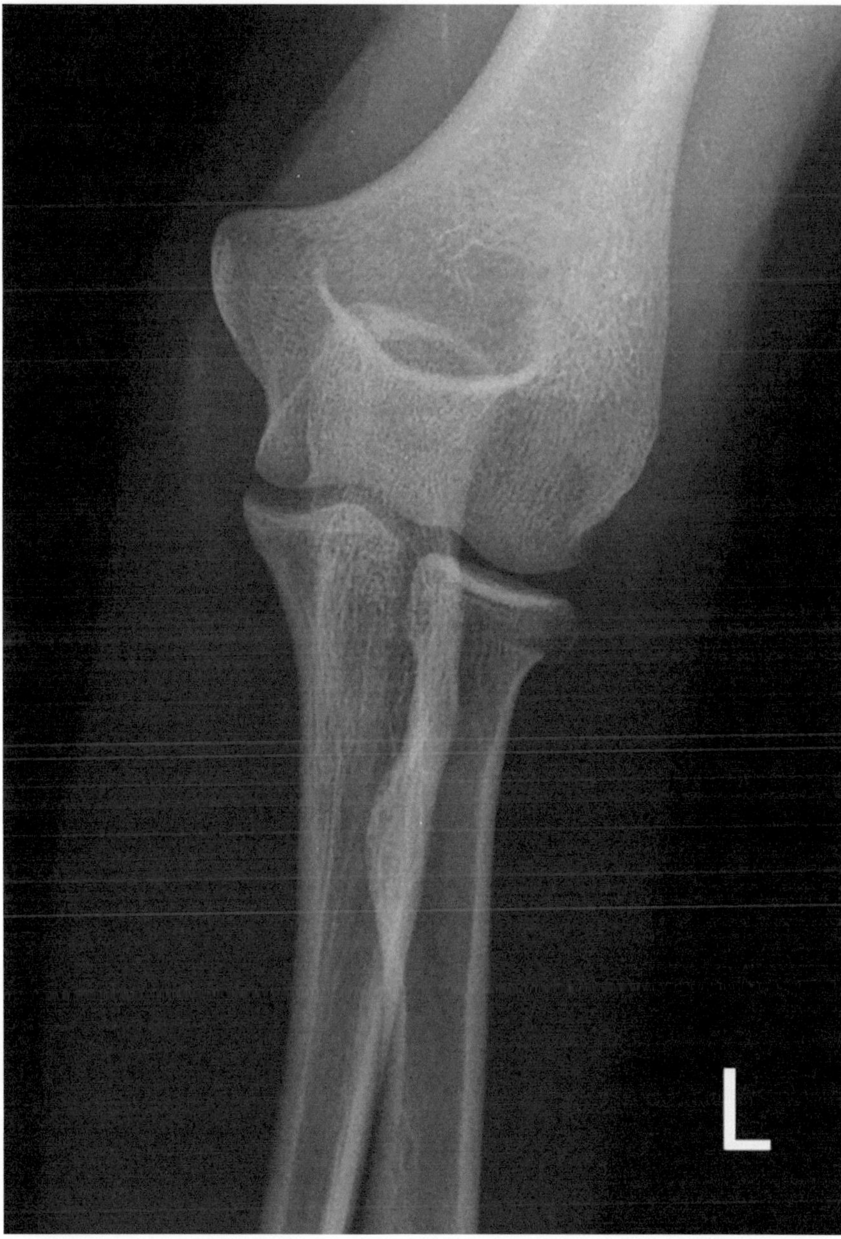

Image 13

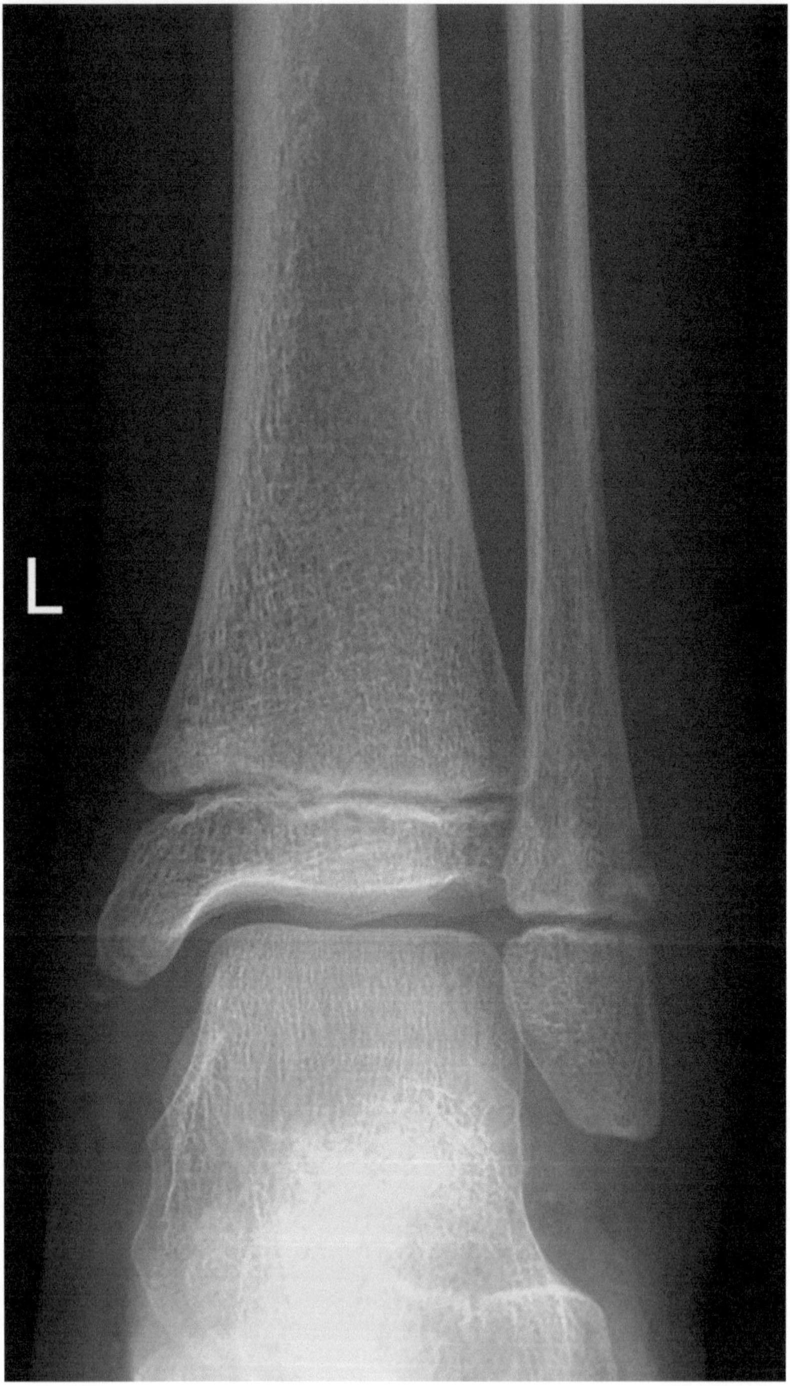

Image 14

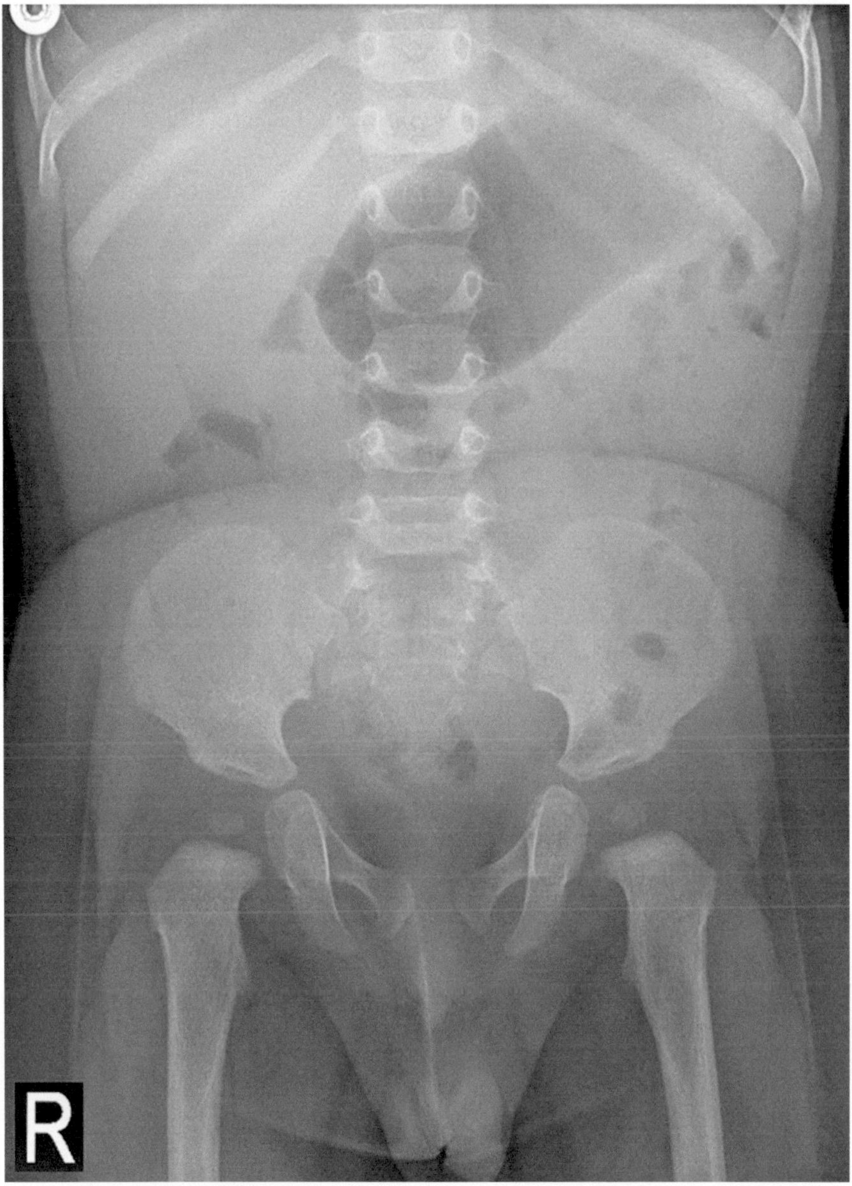

Image 15

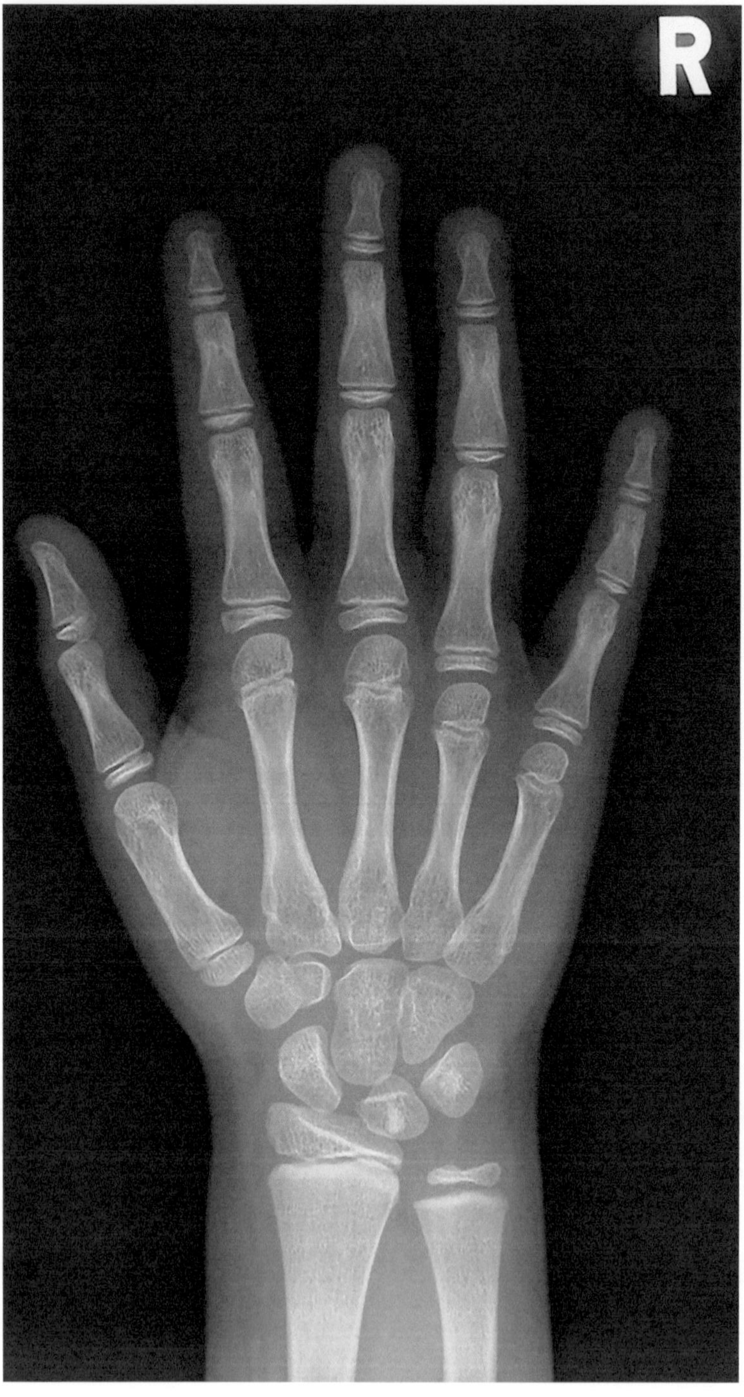

Image 16

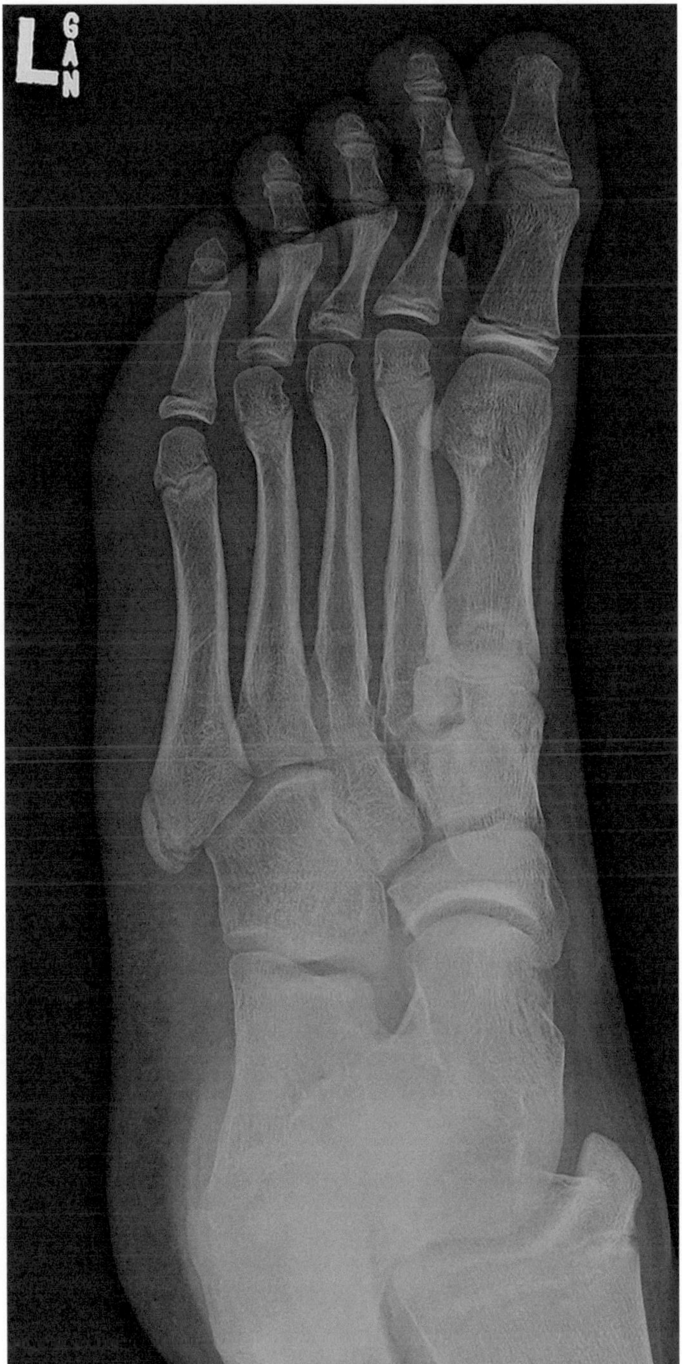

Image 17

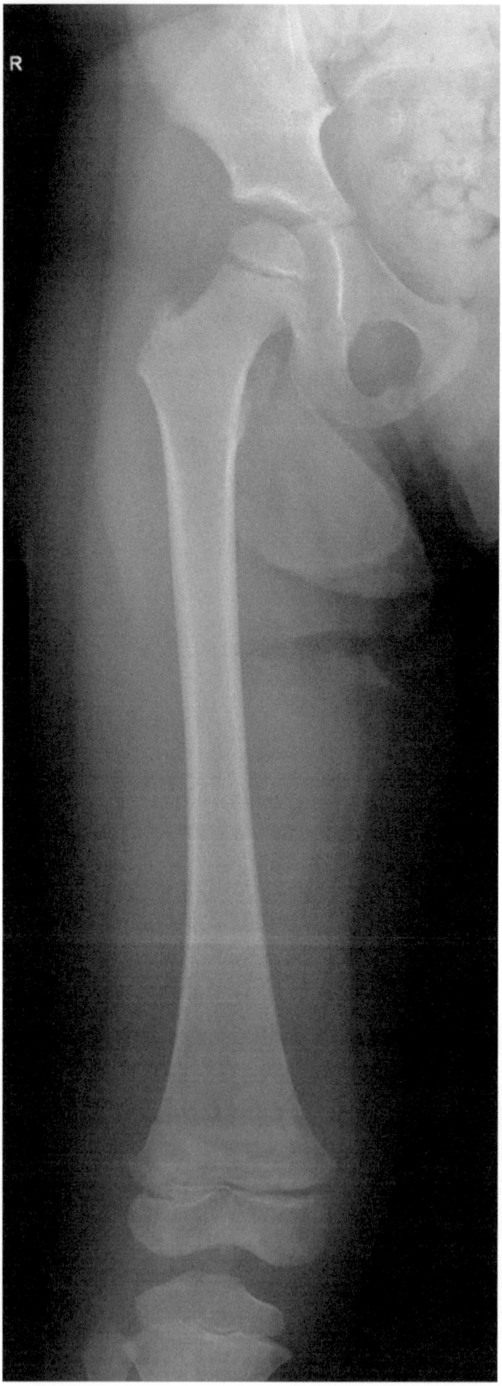

Image 18

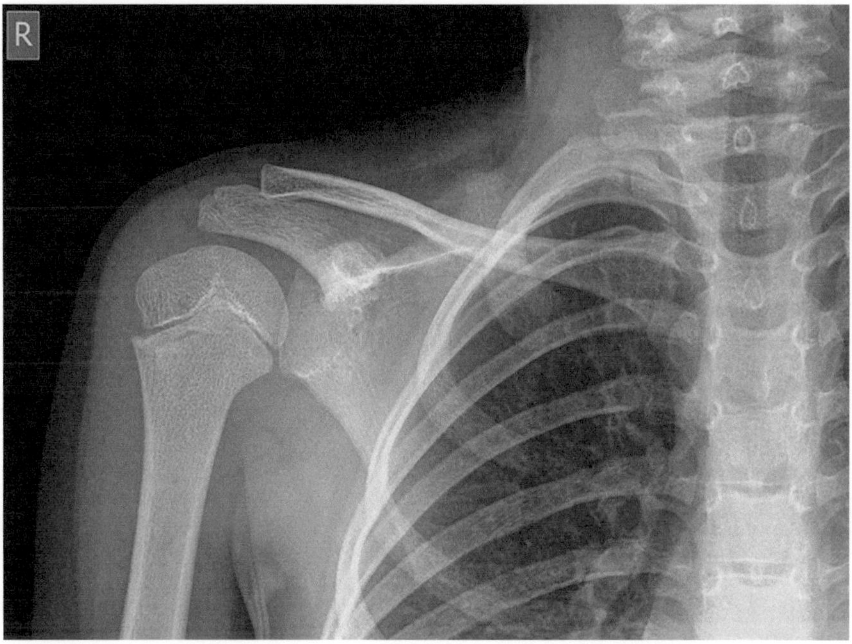

Image 19

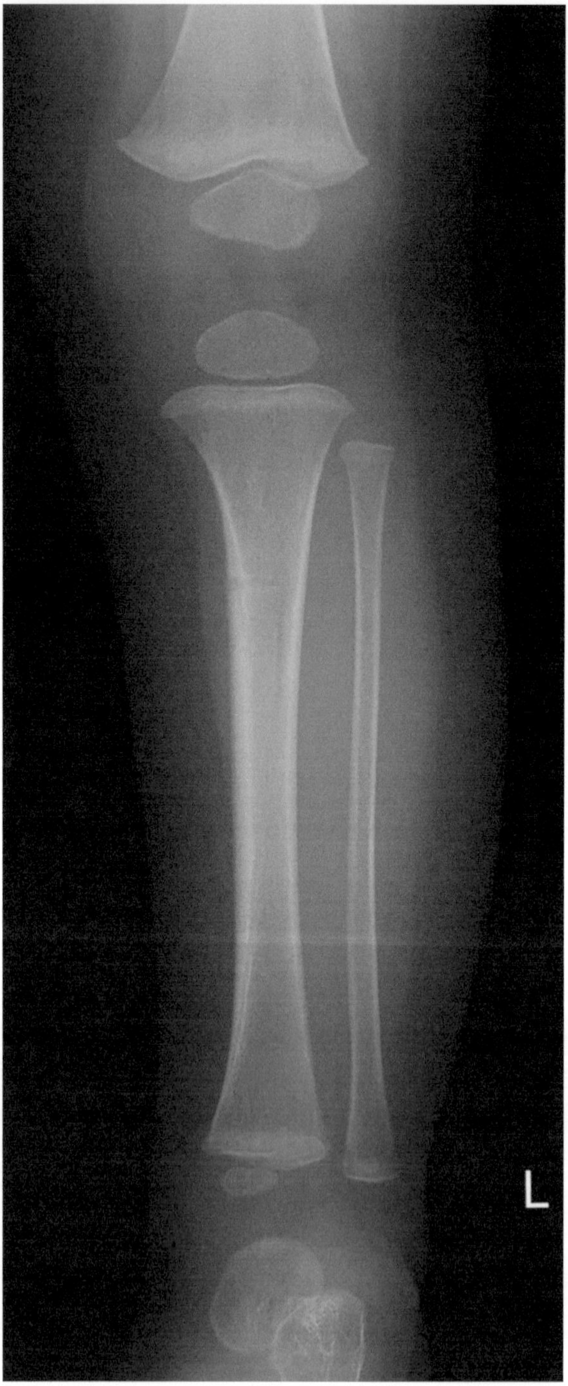

Image 20

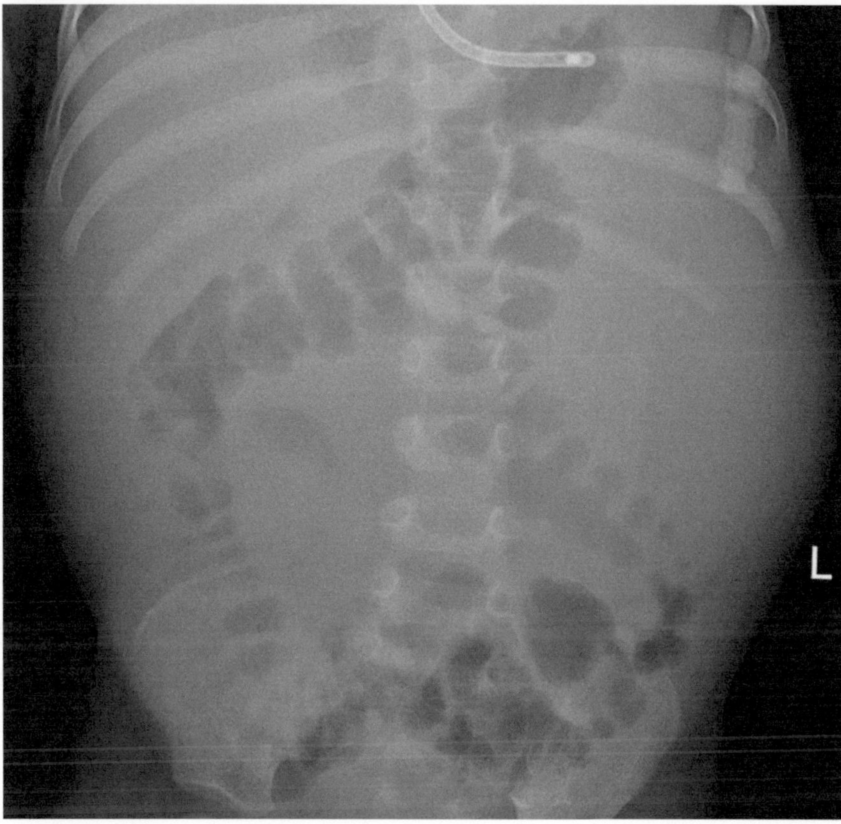

Image 21

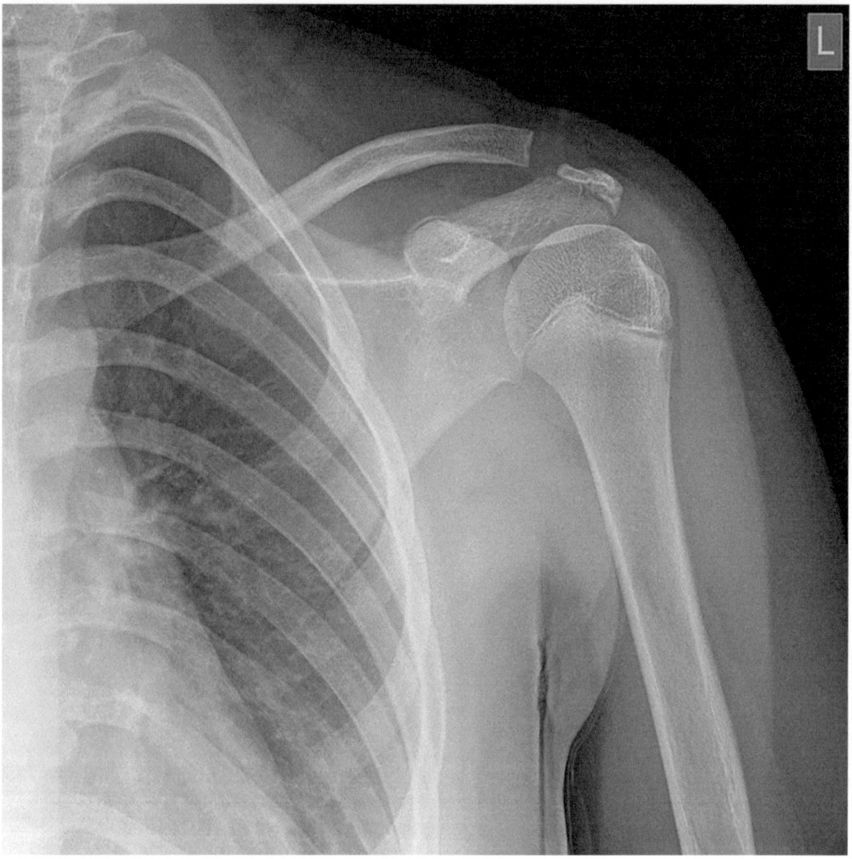

Image 22

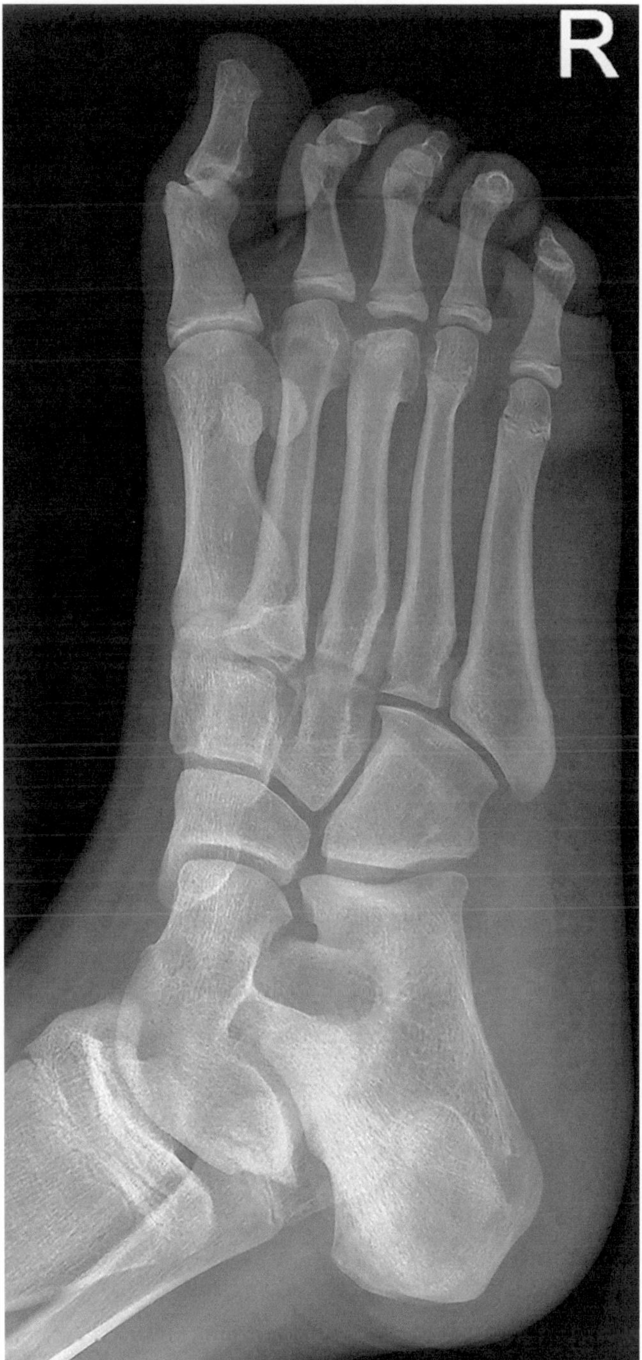

Image 23

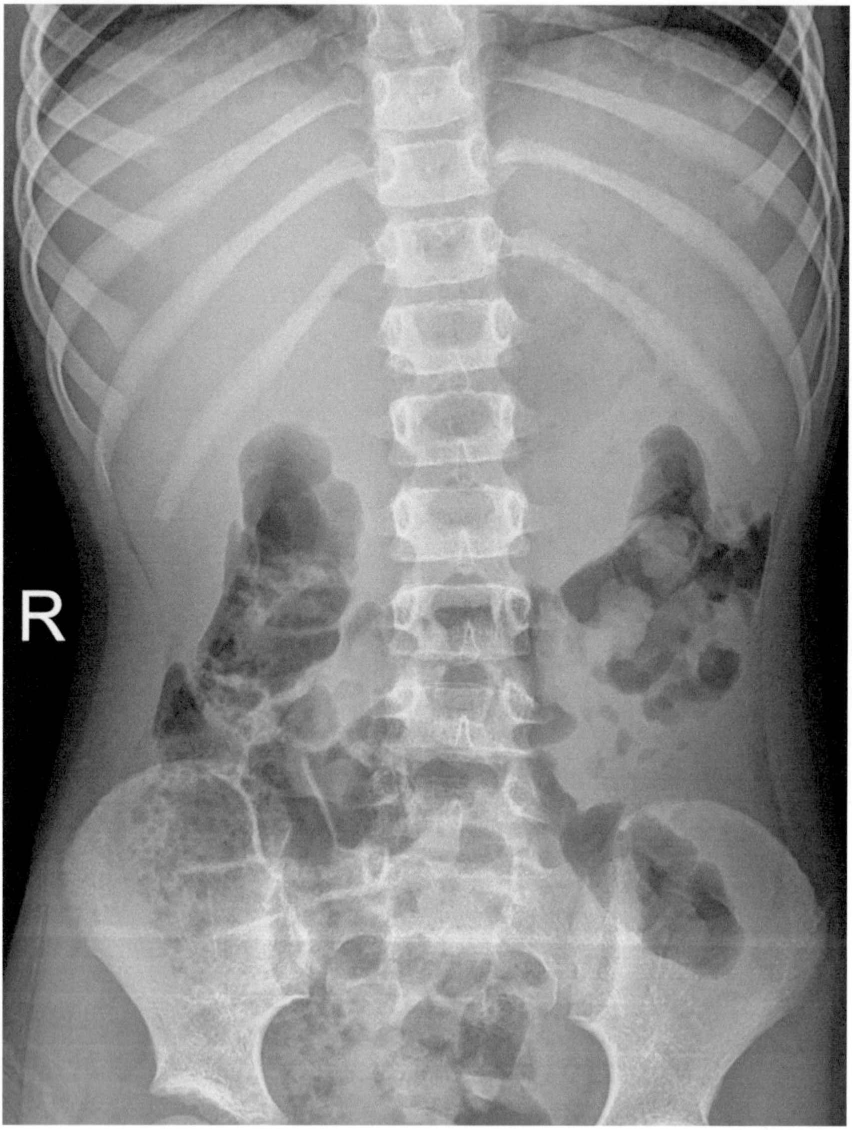

Image 24

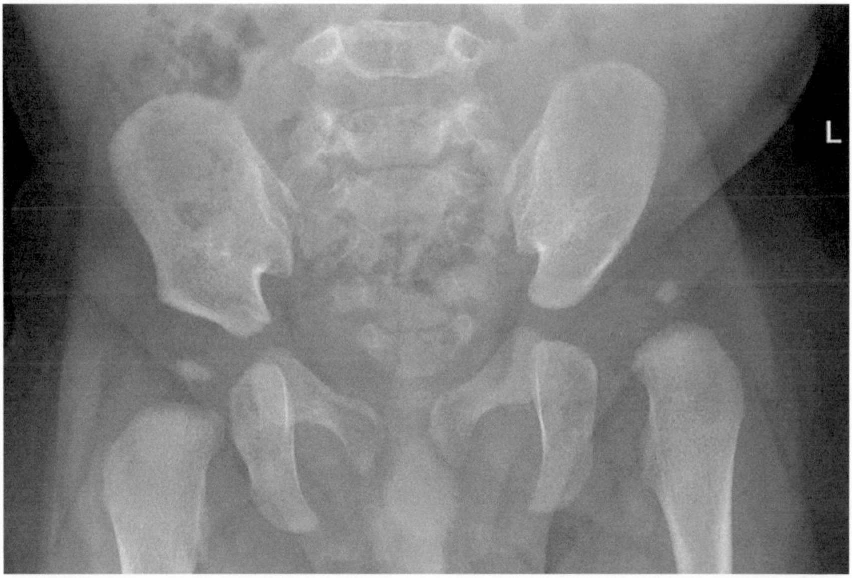

Image 25

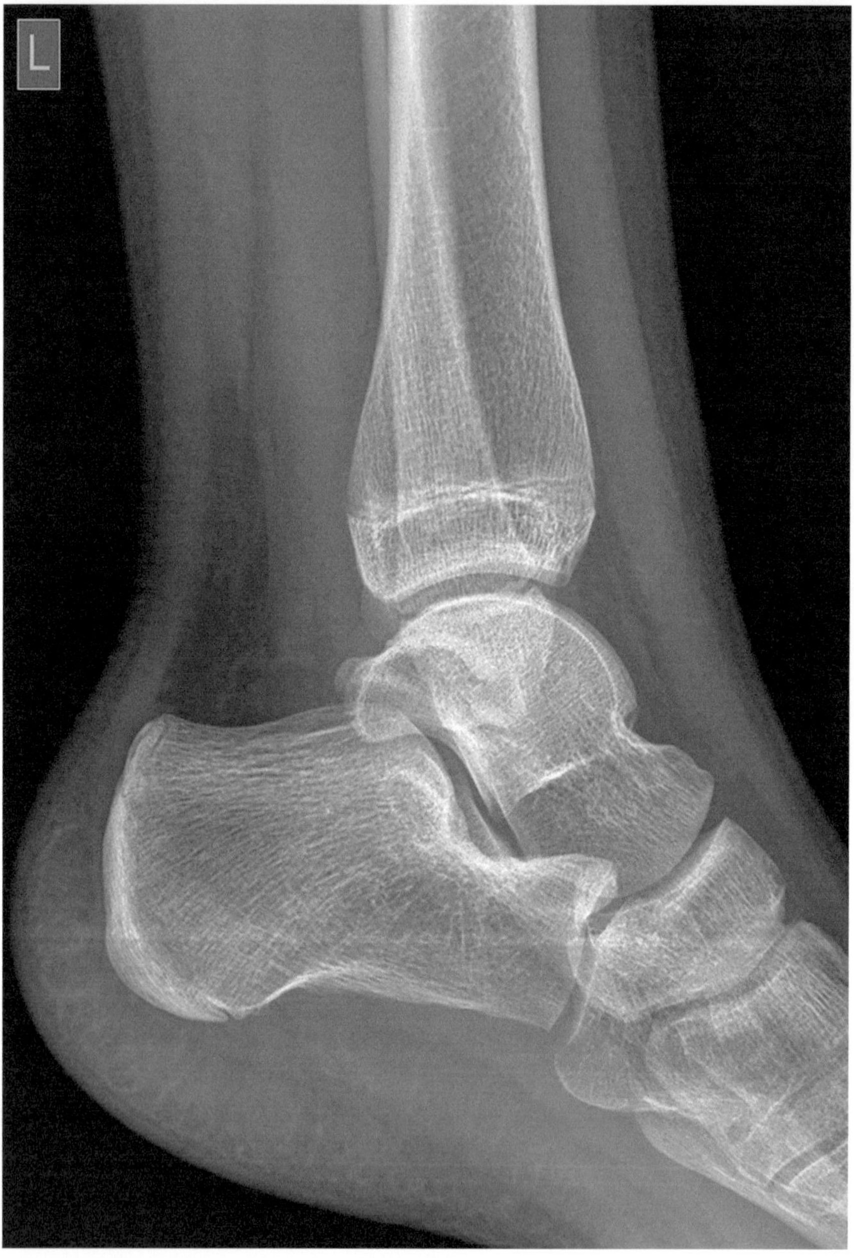

Image 26

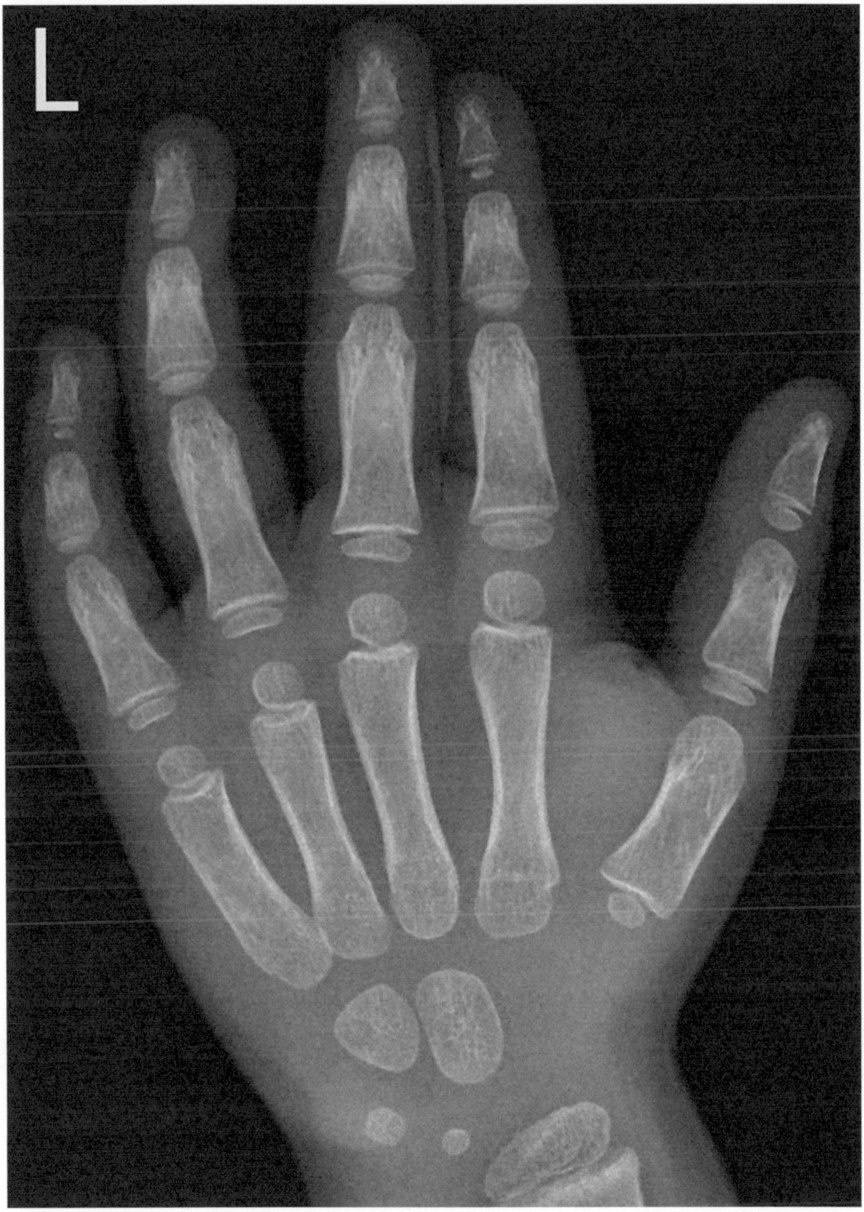

Image 27

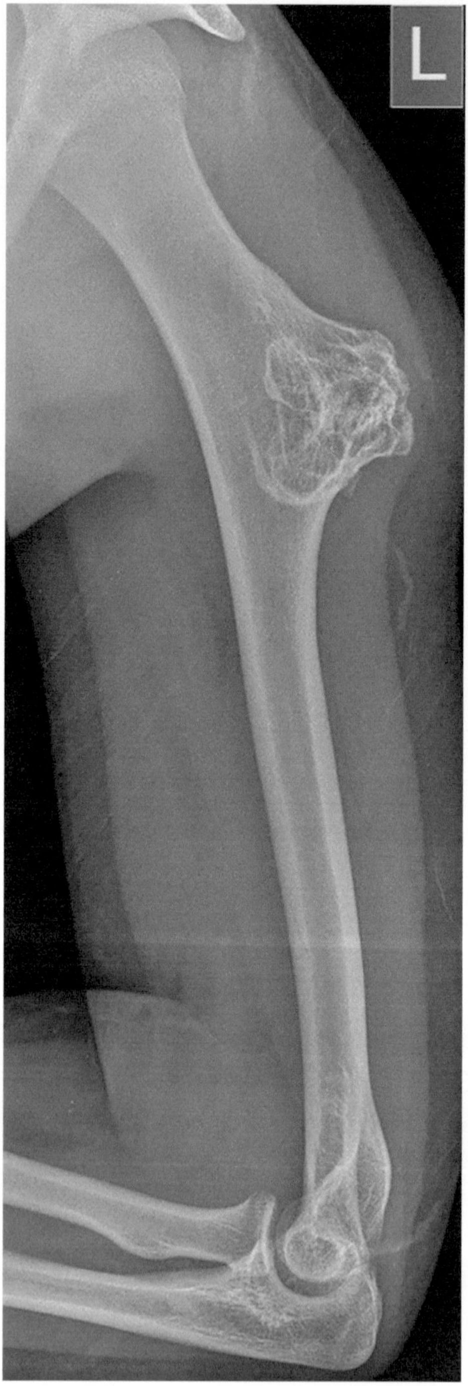

Image 28

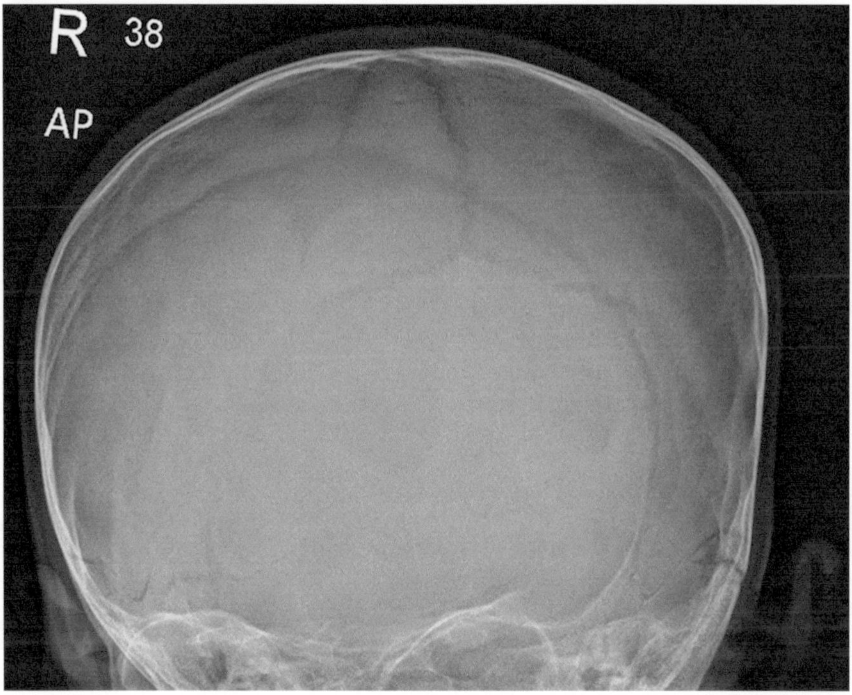

Image 29

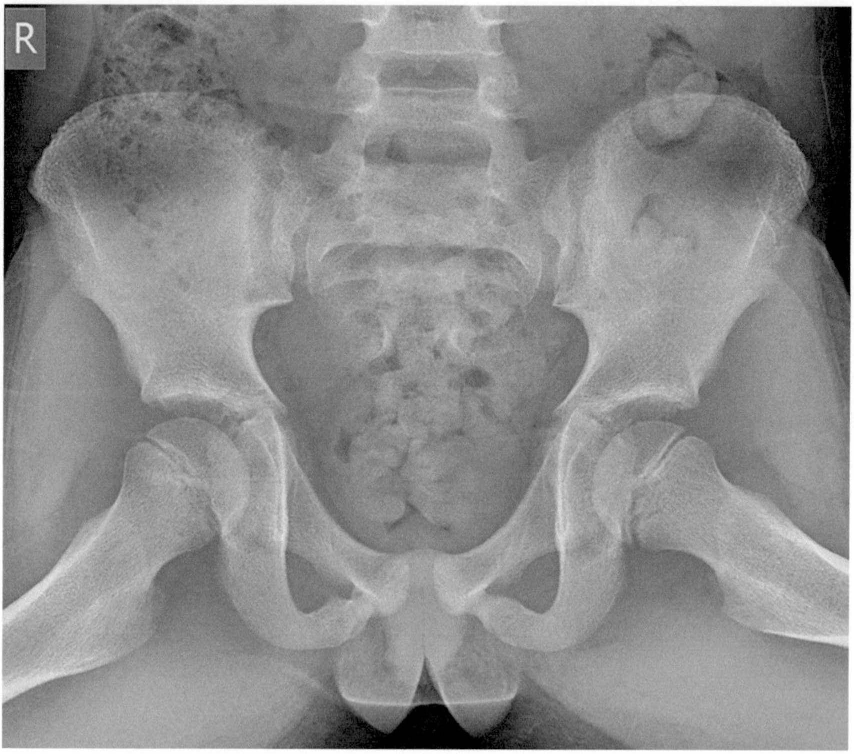

Image 30

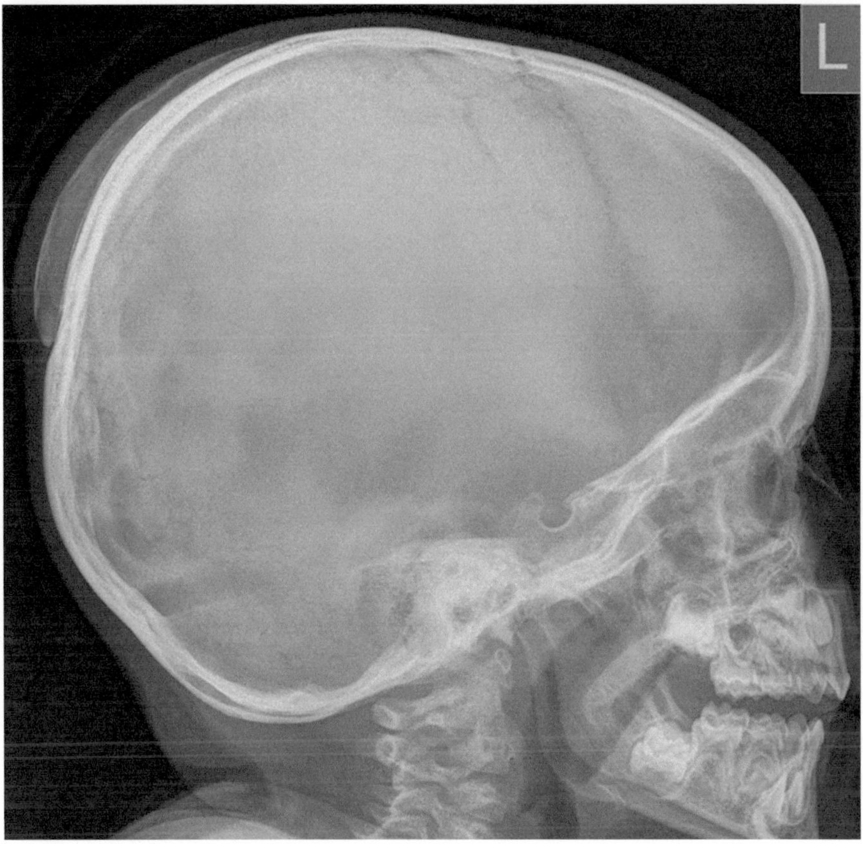

7.2 Answers

Image	Normal	Abnormal	Diagnosis/abnormality (only if abnormal)
1	✓		
2		✓	Healing # R middle finger proximal phalanx
3		✓	# R olecranon
4		✓	Buckle # L distal radial metaphysis
5	✓		
6	✓		
7	✓		
8		✓	Avulsion # R distal clavicle
9		✓	Copper beaten skull
10	✓		
11	✓		
12		✓	# L radial neck
13		✓	Aggressive lesion and periosteal reaction L distal fibula
14	✓		
15	✓		
16		✓	# L fifth metatarsal base
17		✓	SH2 # R distal femur
18	✓		
19		✓	Prior IO needle L proximal tibial diaphysis
20		✓	L upper quadrant mass
21	✓		
22		✓	Osteochondrosis R third metatarsal epiphysis
23	✓		
24		✓	L DDH
25	✓		
26	✓		
27		✓	Exostosis L humeral diaphysis
28	✓		
29	✓		
30		✓	Calcified occipital scalp collection

7.3 Explanations

2. **Healing # R middle finger proximal phalanx**
   There is an incomplete fracture of the radial cortex of the right middle finger proximal phalanx, also known as a greenstick fracture. There is also a buckle fracture of the ulnar cortex. The combination of greenstick and buckle fractures affecting the same bone on opposing cortices is known as a lead pipe fracture due its appearance resembling a lead pipe when it is suddenly bent, i.e. a crack on one side with a bulge on the other. Note the periosteal reaction adjacent to the ulnar cortex buckle fracture in keeping with bony healing.

3. **# R olecranon**
   There is a subtle step of the right olecranon cortex consistent with a minimally displaced fracture. There is an associated elbow joint effusion, typified by elevation of the anterior and posterior fat pads, indicating that this fracture is intraarticular, i.e. it extends to the joint space. The fracture is better visualised in the image below:

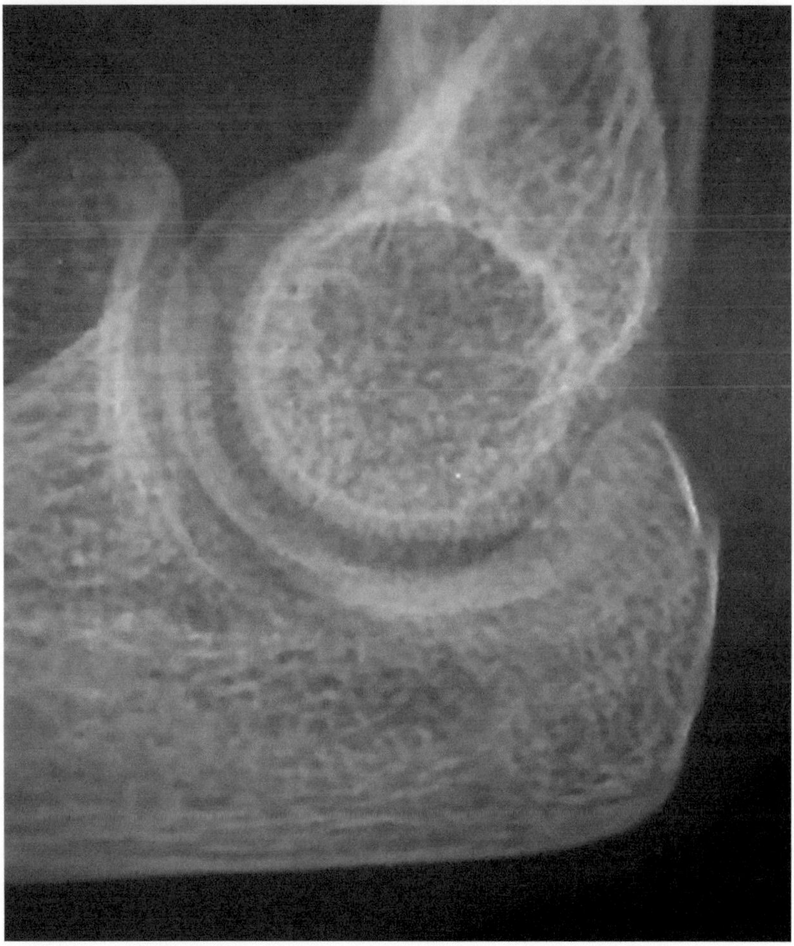

Remember that elbow joint effusions not only result from supracondylar and radial neck fractures (the most and second most common elbow fractures in children, respectively) but from *any* fracture extending to the joint space (even those which are radiographically occult). As discussed previously, elbow joint alignment must be assessed on every radiograph. In this radiograph, the anterior humeral and radiocapitellar alignment are normal. See the explanation for Image 11 of Test 1.

4. **Buckle # L distal radial metaphysis**
   See the explanation for Image 18 of Test 1.

8. **Avulsion # R distal clavicle**
   There is an avulsion fracture of the right distal clavicle which extends to, and involves, the right acromioclavicular joint (ACJ). There is minor cranial displacement of the avulsed fracture fragment. There is no widening of the ACJ, which is normally aligned, and there is no increase in the coracoclavicular distance.

   The irregular ossification adjacent to the acromion represents the *normal* acromion apophysis which has variable appearances at all ages until it fully ossifies and then fuses. The acromion is usually formed by the fusion of several ossification centres between the ages of 15 and 18 years, but which may not be complete until 25 years. An acromion accessory ossification centre which does not fuse results in a fibrocartilaginous connection and is known as an *os acromiale*.

   See the explanation for Image 26 of Test 4 for a discussion of clavicle fractures.

9. **Copper beaten skull**
   This 4-year-old boy with healing rickets has a copper beaten skull appearance on this radiograph. This is due to premature sutural fusion (craniosynostosis) of which healing rickets is an under-recognised cause. This appearance is thought to result from raised intracranial pressure (from the craniosynostosis) which gives rise to the indentations on the inner table of the skull.

10. *Normal right calcaneal apophysis*
    This radiograph is normal. The calcaneal apophysis contributes to the formation of the calcaneal tuberosity and its morphology can be variable across all ages. Secondary ossification usually starts from the plantar third of the apophysis at approximately 7 years of age and progresses dorsally. Physeal fusion begins from around the age of 13 years and finishes at approximately 15 years of age (usually later in boys). The calcaneal apophysis is projected over the body of the calcaneus on this oblique radiograph and its appearance is entirely normal.

11. *Normal right shoulder radiograph*
This axillary view of the right shoulder is normal. The contemporaneous antero-posterior (AP) and dedicated clavicle projections confirmed that there was no fracture: the lucent line medial to the right humeral head is the physis of the coracoid ossification centre which has not yet fused.

12. **# L radial neck**
The cortical step in the left proximal radial metaphysis (neck) in this image is consistent with an acute bony injury. Compare this appearance to that of Image 5 of this test.

13. **Aggressive lesion and periosteal reaction L distal fibula**
There are several radiographic findings in the left distal fibula indicating an aggressive process: irregular lucency; 'moth-eaten'/permeative bone texture; loss of the lateral metaphyseal cortex with scalloping (compare with the normal medial cortex proximally); periosteal reaction of the medial and lateral distal diaphyseal cortices. The periosteal reaction on the lateral cortex has an aggressive appearance consistent with a Codman triangle: see Image 20 of Test 3 for a further example of this, and the explanation for Image 2 of Test 5 for a more general discussion regarding periosteal reaction. There is also significant soft tissue swelling overlying the left distal fibula. The small osseous 'fragment' adjacent to the left distal tibial medial epiphysis represents *normal* ossification for age.

The metaphysis is often the primary site of infection in osteomyelitis, but due to the transphyseal vessels (those which extend across the physis from the metaphysis into the epiphysis) in those less than 18 months of age, direct extension of infection into the epiphysis can result in destruction of the physeal cartilage, physeal arrest, and growth disruption. The epiphyseal extension contributes to the high incidence of septic arthritis. Importantly, one-third of children with osteomyelitis have a history of recent trauma.

The organisms responsible for acute haematogenous osteomyelitis vary with age. The commonest organisms found in neonatal infection are *Staphylococcus aureus* followed by group A *Streptococcus* (GAS) and *Escherichia coli* (and other enteric gram-negative bacilli). *Kingella kingae* is increasingly recognised as a cause of osteomyelitis and septic arthritis worldwide in children less than 5 years of age. Notably, *Salmonella* subspecies (ssp.) infection is a more common cause of osteomyelitis in patients with sickle cell disease.

The radiographic changes of osteomyelitis, all of which are seen in this case, may include focal osteopenia, lysis and/or cortical loss, endosteal scalloping, and loss of bony trabecular architecture. Magnetic resonance imaging (MRI) is the most sensitive and specific imaging modality for detecting osteomyelitis which may be radiographically occult early in its course.

Tip for the viva:

- Normal radiographic appearances do not exclude osteomyelitis as the radiographic features may not be apparent for up to 14 days. If there is ongoing clinical concern, follow-up radiography could be performed 5–7 days following initial radiographs (10–14 days in adults) but ultimately MRI may be required given its increased sensitivity.

14. *Normal abdominal radiograph*
When infants and children cry (a common occurrence when radiography is being performed), they may swallow a lot of air (aerophagia) which distends their stomach as seen in this radiograph. However, there is no air-fluid level to indicate gastric outflow obstruction. The remainder of the bowel gas pattern is normal, as are the bony structures. Both hips are enlocated with normal appearances of both proximal femoral epiphyses.

Tip for the viva:

- The hip joints must be assessed on every abdominal radiograph, particularly when the imaging has been performed for another indication: you may be the first person to detect subluxation resulting from developmental dysplasia of the hip (DDH), slipped upper femoral epiphyses (SUFE), or the early changes of avascular necrosis (AVN) of the proximal femoral epiphyses/Perthes disease.

16. **# L fifth metatarsal base**
The unfused base of the left fifth metatarsal apophysis is aligned vertically (parallel) to the orientation of the metatarsals, as expected. However, there is also a seperate minimally displaced transverse fracture through the proximal base of the left fifth metatarsal which extends through the base of the adjacent apophysis. This is better visualised in the magnified image below:

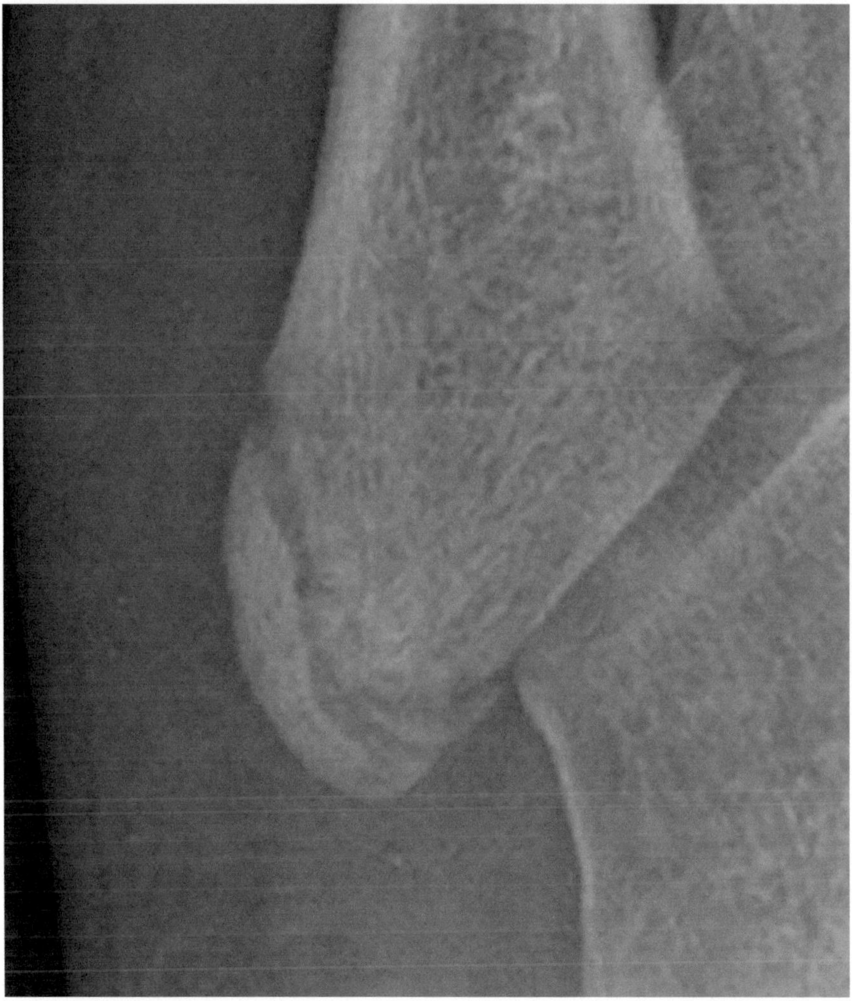

See the explanation for Image 7 of Test 1. Moreover, note the slightly flattened appearance of the second metatarsal head which may be seen in a small proportion of patients: see the explanation for Image 22 of this test.

17. **Salter-Harris 2 # R distal femur**
There is a minimally displaced Salter-Harris 2 fracture of the right distal femoral metaphysis with associated soft tissue swelling. See the explanation for Image 30 of Test 1.

19. **Prior interosseous needle L proximal tibial diaphysis**
The well-defined linear lucency in the medial left proximal tibial diaphysis relates to prior insertion of an interosseous (IO) needle. Note the reactive thickening of the medial tibial cortex. An IO needle is used in emergency situations when intravenous (IV) access is either delayed or difficult to obtain.

This radiograph was obtained as part of a skeletal survey in a 1-month-old boy who was initially presented to the Emergency Department (ED) after becoming unresponsive following a 'fall off the bed'. An IO needle was placed at the time of resuscitation. Subsequent head computed tomography (CT) demonstrated a right parietal skull fracture extending into the occipital bone with diastasis (defined as separation of body parts which are normally joined, i.e. widening) of the right lambdoid suture along with a large underlying extradural haematoma. Given the infant's age and the presenting mechanism, it was felt that these injuries were inflicted.

It is unlikely that this image would appear in the Rapid Reporting component of the examination; however, we have included it just in case it appears in any of the other components.

20. **L upper quadrant mass**
There is a paucity of bowel gas in the left upper quadrant with inferomedial displacement of the splenic flexure of the colon. There is a subtle focus of calcification within the mass just inferior to the anterior end of the left 12th rib. A subsequent ultrasound and MRI were performed which demonstrated a large mass: metaiodobenzylguanidine (MIBG) scintigraphy confirmed the diagnosis of neuroblastoma.

Tip for the viva:

- Be sure to assess the bones for any aggressive features and the imaged lungs for any pulmonary nodules suggesting metastases in the context of an abdominal mass.

22. **Osteochondrosis R third metatarsal epiphysis**
Osteochondrosis of the metatarsal epiphyses (or heads in adults), also known as Freiberg infraction, is thought to result from either acute or repetitive trauma, as in this 11-year-old gymnast presenting with foot pain. It often presents with swelling and pain on weight-bearing, more frequently in active adolescent girls (athletes, dancers, etc.). The radiographic features include flattening of the metatarsal head, sclerosis, cortical thickening, and widening of the affected metatarsophalangeal joint. Typically, the second metatarsal head is affected but the third (as in this case) and fourth metatarsal heads may also be affected. The changes may be bilateral in up to 10% of cases. Remember that flattening of the metatarsal head in the absence of other associated radiographic findings of osteochondrosis may be seen in up to 10% of the *asymptomatic* population: see Image 16 of this test for an example of this.

In general, eponyms should be avoided in the examination except for when this is not possible or cannot be avoided, e.g. in the case of a Monteggia fracture-dislocation or a Tillaux fracture. Under pressure, eponyms with similar names or in similar anatomical locations may get confused, e.g. stating Köhler disease (osteonecrosis of the navicular) instead of Freiberg infraction (as in this case) would be incorrect. The examiner needs to ensure that you have identified the abnormality correctly: for the avoidance of doubt, writing the abnormality out in full, instead of its eponym, ensures that you are clear in your responses.

24. **L developmental dysplasia of the hip**
The left hip is almost completely dislocated with the shallow left acetabulum covering only a portion of left proximal femoral epiphysis. Do not forget that the proximal femoral epiphysis is cartilaginous until it begins to ossify at approximately 6 months of age before which ultrasound is the primary imaging modality employed in the assessment of DDH. There is also coxa valga (an increased angle between the femoral metaphysis and diaphysis). See the explanation for Image 17 of Test 2.

27. **Exostosis L humeral diaphysis**
Exostoses are benign bony outgrowths arising from the surface of the bone. The medullary cavity of the exostosis is usually continuous with the parent bone and is covered by periosteum. They typically arise during childhood but can present at any age and are most frequently encountered incidentally.
When exostoses are capped with cartilage, they are known as osteochondromas and are considered a chondroid neoplasm. Osteochondromas may be congenital or result from previous trauma to the physis. They typically grow *away* from the adjacent joint and given that they represent growth of the physis in an abnormal direction, they usually stop growing once skeletal maturity has been reached, i.e. when the physis has fused. Once present, they do not regress.
Osteochrondromas can be:
- Solitary: these are of low malignant potential if sporadic and solitary (approximately 1%).
- Multiple: (autosomal dominant) hereditary multiple exostoses (HME) account for up to 15% of cases of osteochondromatosis. The cartilage cap can undergo malignant transformation to low grade chondrosarcoma. As the most common associated malignancy, the risk is higher than in cases of solitary osteochondroma (approximately 10% but possibly as high as 25%). Historically, the term 'diaphyseal aclasis' (*aclasis*, from the Greek meaning continuity of structure between normal and pathological tissue) was previously used for what we now refer to as HME and should no longer be used.
- Sessile (attached directly at the base).
- Pedunculated (attached by a stalk or peduncle).

When osteochondromas arise from the epiphysis, consider dysplasia epiphysealis hemimelica as a diagnosis, so termed for its propensity to involve half of an affected limb. This is a rare non-hereditary disease which is eponymously known as Trevor's disease. The lower limb is more commonly affected than the upper limb: the distal femur is a frequent location with the medial and distal aspects typically involved.

Ultrasound accurately assesses the presence of a cartilage cap. While CT may demonstrate the cartilage cap, MRI is the best modality to measure the thickness of any cartilage cap as well as assessing surrounding soft tissue, marrow oedema and malignant degeneration. A cartilage cap measuring over *2 cm* is suspicious for malignant change (MRI has 100% sensitivity for the detection of malignant degeneration when a cut off of 2 cm is used). Remember that in assessment with contrast-enhanced MRI, chondrosarcoma displays internal *septal* enhancement, whereas osteochondroma displays *peripheral* enhancement. The mnemonic **GLADPAST** can be used to remember the features of sarcomatous degeneration of an osteochondroma:

- **G**rowth after skeletal maturity.
- **L**ucency (new).
- **A**dditional scintigraphic activity.
- **D**estruction (cortical).
- **P**ain after puberty.
- **A**nd.
- **S**oft tissue mass.
- **T**hickened cartilage cap greater than 2 cm.

The 14-year-old girl in this case originally presented at the age of 10 years with shoulder pain with radiographs demonstrating the exostosis arising from the left proximal humeral diaphysis. Presentation is usually with pain from local pressure effects, pathological fracture (for which the radiograph should be scrutinised) or malignant degeneration (look for features of an aggressive bone lesion, e.g. cortical irregularity/bone destruction, moth-eaten lucency/permeative texture, a wide zone of transition, an associated soft tissue mass etc.). Once an exostosis has been found, look for others exostoses suggesting a diagnosis of HME.

28. *Normal skull radiograph*

This radiograph is normal. The obliquity of this AP projection allows the cranial sutures to be well visualised. Correlate with the references for Image 26 of Test 2 and compare with Image 9 of this test in which there is a copper beaten skull secondary to craniosynostosis.

30. **Calcified occipital scalp collection**

This child was referred by her General Practitioner (GP) for an ultrasound of her scalp after presenting with a large, non-tender, fluctuant swelling at the vertex. On questioning, she disclosed that she had previously hit her head on a door handle. The ultrasound revealed a compressible subcutaneous fluid collection/haematoma at the location of the calcified occipital scalp collection visualised in this radiograph. Subsequent CT demonstrated the collection to be subgaleal in location. While the location cannot be reliably ascertained from this lateral radiograph, identifying it as a calcified occipital scalp collection would be sufficient in the examination.

When considering the three main types of scalp haematoma (caput succedaneum, subgaleal haematoma, and cephalohaematoma), it is helpful to remember the layers of the scalp in which they lie, which can be best remembered using the mnemonic, **SCALP**:

- **S**kin: a subcutaneous (below the skin) collection of serosanguinous fluid/haematoma is known as *caput succedaneum* (from the Latin, literally meaning 'head' + 'substitute', presumably referring to how the normal head shape is temporarily 'substituted' for another). These collections usually result from pressure on the presenting part of the skull from the dilating cervix and/or bony pelvis during a prolonged second stage of labour. Although they can be ill-defined and may cross the midline if extensive, these are usually simple and self-limiting.
- **C**onnective tissue.
- **A**poneurosis: this tough sheet of fibrous connective tissue is also known as the epicranial aponeurosis or *galea* (from the Latin meaning 'helmet'). Its anterior attachment, the frontalis muscle, inserts on the frontal bone and its posterior attachment, the occipitalis muscle, inserts on the external occipital protuberance of the occipital bone. Subgaleal haematomas are found beneath the galea but above the loose connective tissue and commonly occur following a ventouse/vacuum delivery. Not being bound by sutures, subgaleal haematomas may extend from the orbit to the nape of the neck, i.e. the anterior to posterior aponeurotic insertions, and feel ill-defined on clinical examination. They are potentially lethal and there have been reported neonatal deaths secondary to extensive subgaleal haemorrhage. Neonates can lose a significant amount of their circulating blood volume following a traumatic/difficult delivery: the average circulating volume of a neonate is approximately 300 mL and the aponeurotic space may hold up to 260 mL. Thus, prompt recognition is vital.
- **L**oose connective tissue.
- **P**eriosteum: the periosteum is the outermost layer which covers the bones. Haematomas found in the potential subperiosteal space (the space between the periosteum and the bone) are known as cephalohaematomas and result from rupture of subperiosteal vessels from birth trauma/assisted delivery (e.g. forceps, ventouse/vacuum delivery). Given their location, cephalohaematomas are bound by the periosteum and therefore *cannot* cross suture lines, thus distinguishing them from subgaleal haematomas which *can* cross suture lines. Cephalohaematomas can be thought of as extradural haematomas but on the external side of the skull. They may be unilateral or bilateral and, when long-standing, will usually calcify and gradually resolve by incorporation into the underlying skull (as demonstrated in the radiograph in this case), which may result in deformity.

Representative figures of the various types of scalp collections discussed above are available in the references.

Further Reading

Image 2

Alsmair A et al (2022) Lead pipe fracture. https://radiopaedia.org/articles/lead-pipe-fracture-1. Accessed Sep 2023

Image 9

Forestier-Zhang LY, Arundel P, Gilbey-Cross R et al (2021) Short report: craniosynostosis, a late complication of nutritional rickets. J Pediatr Endocrinol Metab 34(8):1055–1060

Image 10

Murphy A et al (2022) Calcaneal apophysis. https://radiopaedia.org/articles/calcaneal-apophysis. Accessed Aug 2023
Rossi I, Rosenburg Z, Zember J (2016) Normal skeletal development and imaging pitfalls of the calcaneal apophysis: MRI features. Skelet Radiol 45(4):483–493
Vergara AE, Erazo ALM, Moreno GLÁ (2017) Calcaneus normal radiological patterns in children. Revista Cubana de Ortopedia y Traumatología 31(1):1–11

Image 13

Jaramillo D, Dormans JP, Delgado J et al (2017) Haematogenous osteomyelitis in infants and children: imaging of a changing disease. Radiology 283(3):629–643
Thakolkaran N, Shetty AK (2019) Acute hematogenous osteomyelitis in children. Ochsner J 19(2):116–122
Yap J et al (2023) Osteomyelitis. https://radiopaedia.org/articles/osteomyelitis. Accessed Aug 2023

Image 18

Whooley PJ (2021) Proximal humeral fractures. https://dontforgetthebubbles.com/proximal-humeral-fractures/. Accessed Aug 2023
Whooley PJ, Foley J (2022) Shoulder x-ray interpretation. https://dontforgetthebubbles.com/shoulder-x-ray-interpretation/. Accessed Aug 2023

Image 22

Carter KR, Chambers AR, Dreyer MA (2022) Freiberg Infraction. https://www.ncbi.nlm.nih.gov/books/NBK537308/. Accessed Aug 2023
Sheth U et al (2022) Freiberg's disease. https://www.orthobullets.com/foot-and-ankle/7018/freibergs-disease. Accessed Aug 2023
Yap J et al (2023) Freiberg disease. https://radiopaedia.org/articles/freiberg-disease. Accessed Aug 2023

Image 24

Ranchod AI et al (2023) Coxa valga. https://radiopaedia.org/articles/coxa-valga. Accessed Aug 2023

Image 27

Baba Y et al (2023) Osteochondroma. https://radiopaedia.org/articles/osteochondroma. Accessed Aug 2023
Kumar K et al (2023) Hereditary multiple exostoses. https://radiopaedia.org/articles/hereditary-multiple-exostoses. Accessed Aug 2023
Tepelenis K, Papathanakos G, Kitsouli A et al (2021) Osteochondromas: an updated review of epidemiology, pathogenesis, clinical presentation, radiological features and treatment options. In Vivo 35(2):681–691
Weerakkody Y et al (2023) Exostosis. https://radiopaedia.org/articles/exostosis. Accessed Aug 2023
Yap J et al (2023) Dysplasia epiphysealis hemimelica. https://radiopaedia.org/articles/dysplasia-epiphysealis-hemimelica-1. Accessed Aug 2023

Image 30

Al Kabbani A et al (2019) Caput succedaneum. https://radiopaedia.org/articles/caput-succedaneum. Accessed Aug 2023
Chaturvedi A, Chaturvedi A, Stanescu AL et al (2018) Mechanical birth-related trauma to the neonate: an imaging perspective. Insights Imaging 9(1):103–118
Christensen TR, Bahr TM, Henry E et al (2023) Neonatal subgaleal hemorrhage: twenty years of trends in incidence, associations, and outcomes. J Perinatol 43(5):573–577
Howden W et al (2022) Galea aponeurotica. https://radiopaedia.org/articles/galea-aponeurotica. Accessed Aug 2023
Yap J et al (2022) https://radiopaedia.org/articles/cephalohaematoma. Accessed Aug 2023

Test 8

8

M. Paddock et al., *Paediatric Radiology Rapid Reporting*,
https://doi.org/10.1007/978-3-031-48255-7_8

8.1 Images

Image 1

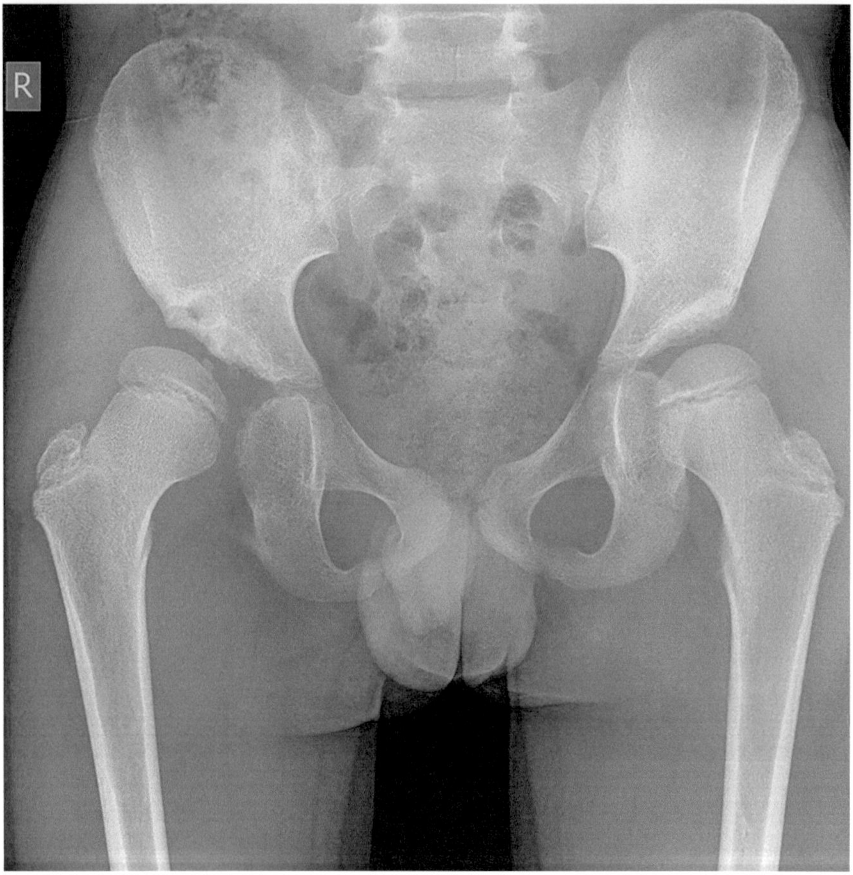

Image 2

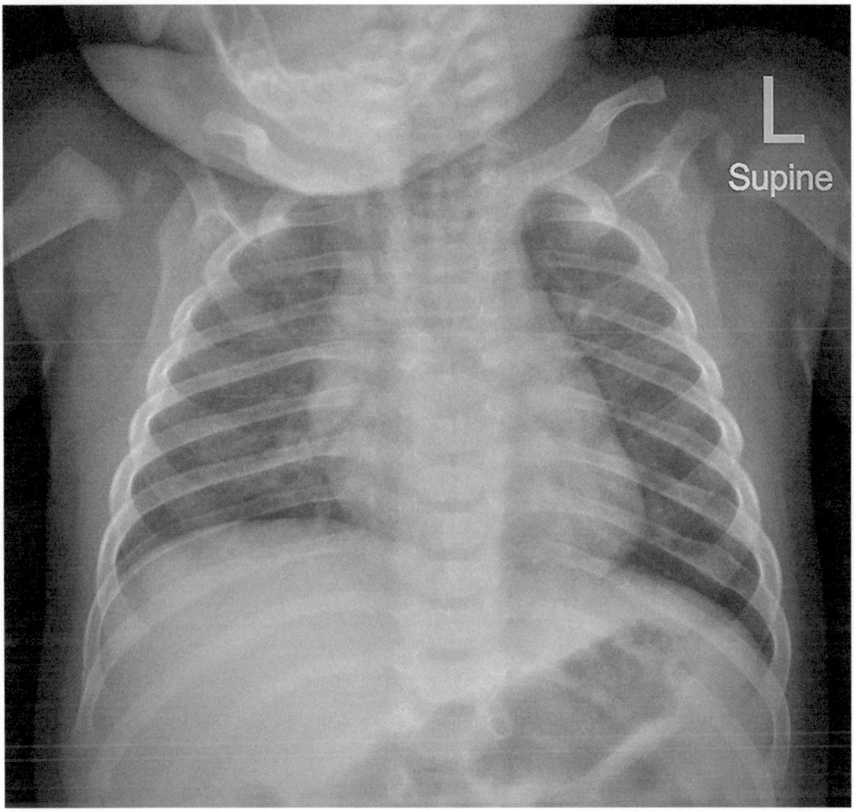

Image 3

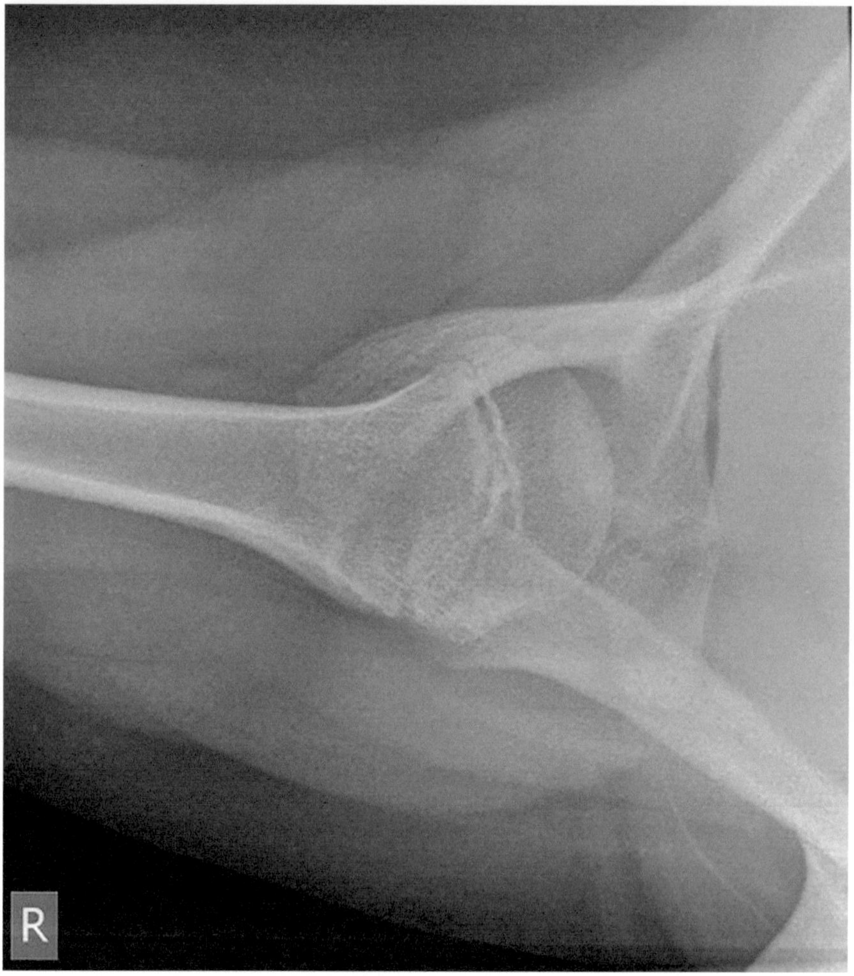

Image 4

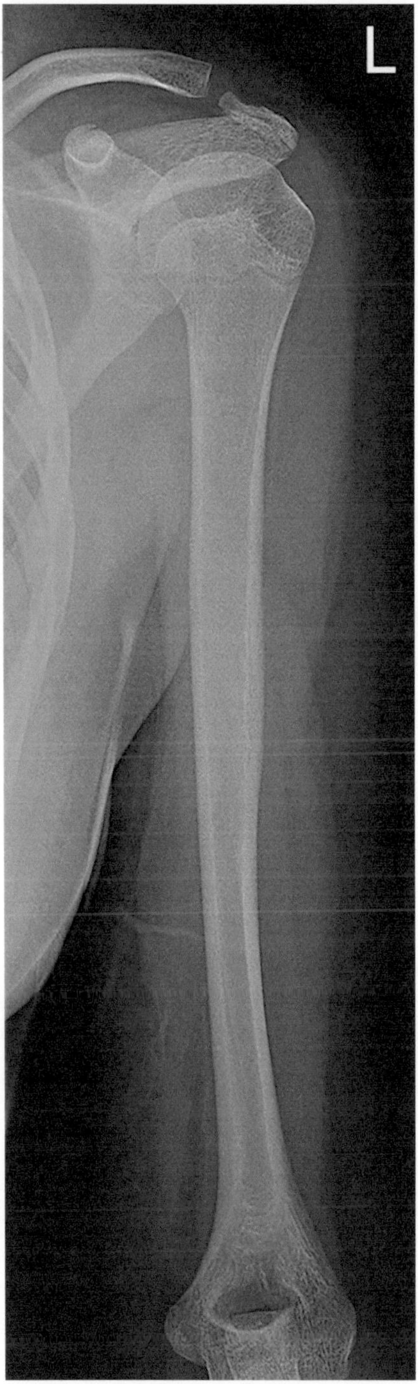

Image 5

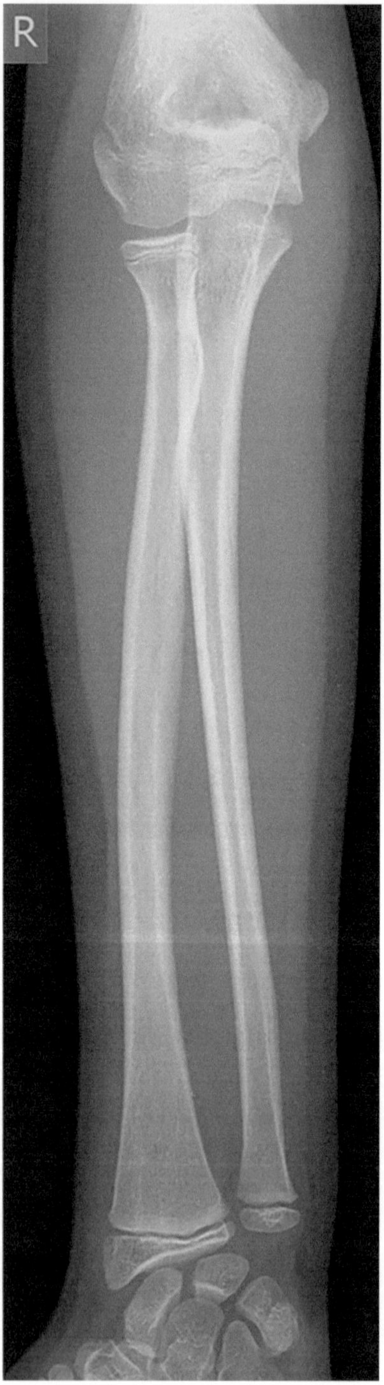

Image 6

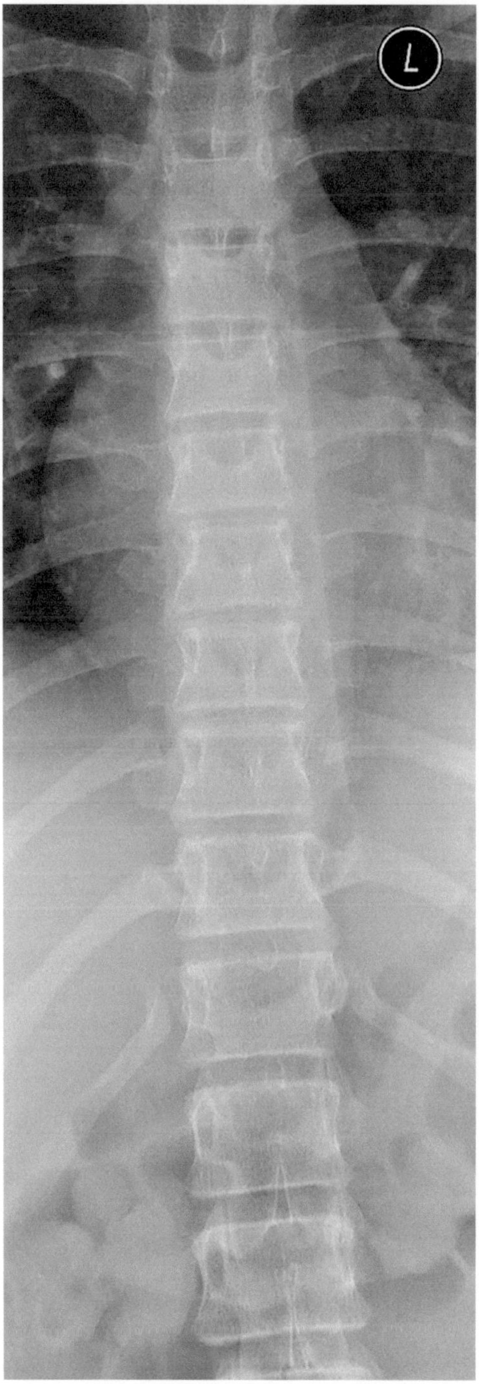

Image 7

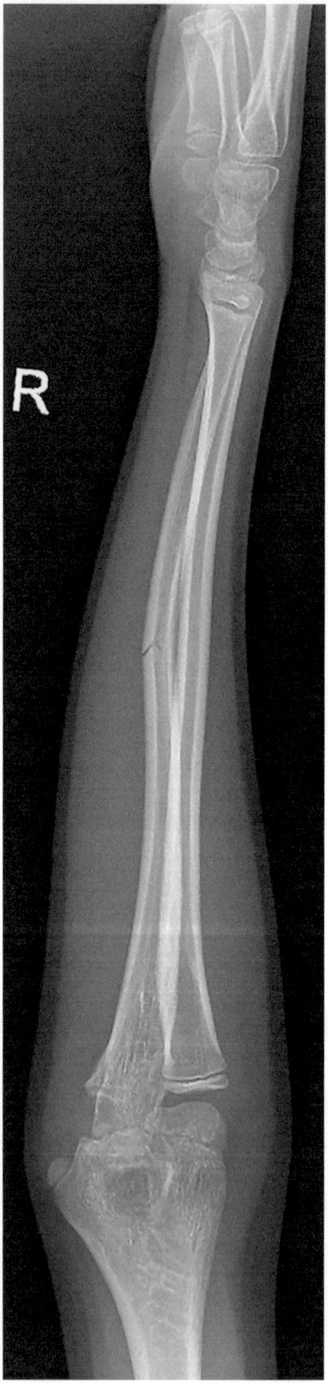

Image 8

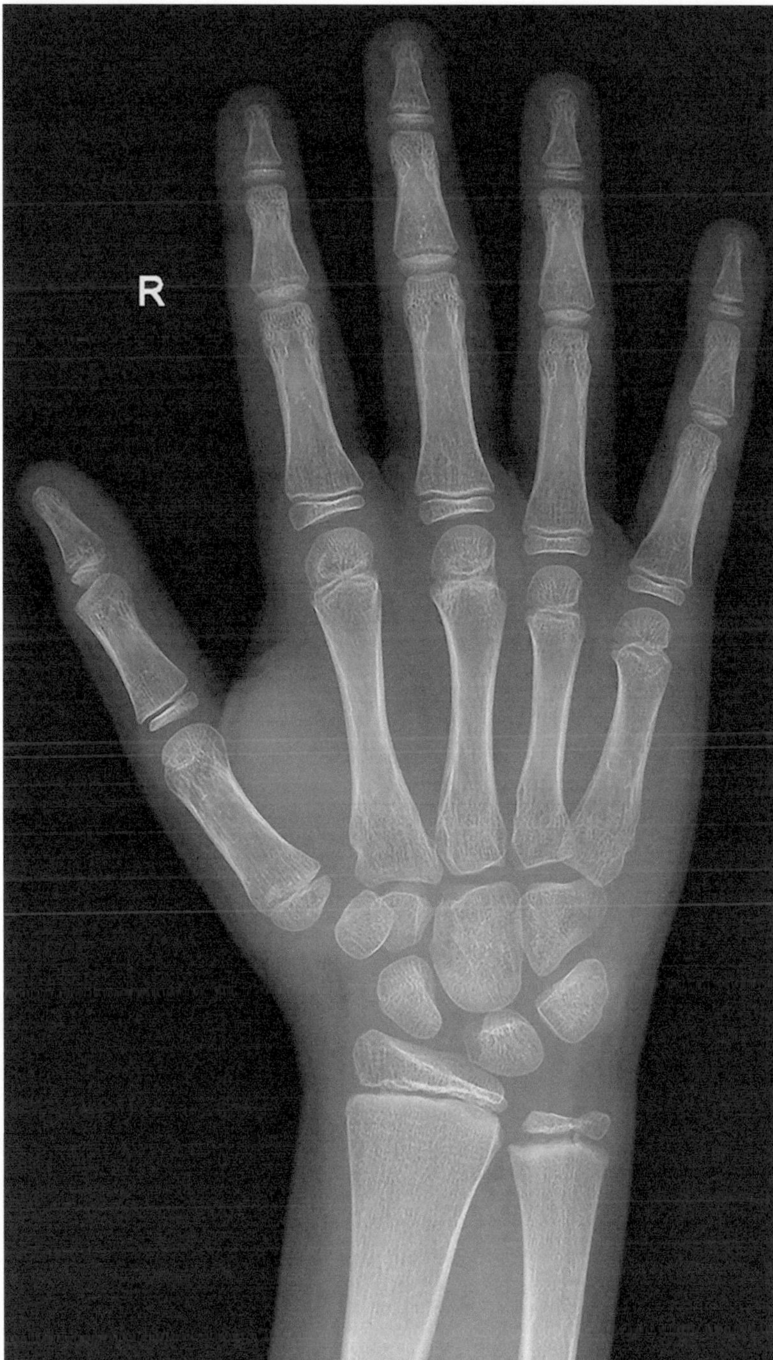

Image 9

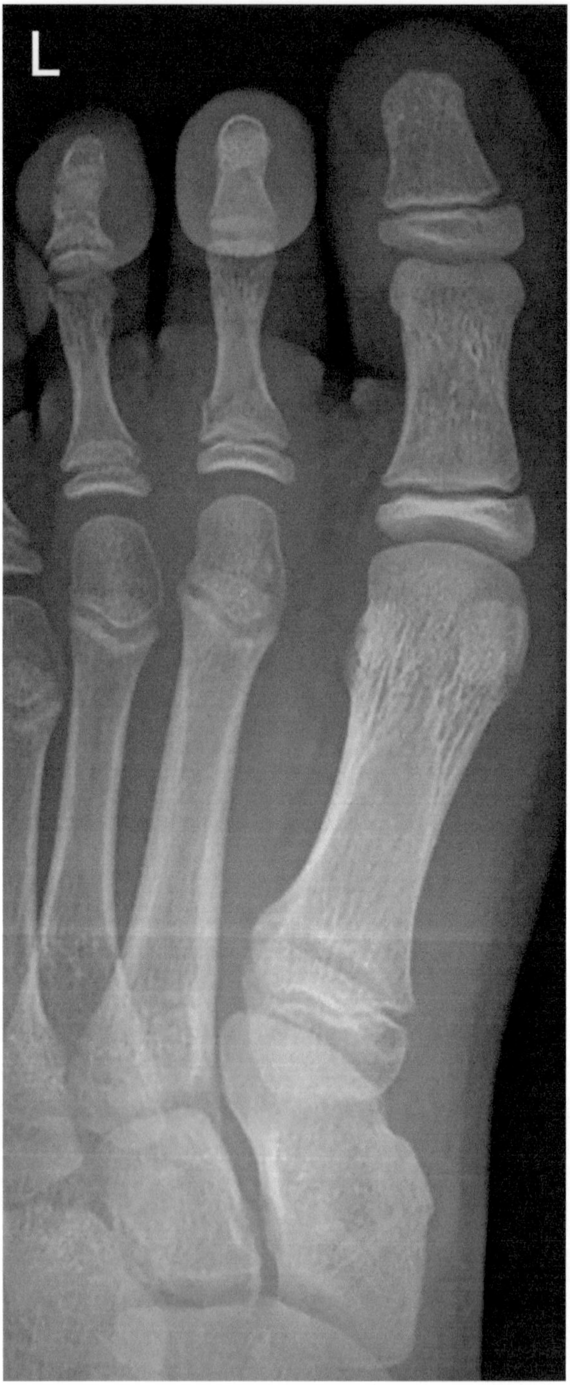

Image 10

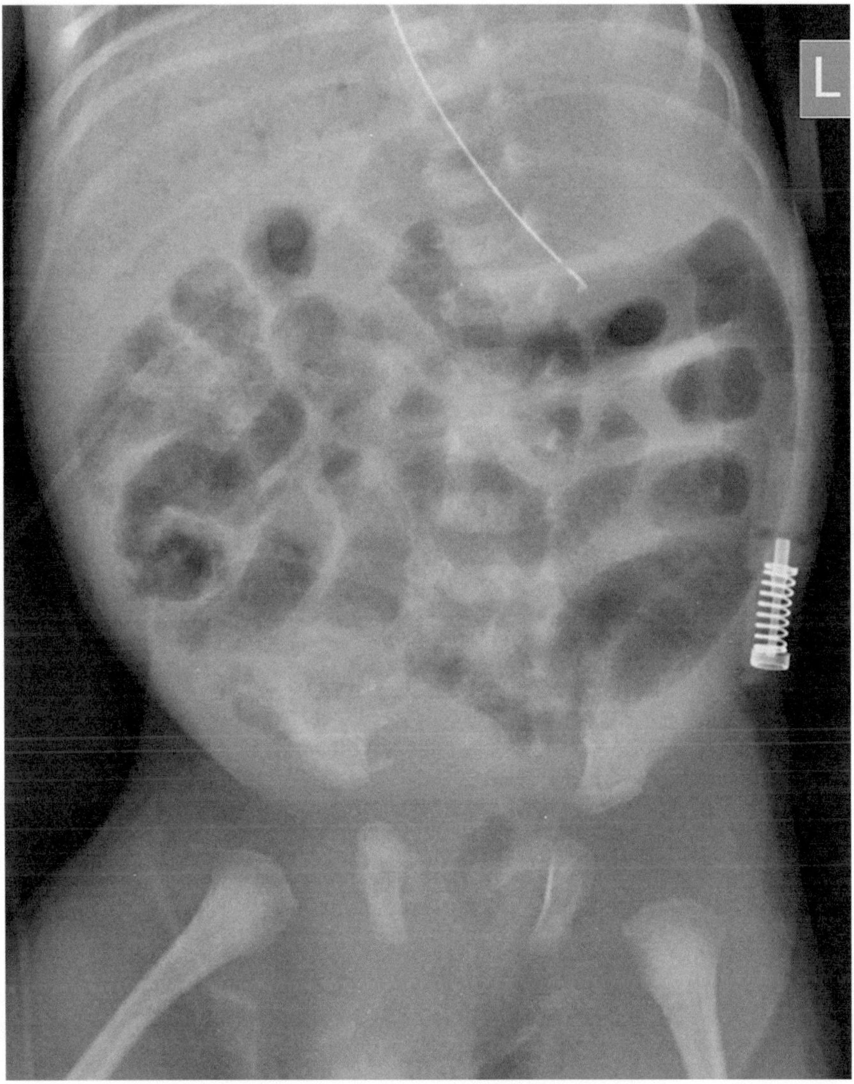

Image 11

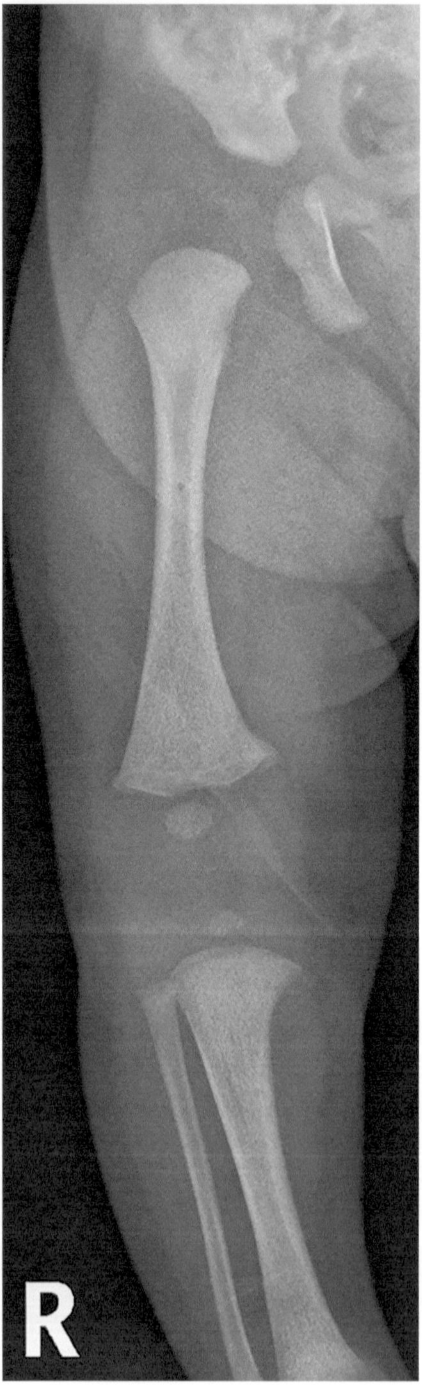

Image 12

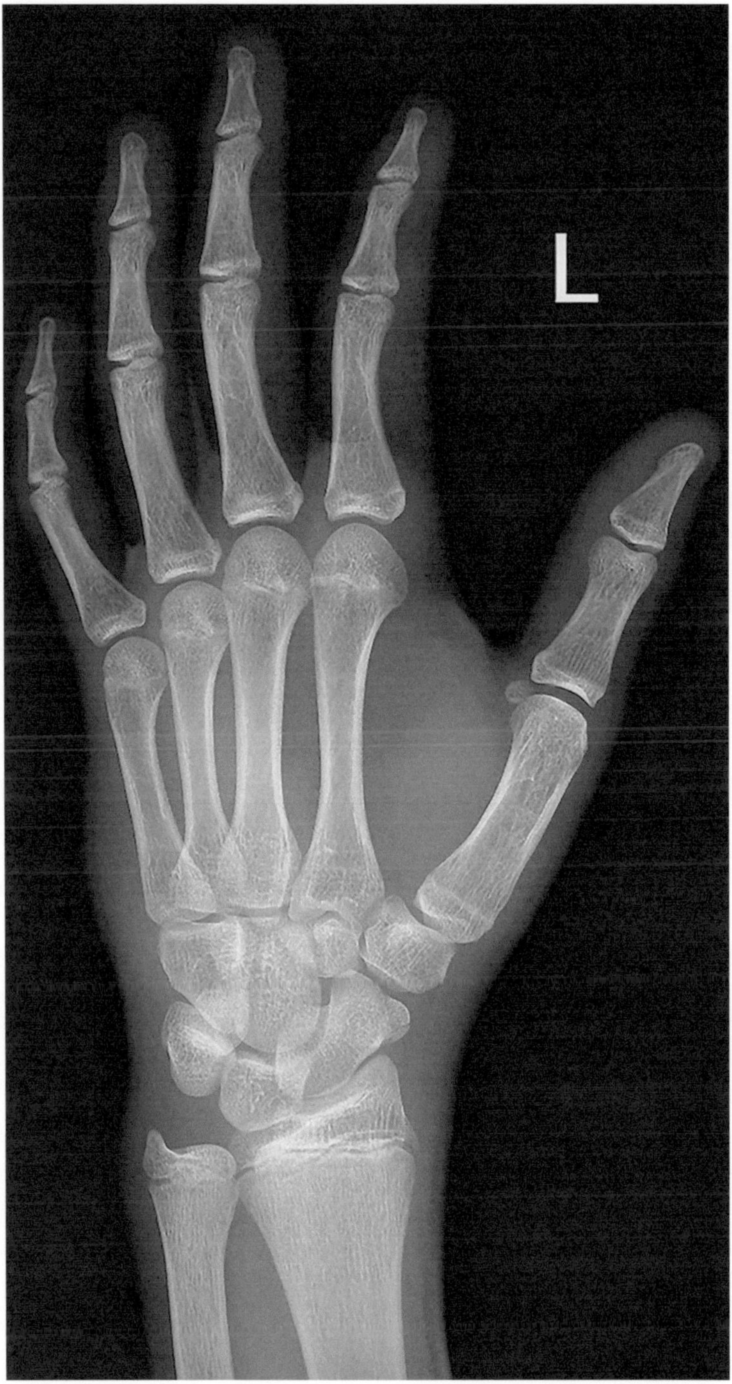

Image 13

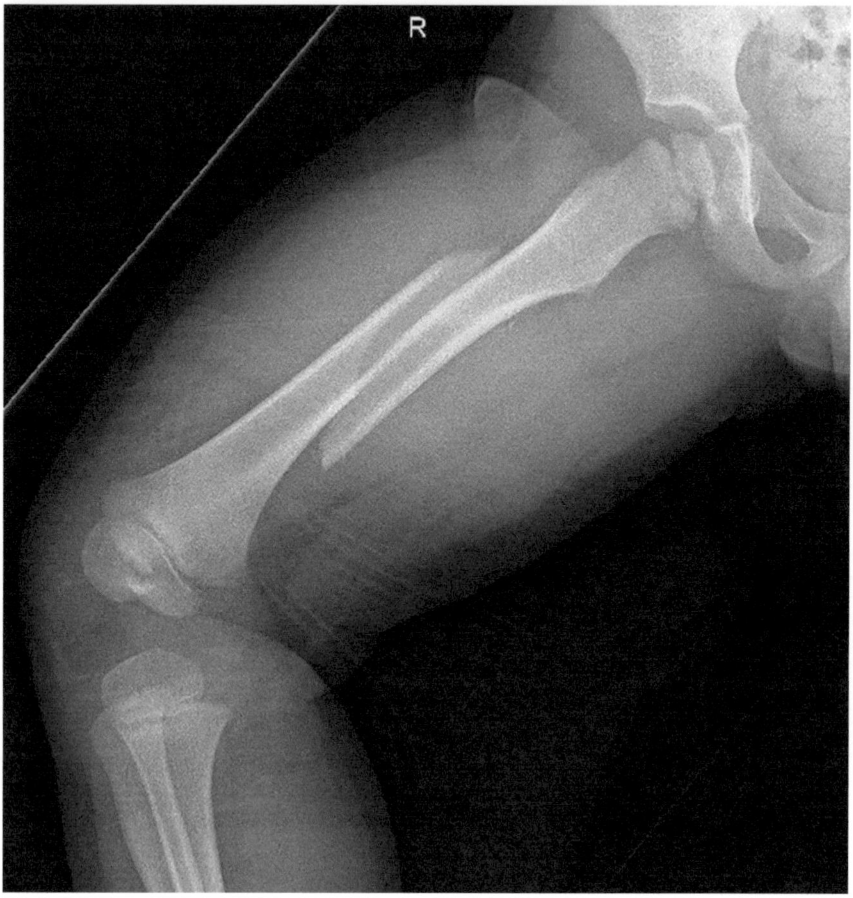

Image 14

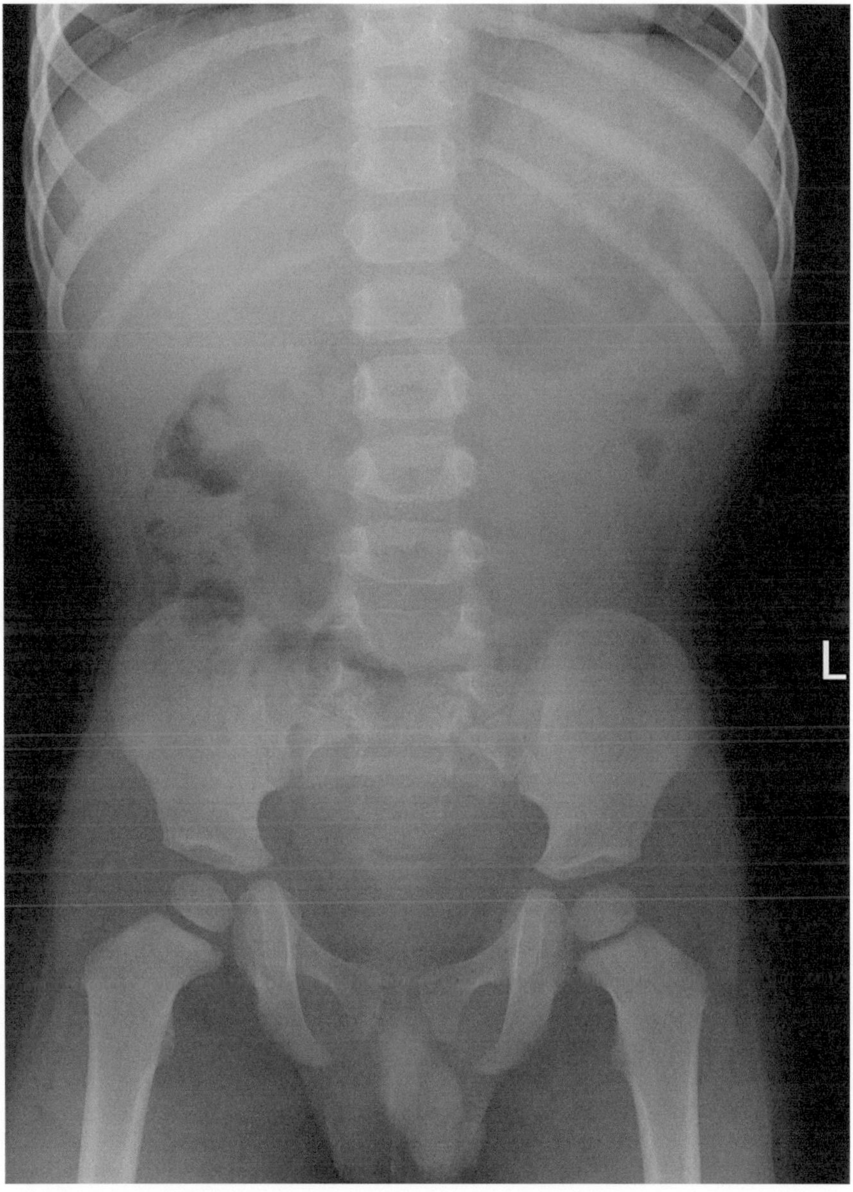

Image 15

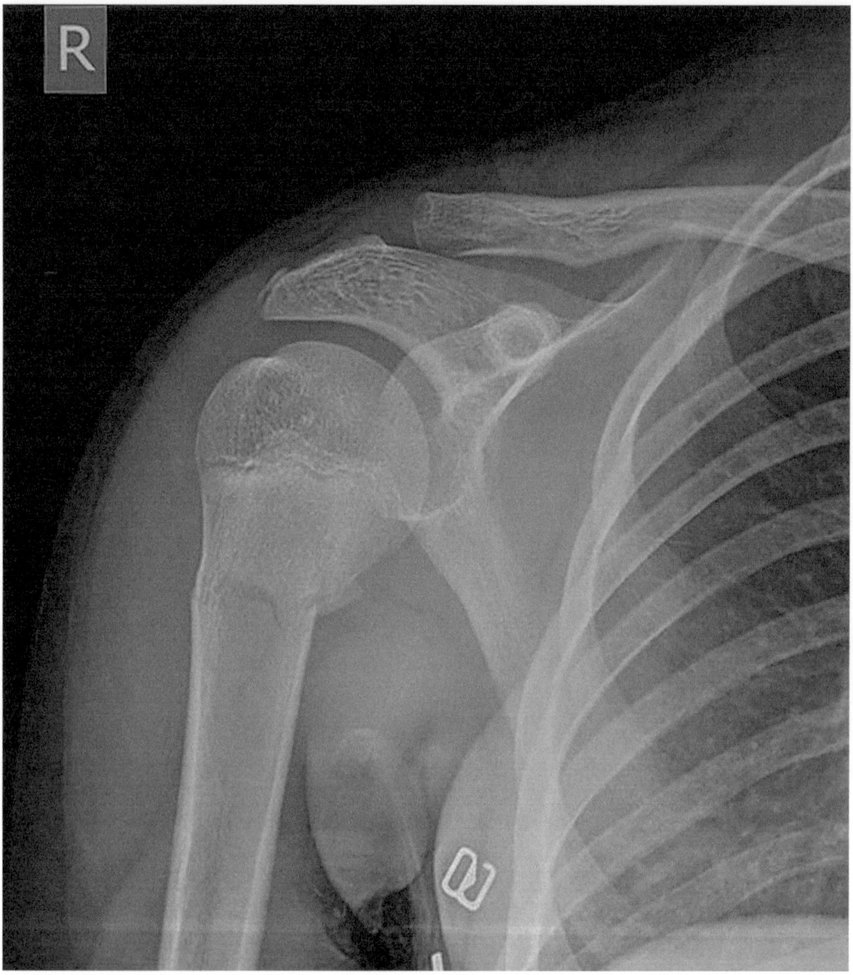

Image 16

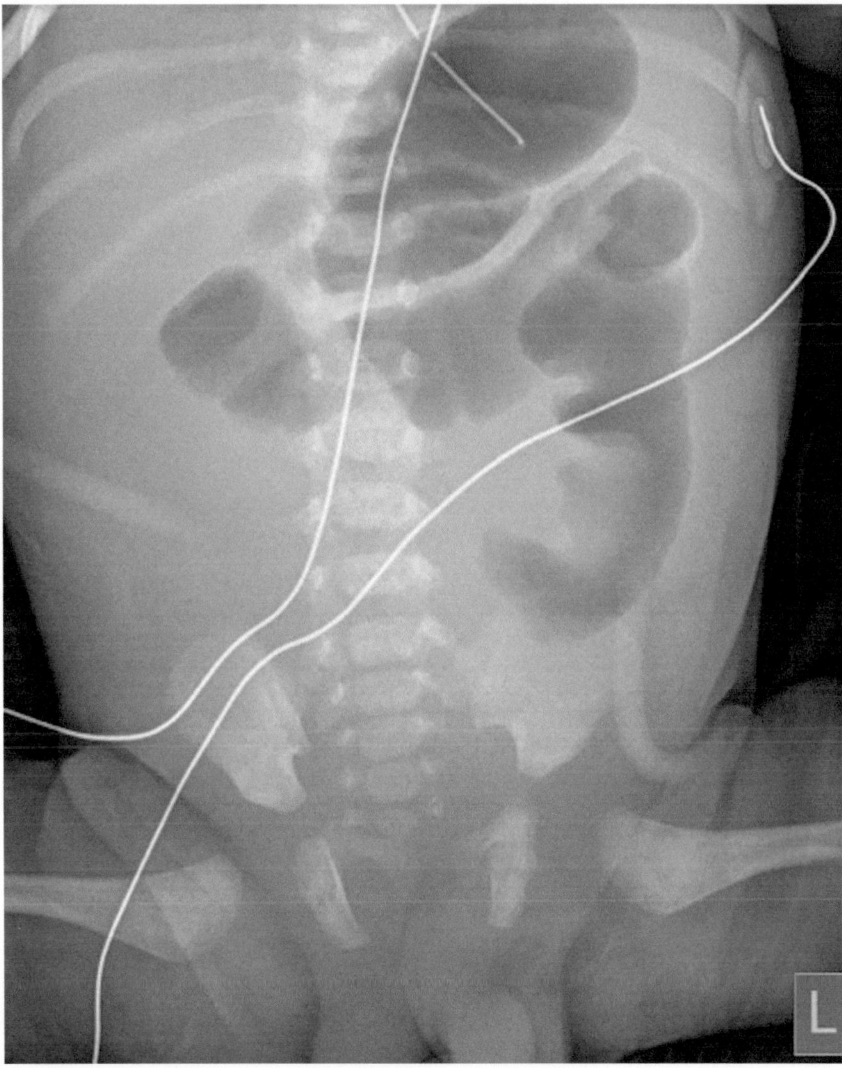

Image 17

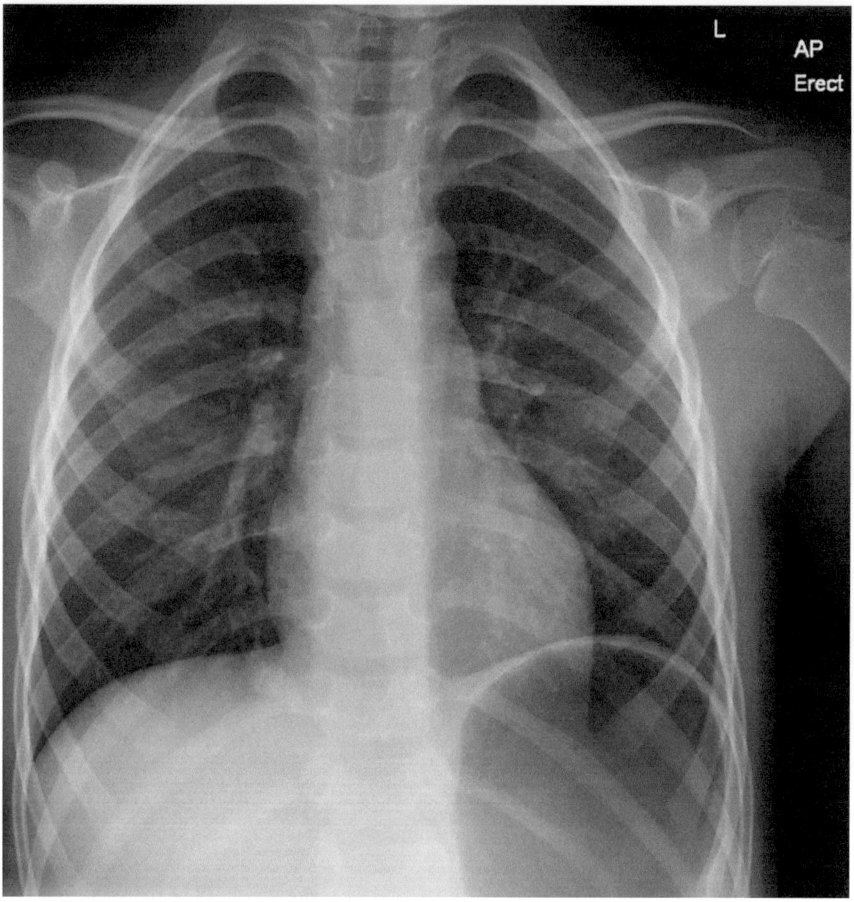

Image 18

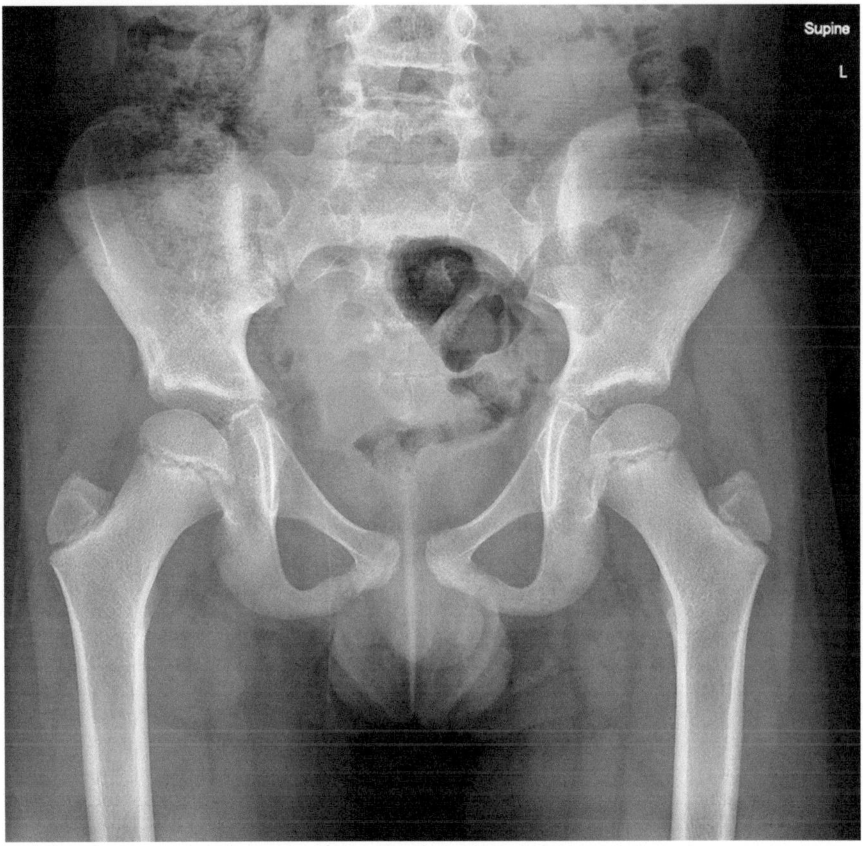

Image 19

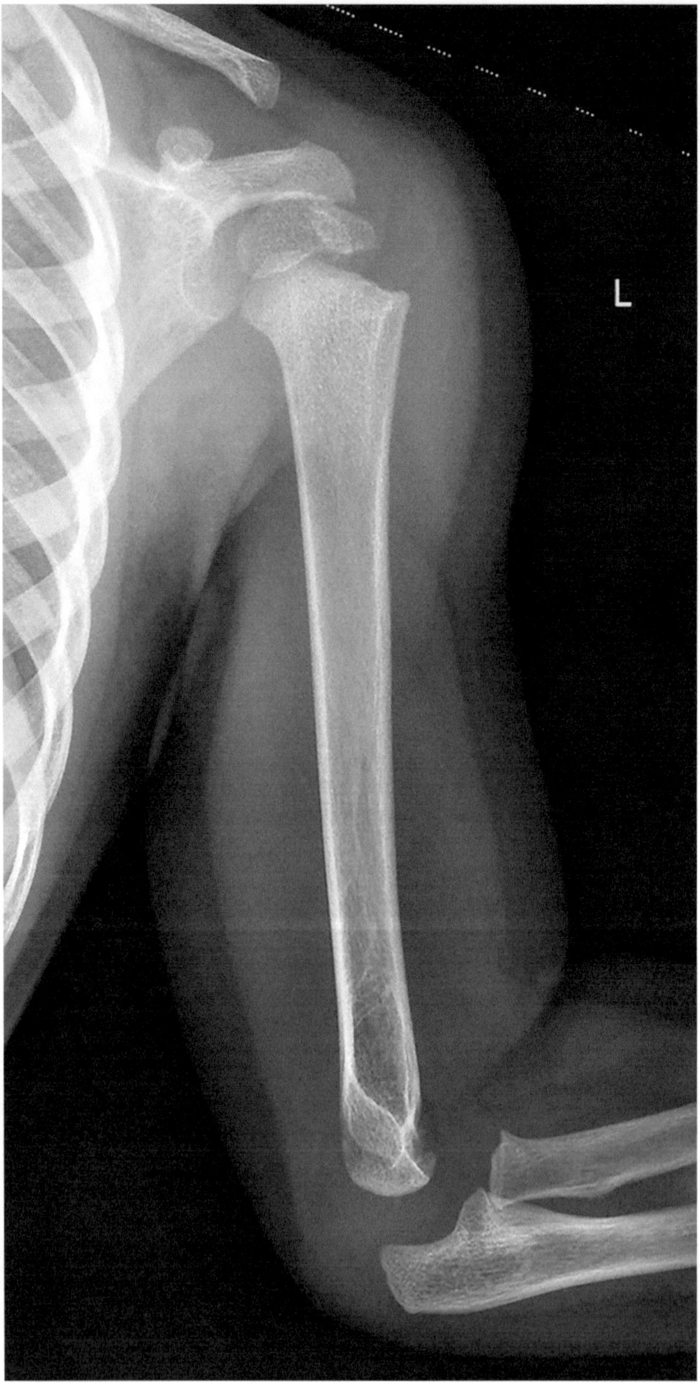

Image 20

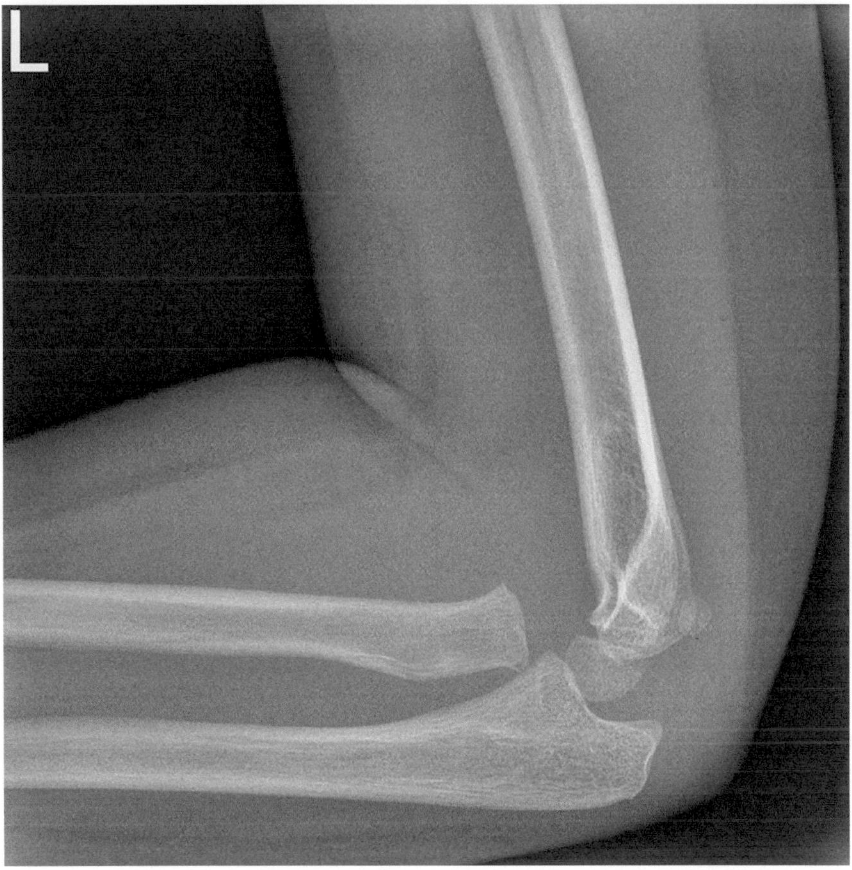

Image 21

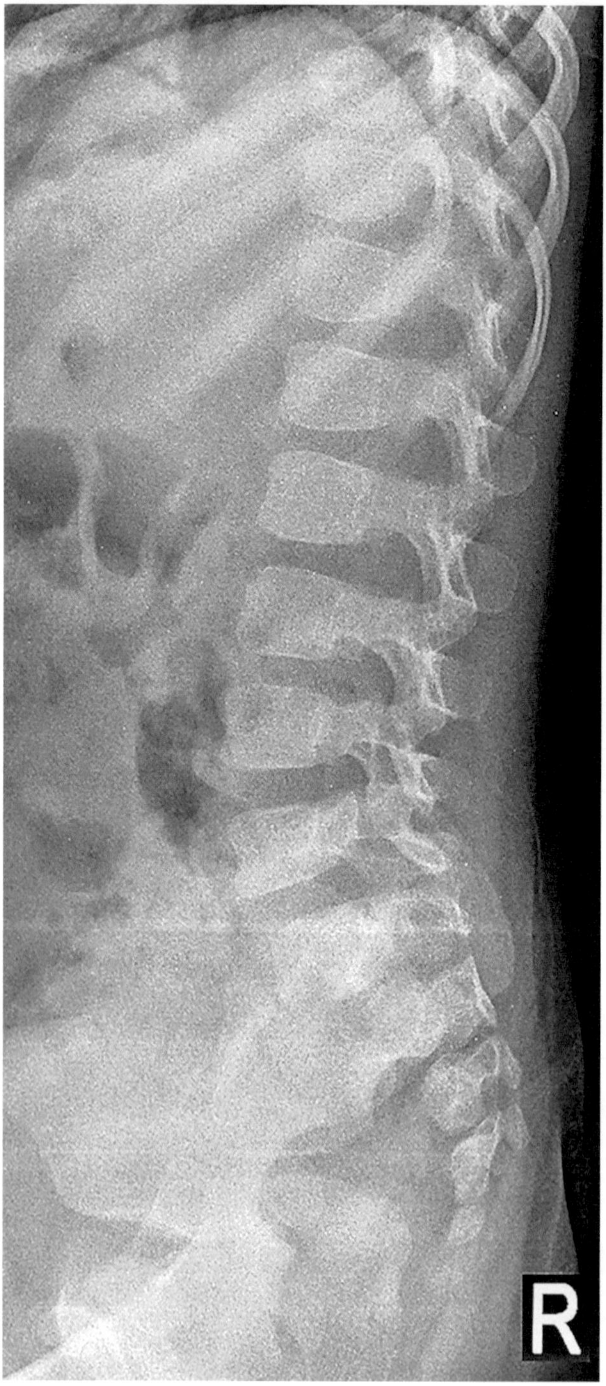

Image 22

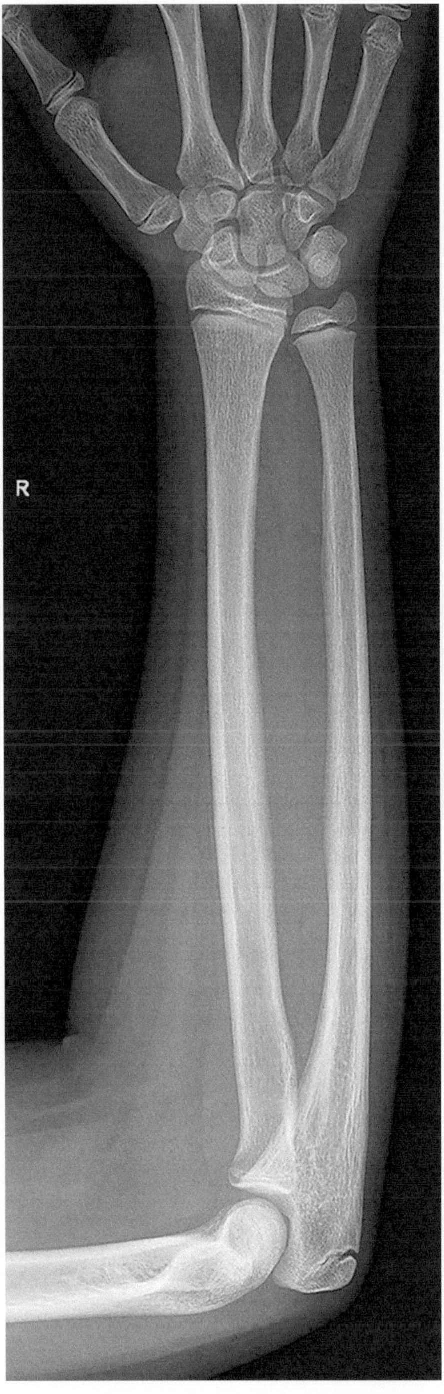

Image 23

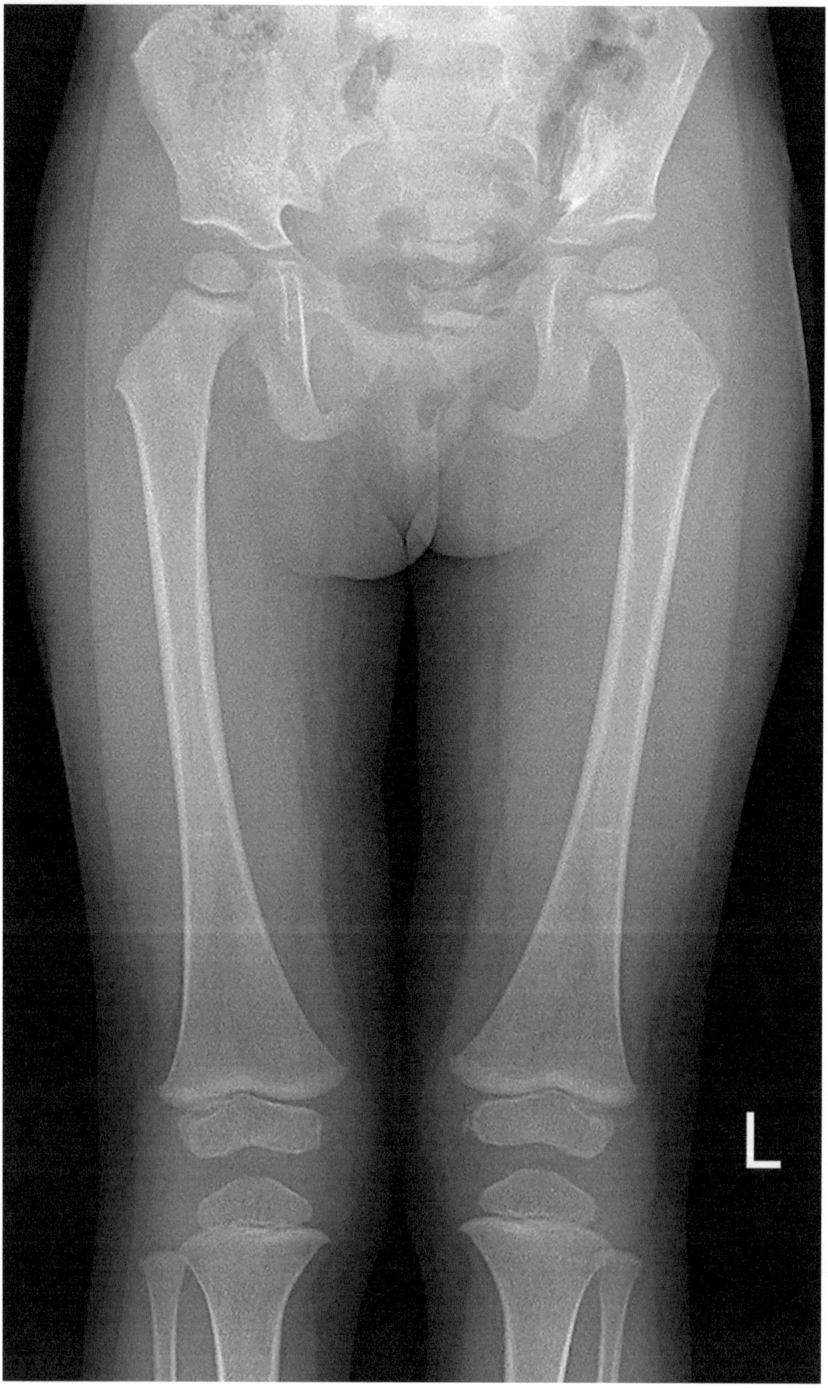

Image 24

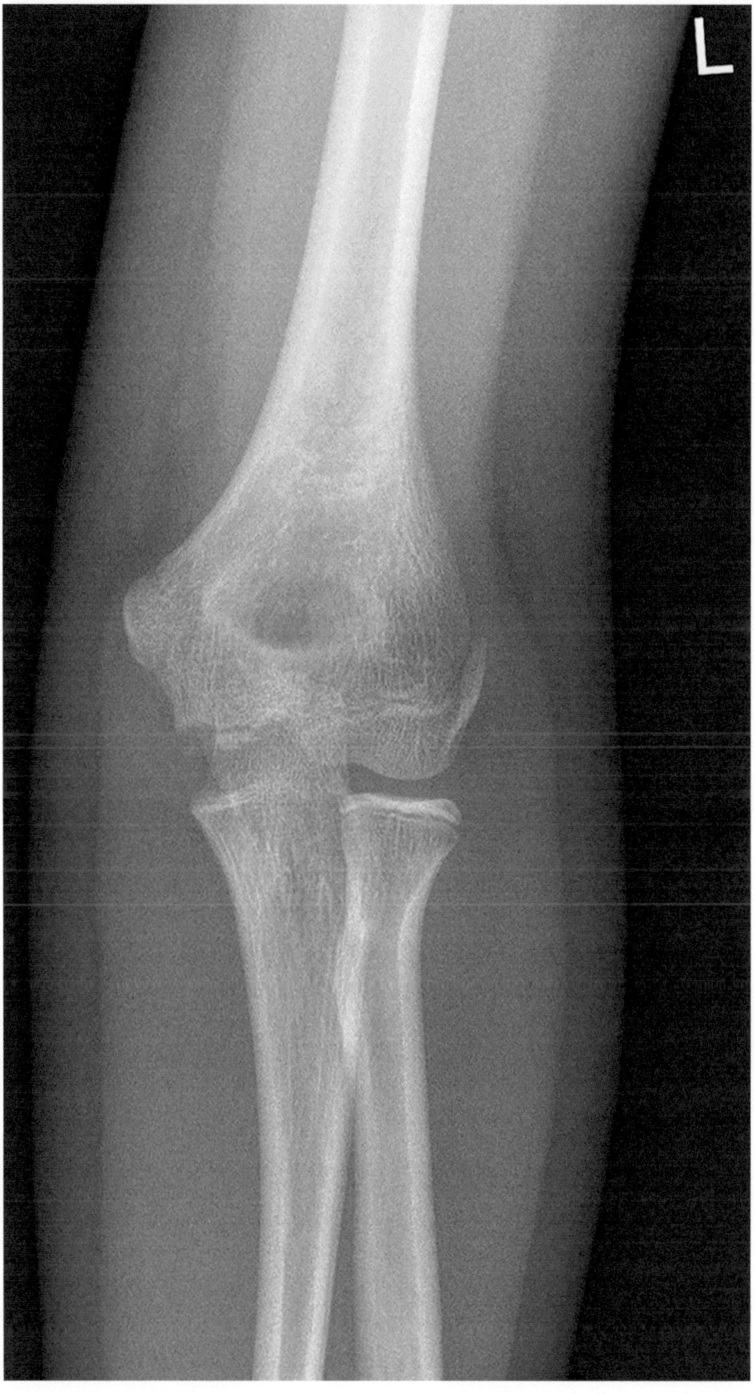

Image 25

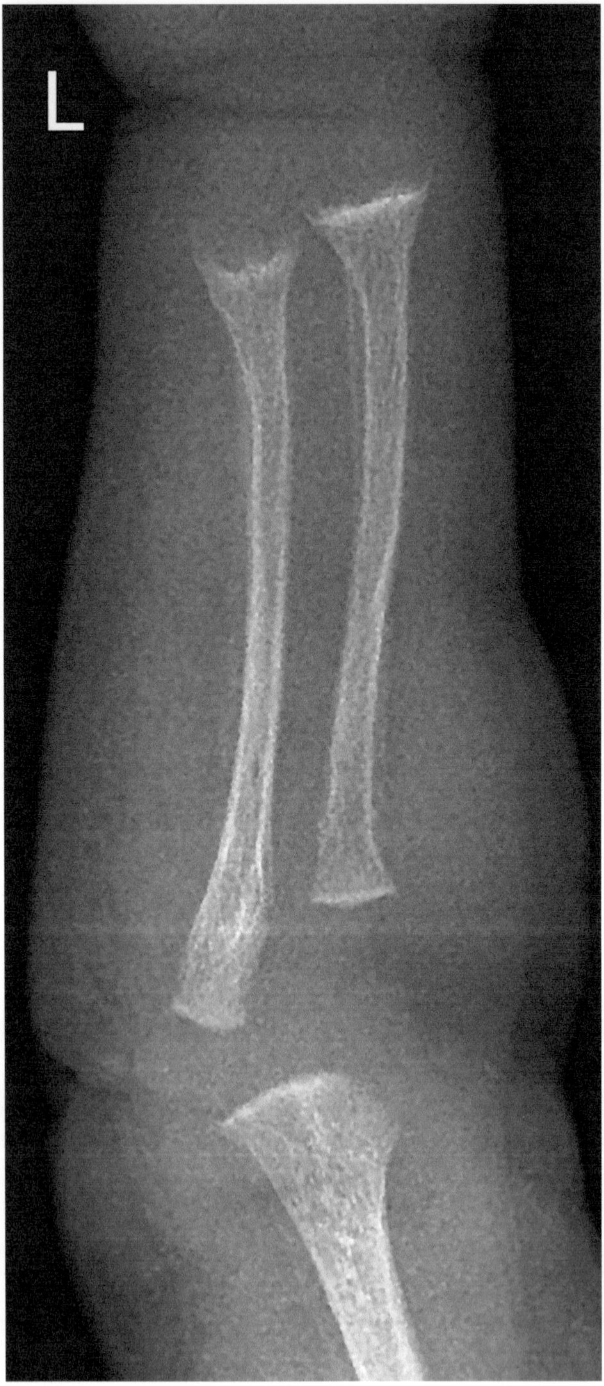

Image 26

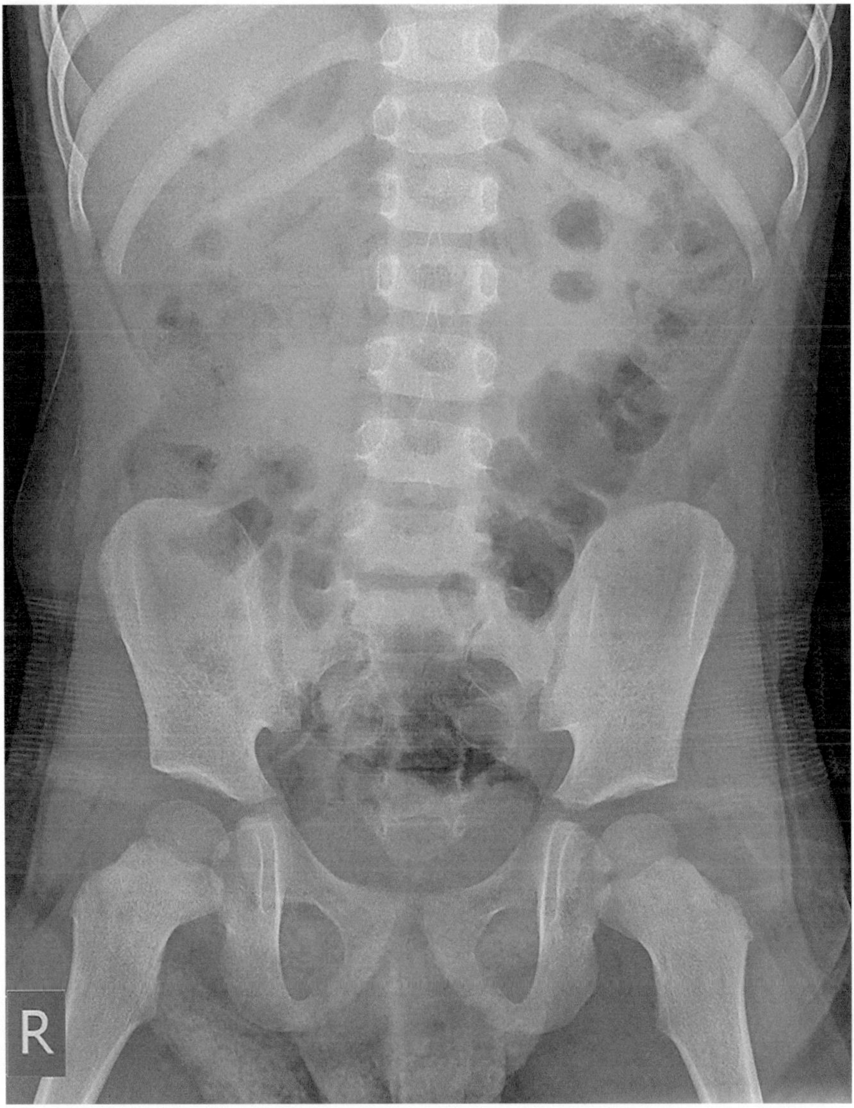

Image 27

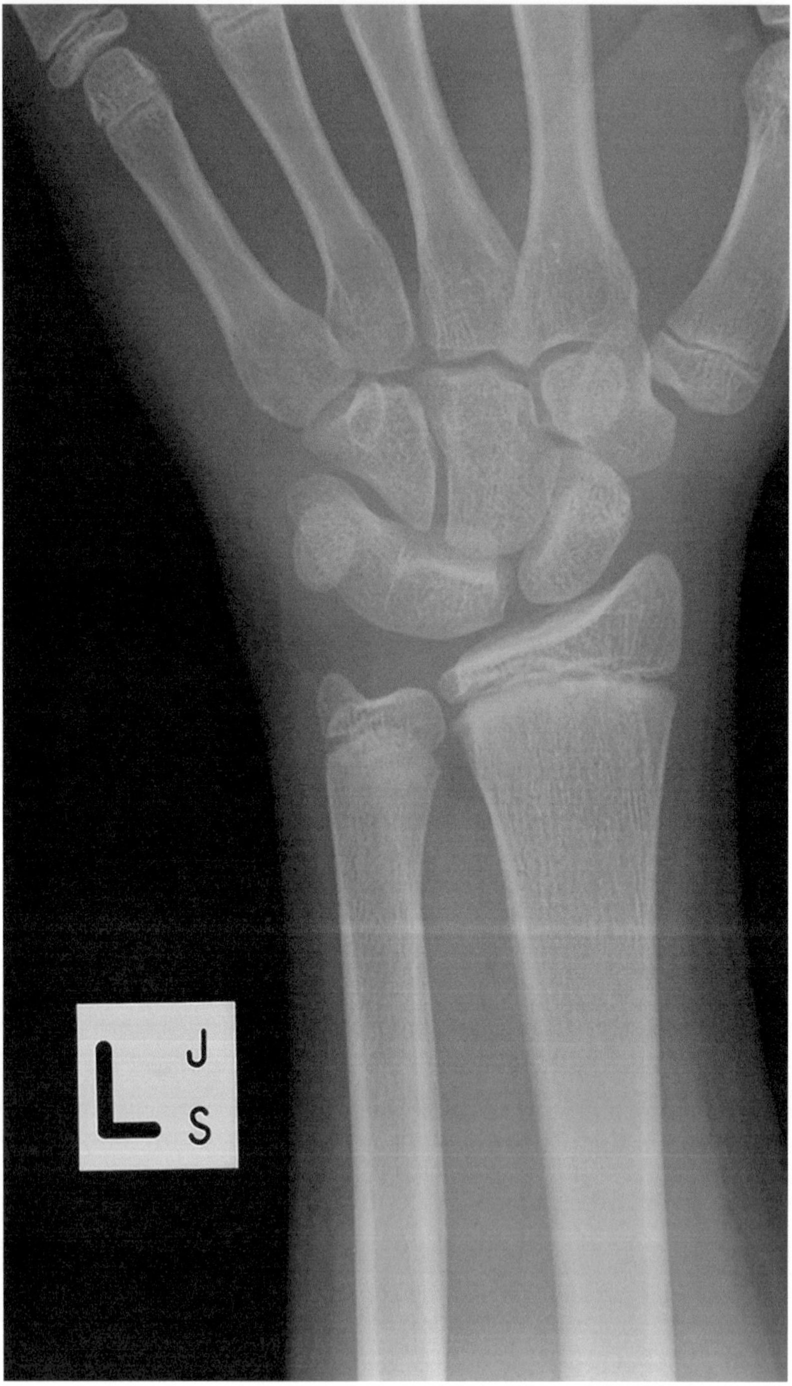

Image 28

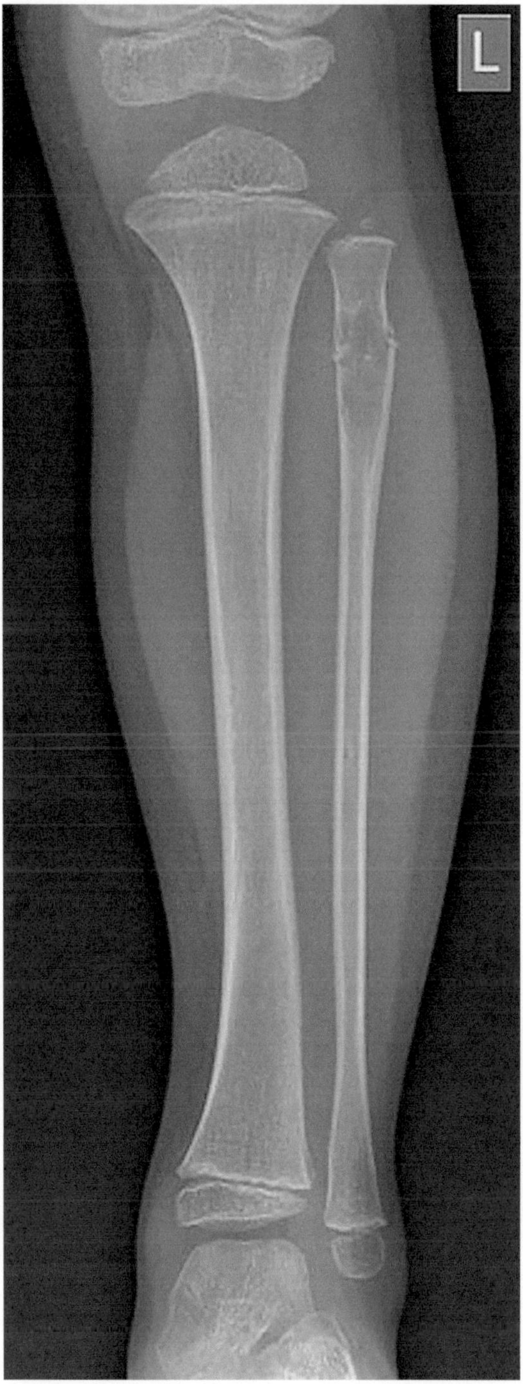

Image 29

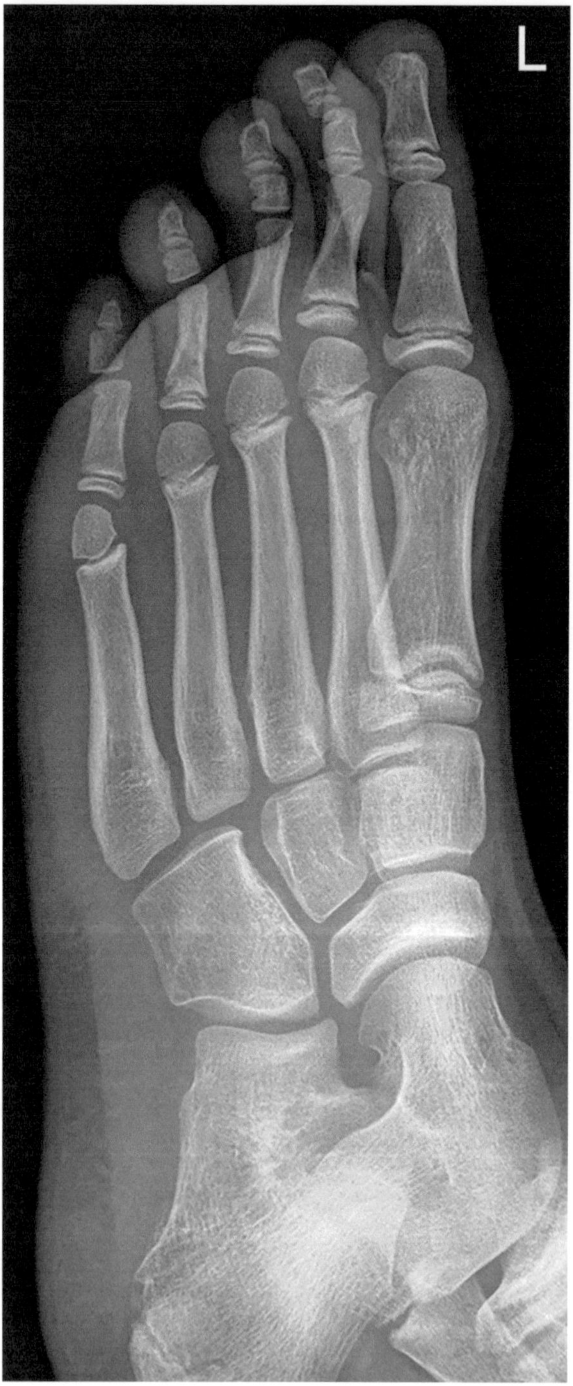

Image 30

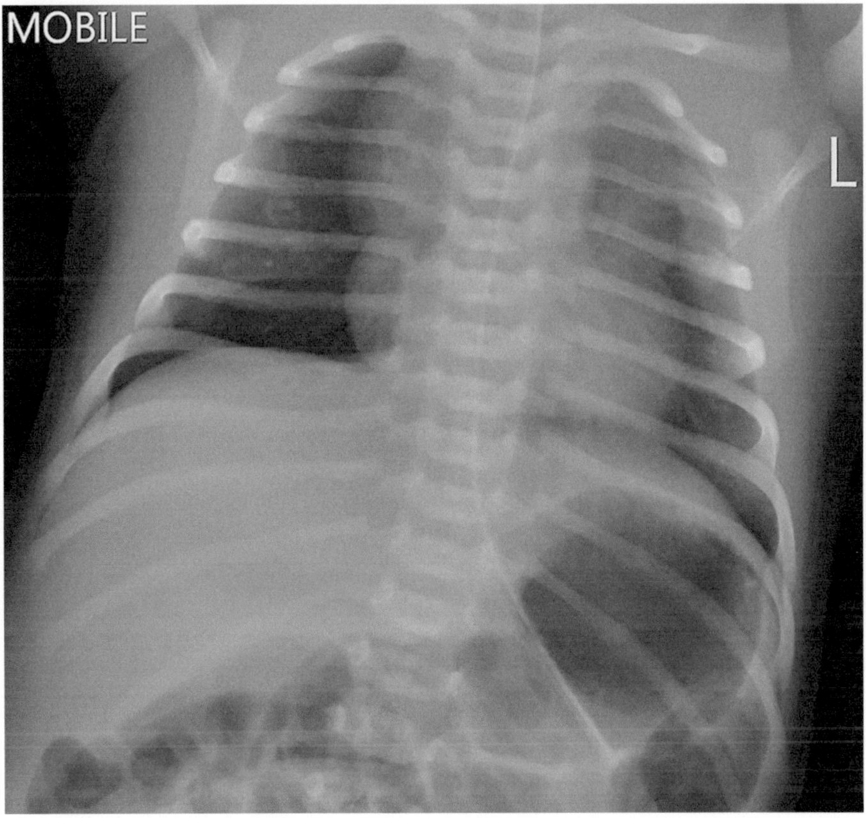

8.2 Answers

Image	Normal	Abnormal	Diagnosis/abnormality (only if abnormal)
1		✓	R DDH
2		✓	Healing #s L seventh and eighth ribs (lateral arcs)
3	✓		
4	✓		
5	✓		
6	✓		
7		✓	# R ulnar diaphysis
8	✓		
9		✓	SH2 # L second toe proximal phalanx
10		✓	NEC
11		✓	Bucket handle # R distal femoral metaphysis
12		✓	# L scaphoid distal pole
13		✓	Spiral # R femoral diaphysis
14	✓		
15		✓	# R humerus surgical neck
16		✓	Proximal bowel obstruction/jejunal atresia
17	✓		
18	✓		
19	✓		
20		✓	L radial head dislocation
21	✓		
22	✓		
23	✓		
24	✓		
25		✓	Rickets
26	✓		
27		✓	L lunotriquetral coalition
28		✓	Pathological # L proximal fibula
29	✓		
30		✓	R pneumothorax

8.3. Explanations

1. **R developmental dysplasia of the hip**
   This radiograph demonstrates features of developmental dysplasia of the right hip (DDH) with flattening of the right proximal femoral epiphysis with lateral uncovering/subluxation, an irregular and sclerotic right acetabulum, and broadening of the right proximal femoral metaphysis. See the explanation for Image 17 of Test 2.

2. **Healing #s L seventh and eighth ribs (lateral arcs)**
   There are healing fractures of the lateral arcs of the left seventh and eighth ribs as evidenced by expansion and periosteal reaction indicating remodelling. The changes are better visualised in the magnified image below:

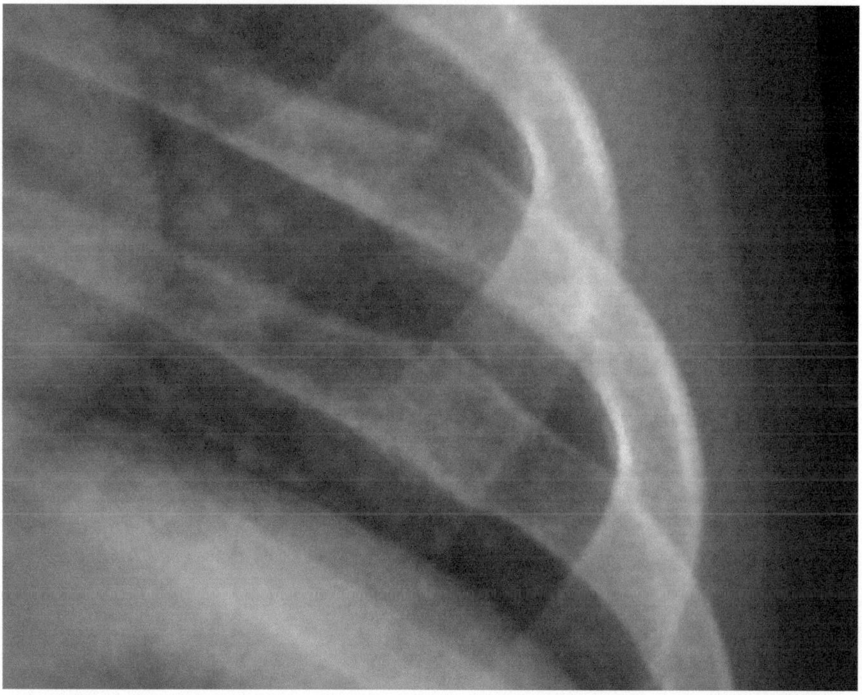

Acute rib fractures are often undetected on chest radiographs because they are usually minimally displaced, incomplete, and may be obscured by overlying structures. Follow-up chest radiographs performed 11–14 days after initial skeletal survey radiographs improve rib fracture detection because of their increased conspicuity from callus formation as they heal. They may also be detected on chest radiography performed for other/unrelated indications as in this case wherein the chest radiograph was performed for *'fever ?cause'*. Vigilance and recognition of these appearances as healing fractures is vital.

7. **# R ulnar diaphysis**
   In the presence of an ulnar shaft fracture, a concomitant radial head dislocation should be sought as part of the Monteggia fracture-dislocation complex, and vice versa. Formal forearm radiographs should be recommended if they have not yet been obtained. In this case, the radial head is enlocated with normal radiocapitellar alignment.

9. **Salter-Harris 2 # L second toe proximal phalanx**
   See the explanation for Image 30 of Test 1.

10. **Necrotising enterocolitis**
    Necrotising enterocolitis (NEC) is the commonest gastrointestinal condition affecting premature neonates. It has an inversely proportional incidence with gestational age: the more premature the infant, the greater the risk of developing NEC. The terminal ileum is the commonest affected location.

    The condition is thought to arise from a number of complex interactions that lead to increased gut wall mucosal permeability. The immune system of a premature neonate allows bacteria and their toxins to permeate the immature bowel wall resulting in mucosal damage and inflammation. The formation of gas within the bowel wall (i.e. intramural gas) as a by-product of bacterial metabolism can progress transmurally until there is eventual compromise of the microvasculature. This then leads to ischaemia, necrosis, mucosal sloughing, bowel wall thinning, and ultimately perforation. The release of bacterial toxins into the systemic circulation can also result in a generalised inflammatory response/sepsis.

    Presentation can be non-specific and should be considered in premature neonates who develop sepsis (discussed above). Other symptoms include the patient 'being unsettled' with temperature and blood pressure instability, episodes of bradycardia, desaturation, and apnoeas. Gastrointestinal symptoms may include feed intolerance, vomiting which may be bile-stained, diarrhoea, blood-stained stools, and rectal bleeding. Clinical examination usually reveals a distended abdomen and there may be discolouration of the overlying skin, which may look tense and 'shiny'. The radiograph in this case was obtained in a 6-day-old premature neonate who became 'unsettled' and developed rectal bleeding. The key radiographic features in this image include:

    - Dilated bowel loops: these are often distributed asymmetrically throughout the abdomen and change very little, if at all, on subsequent radiographs (they are most prominent in the left flank on this radiograph).

- Pneumatosis intestinalis: note the "bubbly" lucencies in the right flank on this radiograph in keeping with pneumatosis (i.e. intramural gas), as described above.
- Portal venous gas: note the branching linear lucencies extending to the periphery of the liver on this radiograph in keeping with portal venous gas, which is distinguished from pneumobilia in which the gas is more central.

Another important radiographic feature is pneumoperitoneum. Whilst not present on this radiograph, it should be actively sought on every neonatal abdominal radiograph, particularly in the setting of sepsis or if there are clinical concerns for NEC. Once the bowel has perforated, the mortality rate increases; thus, prompt recognition of the early radiographic changes of NEC prior to perforation is vital. However, it is important to note that pneumoperitoneum may not be seen on radiographs in an estimated 50–75% of cases, even when perforation has been confirmed (at surgery). A non-exhaustive list of the radiographic signs of pneumoperitoneum includes:

- Rigler sign: this relates to visualisation of both sides of the bowel wall due to the presence of gas both inside (intraluminal) and outside (extraluminal; from the free intraperitoneal gas) the bowel wall.
- Continuous diaphragm sign: a large amount of free gas collects under both the left and right hemidiaphragms creating the appearance of an uninterrupted lucency underneath the hemidiaphragms, i.e. a 'continuous diaphragm'.
- Football sign: seen in massive pneumoperitoneum whereby the abdominal cavity and falciform ligament are outlined by free gas.
- Inverted 'V' sign: free gas outlines the lateral umbilical ligaments creating an inverted 'V' shape projected over the pelvis.
- Urachus sign: free gas outlines the median umbilical ligament creating a vertical line between the bladder and the umbilicus.

We included this radiograph because of the constellation of findings present in one image. You may be presented with one or all of these radiographic findings in any component of the examination and in clinical practice. Thus, awareness and recognition of the radiographic features which support the diagnosis of NEC is paramount. An early paediatric surgical opinion is strongly advised in any neonate in whom there is clinical and/or radiological suspicion of NEC.

See the explanation for Image 19 of Test 1. Also note the tip of the enteric tube projected over the stomach. Remember that all lines and tubes should be assessed for malposition when present.

11. **Bucket handle # R distal femoral metaphysis**
    The 'bucket handle' metaphyseal fracture (classic metaphyseal lesion, CML) of the right distal femur is better visualised in the magnified image below:

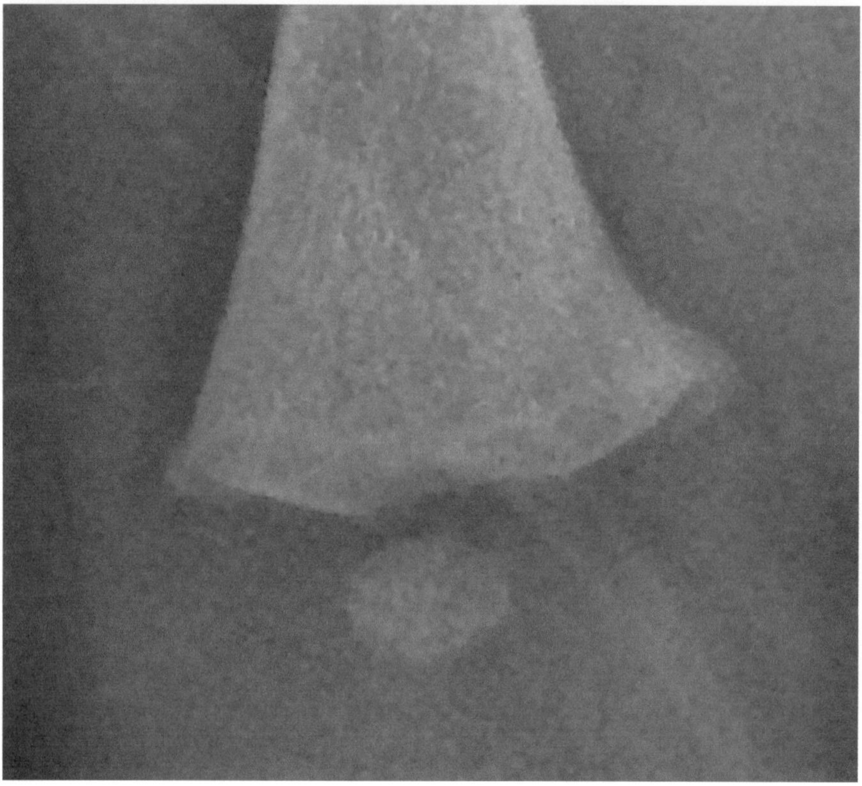

See the explanation for Image 2 of Test 3.

12. **# L scaphoid distal pole**
There is fracture of the distal pole of the left scaphoid which is better visualised in the image below:

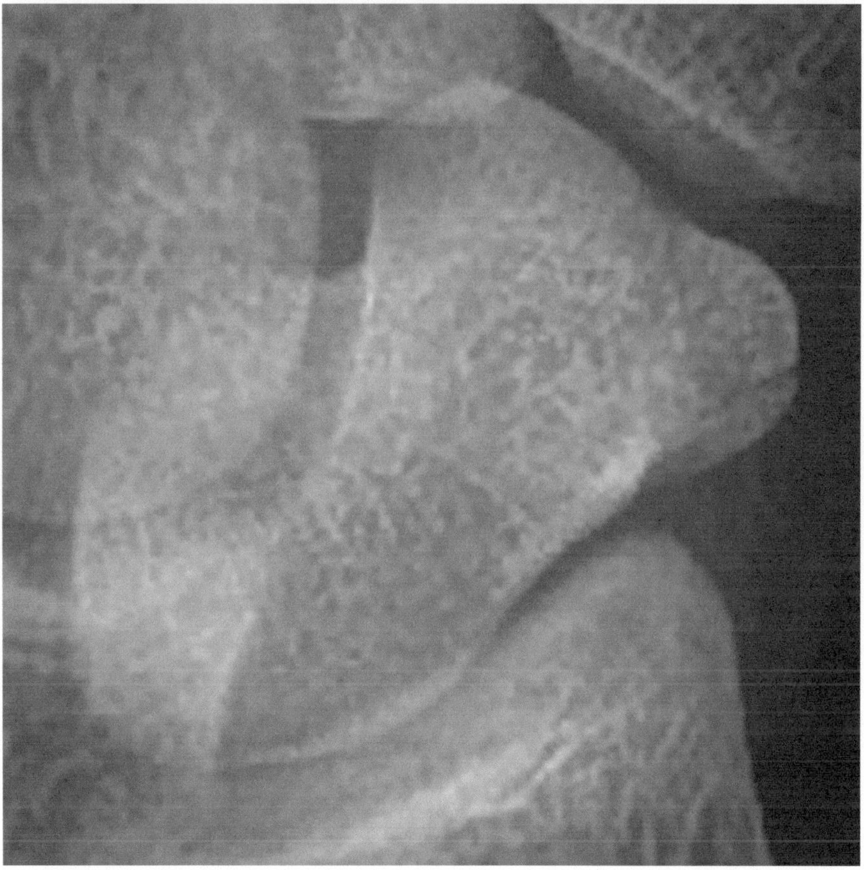

There is currently no evidence on which to propose an imaging algorithm for the diagnosis of suspected scaphoid fractures in children. As such, it is recommended that imaging pathways used in adults should be followed until such a time when high quality evidence is available in the paediatric population. Discuss your local policy with your paediatric and musculoskeletal radiologists.

13. **Spiral # R femoral diaphysis**
This infant with cerebral palsy was presented to the Emergency Department (ED) by his father who heard a 'crack' while changing his nappy. He was not (and may never be) ambulatory. Those children with a physical or developmental impairment, or disability, and those born prematurely are at an increased risk of physical abuse. They are however, also at increased risk of accidental fracture. The initial and follow-up skeletal surveys revealed no other acute or

healing fracture with normal radiographic bone density and modelling. Head computed tomography (CT) demonstrated long-standing ventriculomegaly with a ventriculoperitoneal (VP) shunt in situ but no acute intracranial haemorrhage, specifically no supratentorial or interhemispheric subdural haematoma. It was felt that this mid-diaphyseal spiral femoral fracture was in keeping with the proffered mechanism. See the explanation for Image 23 of Test 3.

The term *inflicted injury* is preferred in these circumstances because it does not necessarily exclude accidental injury and is more accurate in describing the causal mechanism of injury, i.e. an injury that was consequent upon the caregiver's actions but without ascribing a malicious intent to cause harm (which is the case when the term "non-accidental injury" is used). This is a subtle but important difference, particularly from a medicolegal perspective.

15. **# R humerus surgical neck**
The surgical neck of the proximal humerus is the 'line' inferior to the greater and lesser tuberosities, i.e. the start of the proximal humeral diaphysis. It is much more commonly fractured than the anatomical neck which represents the physis in children and the old fused physeal plate in adults. Note the linear ossific fragment adjacent to the right acromion; this is the normal ossification centre which can have variable/fragmented appearances at all ages.

16. **Proximal bowel obstruction/jejunal atresia**
The radiographic appearances are in keeping with a proximal (high) bowel obstruction. The distended gas-filled stomach (first bubble), duodenum (second bubble), and the duodenojenunal (DJ) flexure are visualised in the left upper quadrant with only a short, but dilated, segment of proximal jejunum (third bubble). There is an abrupt cut-off and an absence of bowel gas distal to the proximal jejunum in keeping with the 'triple bubble sign' seen in jejunal atresia. The atresia can be anywhere from the DJ flexure to the jejunoileal junction. Additionally, there may be more than one atretic jejunal segment. Note the appropriately sited tip of the enteric tube projected over the stomach.

Tip for the viva:

- You would be expected to be able to categorise the pattern of obstruction as either proximal (high) or distal (low) and offer an appropriate differential diagnosis depending on the age of the child and the clinical context. See the explanations for Image 19 of Test 1 and Image 30 of Test 5.

20. **L radial head dislocation**
See the explanation for Image 28 of Test 1.

24. *Normal left elbow radiograph*
This radiograph is normal. All the elbow ossification centres are present in this 11-year-old girl (note that the olecranon ossification centre is not well visualised on anteroposterior (AP) projections and is typically better visualised on

contemporaneous lateral projections). Note the normal lateral epicondyle projecting over the capitellum inferiorly.

The trochlear ossification centre may have two or more ossific nuclei (i.e centres of ossification), which can often lead to a variable and fragmented appearance during ossification. On the lateral projection, they may also appear as 'fragments' projecting into the joint space, simulating intra-articular loose bodies. It is important to remember that an avulsed medial epicondyle ossification centre may be displaced into the elbow joint space mimicking the normal trochlear ossification centre: a serious finding not to be overlooked. See the explanation for Image 9 of Test 6.

It is imperative that when evaluating any paediatric elbow radiograph, you should establish the age of the child and actively consider the expected pattern of ossification centres on *both* orthogonal projections.

Tip for the viva:

- Search for elbow radiographs in children aged 10–14 years of age on your local picture archive and communications system (PACS) and familiarise yourself with the normal (and variable) appearances of all the elbow ossification centres, in particular the trochlear ossification centre. Look out for examples of avulsion fractures with which you can compare.

25. **Rickets**

Rickets is a condition of physeal demineralisation with abnormal growth in children who are vitamin D deficient (the most common cause of calcipenic rickets). The metaphyseal irregularity in this radiograph is typical for rickets with:

- Cupping: concave appearance of the metaphysis.
- Flaring/splaying: widening of the metaphyseal ends.
- Fraying: indistinct metaphyseal margins/irregularity.

There is also coarsened bony trabeculation and periosteal reaction along both radial and ulnar diaphyses. Bowing deformities occur with continued growth in weight-bearing children. The radiographic features of rickets can be best remembered using the mnemonic, **RICKETS**:

- **R**eaction of the periosteum (i.e. periosteal reaction, which may also be present in the context of healing fractures).
- **I**ndistinct cortex.
- **C**oarse trabeculation.
- **K**nees, wrists, and ankles mainly affected (the sites of most rapid growth).
- **E**piphyseal widening and irregularity.
- **T**remendous metaphyses (concave and widened).
- **S**pur (cortical spurs projected at right angles to the metaphysis).

The metaphyses may be fragmented which may sometimes be mistaken for fractures i.e. CMLs. Whilst the above features are evident in this example, recognition of the subtle radiographic features of rickets is imperative so that they are not mistaken as suspicious/abusive fractures.

Osteomalacia (from the Latin and Greek meaning *bone* + *softness*, respectively) is the result of bone matrix demineralisation, most commonly due to vitamin D deficiency and can occur in adults after the physes have fused.

Tips for the viva:

- In the context of unexplained fractures, a low vitamin D level in the absence of other biochemical and radiological features of rickets does *not* account for the fractures.
- Do not mistake *isolated* ulnar cupping in infants, a normal radiographic appearance in this age group, for the changes of rickets.

27. **L lunotriquetral coalition**
    This is the commonest carpal coalition and results from a congenital lack of separation of the lunate and triquetral bones. It is commonly bilateral and there is a female predominance. The thin sclerotic line visualised in the centre of this lunotriquetral osseous coalition represents the site of failed separation. It is usually discovered incidentally when imaging is performed for another indication given that osseous lunotriquetral coalitions are known to be asymptomatic. However, fibrocartilagenous lunotriquetral coalitions may present as an uncommon cause of ulnar-sided wrist pain, often from the pseudoarthrosis or from disruption following trauma. Cross-sectional imaging will better elucidate the exact nature of the coalition. Remember, coalitions (any location) can be osseous, fibrous, cartilaginous, or a combination of these types.

28. **Pathological # L proximal fibula**
    There is a lucent, expansile lesion in the left proximal fibular metadiaphysis with associated cortical thinning suggestive of an aneurysmal bone cyst through which there is a pathological fracture. These fractures are secondary to normal stresses on abnormal bones (in this case, the aneurysmal bone cyst).

30. **R pneumothorax**
    There is a right pneumothorax. There is no mediastinal tension, left-sided pneumothorax or pneumomediastinum for which the radiograph should be scrutinised when a pneumothorax has been detected. Do not forget to assess the positions of all the lines and tubes. The tip of the nasogastric tube (NGT) is appropriately sited in this image.

Further Reading

Image 10

Awolaran OT (2015) Radiographic signs of gastrointestinal perforation in children: a pictorial review. Afr J Paediatr Surg 12(3):161–166
Menashe SJ, Iyer RS, Parisi MT et al (2017) Pediatric abdominal radiographs: common and less common errors. Am J Roentgenol 209(2):417–429
Shah V et al (2018) Pneumoperitoneum. https://radiopaedia.org/articles/pneumoperitoneum. Accessed Aug 2023
Zhang H, Guo L, Ling K et al (2014) Specific imaging features of intestinal perforation on supine abdominal X-ray evaluation in infants with necrotizing enterocolitis. World J Pediatr Surg 4:e000255

Image 12

Offiah AC, Burke D (2018) The diagnostic accuracy of cross-sectional imaging for detecting acute scaphoid fractures in children: a systematic review. Br J Radiol 91(1086):20170883

Image 15

Watts E, Shirley E, Skaggs DL (2022) Proximal humerus fracture—pediatric. https://www.orthobullets.com/pediatrics/4004/proximal-humerus-fracture%2D%2Dpediatric. Accessed Aug 2023

Image 16

Rasuli B et al (2021) Jejunal atresia. https://radiopaedia.org/articles/jejunal-atresia. Accessed Aug 2023
Sharma R et al (2019) Triple bubble sign. https://radiopaedia.org/articles/triple-bubble-sign. Accessed Aug 2023

Image 24

Smithuis R (2018) Elbow—fractures in children. https://radiologyassistant.nl/pediatrics/hip/fractures-in-children-1. Accessed Aug 2023

Image 25

Karmazyn B, Marine MB, Jones RH et al (2022) Radiologists' diagnostic performance in differentiation of rickets and classic metaphyseal lesions on radiographs: a multicenter study. Am J Roentgenol 219(6):962–972
Sriselvakumar S et al (2023) Rickets. https://radiopaedia.org/articles/rickets. Accessed Aug 2023

Image 27

Fagbohun AO et al (2023) Lunotriquetral coalition. https://radiopaedia.org/articles/lunotriquetral-coalition-2. Accessed January 2024

Test 9

9

M. Paddock et al., *Paediatric Radiology Rapid Reporting*,
https://doi.org/10.1007/978-3-031-48255-7_9

9.1 Images

Image 1

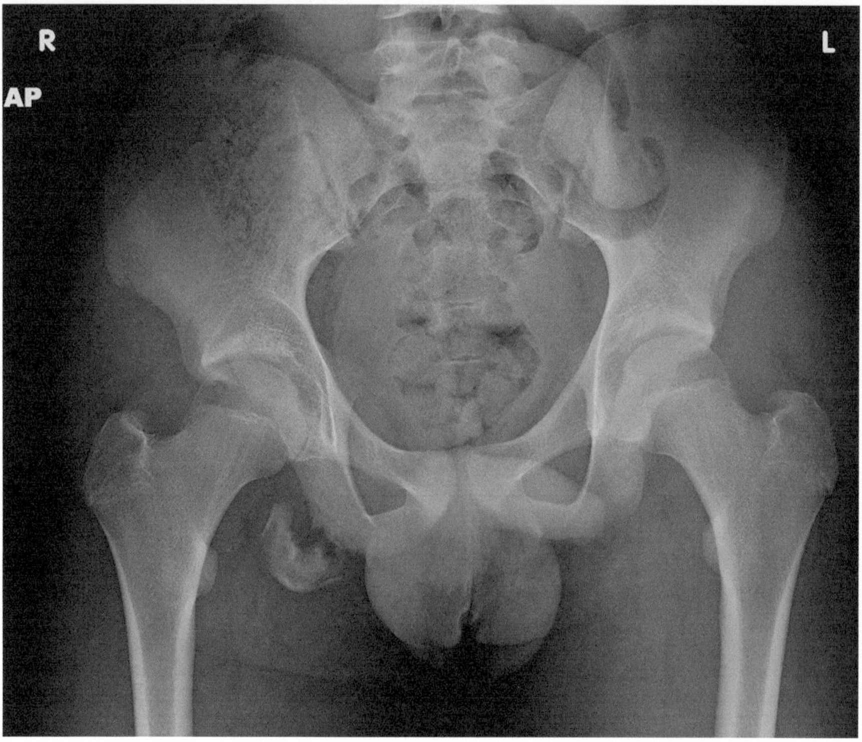

Image 2

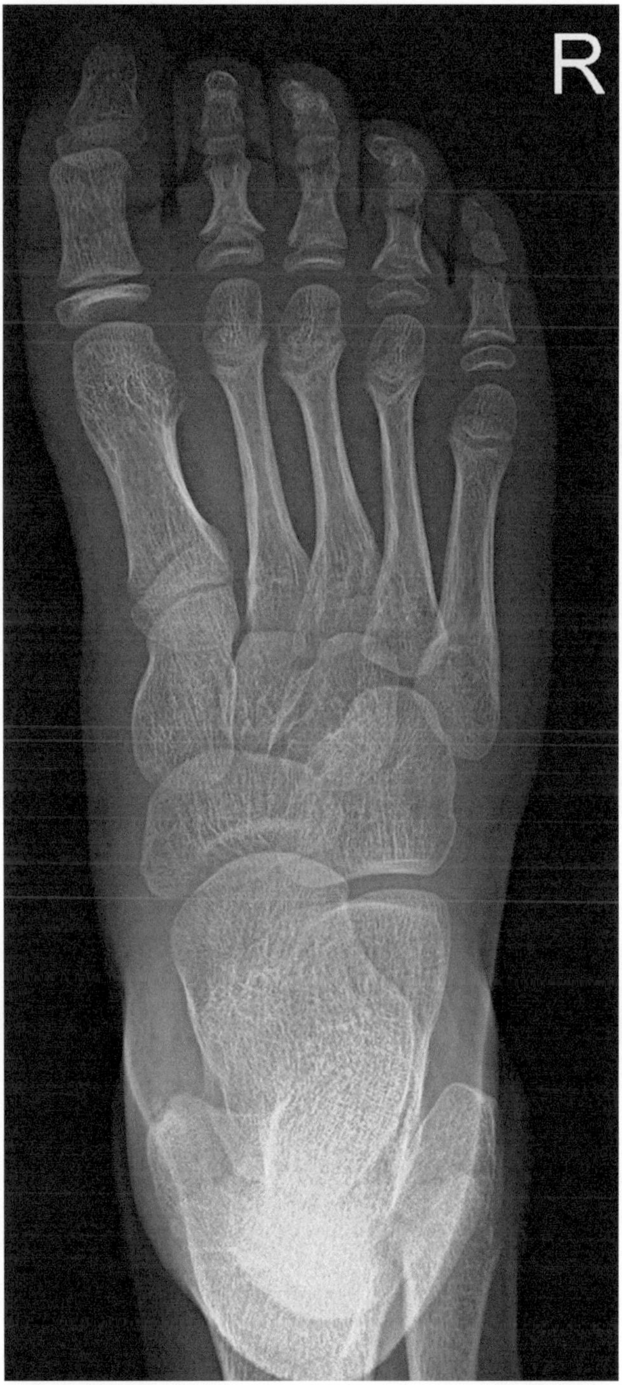

Image 3

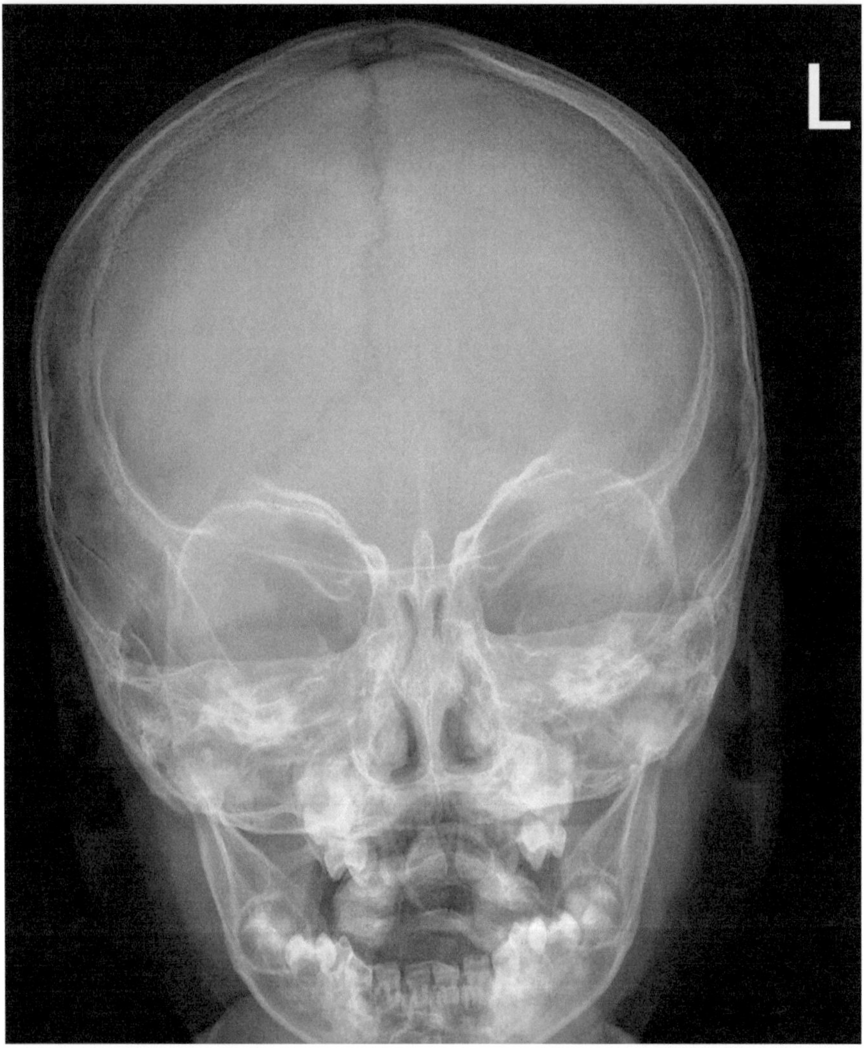

Image 4

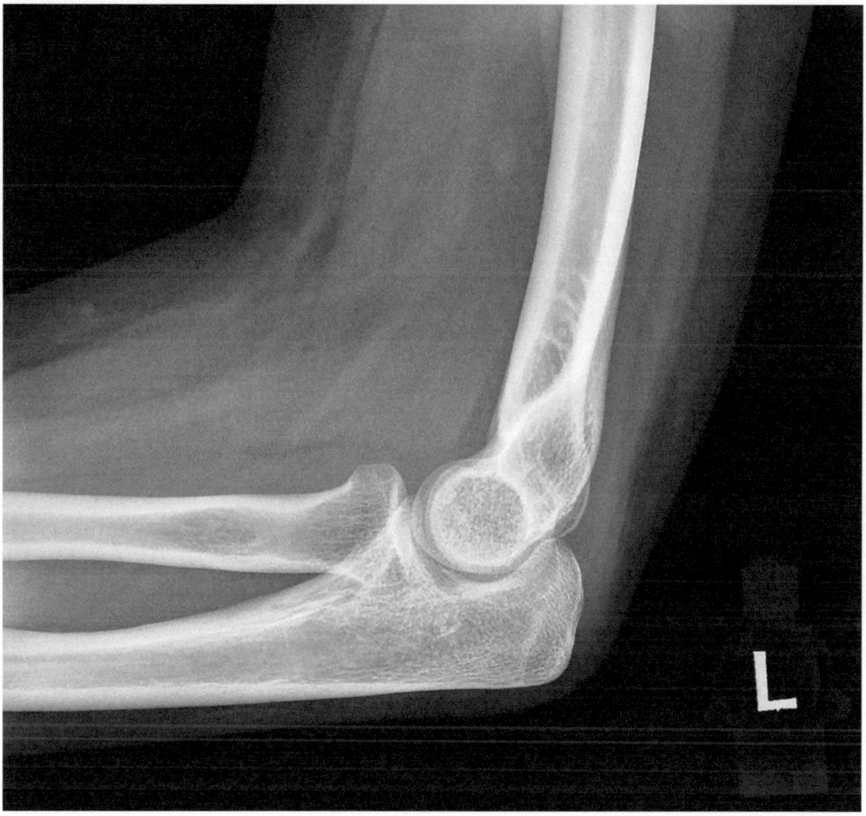

Image 5

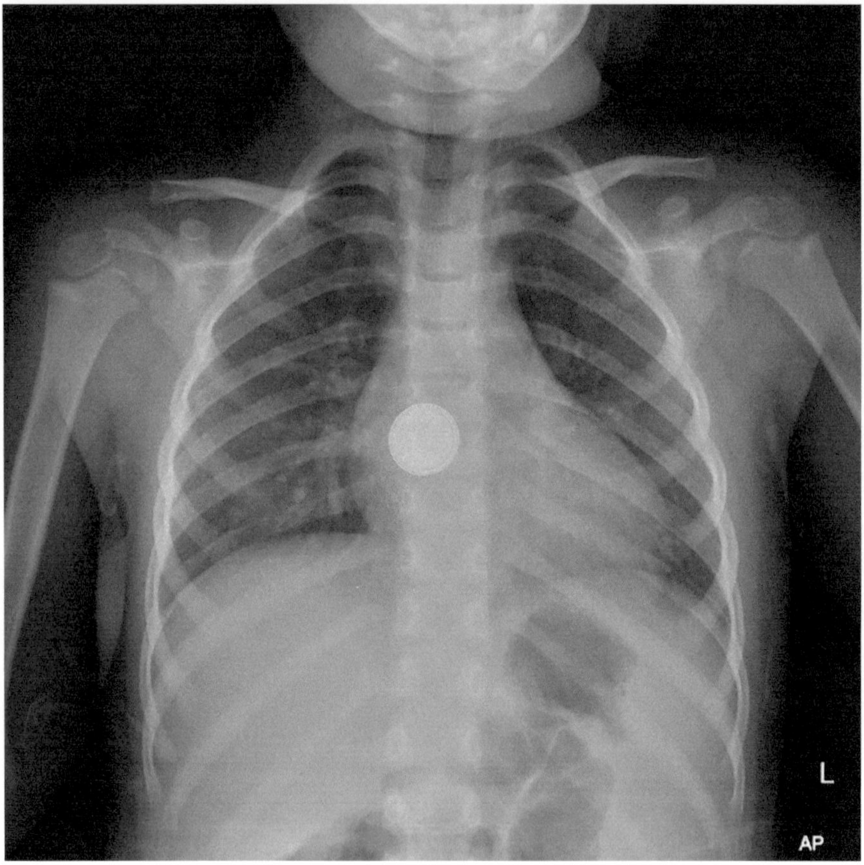

Image 6

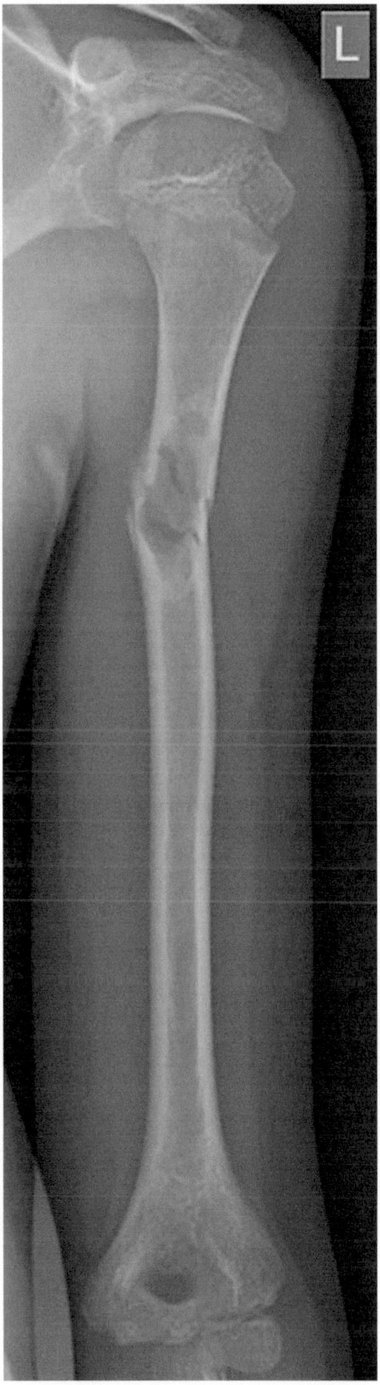

Image 7

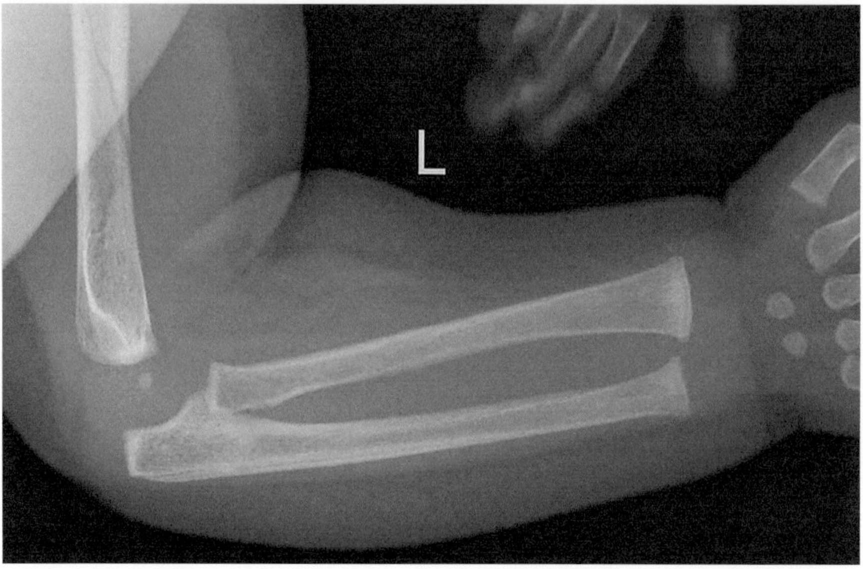

Image 8

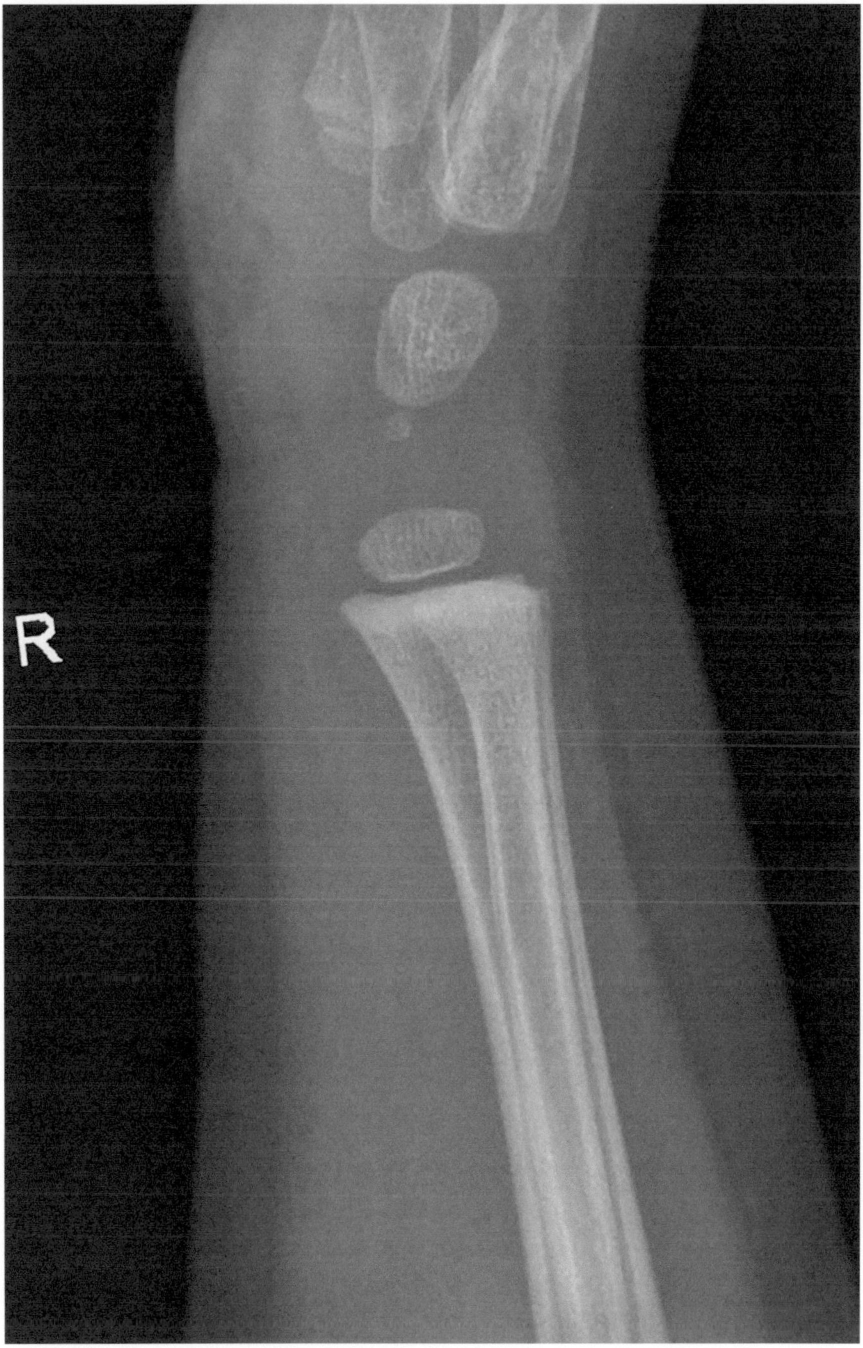

Image 9

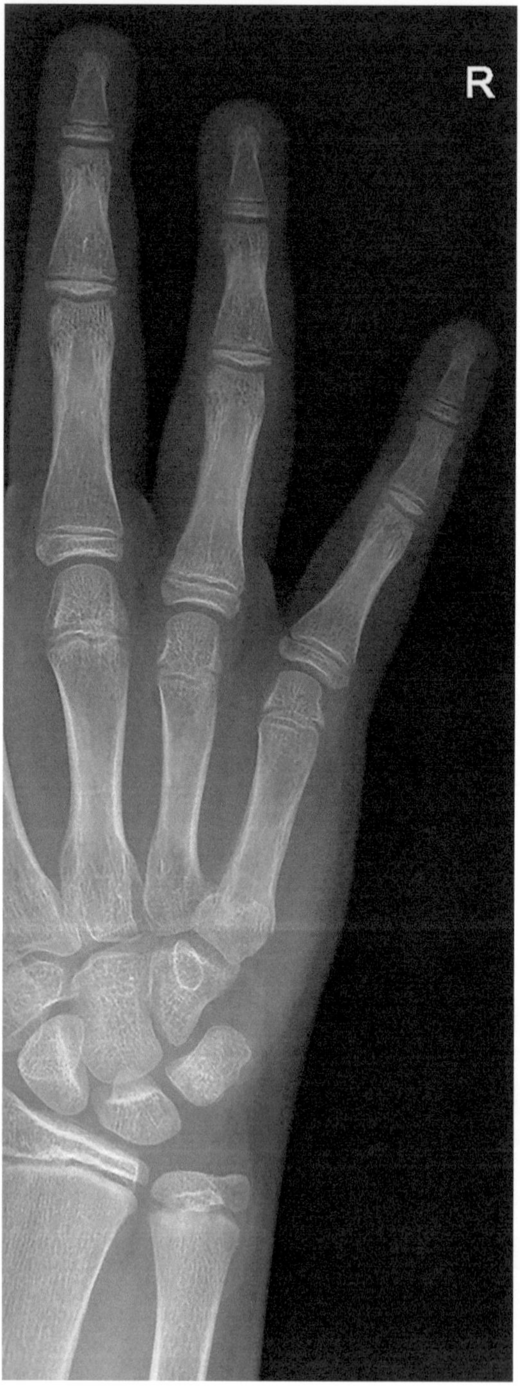

Image 10

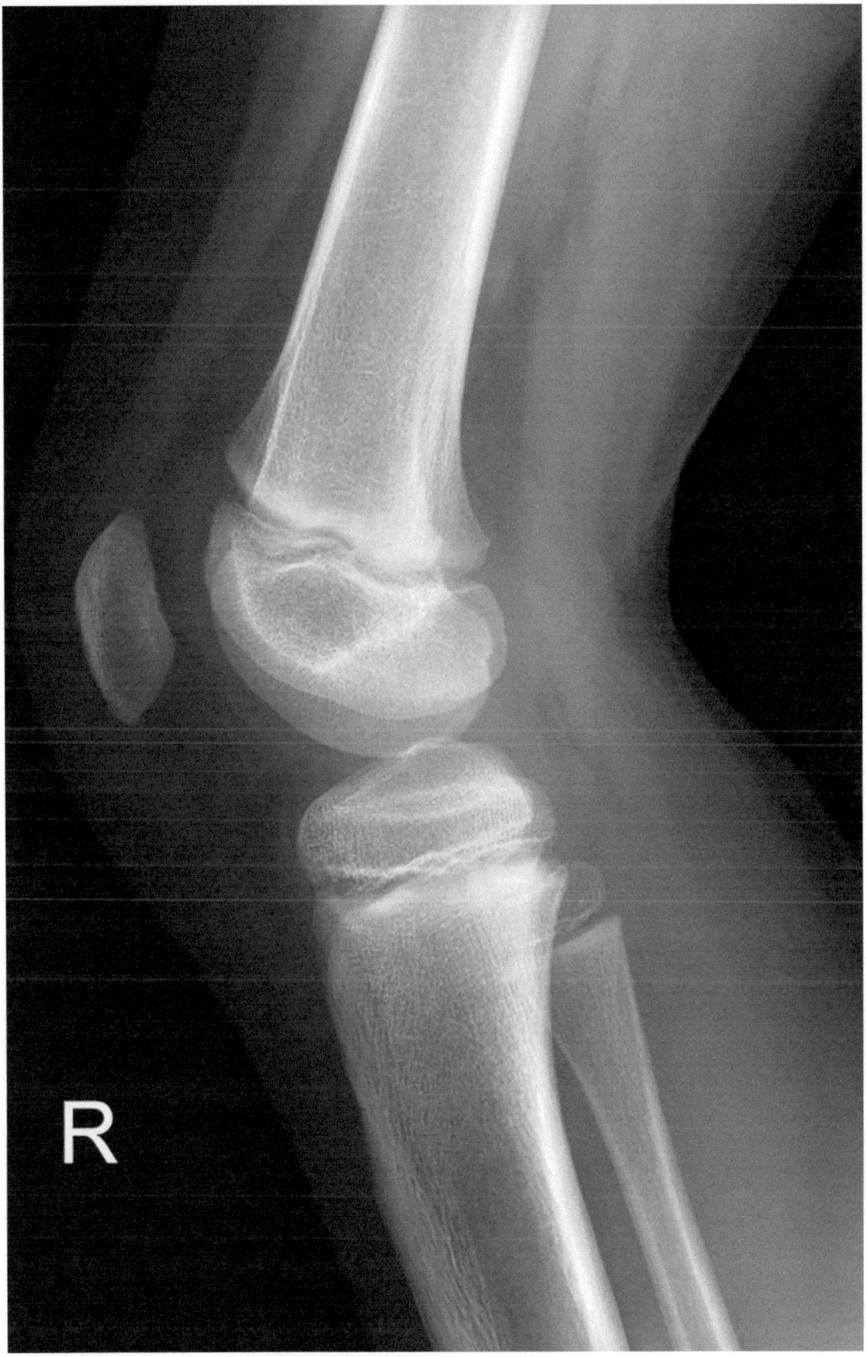

Image 11

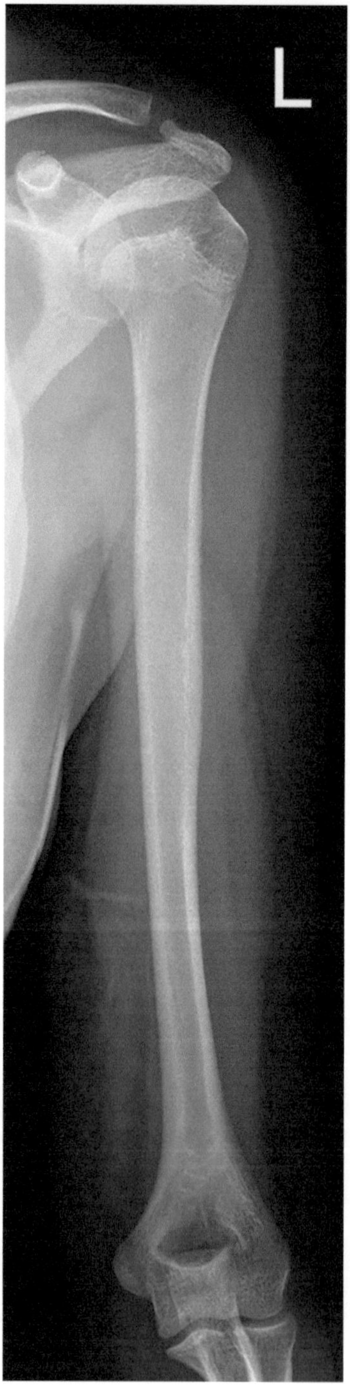

Image 12

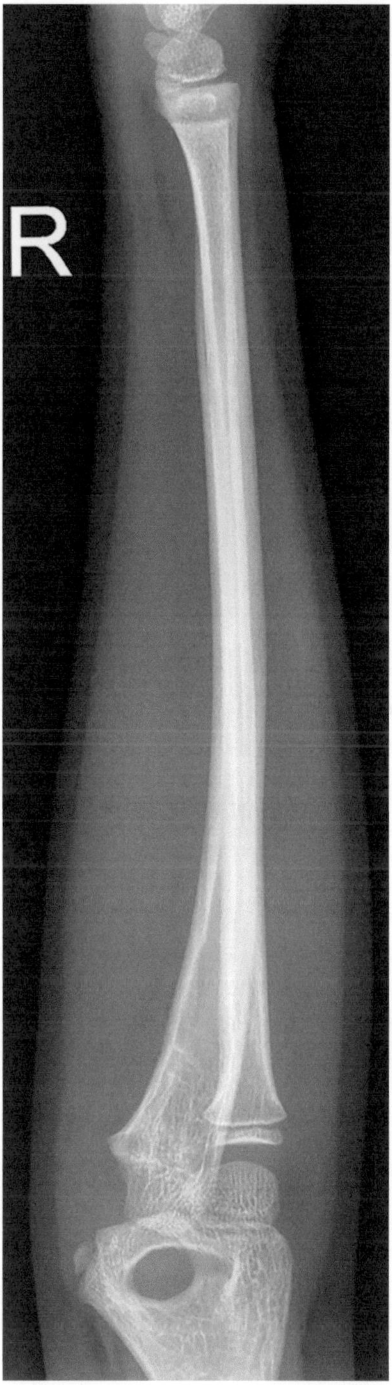

Image 13

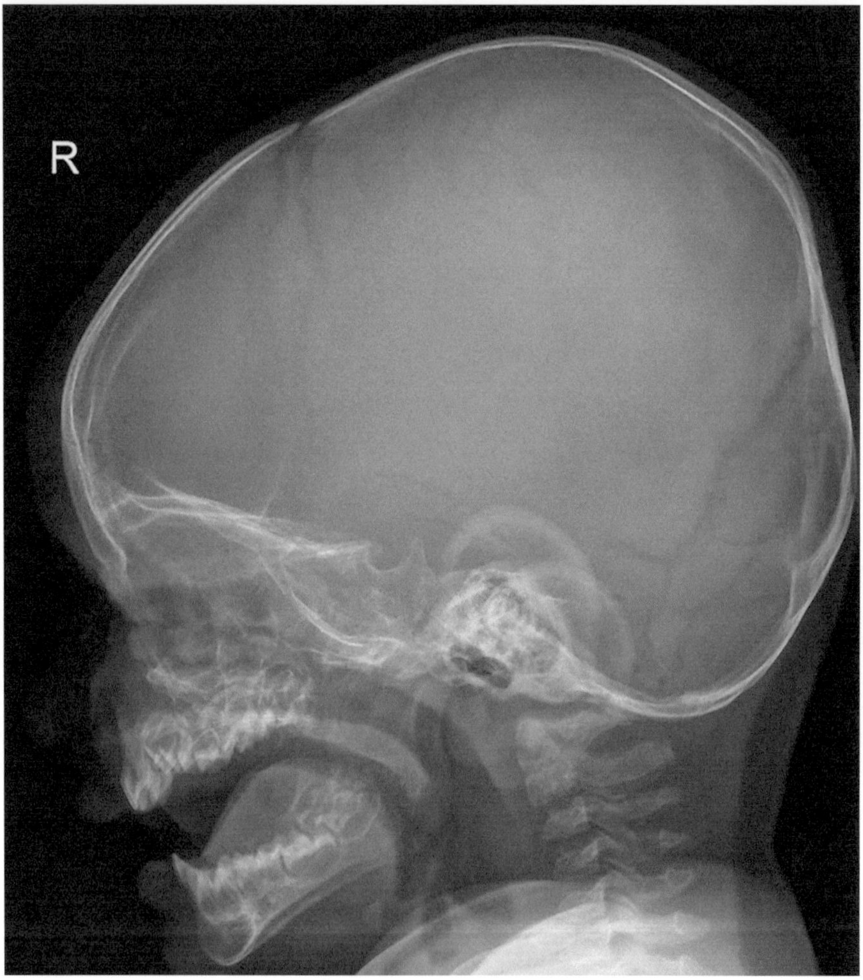

Image 14

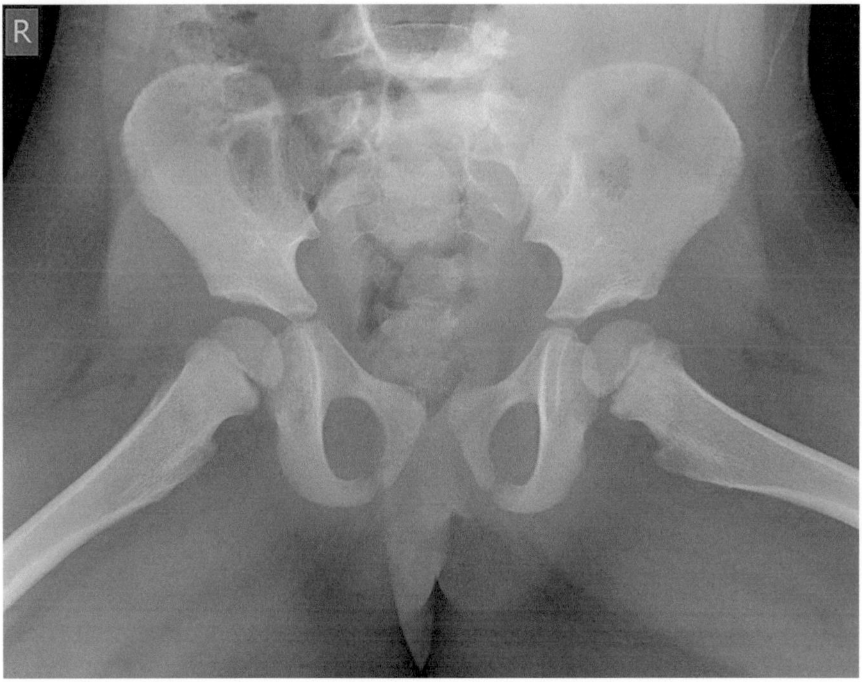

Image 15

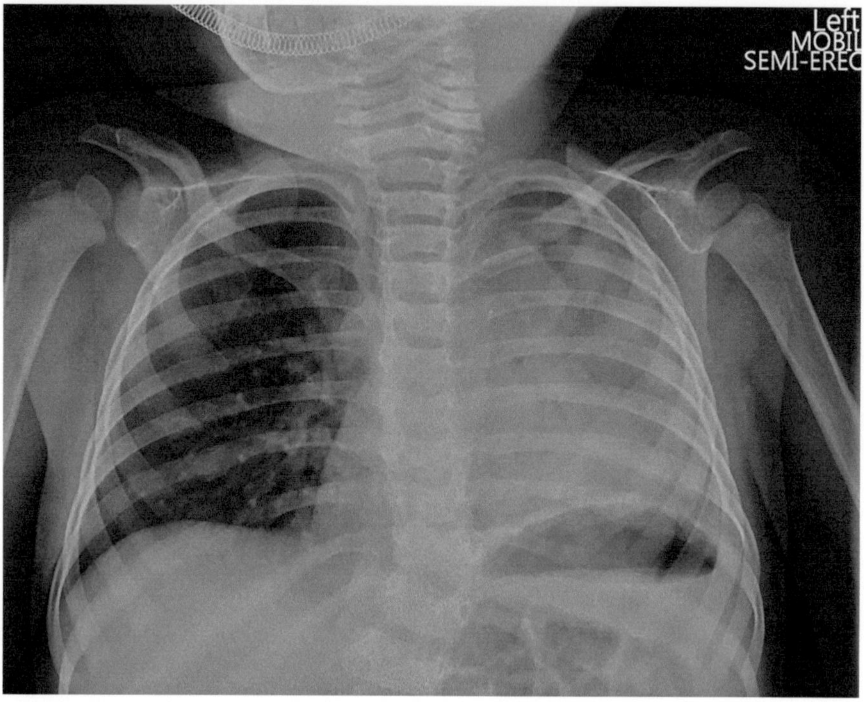

Image 16

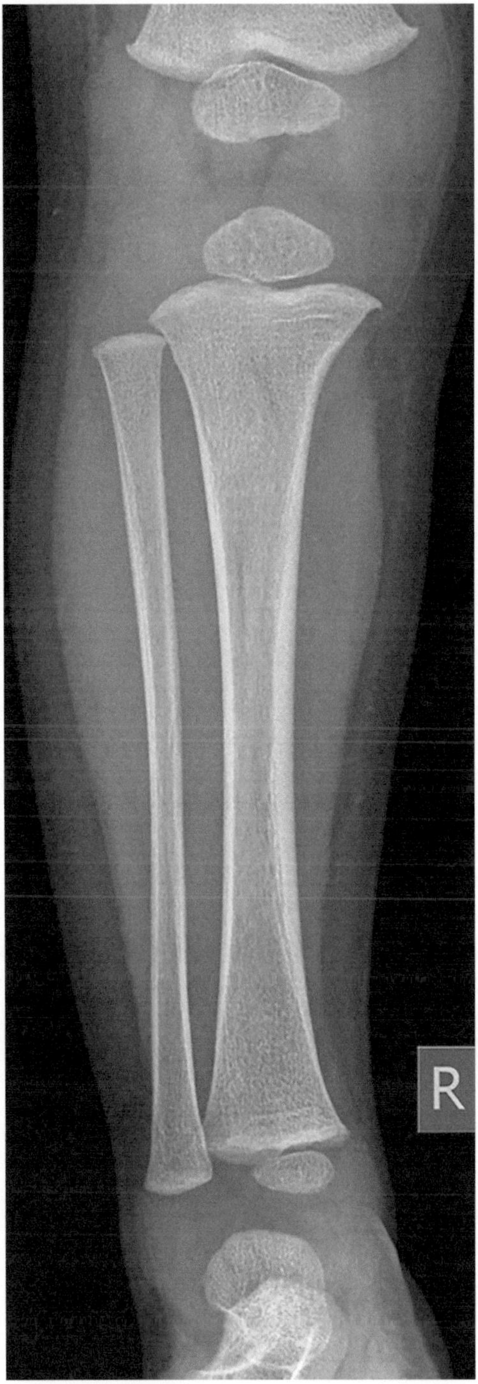

Image 17

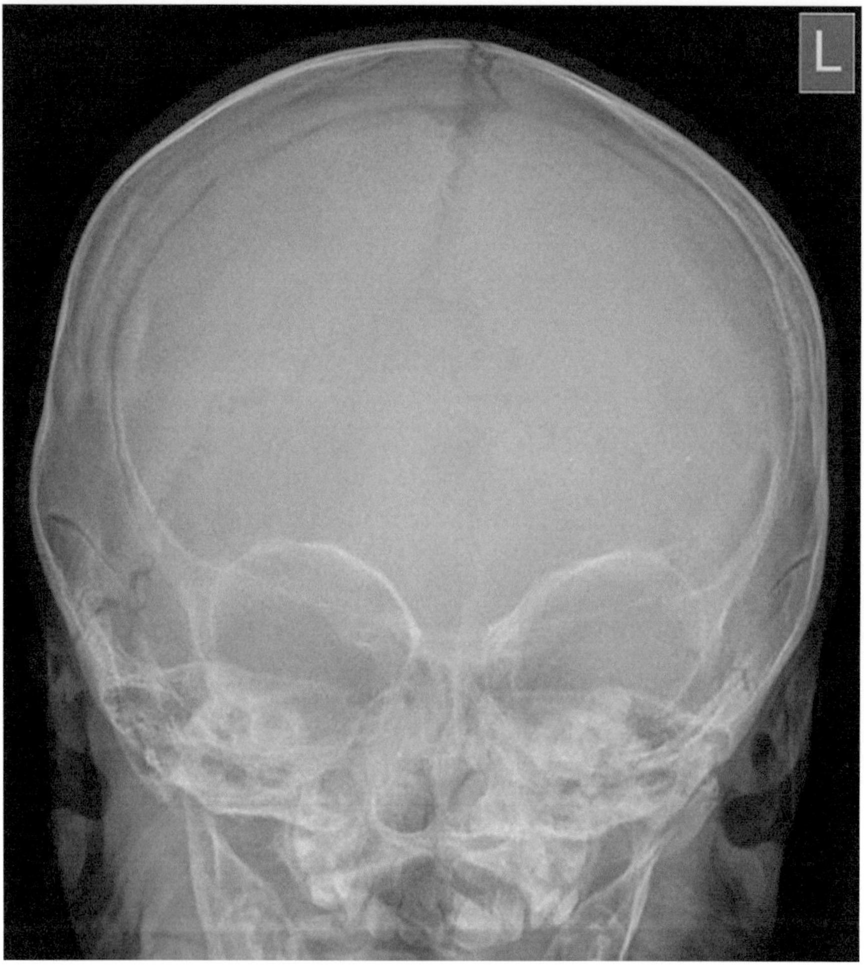

Image 18

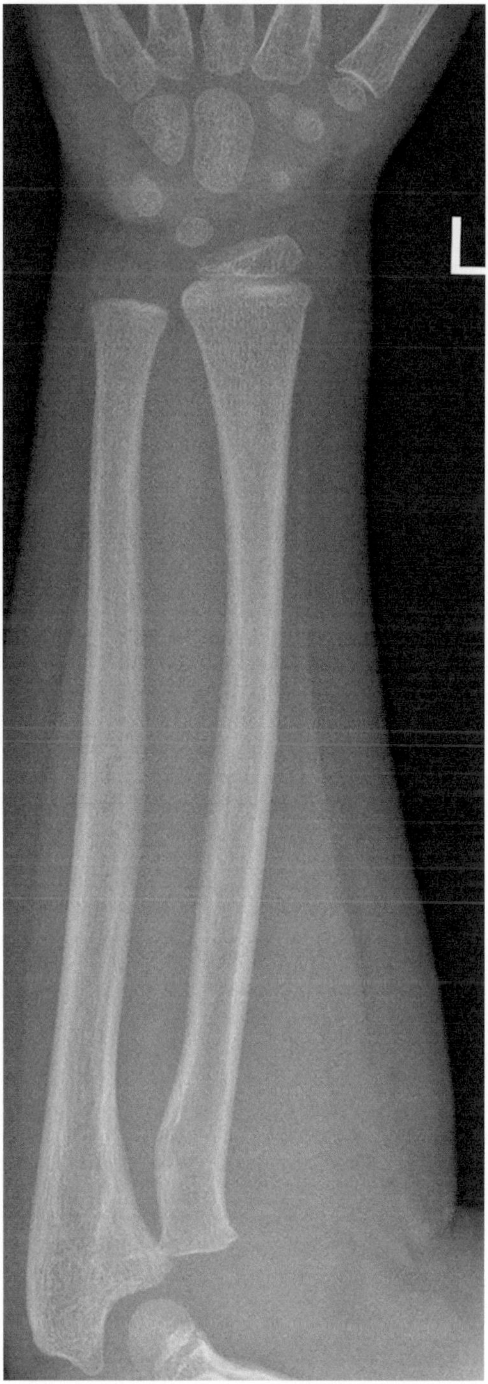

Image 19

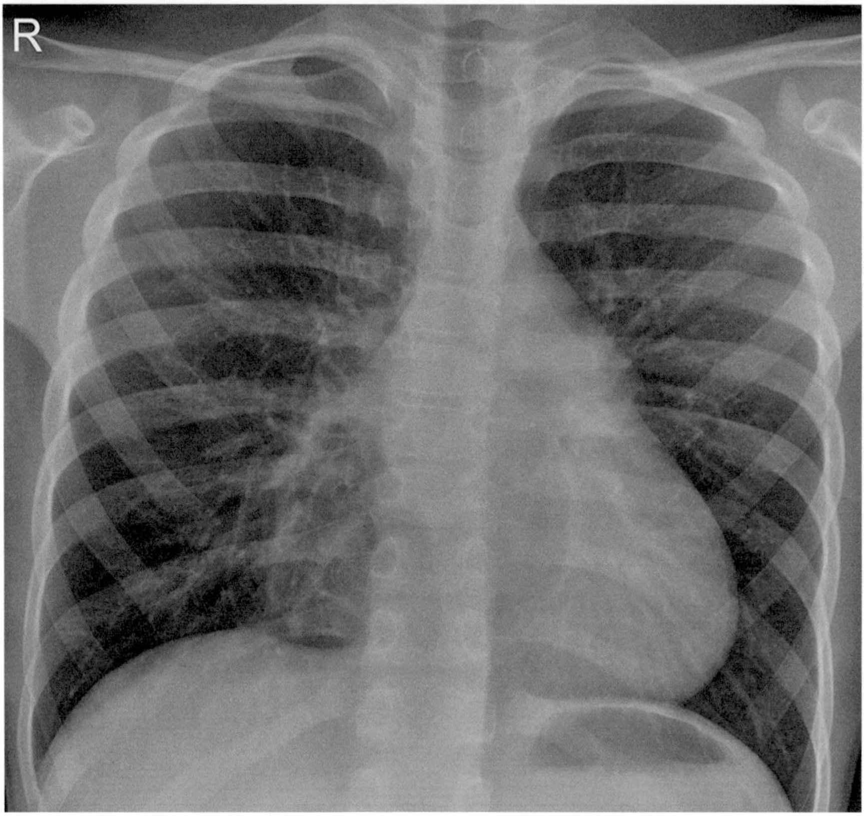

Image 20

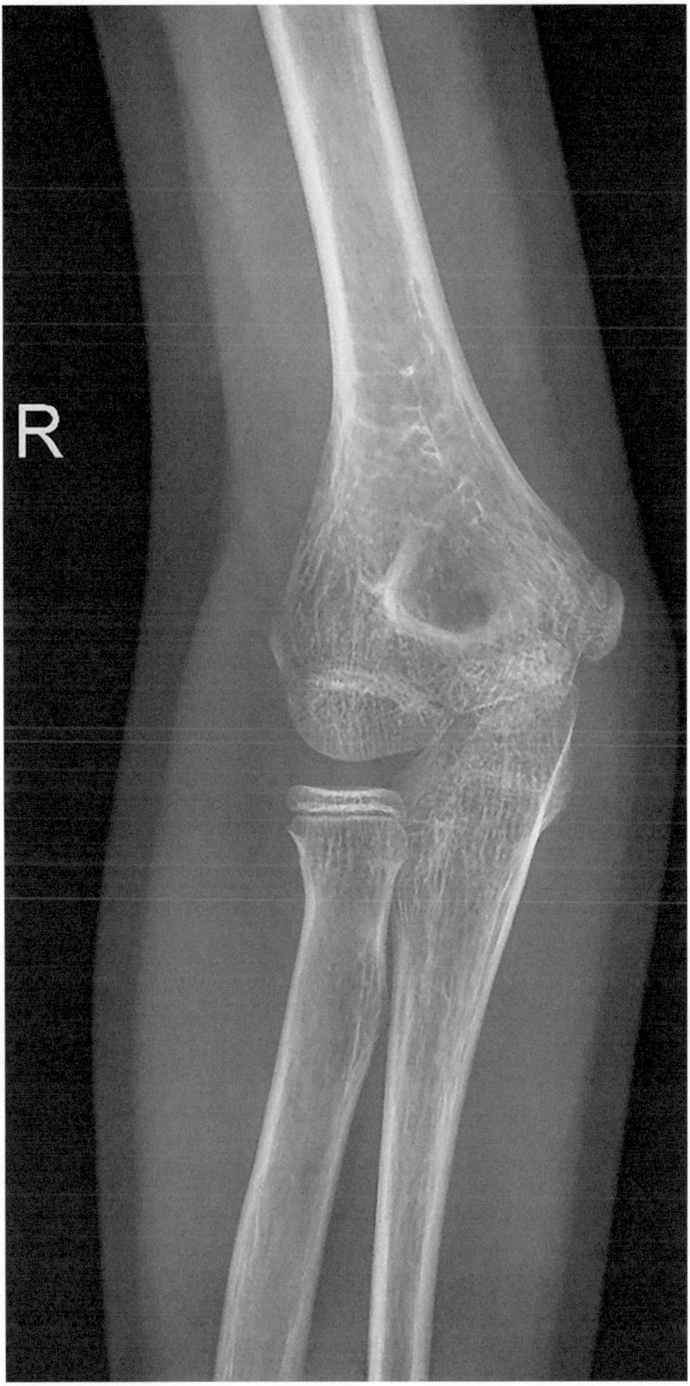

Image 21

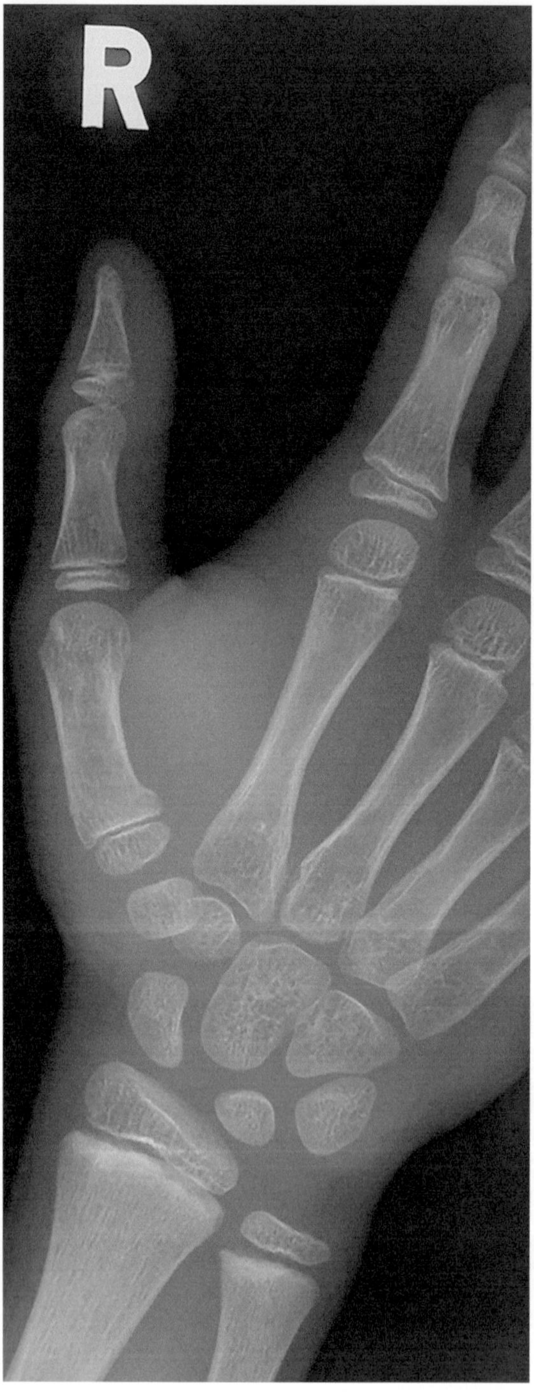

Image 22

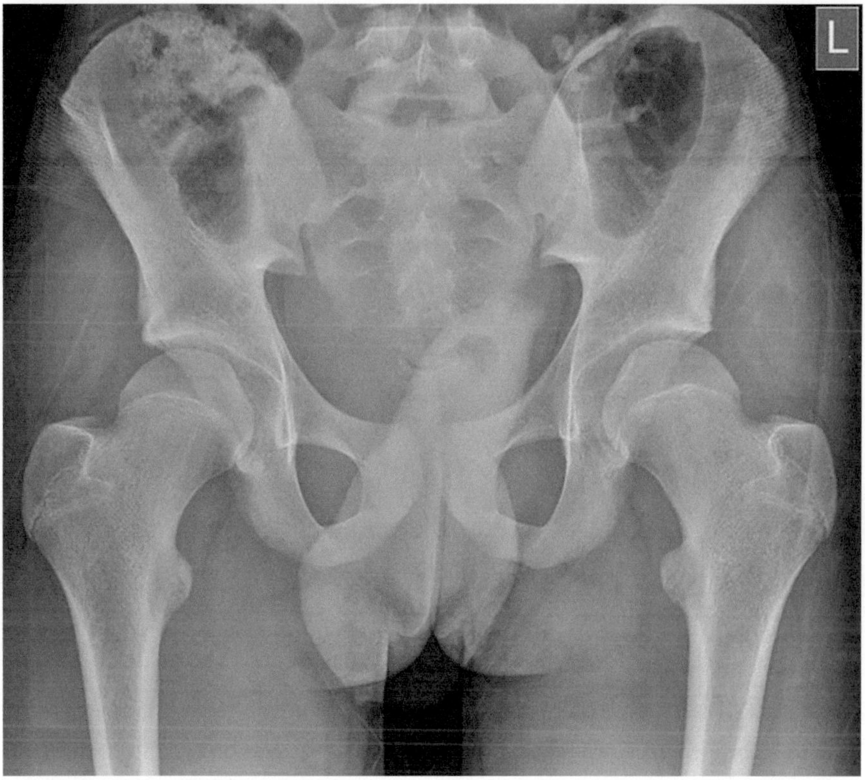

Image 23

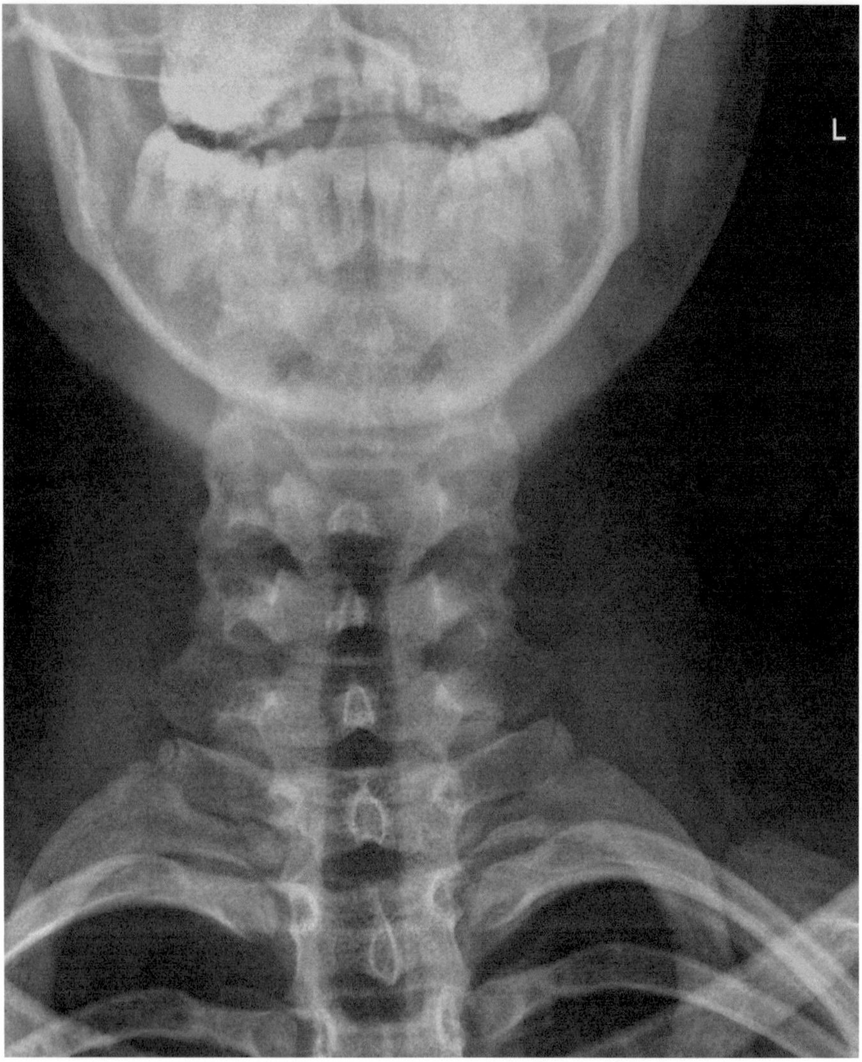

Image 24

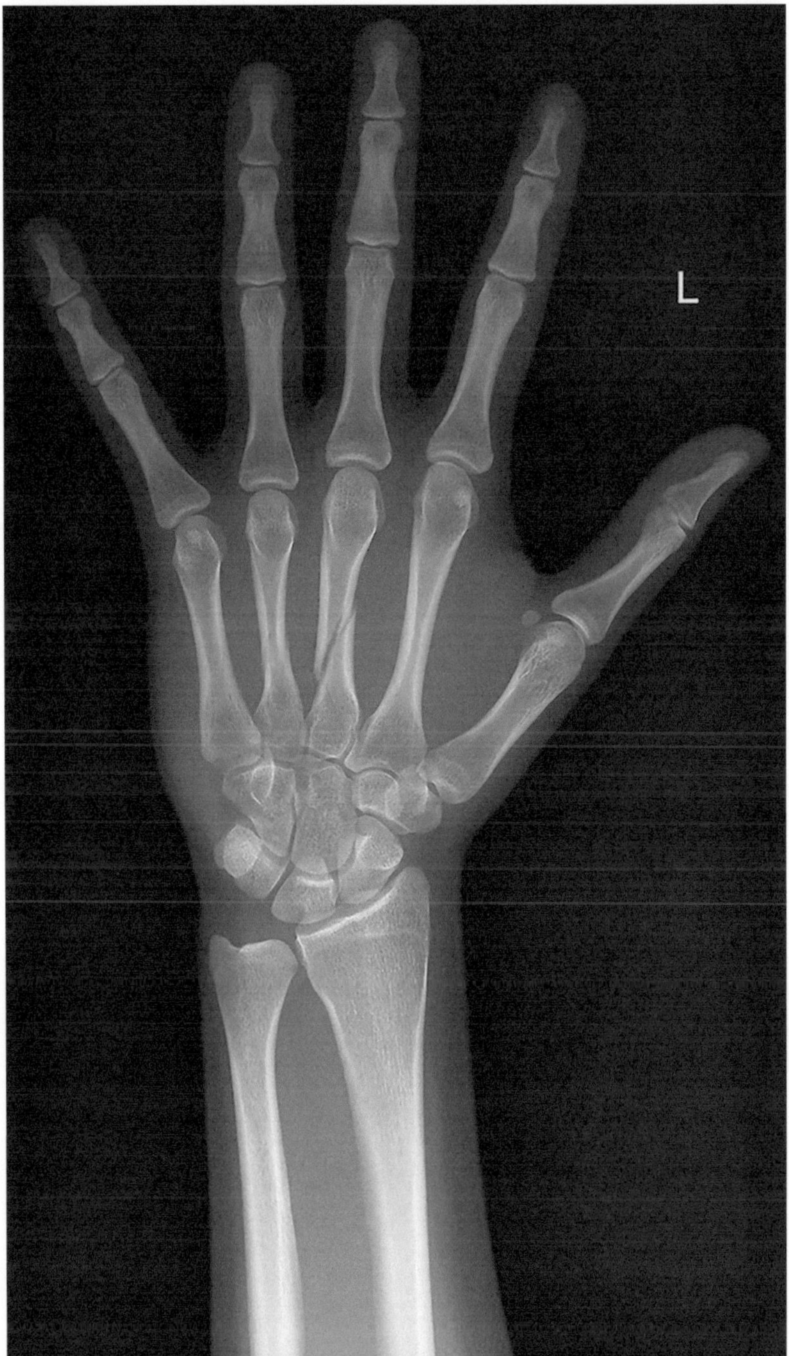

Image 25

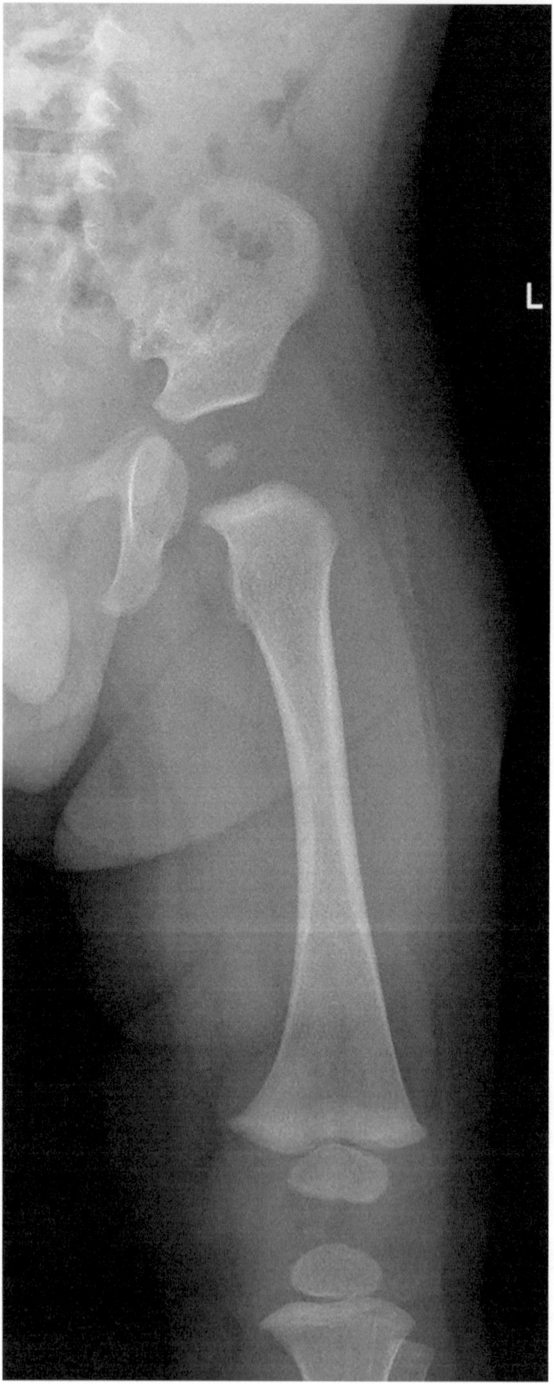

Image 26

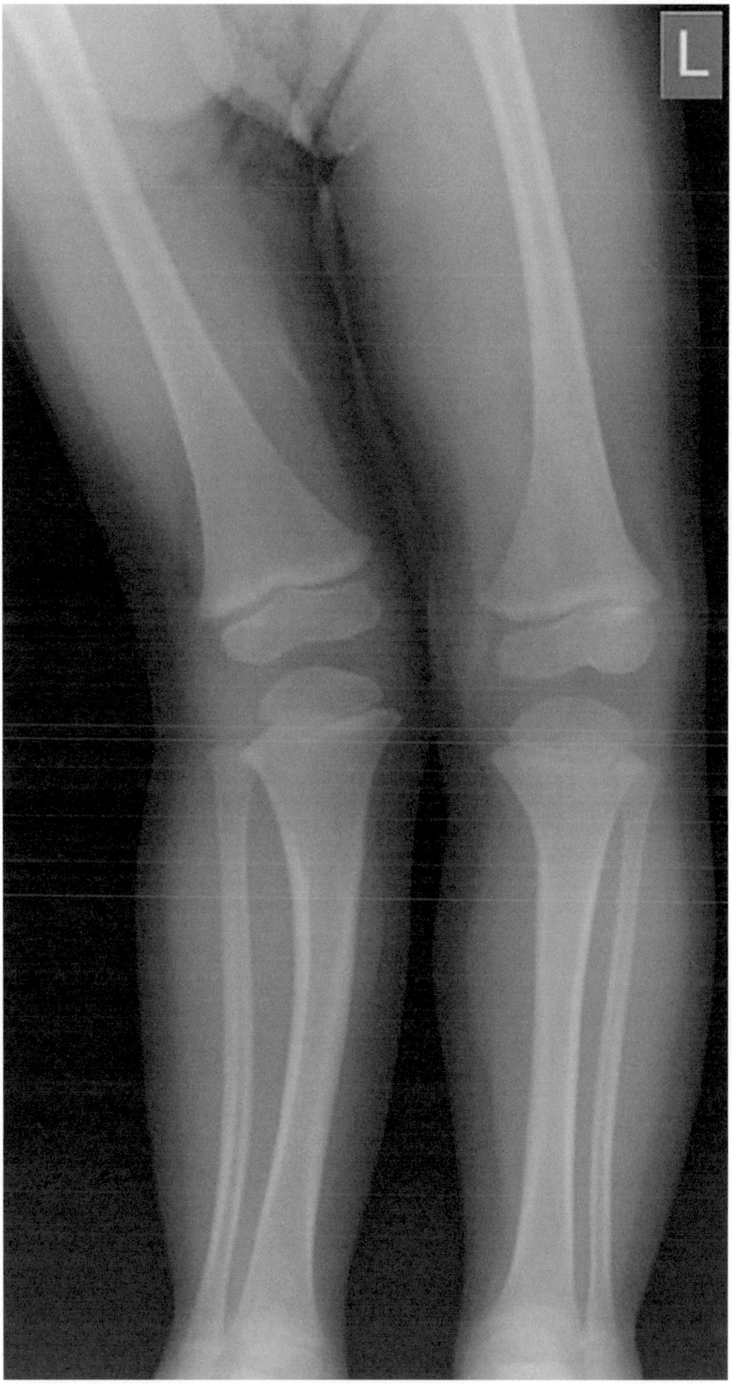

Image 27

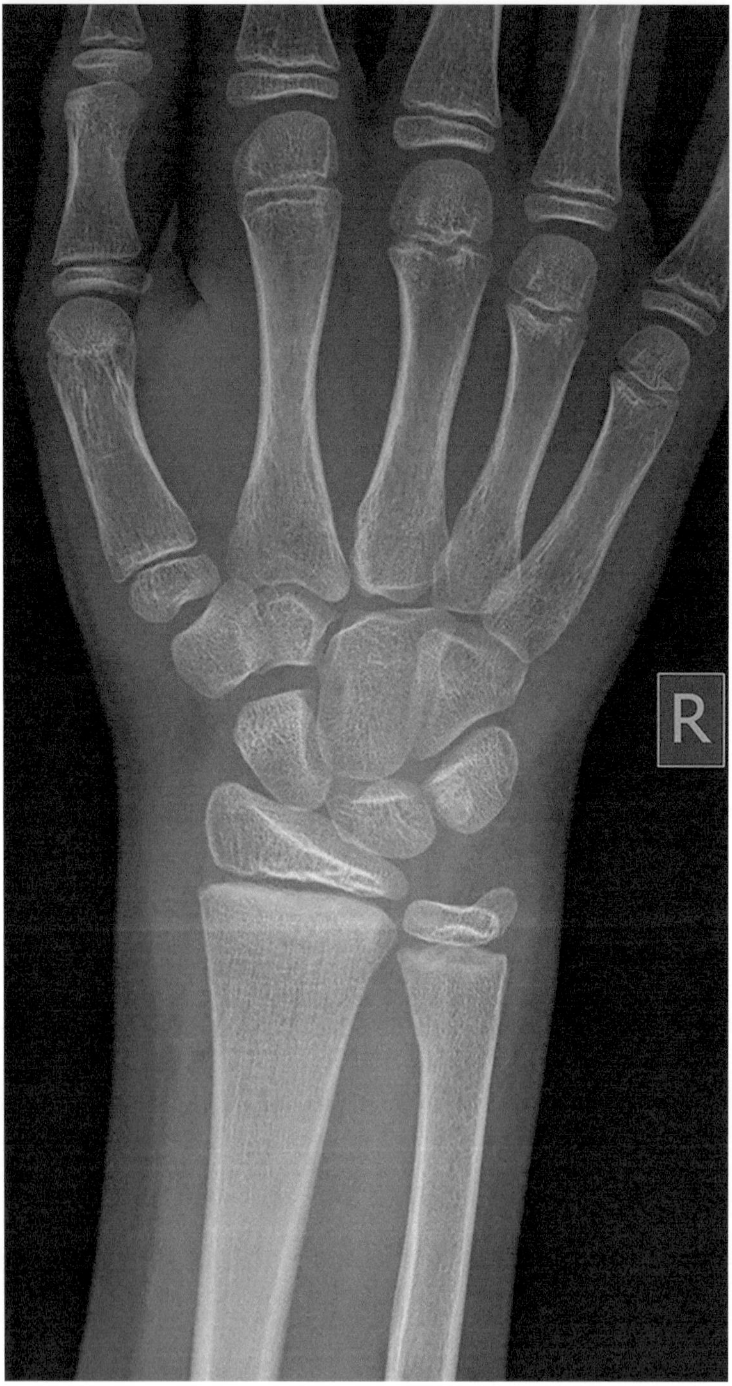

Image 28

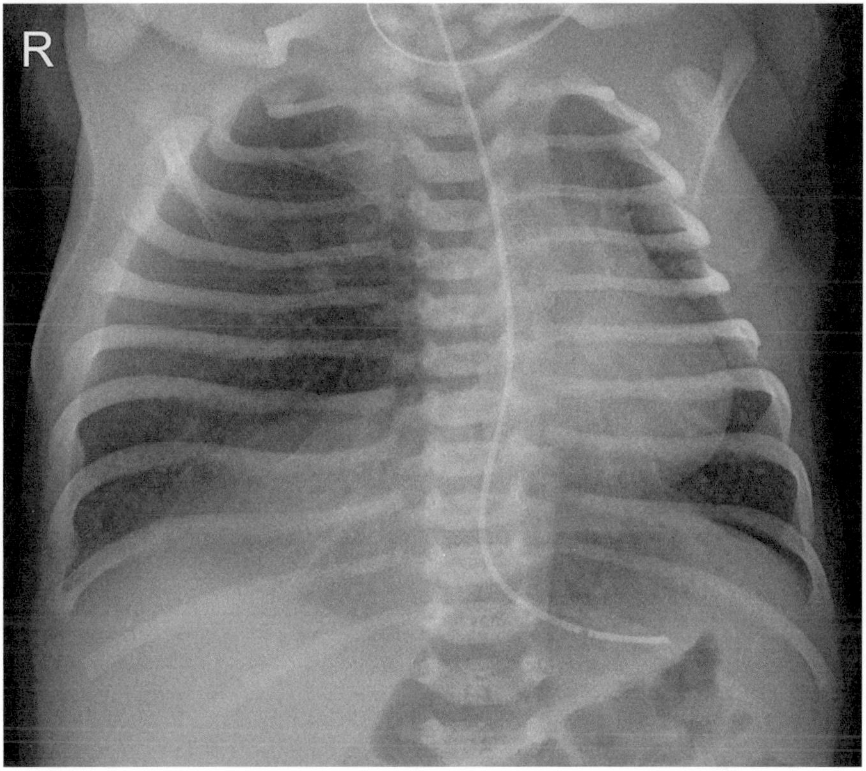

Image 29

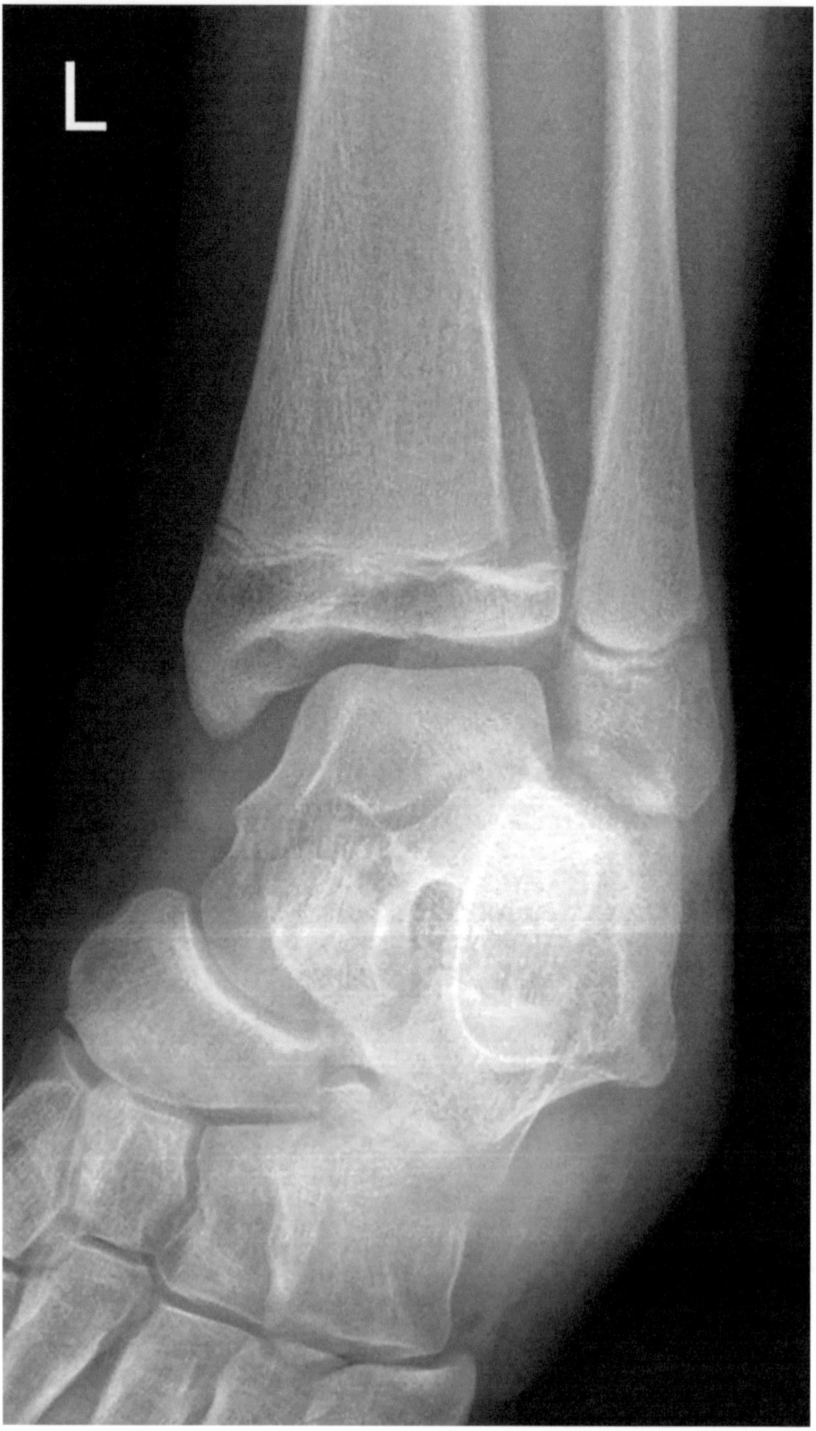

Image 30

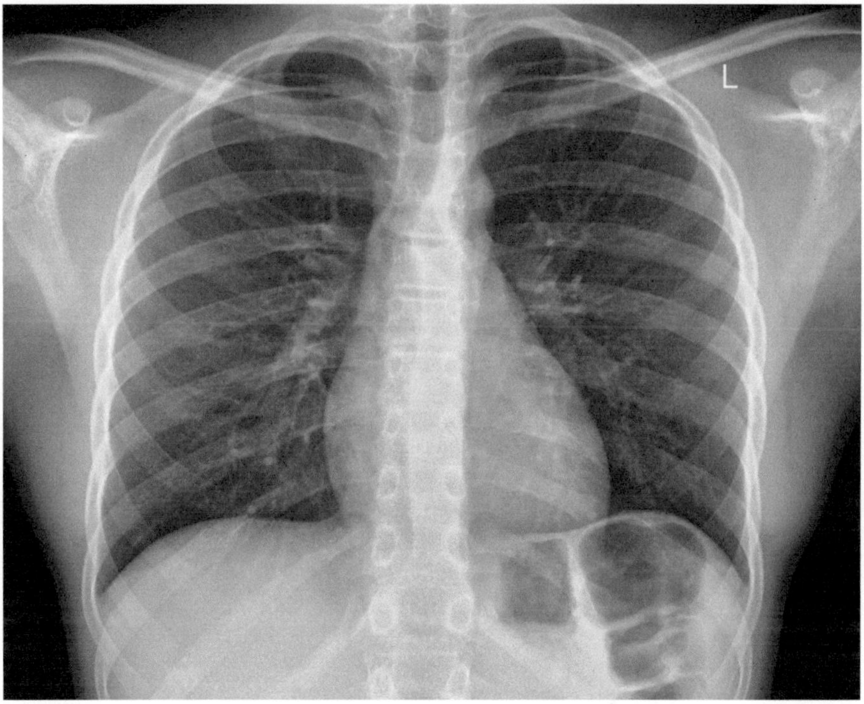

9.2 Answers

Image	Normal	Abnormal	Diagnosis/abnormality (only if abnormal)
1		✓	Healing/chronic avulsion # R ischial tuberosity
2	✓		
3	✓		
4	✓		
5		✓	Ingested radiopaque foreign body
6		✓	Pathological # L humeral diaphysis
7		✓	Spiral # L humeral diaphysis
8	✓		
9		✓	Transverse # R little finger metacarpal base
10	✓		
11	✓		
12	✓		
13	✓		
14	✓		
15		✓	L upper lobe collapse
16		✓	Buckle # R proximal tibial metaphysis
17	✓		
18		✓	L radial head dislocation
19		✓	Pectus excavatum
20	✓		
21		✓	SH2 # R thumb metacarpal base
22	✓		
23		✓	L apical pneumothorax
24		✓	Spiral # L middle finger metacarpal diaphysis
25	✓		
26		✓	R genu valgum/Cozen phenomenon
27		✓	Buckle # R distal ulnar metaphysis
28		✓	R middle lobe congenital lobar overinflation
29		✓	L triplanar #
30	✓		

9.3 Explanations

1. **Healing/chronic avulsion # R ischial tuberosity**
The ischial tuberosity is the insertion for the hamstring tendons. This image shows a displaced and fragmented healing avulsion fracture. See the explanation for Image 13 of Test 4.

5. **Ingested radiopaque foreign body**
Whilst the abnormality may be obvious, we have included this radiograph so that you are able to recognise this foreign body as a *button battery*. They account for approximately 2% of all ingested foreign bodies in children with a peak incidence between 6 months and 3 years of age. Given its shape, size and contour, a button battery may be mistaken for a coin. Significant sequelae can result from button battery ingestion (BBI) including reported cases of death. This necessitates that *any* suspected coin or ingested well-circumscribed radiopaque foreign body be scrutinised on radiographs. Button batteries have a distinctive appearance on anteroposterior (AP) radiographs described as a 'double ring', 'double halo', or 'double density', as seen in the magnified image below:

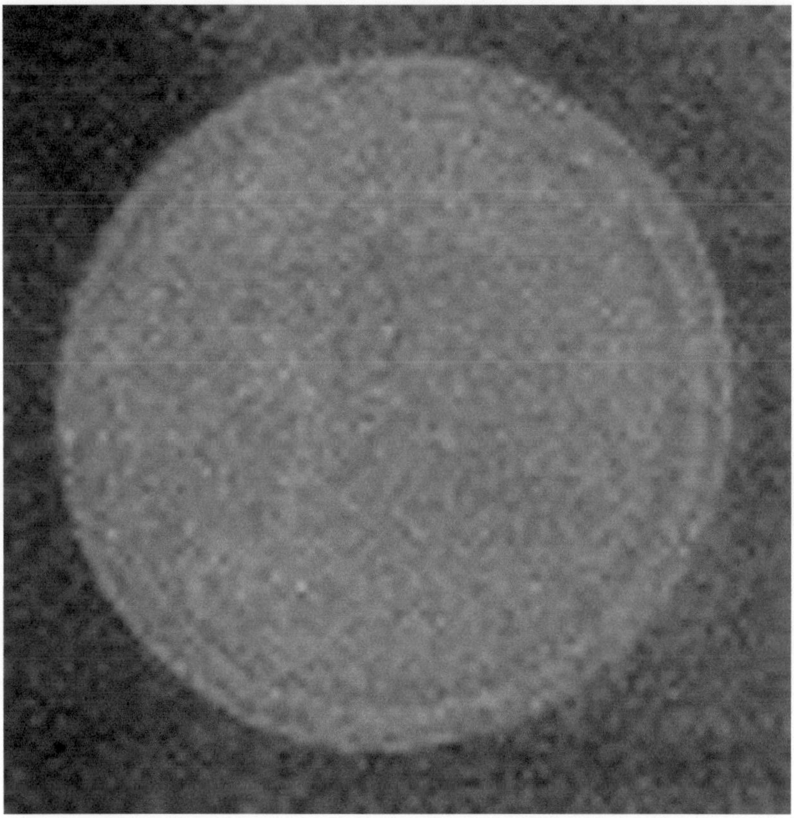

Severe tissue damage can result from BBI from as little as 2 h post-ingestion. The mechanism is that of electrolysis of fluid in the local oesophageal tissue which generates a current, and subsequently hydroxide, at the negative pole of the battery. The type of button battery is also important: the ubiquitous lithium button batteries have a higher voltage and capacitance than other types resulting in an increased production of hydroxide, and therefore, more tissue damage. Other mechanisms include pressure necrosis and leakage of alkaline electrolytes from the battery itself; this is supposedly less of a problem with lithium batteries resulting in less mucosal irritation. Delayed complications include but are not limited to:

- Oesophageal perforation.
- Tracheo-oesphageal fistula.
- Exsanguination after fistulation into a major blood vessel, e.g. aorto-oesophageal fistula.
- Vocal cord paralysis.
- Oesophageal stricture.

Given the importance of identifying this finding, we have also included a lateral soft tissue neck projection from a different patient which may also be obtained in the investigation of '*?foreign body*':

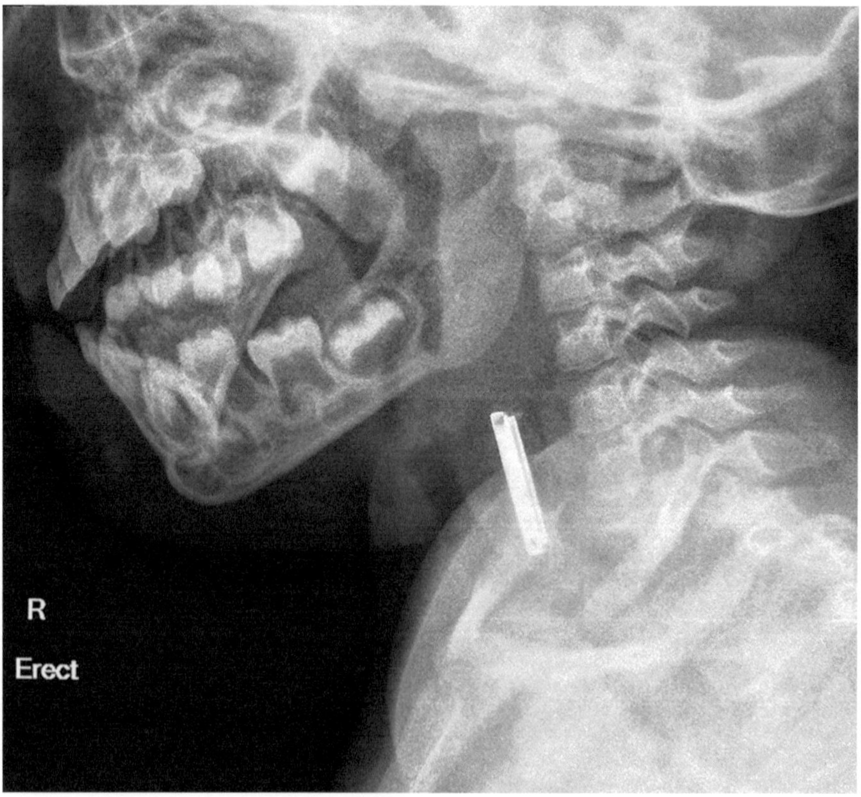

The button battery in the above lateral projection lies in the oesophagus, *posterior* to the gas-filled trachea.

Urgent surgical opinion should be sought alongside maintaining close liaison with Emergency Department (ED) colleagues. If the battery is located in the stomach or beyond, management (conservative or surgical) is dictated by the age of the child, the size of the battery, and whether or not there is concern for concurrent oesophageal injury.

6. **Pathological # L humeral diaphysis**

This child was presented to the ED with arm pain following a fall at a trampoline park. There is a well-defined lucency in the left proximal humeral diaphysis with surrounding sclerosis and associated cortical thinning/scalloping consistent with a simple bone cyst through which there is a pathological fracture.

Non-aggressive lucent bone lesions such as these, also known as unicameral (from the Latin meaning *one* + *chamber*) bone cysts (UBCs), are usually asymptomatic. Their most frequent presentation is due to pathological fracture which may be discovered incidentally when imaging is performed for another indication. These cysts are intramedullary in location and are usually found in the metaphyses of long bones adjacent to the physis. The proximal humerus is the most common location accounting for up to approximately 60% of cases, followed by the proximal femur (up to 30%). As the bone grows, UBCs migrate toward the diaphysis and heal.

The diagnosis is usually made on radiographs: their typical imaging features include a narrow zone of transition with a thin sclerotic margin and thinning of the endosteum (scalloping). There is no soft tissue component or associated periosteal reaction unless there is healing from a pathological fracture. A dependent bony fragment may be visualised in the context of a fracture, known as the 'fallen fragment' sign. UBCs may appear multiloculated following repeated pathological fractures.

7. **Spiral # L humeral diaphysis**
   The humeral fracture at the edge of the image is magnified below:

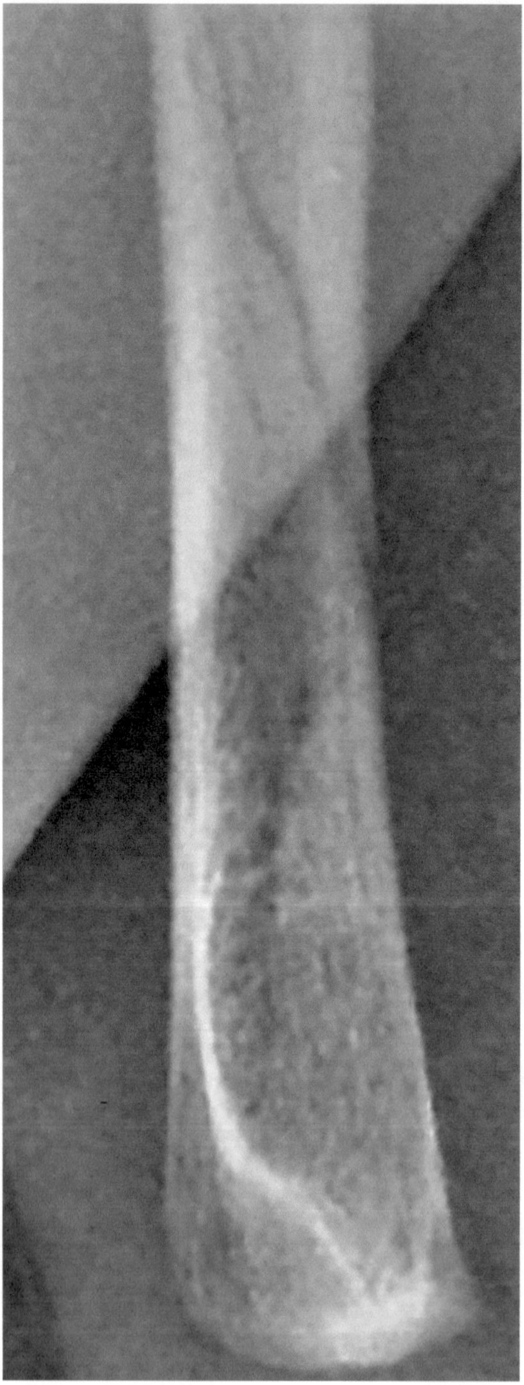

9. **Transverse # R little finger metacarpal base**
   Base of little finger metacarpal fractures usually occur as a result of axial loading forces to a flexed hand and so are often seen as a result of injuries with a clenched fist such as punching. It is important that alignment is carefully assessed in the presence of these injuries as fractures extending to the carpometacarpal joint are unstable due to the unopposed action of extensor carpi ulnaris, resulting in ulnar and dorsal subluxation.

15. **L upper lobe collapse**
   This portable chest radiograph demonstrates the distinctive 'veil-like opacity' of left upper lobe collapse in which the left upper lobe collapses anteriorly, is apposed to the anterior chest wall and results in both volume loss and increased radiographic density of the left hemithorax. Other features of left upper lobe/hemithorax volume loss include:
   - Mediastinal shift to the left.
   - Superior displacement of the left hilum.
   - Elevation of the left hemidiaphragm, which may be 'tented' or 'peaked'.
   - Crowding of the left-sided ribs (compare to the normally spaced right-sided ribs).

   Other radiographic features of left upper lobe collapse include:
   - Obscuration of the anterior portion of the left heart border which reflects where the collapsed lingular segments of the left upper lobe abut the left heart border.
   - Luftsichel sign: from the German meaning 'air + sickle' which describes the 'air crescent' seen between the aortic arch and the medial border of the collapsed left upper lobe. This 'classic' appearance results from the interposition of the hyperinflated superior segment of the left lower lobe between the mediastinum and the collapsed left upper lobe.

   A common cause of lobar collapse in children is mucous plugging due to asthma, bronchiolitis (which often results in multifocal atelectasis), or endobronchial infection. A very important cause not to be forgotten is foreign body inhalation or aspiration, usually in younger children but also possibly in zealous older children!

   Tip for the viva:
   - This is a classic starter case in the *viva voce* examination, typically in an adult patient with left upper lobe collapse from an underlying bronchogenic carcinoma.

16. **Buckle # R proximal tibial metaphysis**
   There is a subtle buckle fracture of the lateral cortex of the right proximal tibial metaphysis, better visualised in the magnified image below:

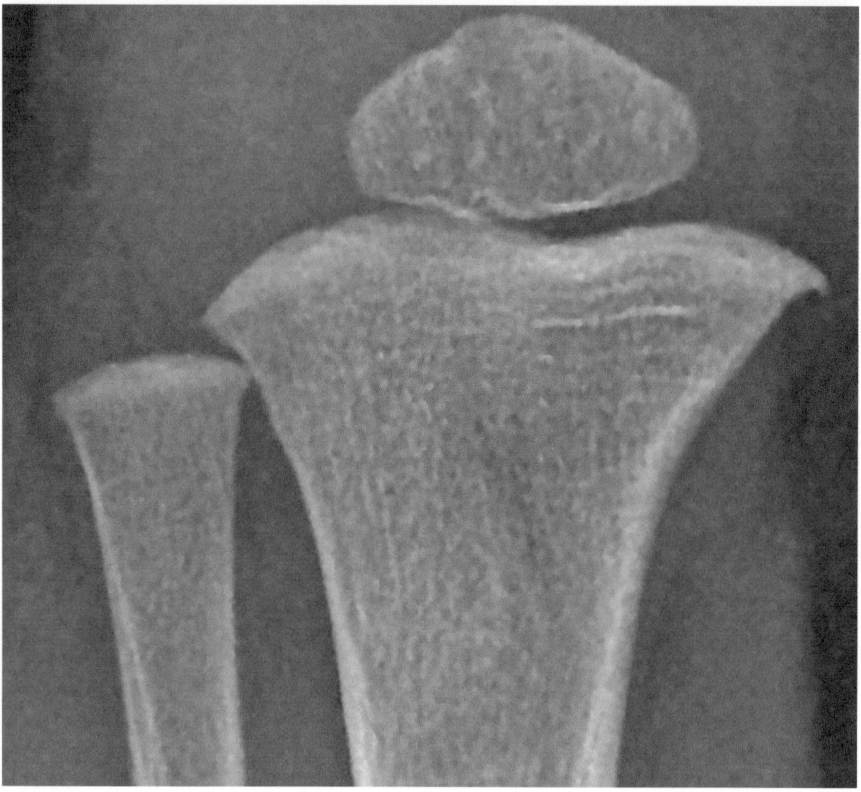

Whilst this fracture is subtle, it is genuine. It is important that these injuries are not missed: add the proximal tibial metaphysis to your review checklist when reporting paediatric tibia/fibula and knee radiographs. See the explanation for Image 24 of Test 4.

18. **L radial head dislocation**
    Did you spot the radial head dislocation at the edge of the image? Remember that elbow joint alignment must be assessed on every forearm and elbow radiograph. See Image 11 of Test 1 for a detailed discussion on the radiographic assessment of elbow joint alignment and Image 28 of Test 1 for a further example of radial head dislocation.

19. **Pectus excavatum**
    This image demonstrates the typical radiographic features of pectus excavatum which include:
    - Horizontal posterior ribs with vertical anterior ribs creating the classic '7' rib configuration.
    - Blurring/obscuration of the right heart border.
    - Increased density of the right inferomedial lung zone.
    - Displacement/shift of the cardiac silhouette to the left.
    - Decreased visualisation/absence of the descending aortic interface.

Tip for the viva:

- Pectus excavatum is a common viva case because at a first or quick glance, the radiograph may appear normal. It is only on further inspection that the radiographic features of pectus excavatum described above are appreciated.

21. **Salter-Harris 2 # R thumb metacarpal base**
See the explanation for Image 30 of Test 1.

22. *Normal pelvic radiograph*
Note the normal iliac crest and anterior inferior iliac spine (AIIS) apophyses which have not yet fused and are normal for age.

23. **L apical pneumothorax**
Careful inspection reveals a small volume left apical pneumothorax. Be vigilant and comprehensive in your imaging evaluation.

24. **Spiral # L middle finger metacarpal diaphysis**
Metacarpal fractures may result from a direct blow to the hand or from a rotational injury with axial loading.

26. **R genu valgum/Cozen phenomenon**
This radiograph demonstrates a right genu valgum deformity following a right proximal tibial fracture 12 months previously; this is known as Cozen's phenomenon. See the explanation for Image 24 of Test 4.

27. **Buckle # R distal ulnar metaphysis**
There is an acute angulation of the radial aspect of the right distal ulnar metaphyseal cortex, which is consistent with a buckle fracture. This finding is subtle but does represent a genuine bony injury. There is no concurrent acute bony injury of the right distal radius and there is normal alignment of the right distal radioulnar joint. See the explanation for Image 18 of Test 1.

28. **R middle lobe congenital lobar overinflation**
Congenital lobar overinflation (CLO), previously known as congenital lobar emphysema (CLE), is a congenital progressive overinflation of a lung lobe (or less frequently lobes) with a male predominance.

CLO occurs due to bronchial obstruction with a resultant 'one way valve' effect and distal air trapping. It is more frequent in the left upper lobe (up to 45% of cases) > right middle lobe > right upper lobe (and rarely in the lower lobes). Interestingly, whilst the left upper lobe is the commonest affected lobe, the right hemithorax is more frequently involved than the left. This chest radiograph demonstrates the typical features of an overinflated right middle lobe:

- Hyperlucency with a paucity of blood vessels (pulmonary oligaemia).
- Resultant mediastinal shift to the left.
- Tenting of the right horizontal fissure which has been displaced superiorly between the right second and third rib spaces medially.

The right hemidiaphragm is not depressed and lies slightly higher than the left hemidiaphragm, inferring that the right lower lobe is not overinflated, in which case the right hemidiaphragm would be depressed. Thus, the overinflation can be localised to the right middle lobe.

CLO may be suggested on antenatal imaging. Immediate postnatal radiographs may be normal, or the affected lobe may be fluid-filled with increased lobar opacity representing fetal lung fluid that has yet to clear. Serial radiographs may show progressive distension. Alternatively, as in this case, an initial radiograph taken after birth (in the first few days or months of life depending on severity) when respiratory distress develops (i.e. grunting, increased work of breathing, new or progressive oxygen requirement) may reveal the lobar inflation. This signifies that the normal ipsilateral lobes and contralateral normal lung can no longer compensate for the overinflated lobe(s).

Investigation with computed tomography pulmonary angiogram (CTPA) will not only delineate the lobe(s) affected but also help to differentiate from other pathologies such as congenital pulmonary airway malformation (CPAM), bronchial atresia, and bronchogenic cyst (the differential for this radiographic appearance). Furthermore, this allows the mediastinum and vascular anatomy to be evaluated for an anatomical defect such as an aberrant left pulmonary artery, a known abnormality associated with CLO. Associated cardiac defects include ventricular septal defect (VSD), patent ductus arteriosus (PDA), and tetralogy of Fallot, for which formal evaluation with echocardiography would be advised. As with CPAM, CLO is hyperechoic on fetal ultrasound and T2 hyperintense on *in utero* magnetic resonance imaging (MRI).

Management is determined by the symptom burden and may be conservative or surgical; emergent surgical resection may be required in symptomatic neonatal patients.

29. **L triplanar #**

A triplanar fracture is usually seen in younger children before distal tibial physeal fusion has begun, i.e. when the physis is completely ‘open’. These fractures are complex Salter-Harris 4 injuries, and as the name suggests, involve three planes centred around the distal tibial physis:

- A vertical fracture through the lateral aspect of the epiphysis.
- A horizontal fracture through the physis.
- An oblique (posteriorly oriented) fracture through the metaphysis.

A contemporaneous lateral/orthogonal projection *must* be carefully evaluated for fracture extension through the posterior distal tibial metaphysis. By contrast, a Salter-Harris 3 fracture through the *lateral* aspect of the distal tibial epiphysis is known as a Tillaux fracture (see the explanation for Image 1 of Test 6). If there is *any* uncertainty regarding the type of fracture sustained, evaluation with computed tomography (CT) is indicated, particularly given that small vertically oriented fractures of the posterior distal tibial metaphysis may be overlooked on radiography. The degree of fracture fragment displacement determines the management: open reduction and internal fixation (ORIF) is indicated when lateral talar displacement is greater than 1 mm.

See the explanations for Image 1 of Test 6 for a discussion of Tillaux fractures and Image 30 of Test 1 for a discussion regarding the Salter-Harris classification.

Further Reading

Image 5

Kipiki PE, Chussi D, Shija P et al (2023) Button battery ingestion: a serious pitfall of diagnosis of ingested foreign bodies in children from resource-limited settings—a case report. Int J Surg Case Rep 109:108593

Lorenzo M, Beno S (2023) Evolving threat of pediatric ingestions: a discussion of cannabis and button batteries and their implications for children. Curr Opin Pediatr 35(3):316–323

Image 15

Dembla SR et al (2022) Left upper lobe collapse. https://radiopaedia.org/articles/left-upper-lobe-collapse. Accessed Aug 2023

Gaillard F et al (2023) Luftsichel sign (lungs). https://radiopaedia.org/articles/luftsichel-sign-lungs. Accessed Aug 2023

Image 19

Ashraf A et al (2023) Pectus excavatum. https://radiopaedia.org/articles/pectus-excavatum. Accessed Sep 2023

Image 28

El-Ali AM, Strubel NA, Lala SV (2022) Congenital lung lesions: a radiographic pattern approach. Pediatr Radiol 52(4):622–636

Sintim-Damoa A, Cohen HL (2022) Fetal imaging of congenital lung lesions with postnatal correlation. Pediatr Radiol 52(10):1921–1934

Image 29

Bell D et al (2022) Triplane fracture. https://radiopaedia.org/articles/triplane-fracture. Accessed Aug 2023

Smithius R (2018) Special cases of ankle fracture. Detection of 'not so obvious' fractures. https://radiologyassistant.nl/musculoskeletal/ankle/special-fracture-cases. Accessed Aug 2023

Image 30

Bell DJ et al (2021) Thymic sail sign. https://radiopaedia.org/articles/thymic-sail-sign. Accessed Sep 2023

Test 10

10

M. Paddock et al., *Paediatric Radiology Rapid Reporting*,
https://doi.org/10.1007/978-3-031-48255-7_10

10.1 Images

Image 1

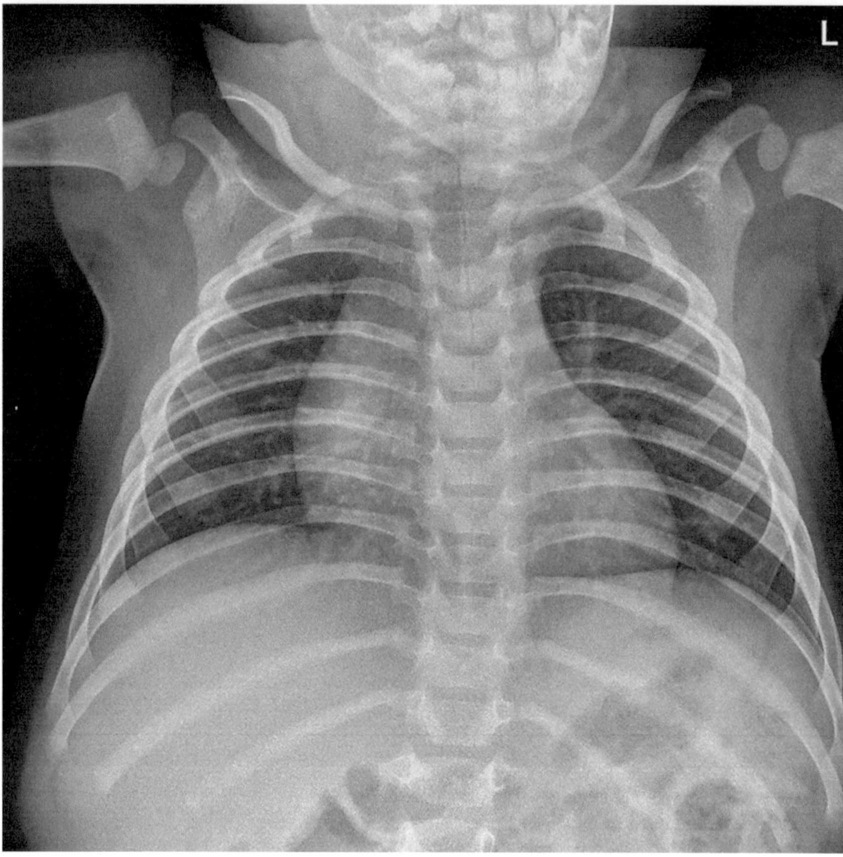

Image 2

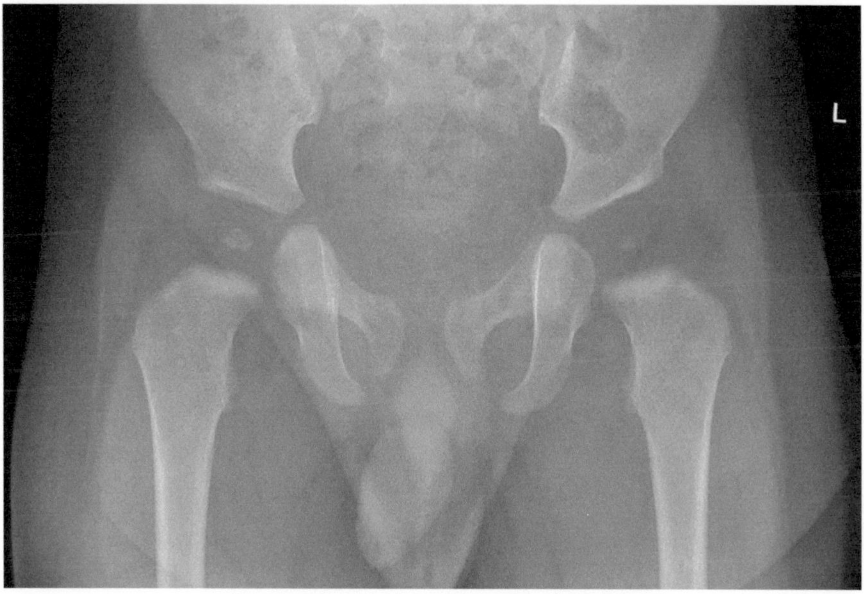

Image 3

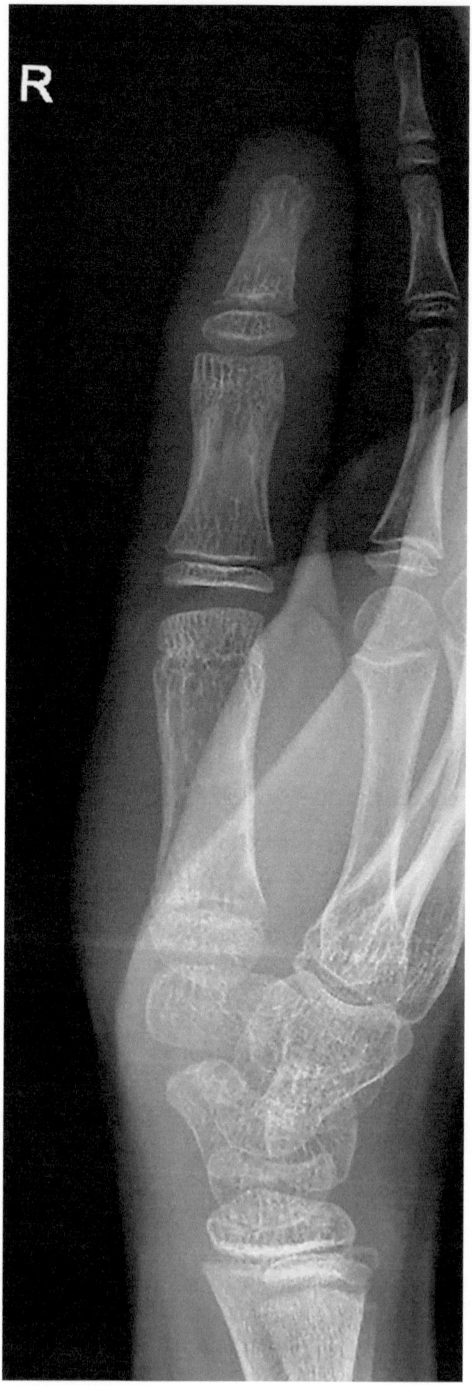

Image 4

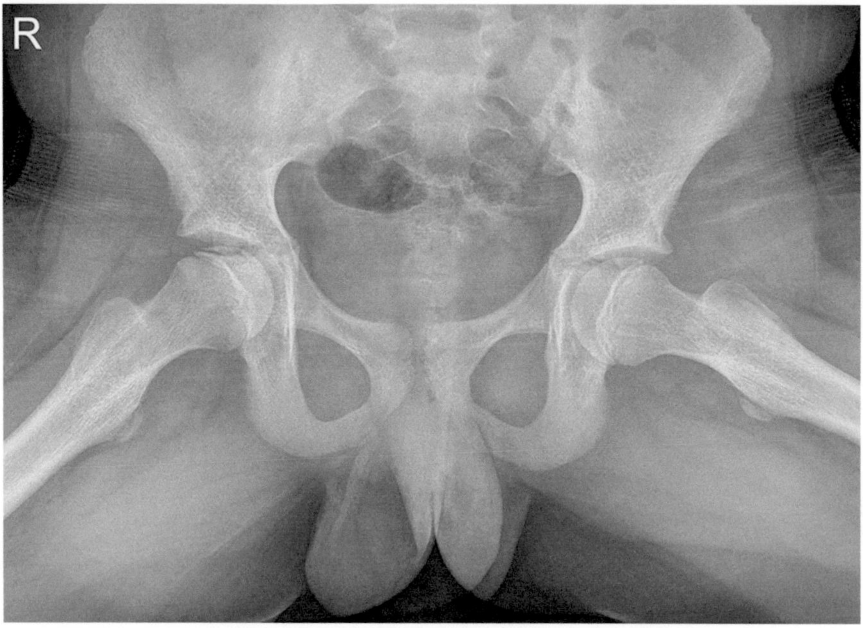

Image 5

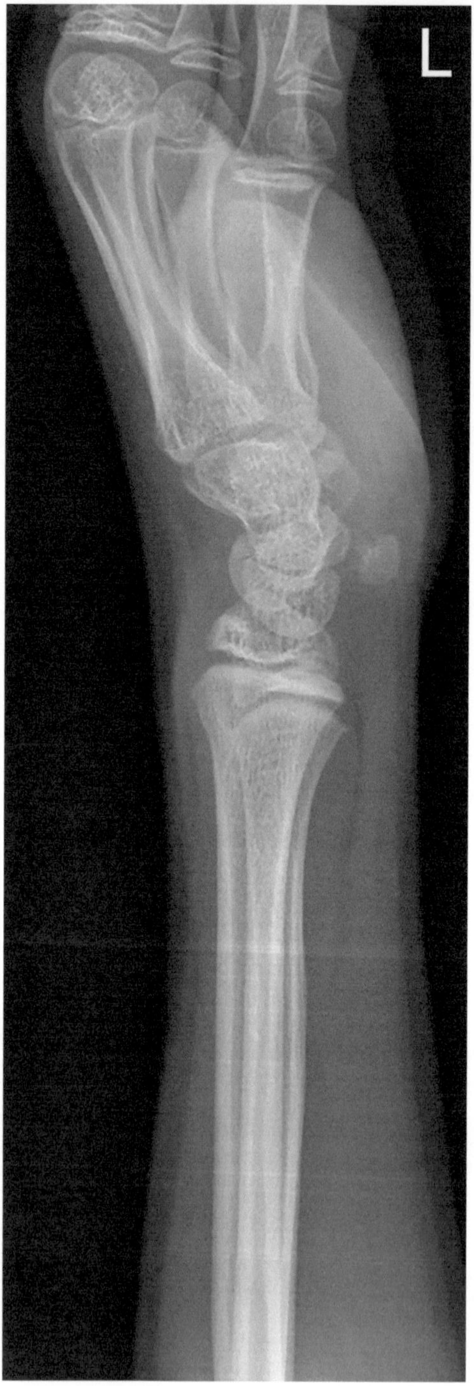

Image 6

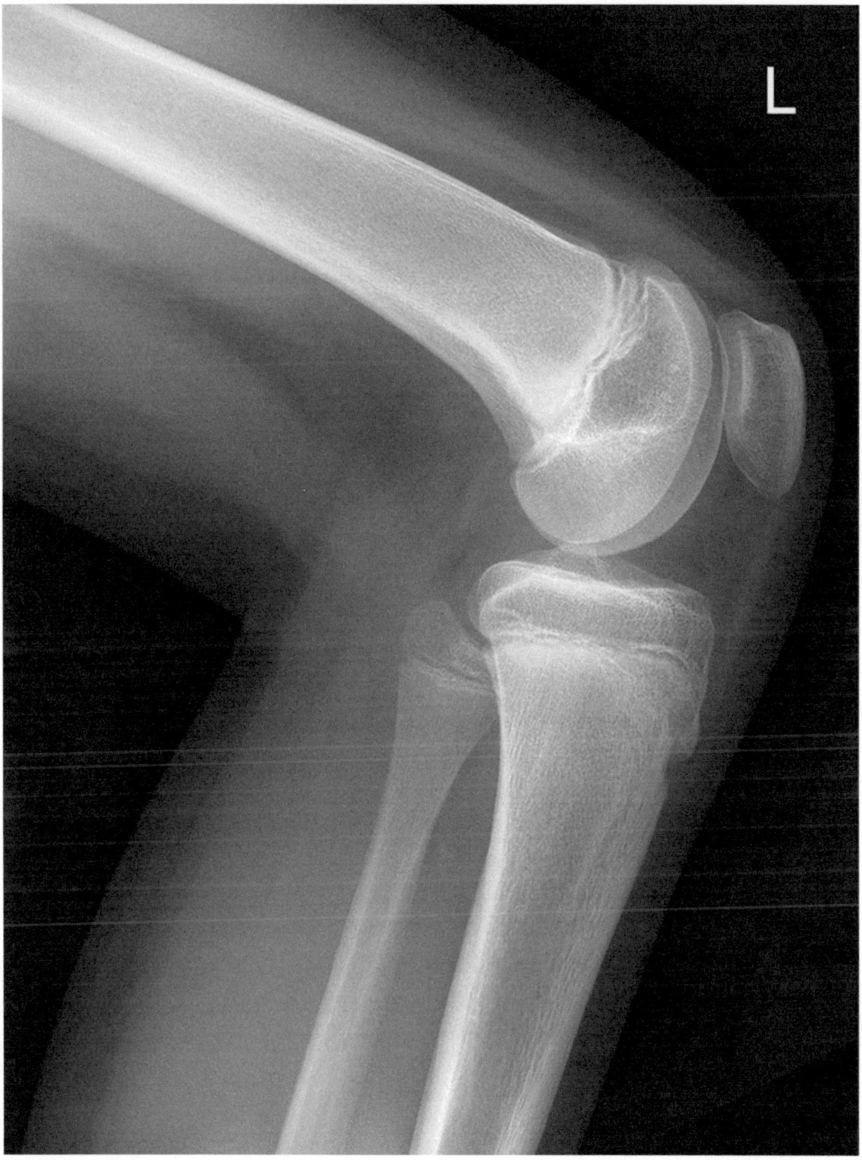

Image 7

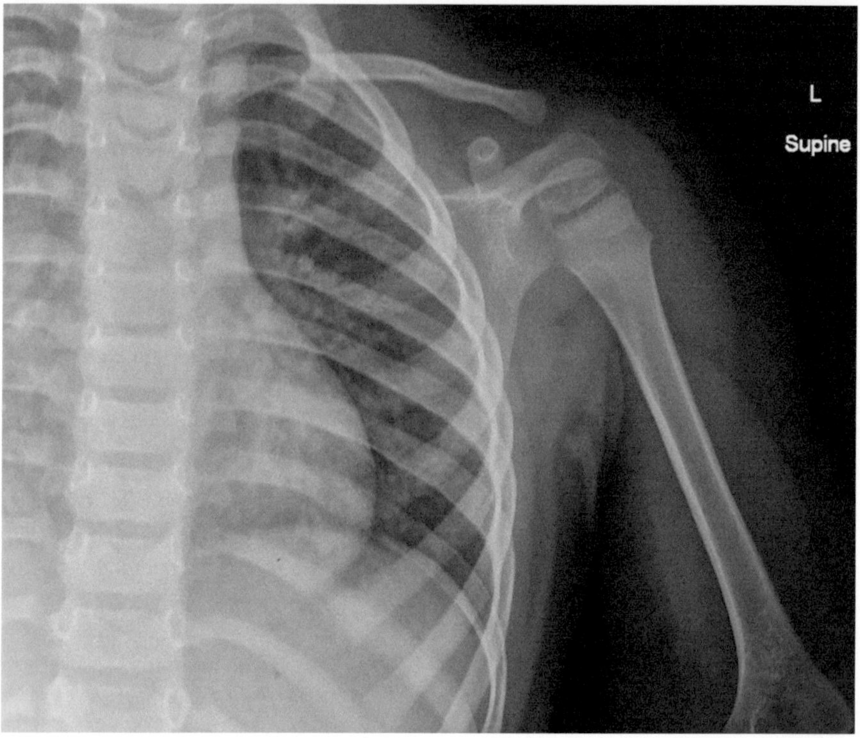

Image 8

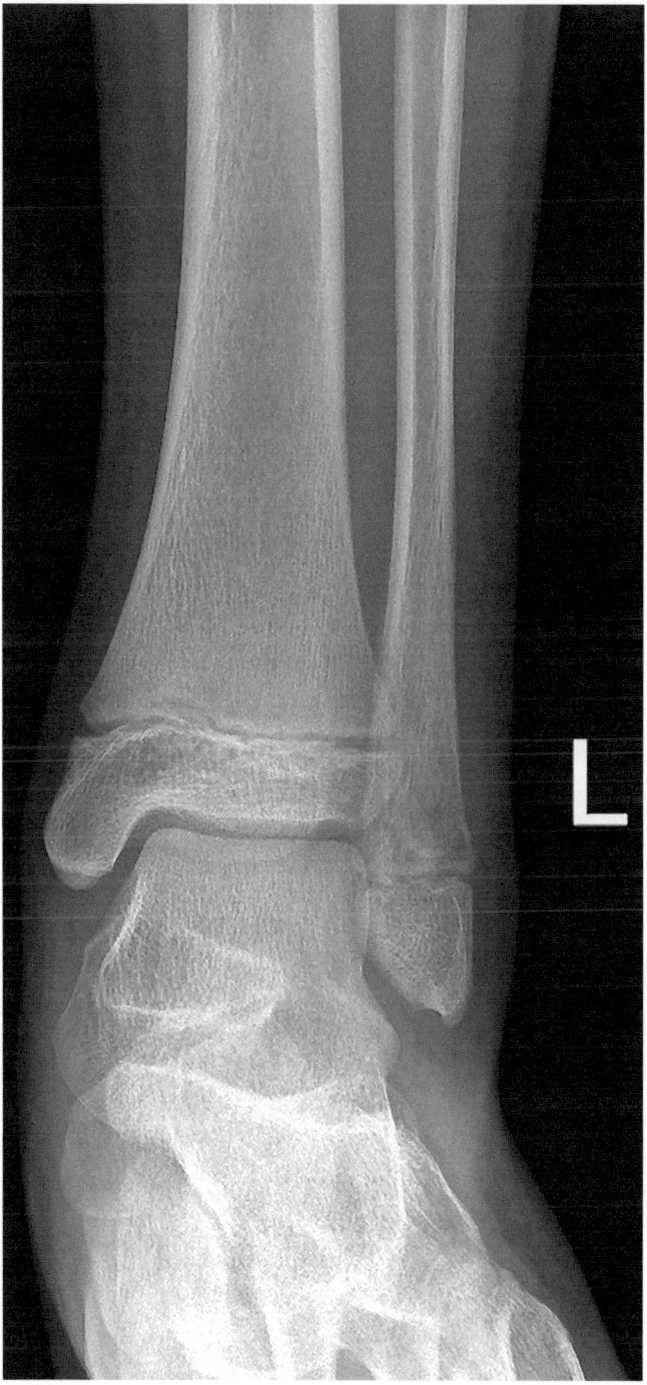

Image 9

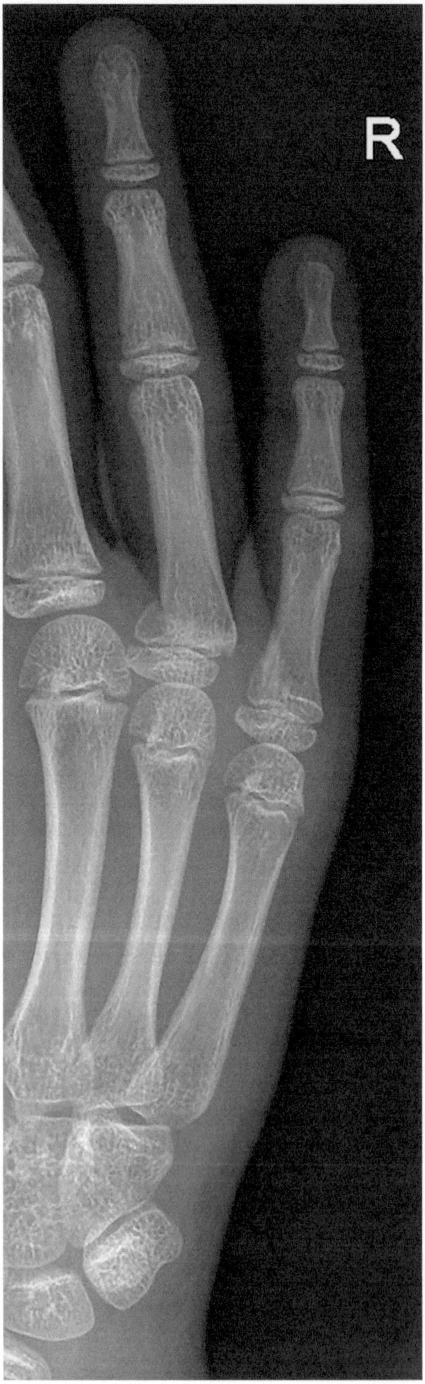

Image 10

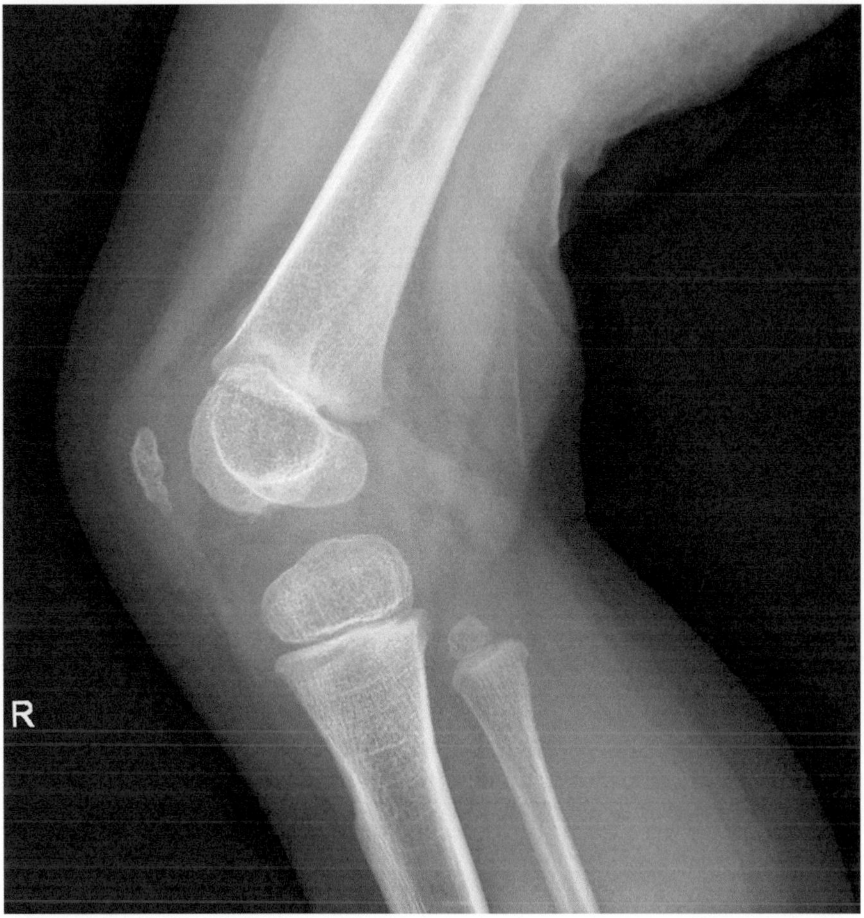

Image 11

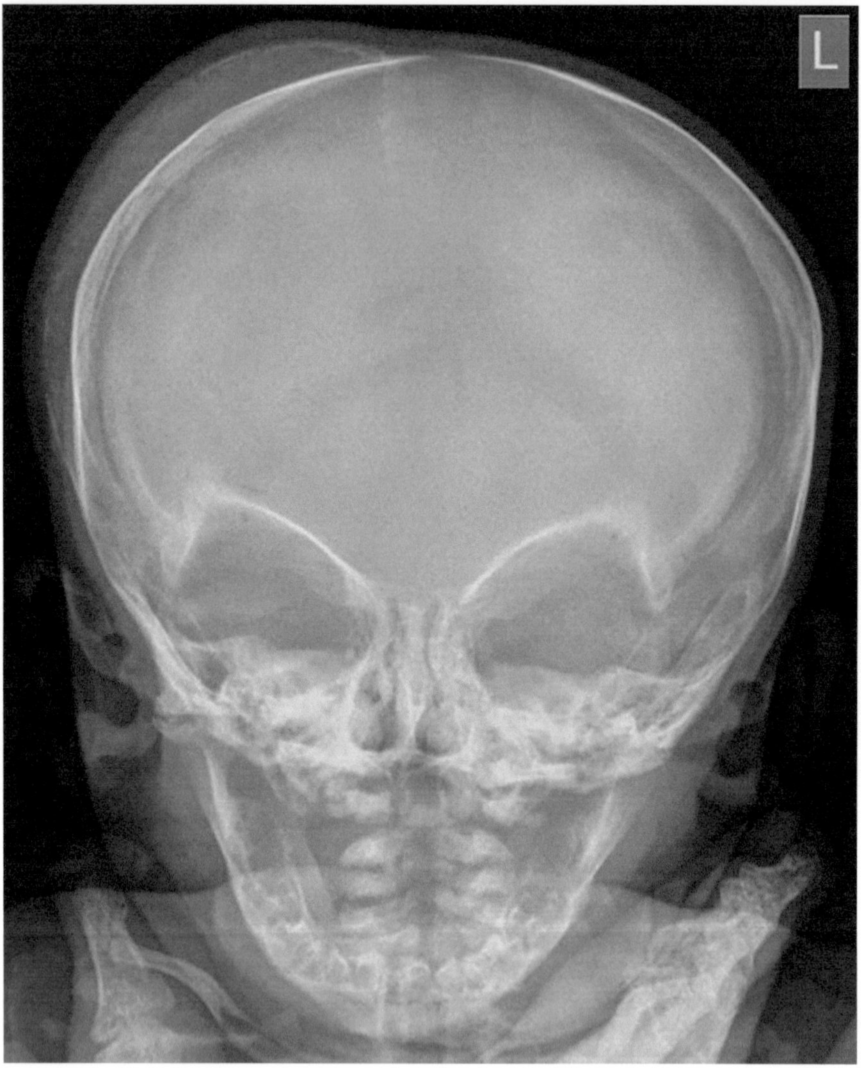

Image 12

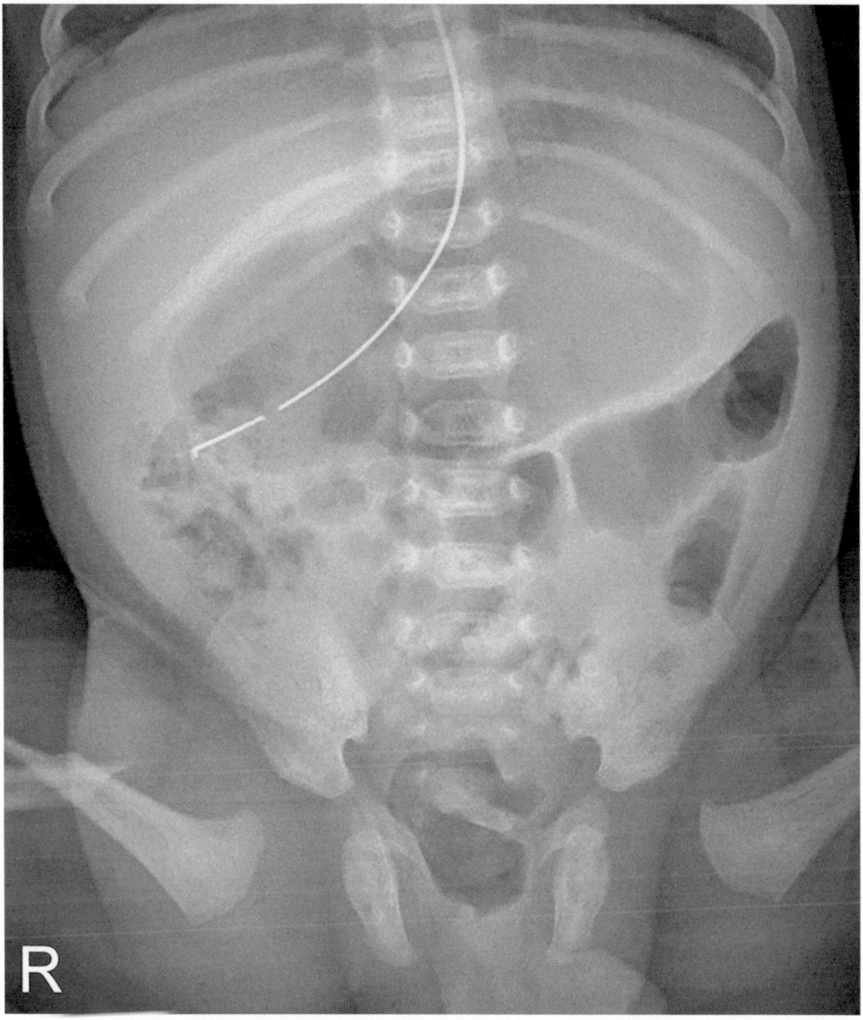

Image 13

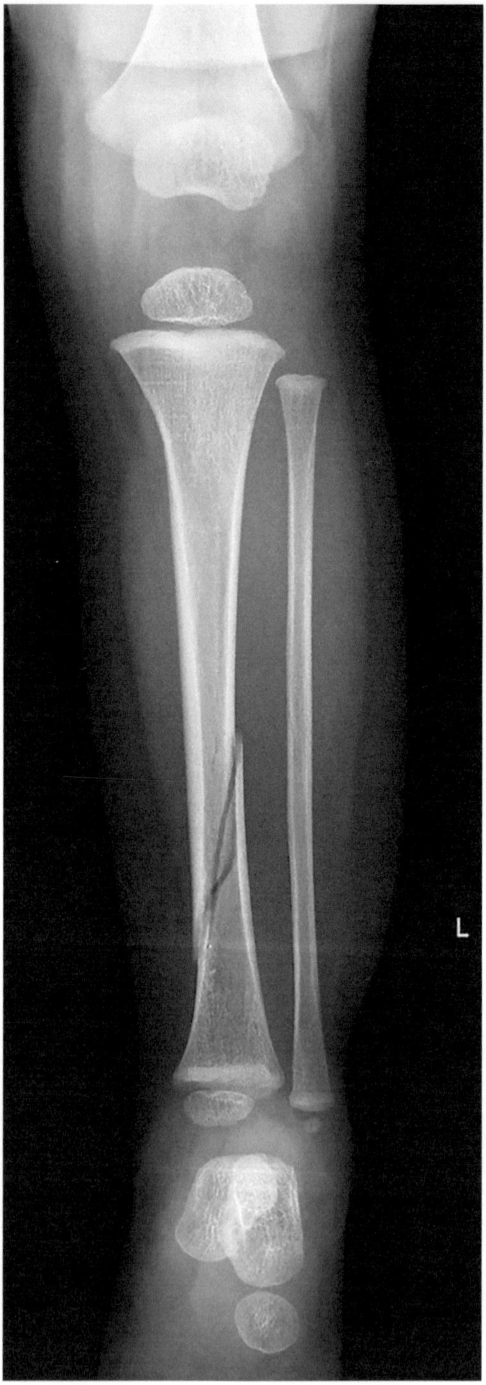

Image 14

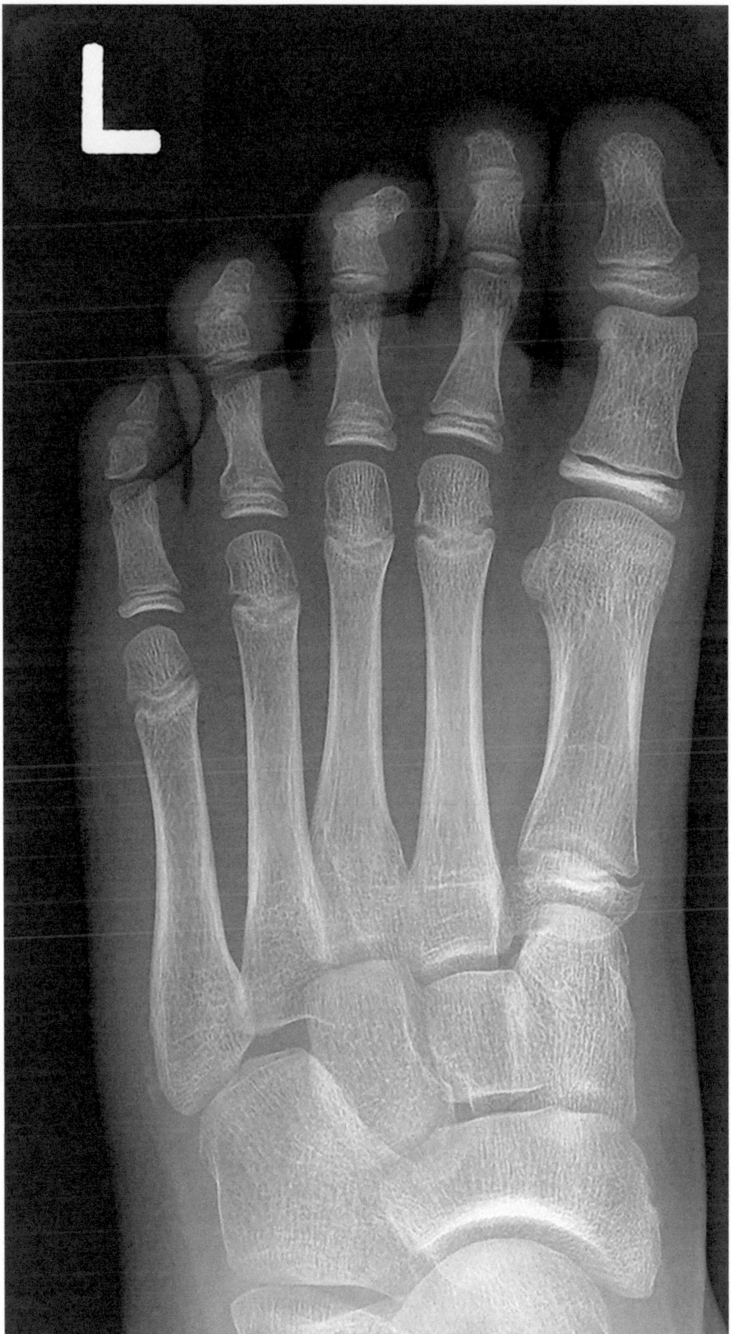

Image 15

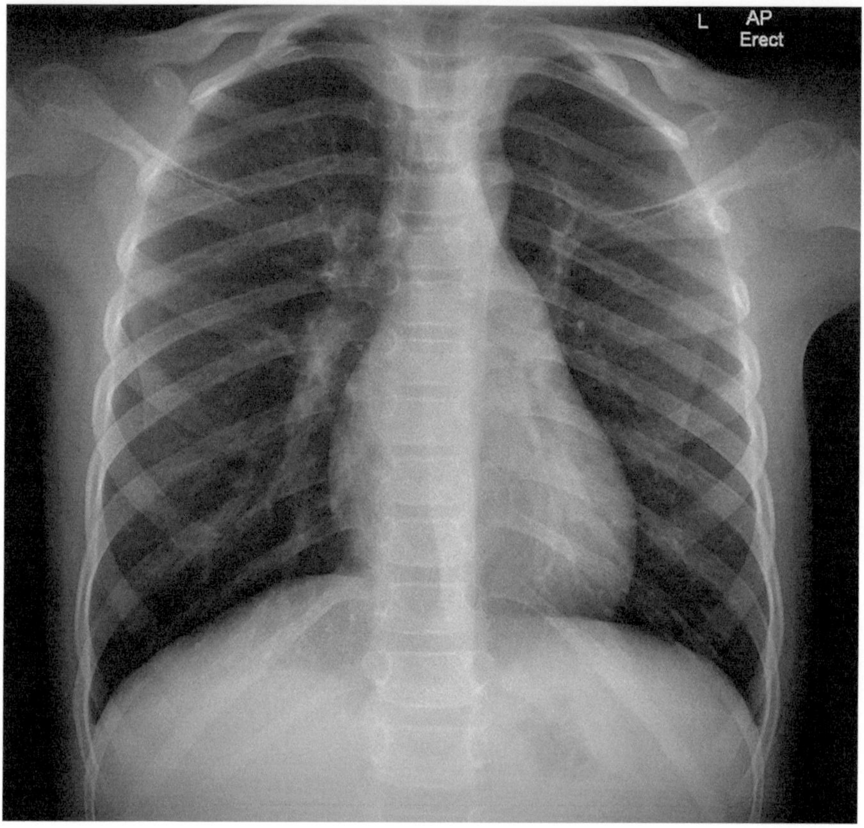

Image 16

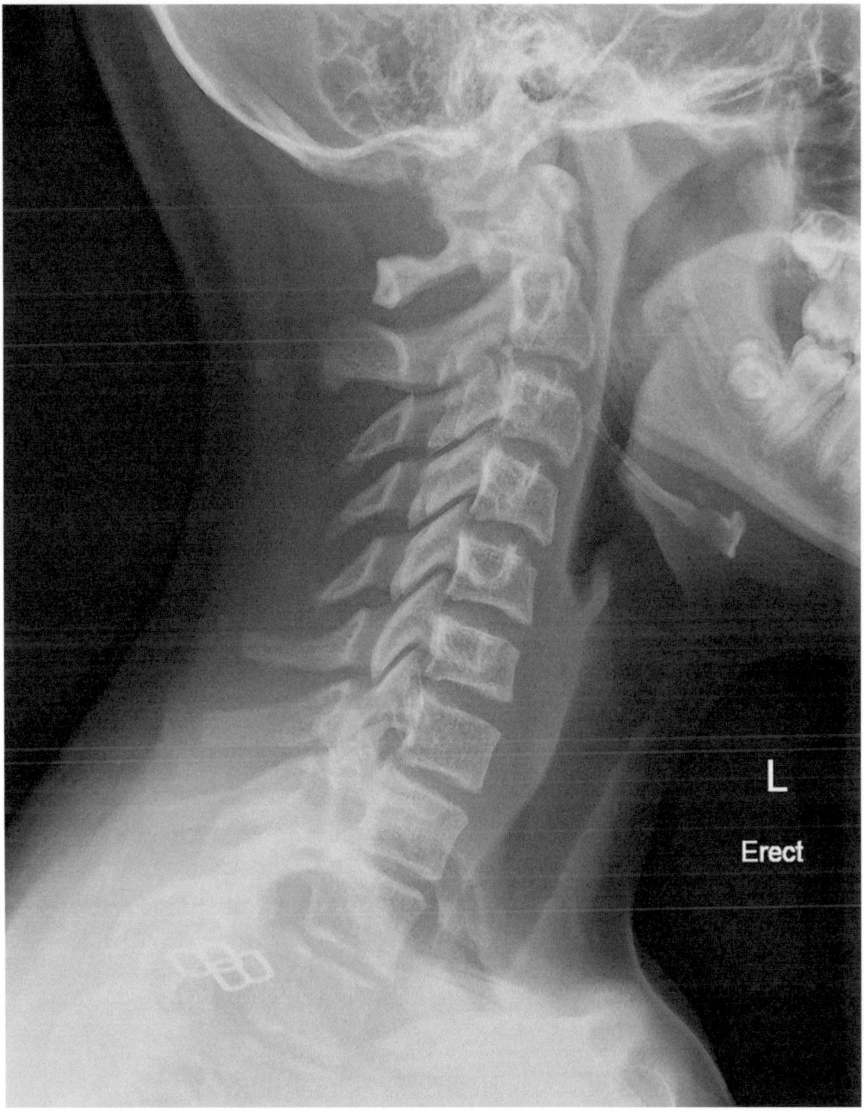

Image 17

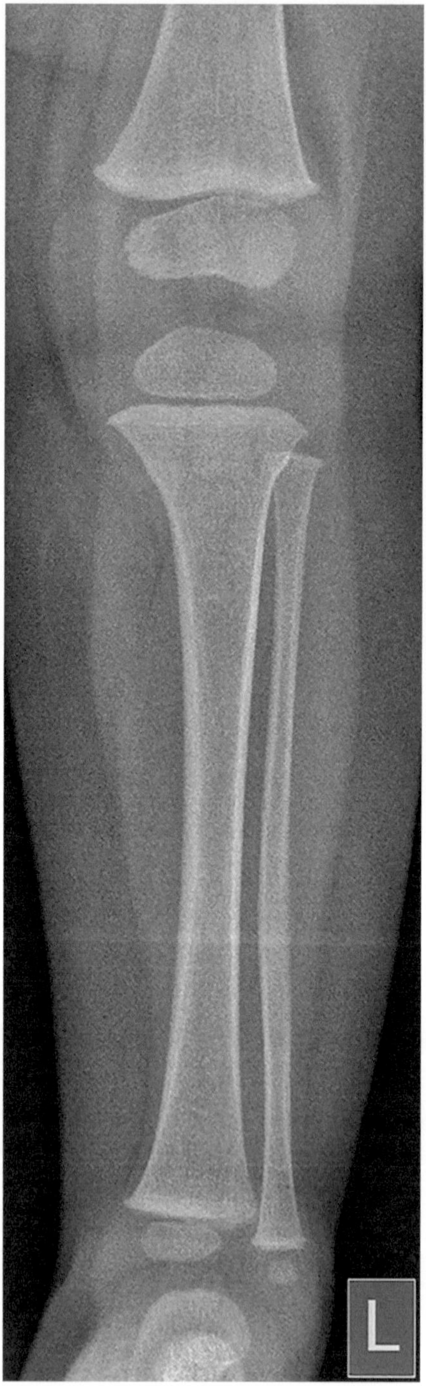

Image 18

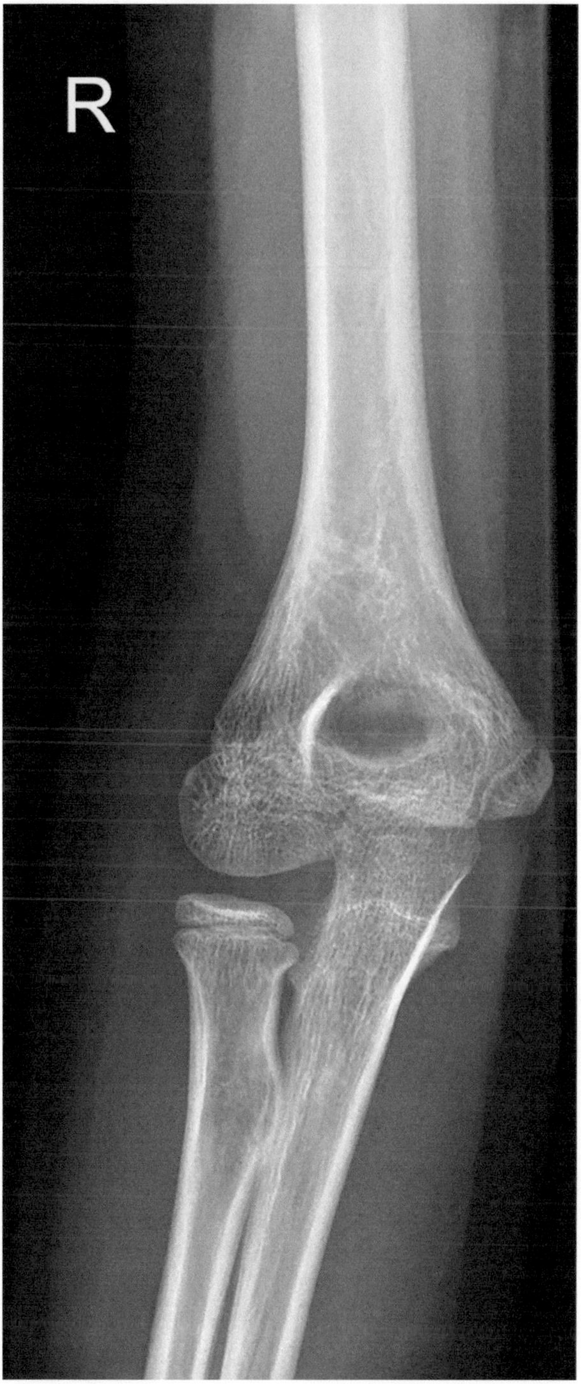

Image 19

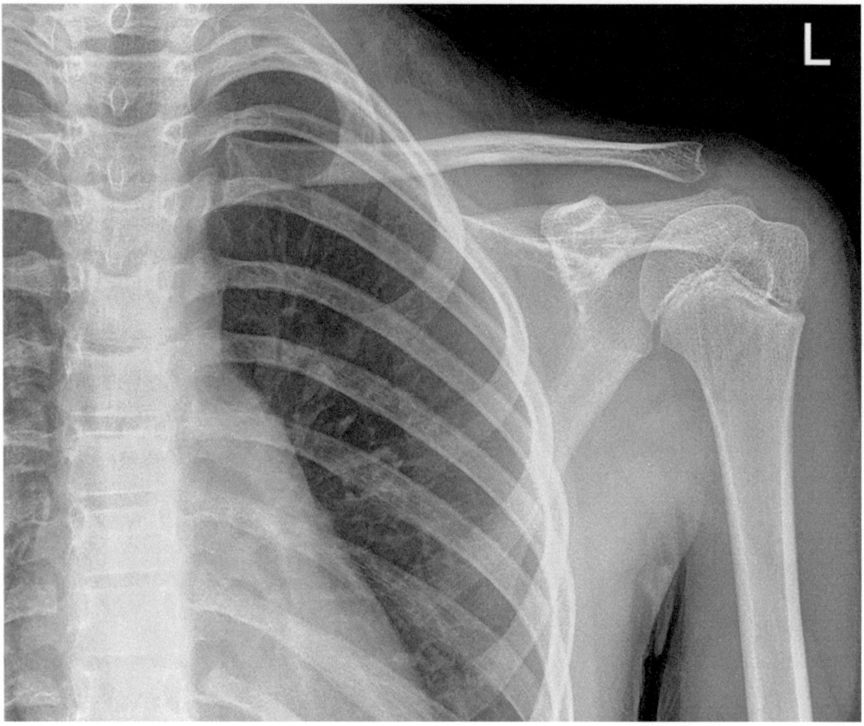

Image 20

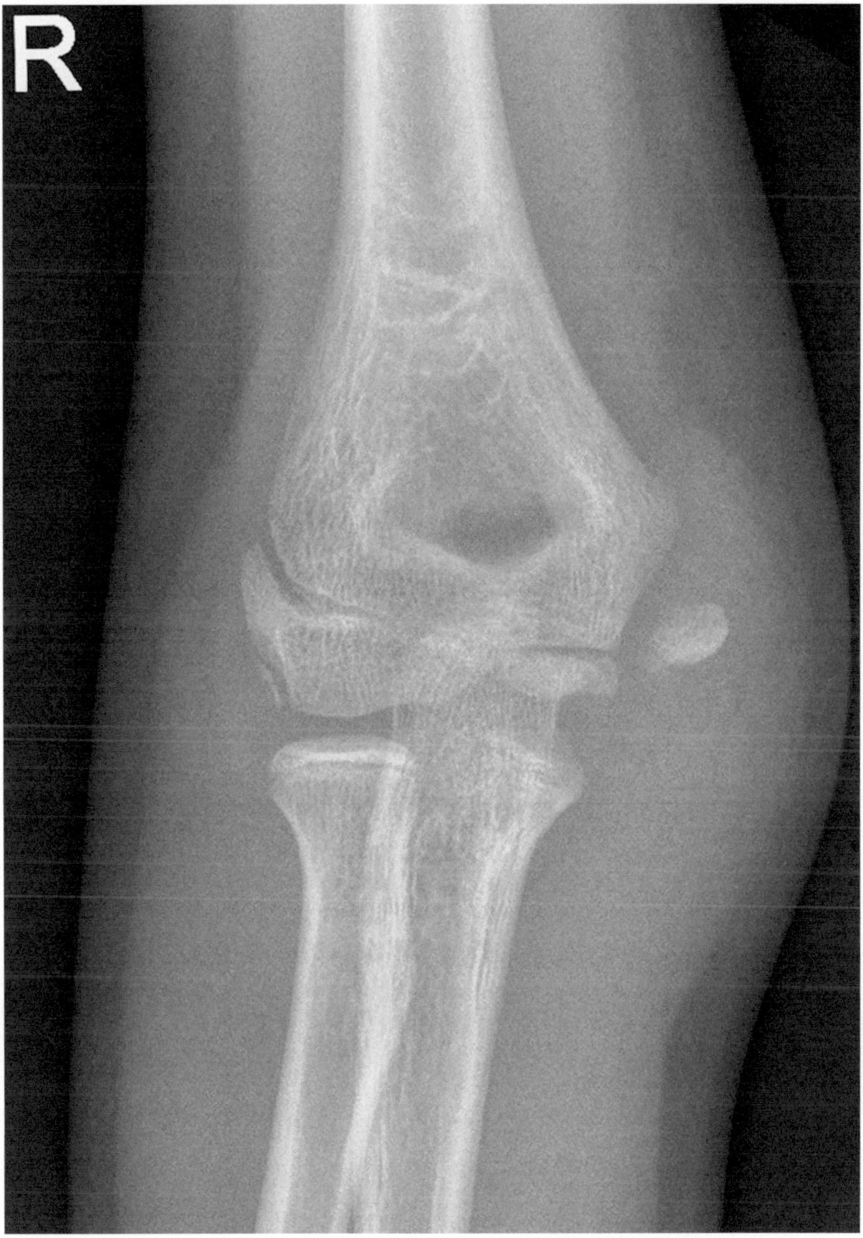

Image 21

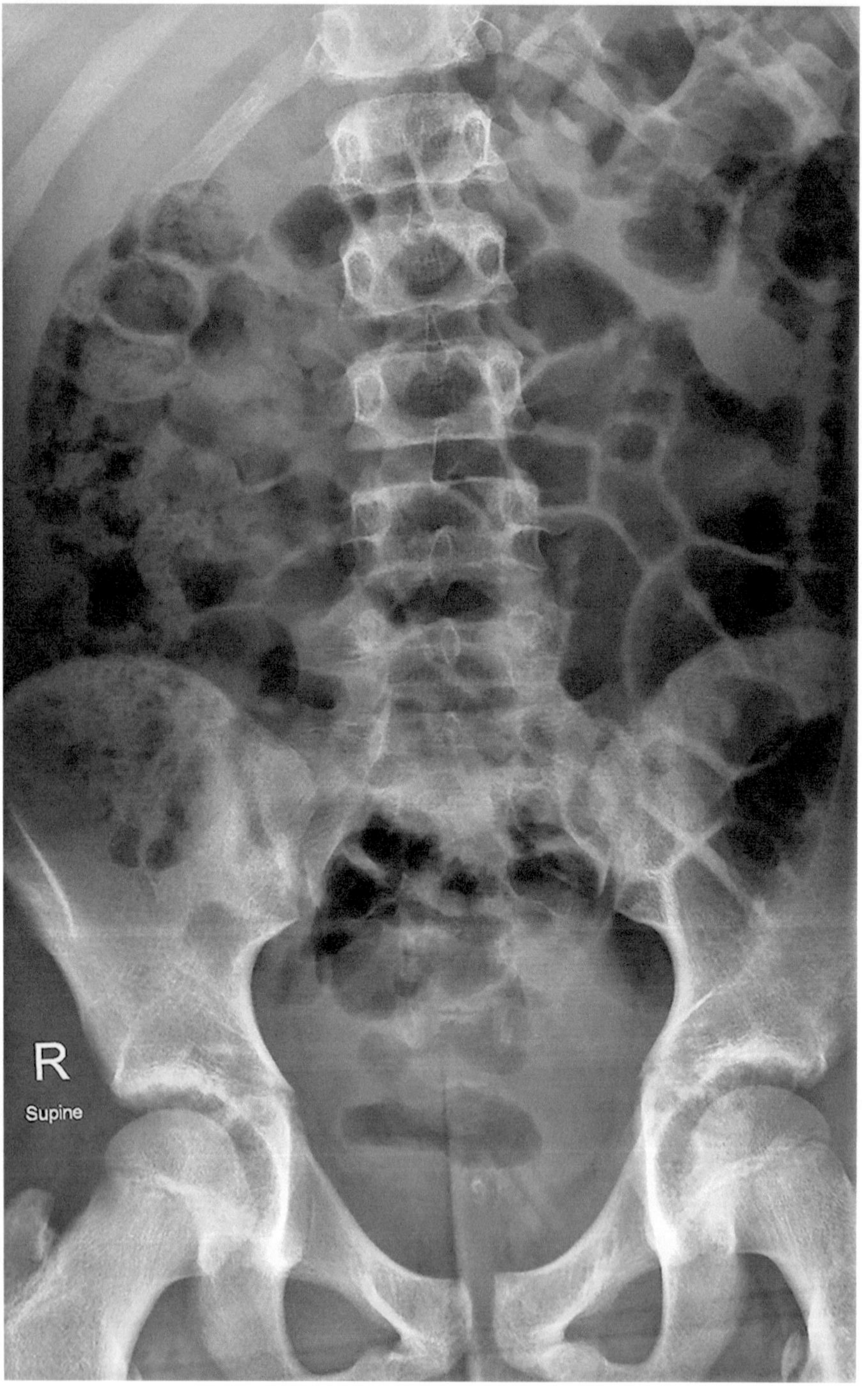

Image 22

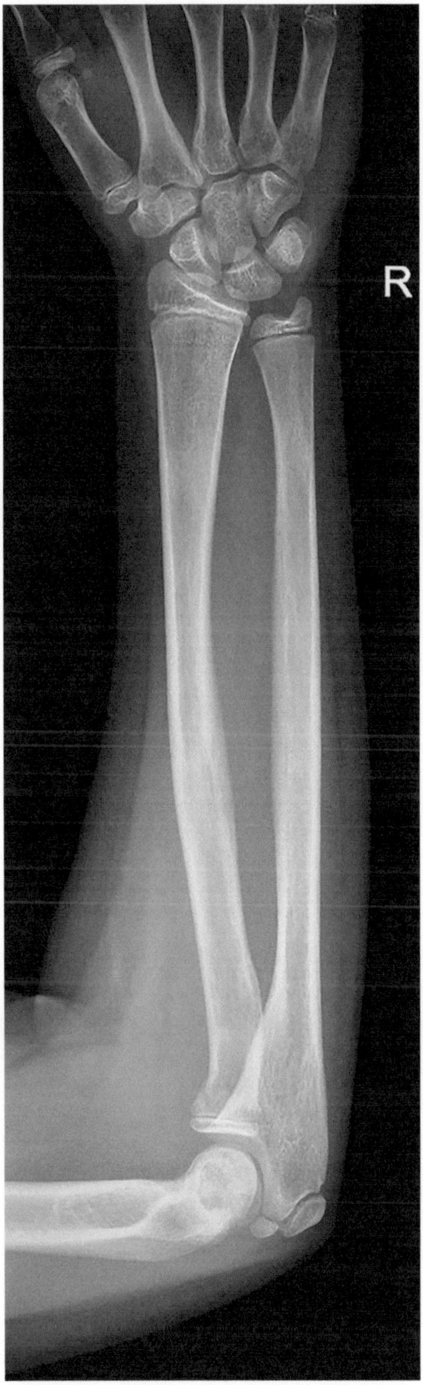

Image 23

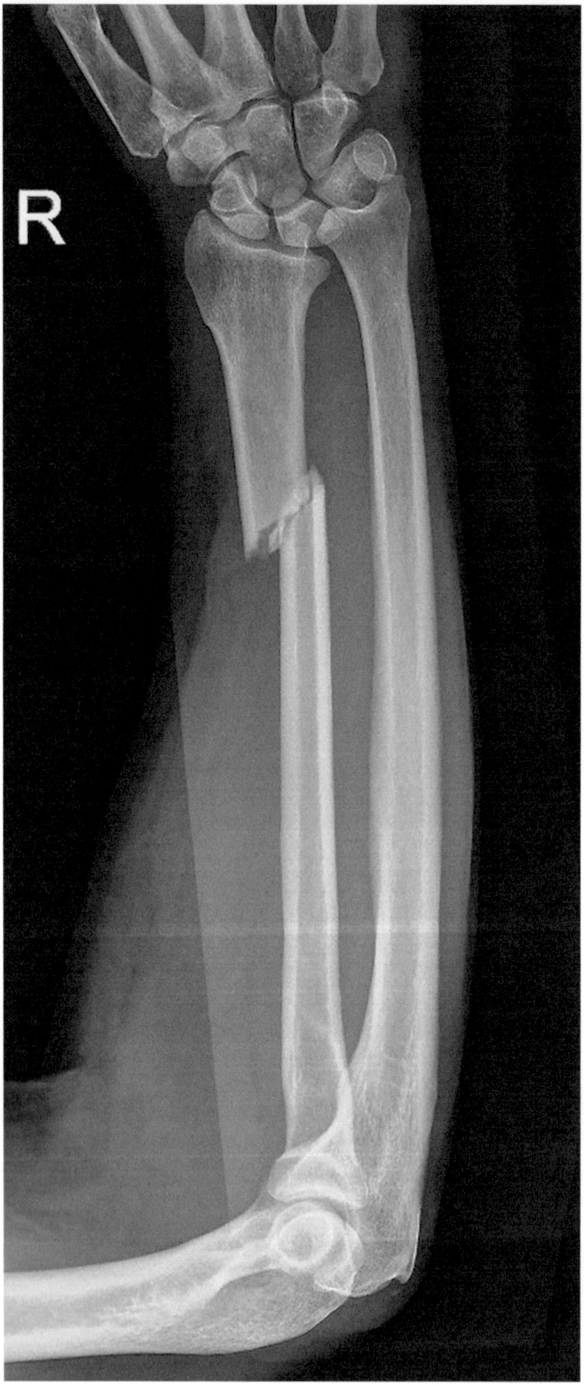

Image 24

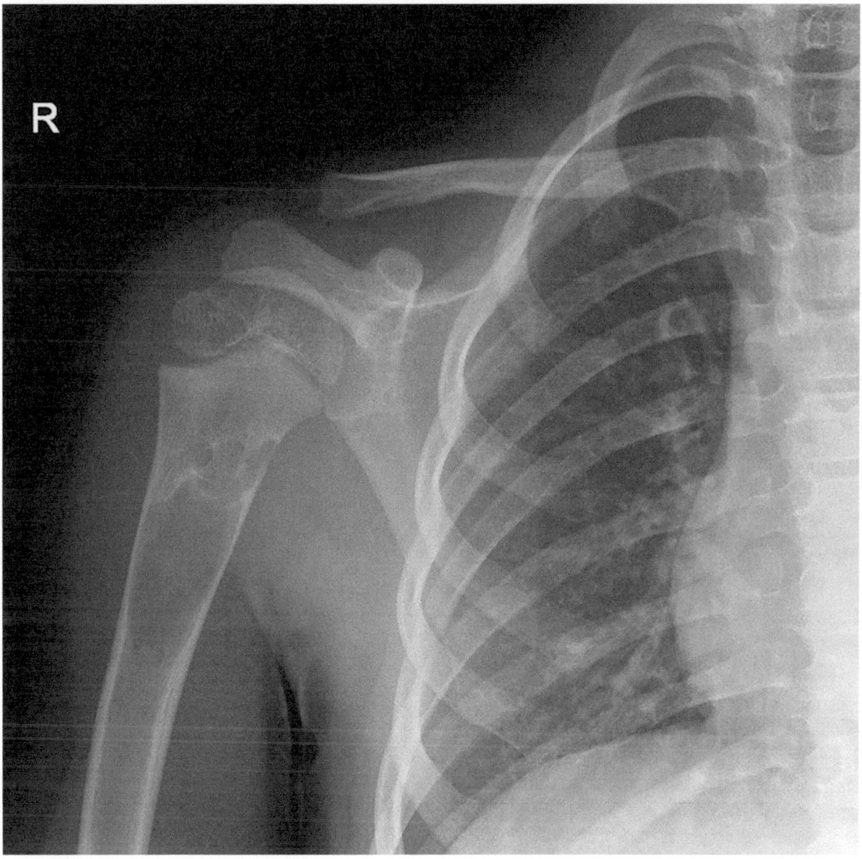

Image 25

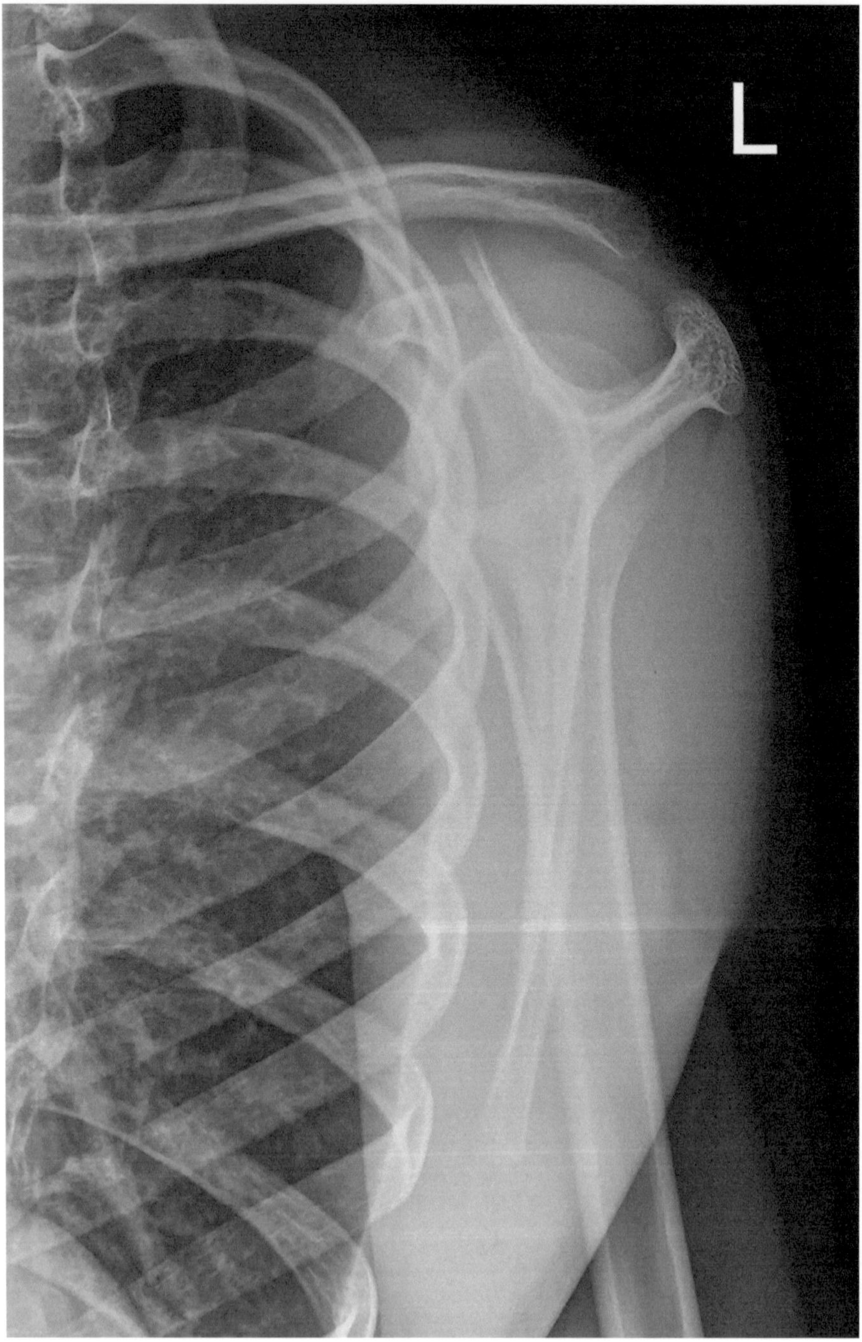

Image 26

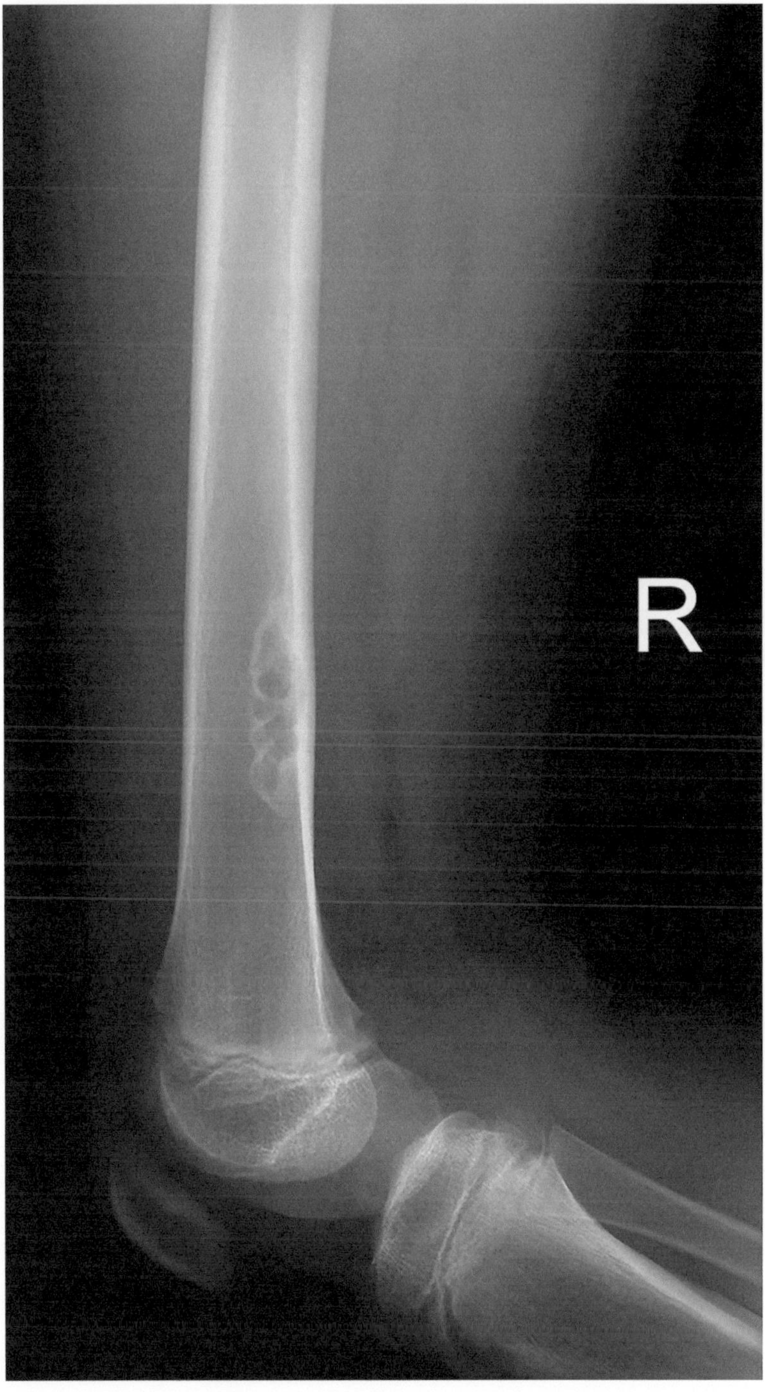

Image 27

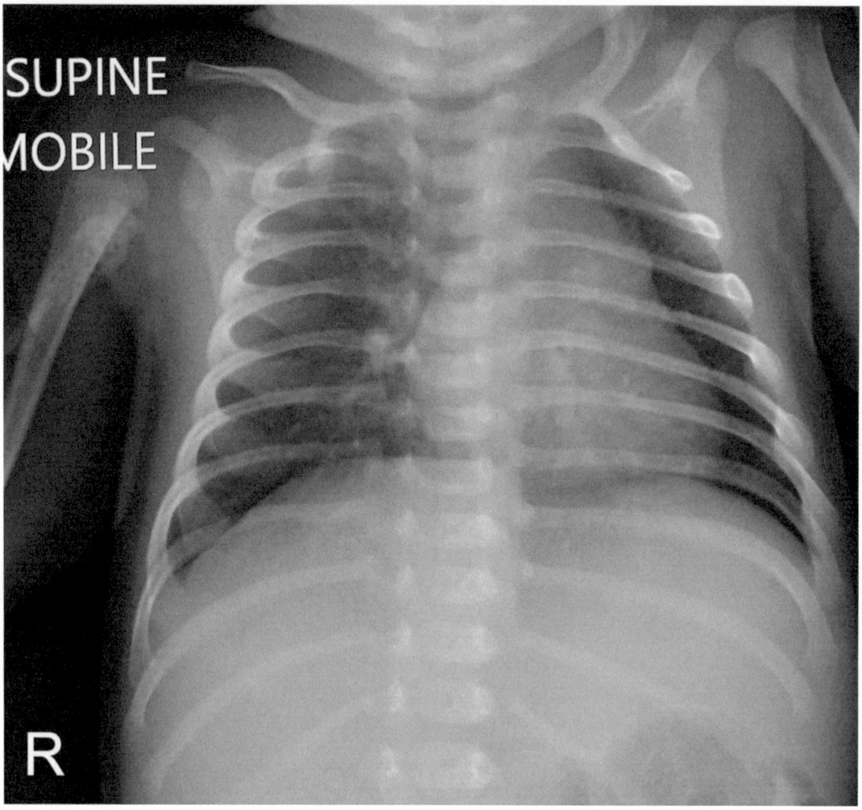

Image 28

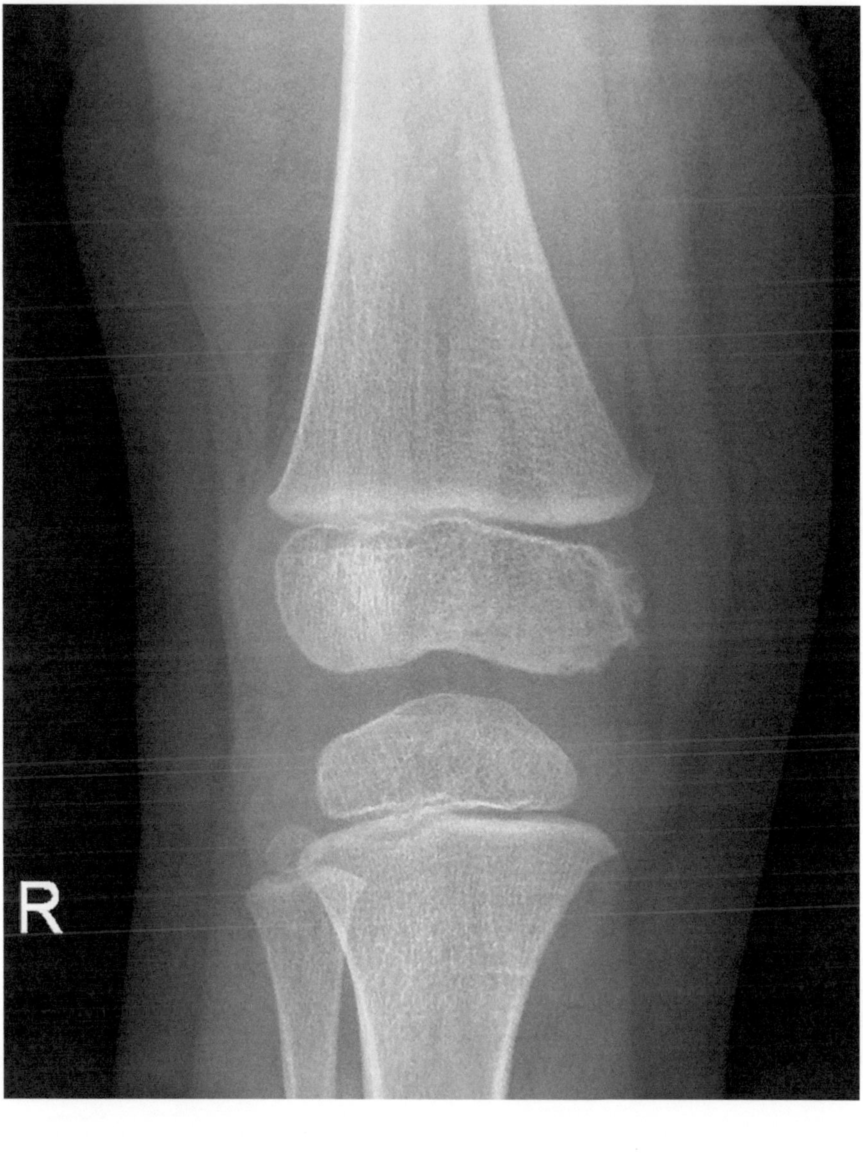

Image 29

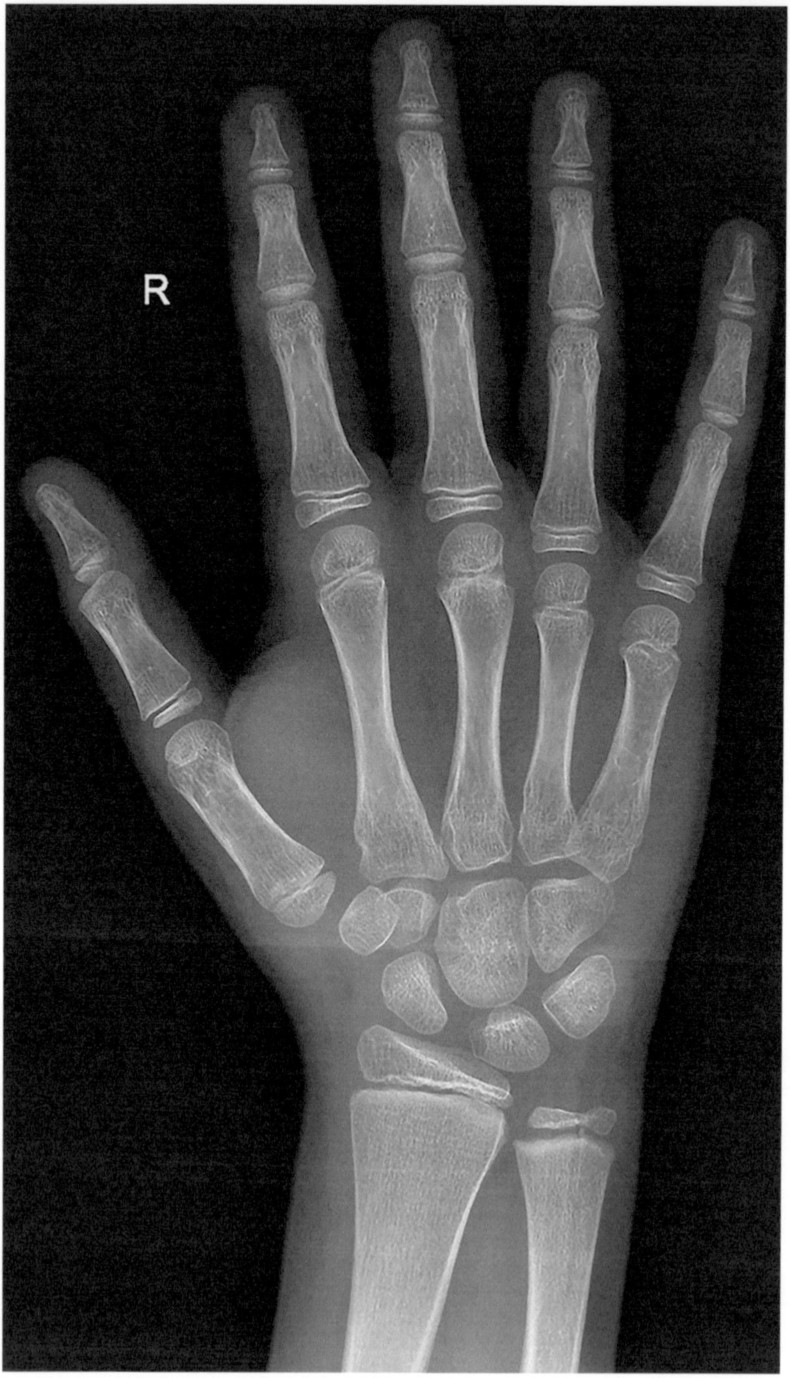

Image 30

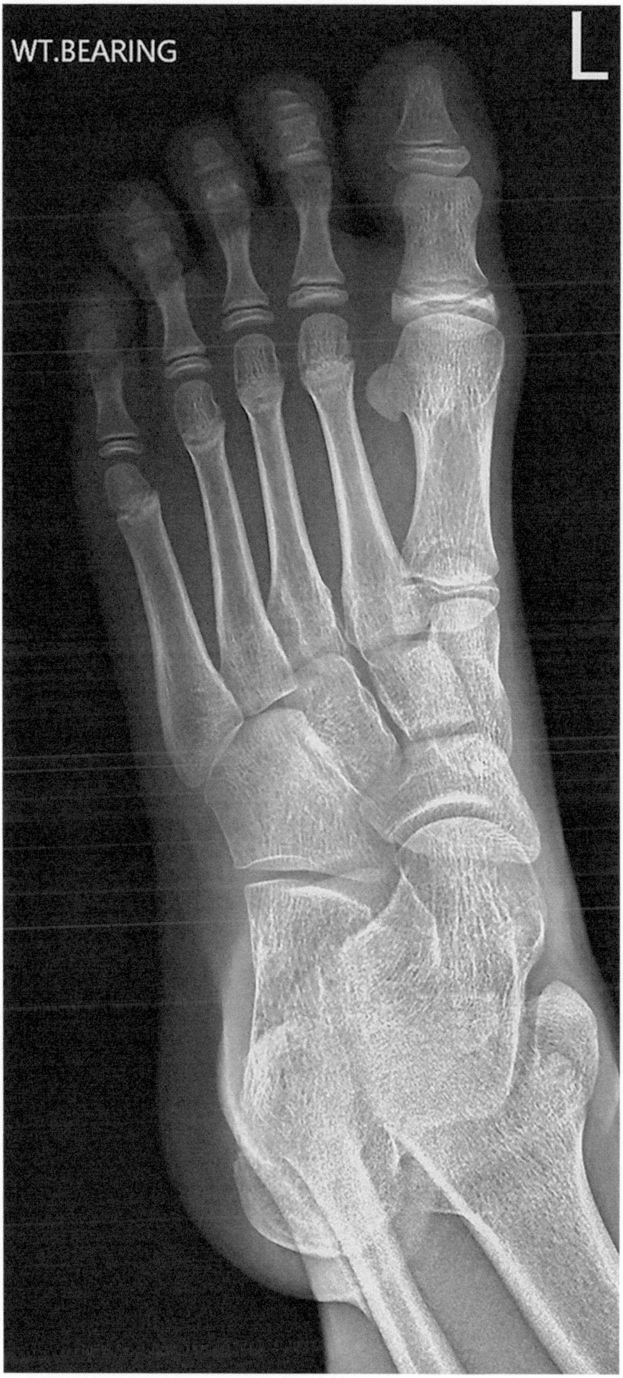

10.2 Answers

Image	Normal	Abnormal	Diagnosis/abnormality (only if abnormal)
1	✓		
2		✓	L DDH
3		✓	SH2 # R thumb distal phalanx
4		✓	AVN R proximal femoral epiphysis
5	✓		
6	✓		
7	✓		
8		✓	Aggressive lesion L distal fibula
9		✓	SH2 # R ring and little finger proximal phalanges
10	✓		
11		✓	R parietal calcified cephalohaematoma
12		✓	Displaced angulated # R femoral shaft
13		✓	Spiral # L distal tibial diaphysis
14		✓	Buckle # L fourth toe proximal phalanx
15	✓		
16	✓		
17		✓	Buckle # L proximal tibial metaphysis
18	✓		
19	✓		
20		✓	Avulsion # R medial epicondyle
21	✓		
22		✓	# R radial neck
23		✓	R Galeazzi #-dislocation
24		✓	UBC R proximal humeral diaphysis
25	✓		
26		✓	NOF R distal femoral diaphysis
27		✓	Healing # L midshaft clavicle
28	✓		
29	✓		
30	✓		

10.3 Explanations

2. **Left developmental dysplasia of the hip**
   See the explanation for Image 17 of Test 2.

3. **Salter-Harris 2 # R thumb distal phalanx**
   See the explanation for Image 30 of Test 1.

4. **Avascular necrosis R proximal femoral epiphysis**
   This radiograph demonstrates a well-defined subchondral lucency in the lateral aspect of the right proximal femoral epiphysis, also known as the 'crescent sign' of avascular necrosis (AVN). See the explanation for Image 1 of Test 1. The lucency projected over the left posterosuperior proximal femoral epiphysis is the unfused triradiate cartilage and is normal for age.

5. *Normal left wrist radiograph*
   The rounded opacity at the volar aspect of the carpus is the left pisiform bone. If the radiograph is not obtained in a true lateral position, the pisiform can be projected volar to, as opposed to over, the scaphoid.

8. **Aggressive lesion L distal fibula**
   This child was presented to the Emergency Department (ED) with atraumatic left ankle swelling and redness. This radiograph demonstrates a 'moth-eaten'/ permeative bone texture in the left distal fibula with heterogenous lucency of the metaphysis and focal lysis of the lateral metaphyseal cortex. Appearances are in keeping with an aggressive lesion. There is associated overlying soft tissue swelling. The distal fibular epiphysis and distal tibia appear radiographically normal. Subsequent magnetic resonance imaging (MRI) demonstrated features consistent with osteomyelitis. See Image 13 of Test 7 for a further example of an aggressive bony lesion with similar appearances in a different patient.

   Tip for the viva:
   - Whilst not present in this case, it is important to look for a pathological fracture in the context of abnormal radiographic bone texture.

9. **Salter-Harris 2 # R ring and little finger proximal phalanges**
   See the explanation for Image 30 of Test 1.

11. **R parietal calcified cephalohaematoma**
    This 3-week-old girl was born by normal vaginal delivery. She was referred by her General Practitioner (GP) for a head swelling that had been present from birth, but which had not resolved. This radiograph demonstrates a calcified collection overlying the right parietal bone bound by the sagittal suture superiorly and the right squamous suture inferiorly which localises the collection to the subperiosteal space. Collections in this potential space *cannot* cross suture lines, making it a cephalohaematoma. This is distinguished from a subgaleal haematoma which *can* cross suture lines. See the explanation for Image 30 of Test 7 for a more detailed discussion of scalp collections.

12. **Displaced angulated # R femoral shaft**
There is a displaced and angulated right femoral diaphyseal fracture at the edge of the image (this abdominopelvic radiograph was taken as part of an initial skeletal survey for suspected inflicted injury). The enteric tube tip is appropriately sited within the gas filled stomach (aerophagia). See Image 23 of Test 3 for another example of and discussion around femoral diaphyseal fractures.

13. **Spiral # L distal tibial diaphysis**
See the explanation for Image 4 of Test 1.

14. **Buckle # L fourth toe proximal phalanx**
This buckle fracture of the lateral cortex of the left fourth toe proximal phalanx is better appreciated in the magnified image below:

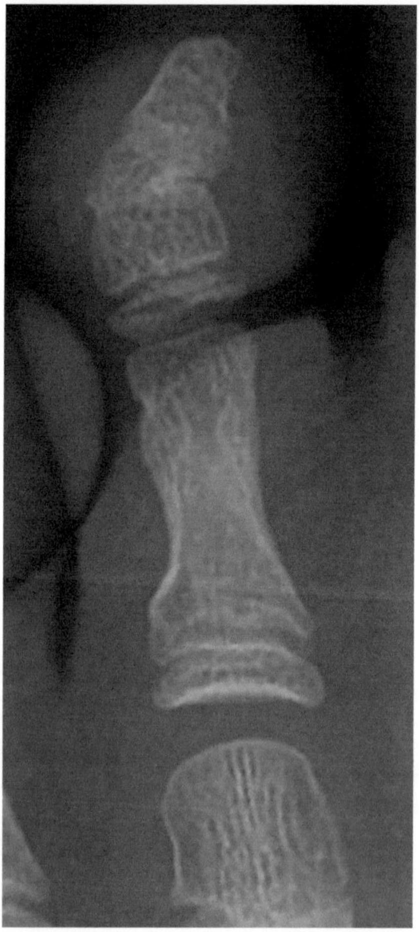

17. **Buckle # L proximal tibial metaphysis**
This is another example of a 'trampoline fracture'. See the explanation for Image 24 of Test 4 and the longer-term complication in Image 26 of Test 9.

20. **Avulsion # R medial epicondyle**
The medial epicondyle ossification centre is displaced from its normal position with significant associated soft tissue swelling in keeping with an acute avulsion fracture. Note the small linear fragmented ossification at the inferolateral aspect of the capitellar ossification centre which represents normal ossification for age. See the explanation for Image 9 of Test 6.

22. **# R radial neck #**
Note the acute angulation of the right radial neck in keeping with a minimally displaced fracture. Upon scrutiny, the fracture line extends from the volar cortex through the proximal radial metaphysis (neck) to the physis; as such, this fracture is technically a Salter-Harris 2 injury. The fracture is better visualised in the magnified image below:

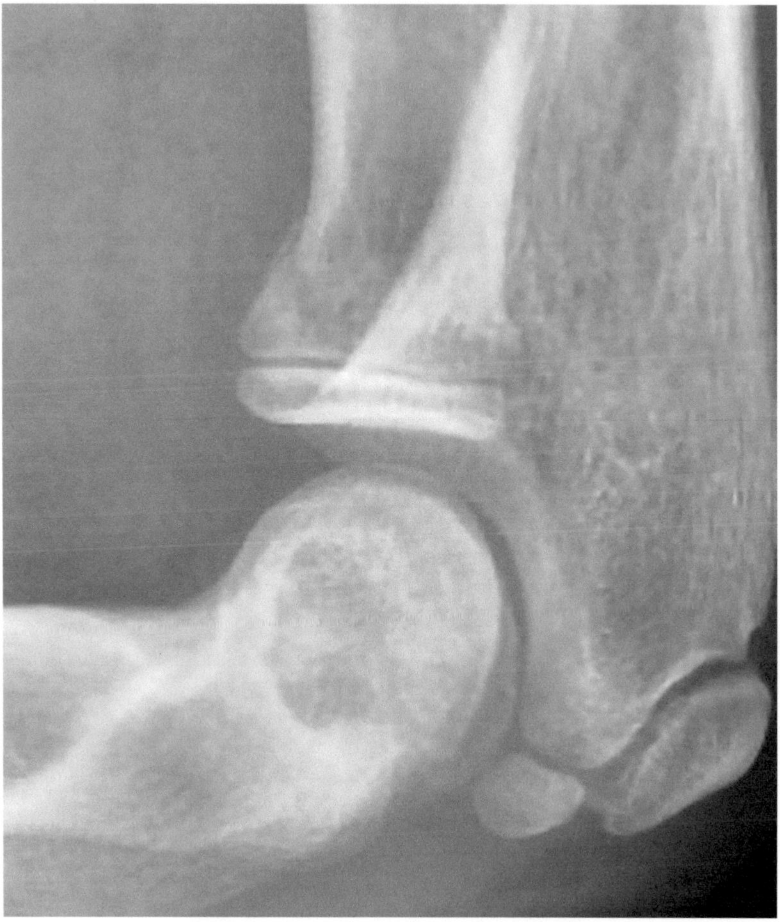

23. **R Galeazzi #-dislocation**
In the context of a distal radial fracture, typically at the junction of the middle and distal thirds as in this case, one must carefully assess the distal radioulnar joint (DRUJ) for dislocation as part of the Galeazzi fracture-dislocation pattern. Inspection of the right DRUJ on this anteroposterior (AP) projection reveals the dislocation alongside radial shortening (>10 mm suggests complete disruption of the interosseous membrane) with confirmation of the Galeazzi fracture-dislocation complex on the contemporaneous lateral projection as visualised in the image below:

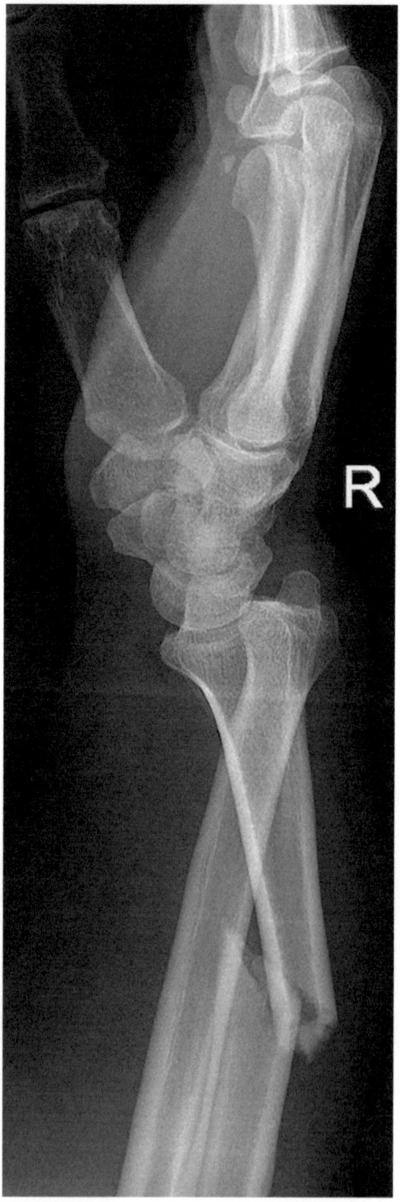

This pattern typically occurs following a fall onto an outstretched hand (FOOSH) with the elbow held in flexion at the time of the injury.

Galeazzi fracture-dislocations are unstable injuries which often require open reduction and internal fixation (ORIF) of the radial fracture, assessment and reduction/stabilisation of the DRUJ, and exploration of the triangular fibrocartilage complex (TFCC). In children, remember that Galeazzi-equivalent fractures are those in which there is a distal radius fracture alongside a concomitant (Salter-Harris) fracture of the distal ulnar physis. Recovery may be complicated by physeal arrest of the ulna.

Tip for the viva:

- Formal forearm radiographs should be recommended if they have not yet been obtained: ensure that *both* the wrist and elbow joints have been imaged.

24. **Unicameral bone cyst R proximal humeral diaphysis**
See the explanation for Image 6 of Test 9 and the images below for an example of a pathological fracture through a unicameral bone cyst (UBC) with the 'fallen fragment' sign in a different patient:

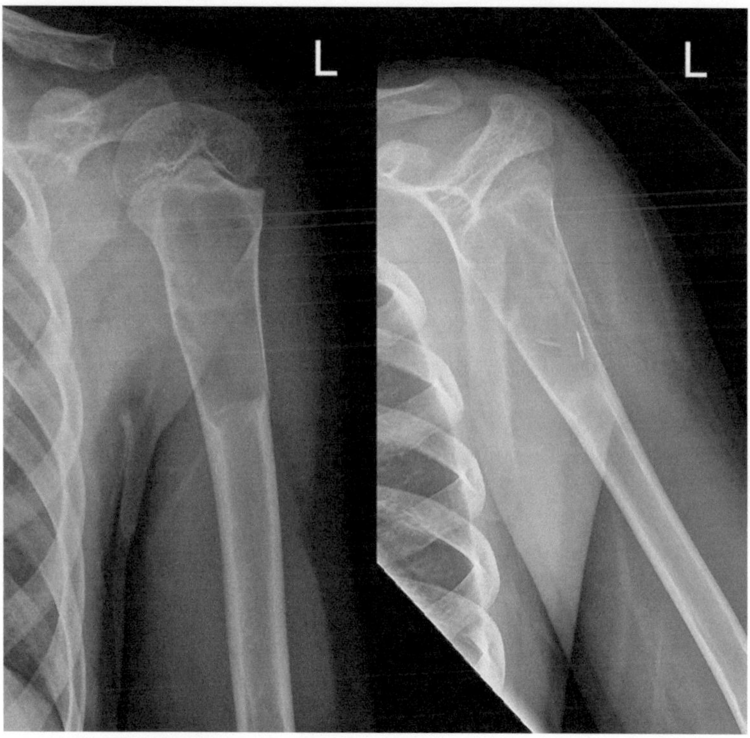

26. **Non-ossifying fibroma R distal femoral diaphysis**
Given the apparent septations/multilocations, the differential diagnosis for this appearance includes an aneurysmal bone cyst (ABC). See the explanation for Image 5 of Test 5 for a discussion on fibrous cortical defects (FCDs) and non-ossifying fibromas (NOFs).

27. **Healing # L midshaft clavicle**
This chest radiograph demonstrates a healing fracture of the left clavicle at the edge of the image with callus formation and remodelling. Compare with the normal appearances of the right clavicle. The dedicated clavicle radiograph confirms the healing left clavicle fracture:

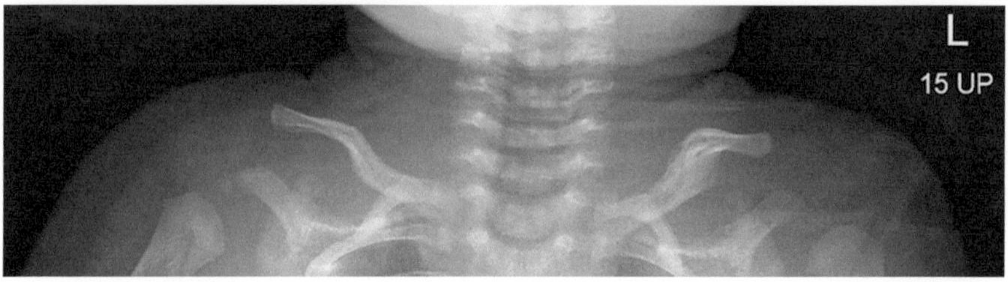

Images were obtained in a 6-week-old boy following presentation to ED after a brief resolved unexplained event (BRUE), previously termed an apparent life-threatening event (ALTE). These events are typified by a combination of apnoea (or absent, decreased or irregular breathing), colour change (cyanosis or pallor), marked change in muscle tone (often hypotonia, or 'floppy baby', but also hypertonia), altered level of consciousness and choking. The mean age of presentation is 1–3 months of age. These events are frightening for parents/ caregivers who observe and report this presentation to clinicians.

Aetiologies include:

- Gastrointestinal: typically gastro-oesophageal reflux.
- Neurological: seizure is the most common disorder associated with BRUE/ALTE.
- Respiratory: infection, such as bronchiolitis, or lung disease of prematurity.
- Cardiovascular: structural/congenital heart disease (CHD).
- Metabolic and endocrine: hypoglycaemia or inborn errors of metabolism.
- Inflicted injury/physical abuse.

Whilst less than 3% are reported to result from physical abuse, this must be ever present in the mind of all clinicians who assess infants presenting with BRUE/ ALTE. Similarly, as clinical radiologists reporting imaging performed for 'BRUE/ALTE', 'blue episode', 'collapse', or 'apnoea', physical abuse should always be considered, particularly if there is evidence of an acute or healing bony injury (as in this case). Close liaison with paediatric colleagues is advised, particularly given that published guidance recommends that chest radiography should *not* be performed for this indication—please see the references.

The initial and follow-up skeletal survey did not reveal any further acute or healing fractures. There was normal radiographic bone density and modelling, i.e. no radiographic evidence of a skeletal dysplasia. Head computed tomography (CT) was normal with no skull fracture or acute intracranial haemorrhage. Whilst the healing fracture was unexplained, it was felt that the fracture was likely sustained at the time of delivery (normal vaginal delivery). Note that any birth injury should have healed completely by the age of 3 months.

Further Reading

Image 23

El-Feky M et al (2023) Galeazzi fracture-dislocation. https://radiopaedia.org/articles/galeazzi-fracture-dislocation. Accessed Jul 2023
Lustosa L et al (2022) Bado classification of Monteggia fracture-dislocations. https://radiopaedia.org/articles/bado-classification-of-monteggia-fracture-dislocations-1. Accessed Jul 2023
Yap J et al (2023) Monteggia fracture-dislocation. https://radiopaedia.org/articles/monteggia-fracture-dislocation. Accessed Jul 2023

Image 24

Ashraf A et al (2023) Unicameral bone cyst. https://radiopaedia.org/articles/unicameral-bone-cyst-1. Accessed Sep 2023

Image 27

Kondamudi NP, Virji M (2023) Brief resolved unexplained event. https://www.ncbi.nlm.nih.gov/books/NBK441897/. Accessed Sep 2023
Tate C, Sunley R (2018) Brief resolved unexplained events (formerly apparent life-threatening events) and evaluation of lower-risk infants. Arch Dis Child Educ Pract Ed 103(2):95–98

Test 11

11

M. Paddock et al., *Paediatric Radiology Rapid Reporting*,
https://doi.org/10.1007/978-3-031-48255-7_11

11.1 Images

Image 1

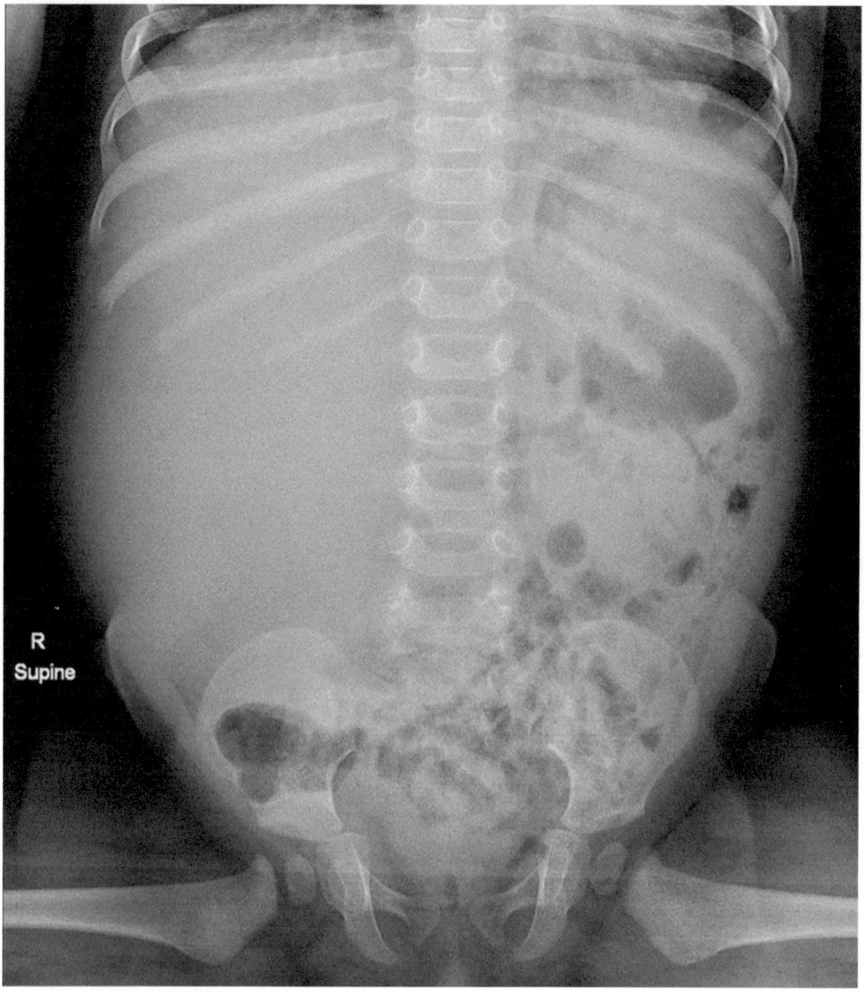

Image 2

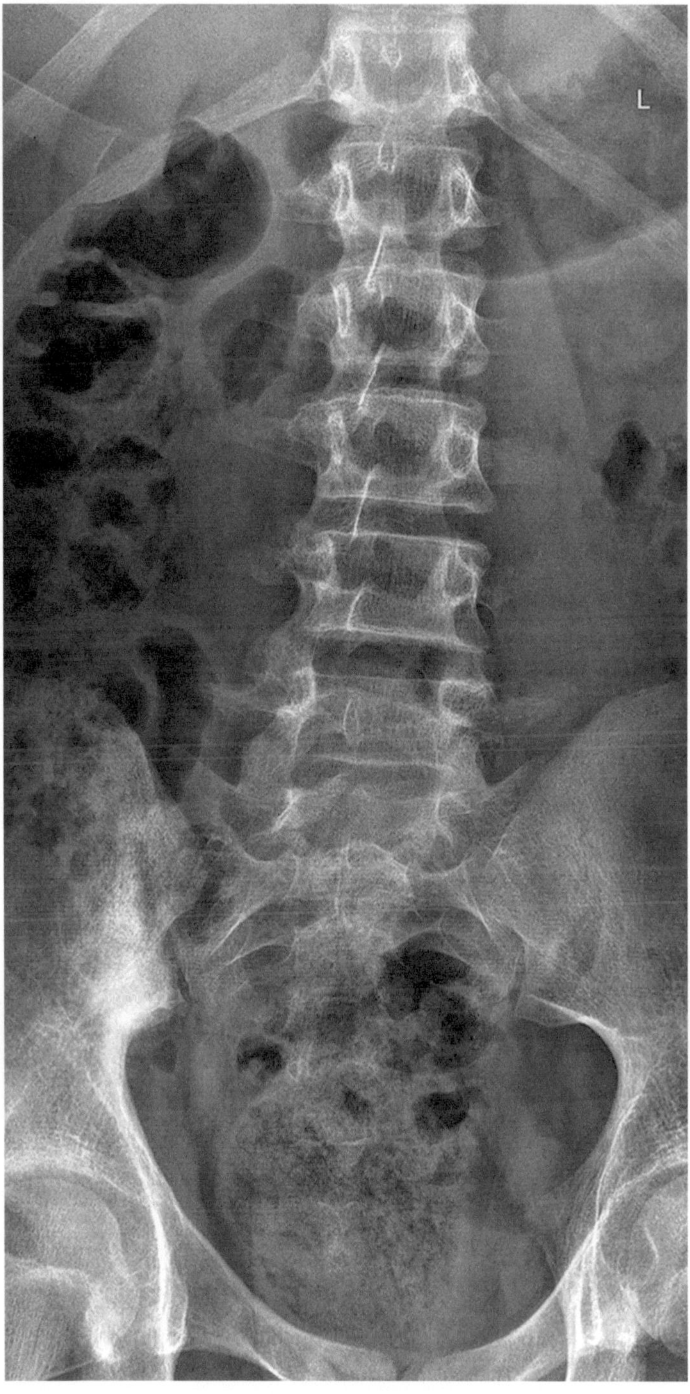

Image 3

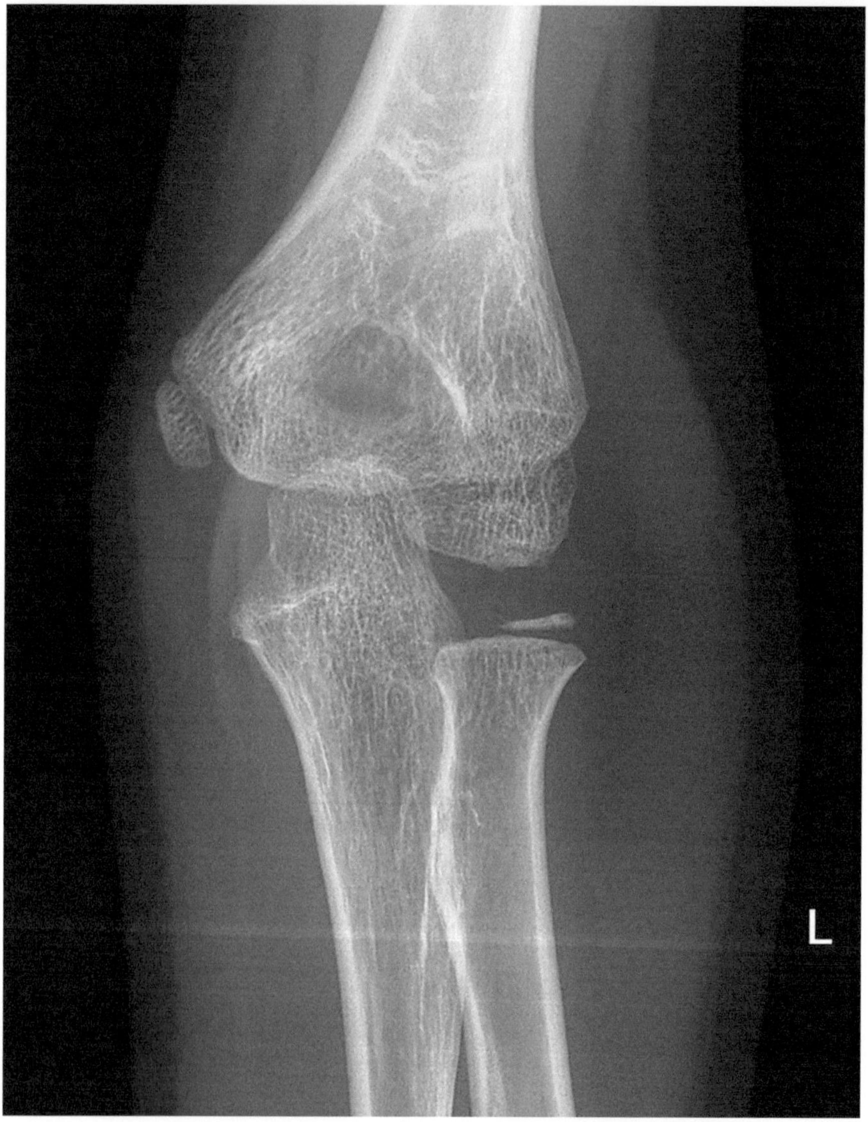

Image 4

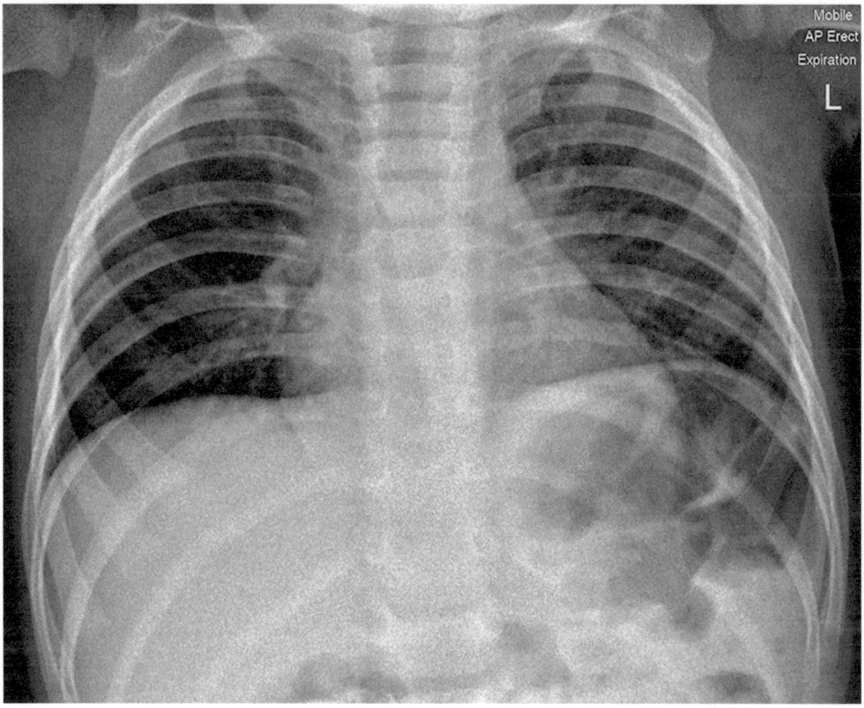

Image 5

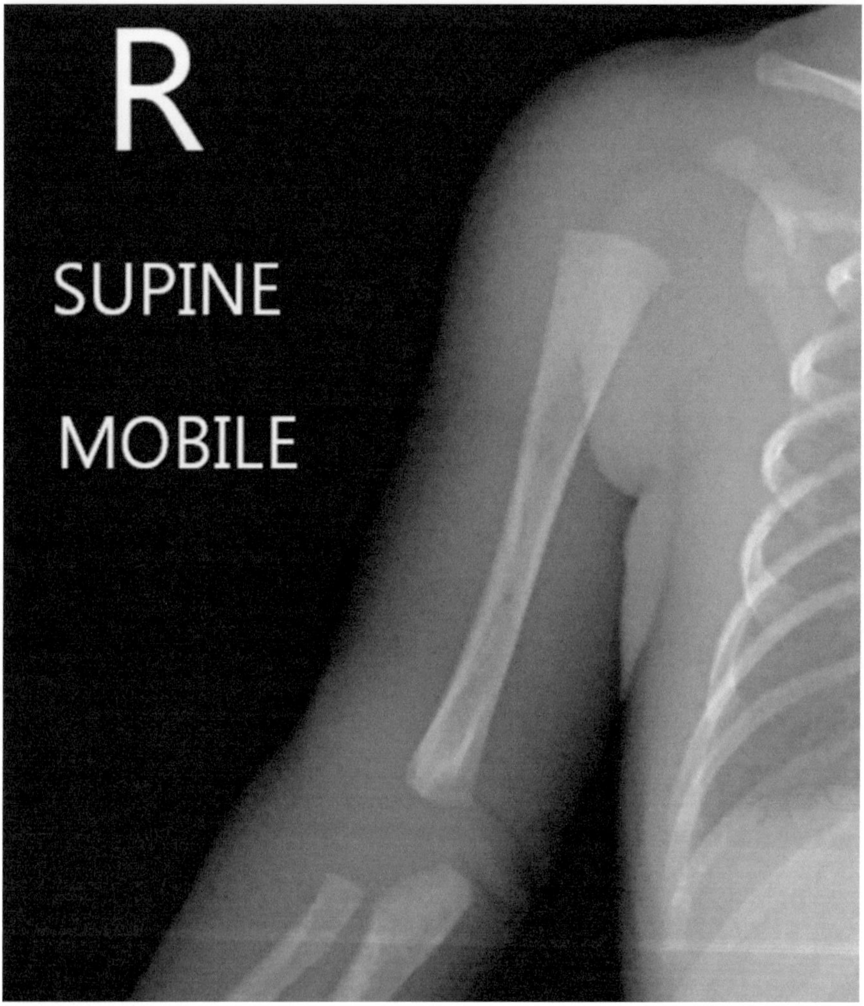

Image 6

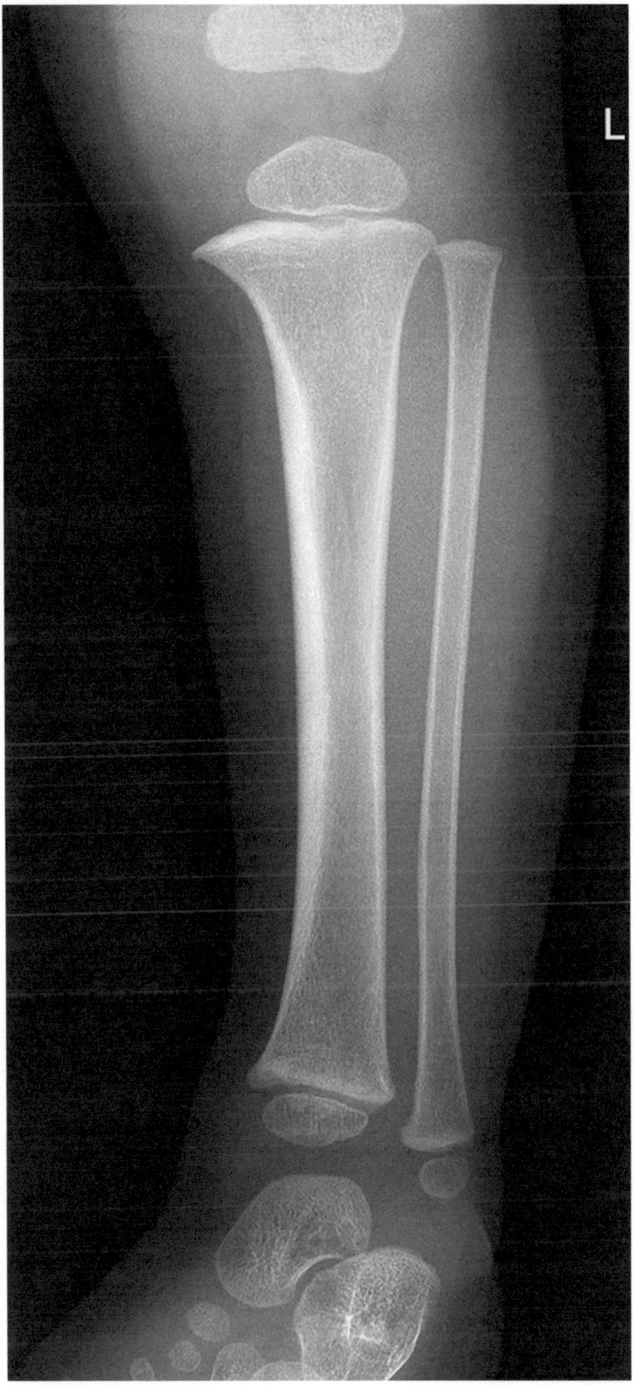

Image 7

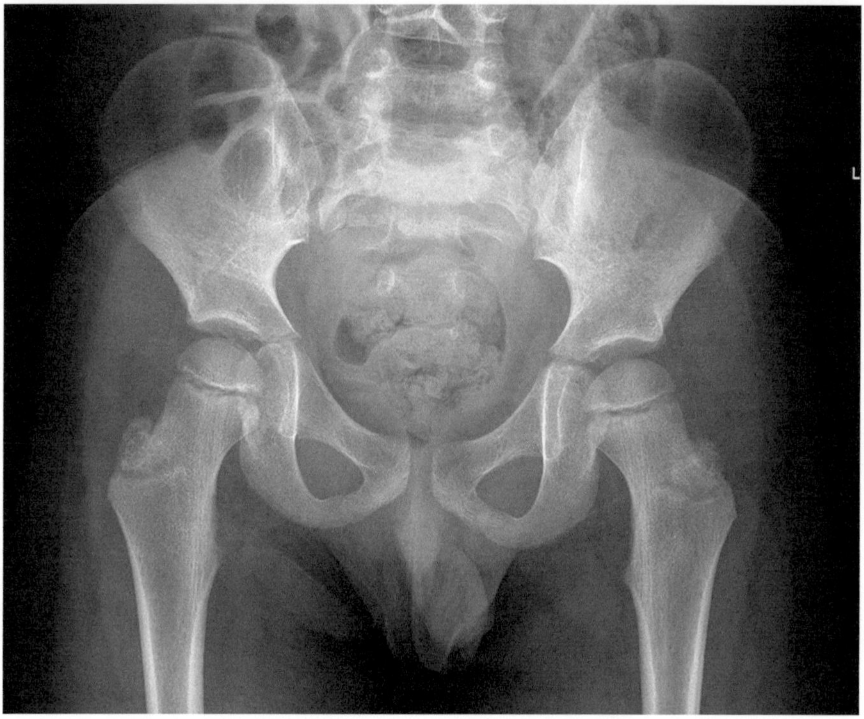

Image 8

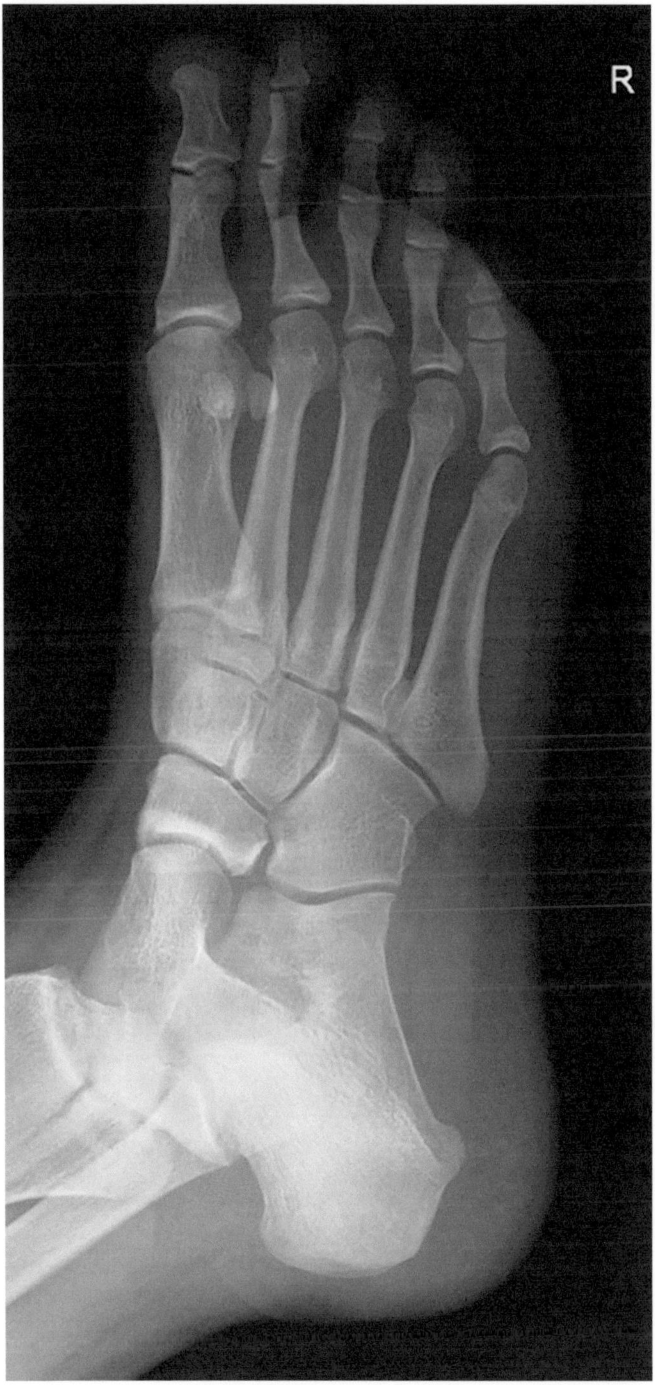

Image 9

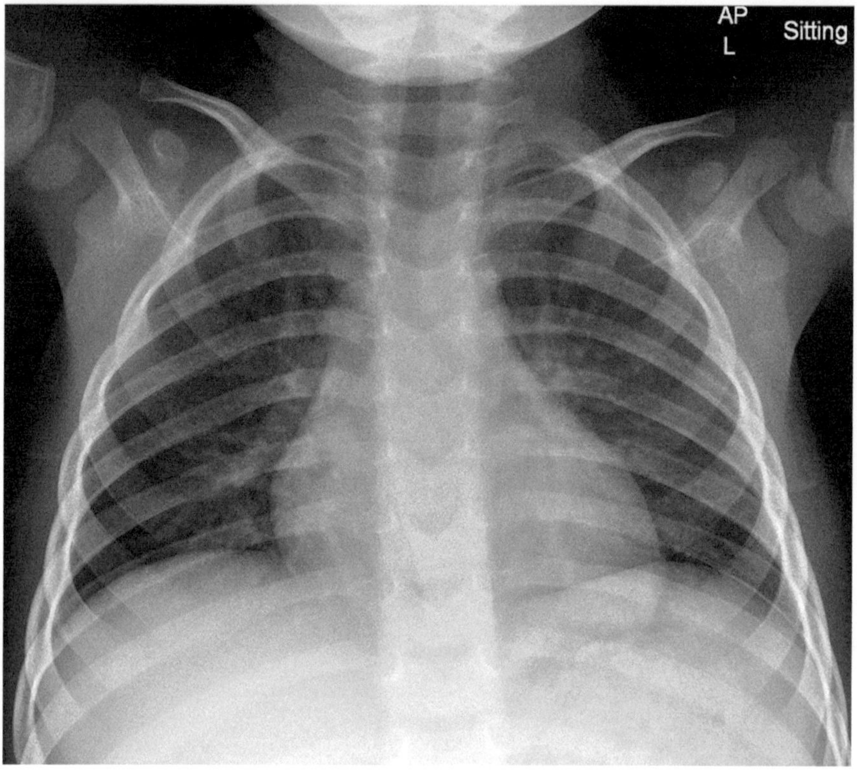

Image 10

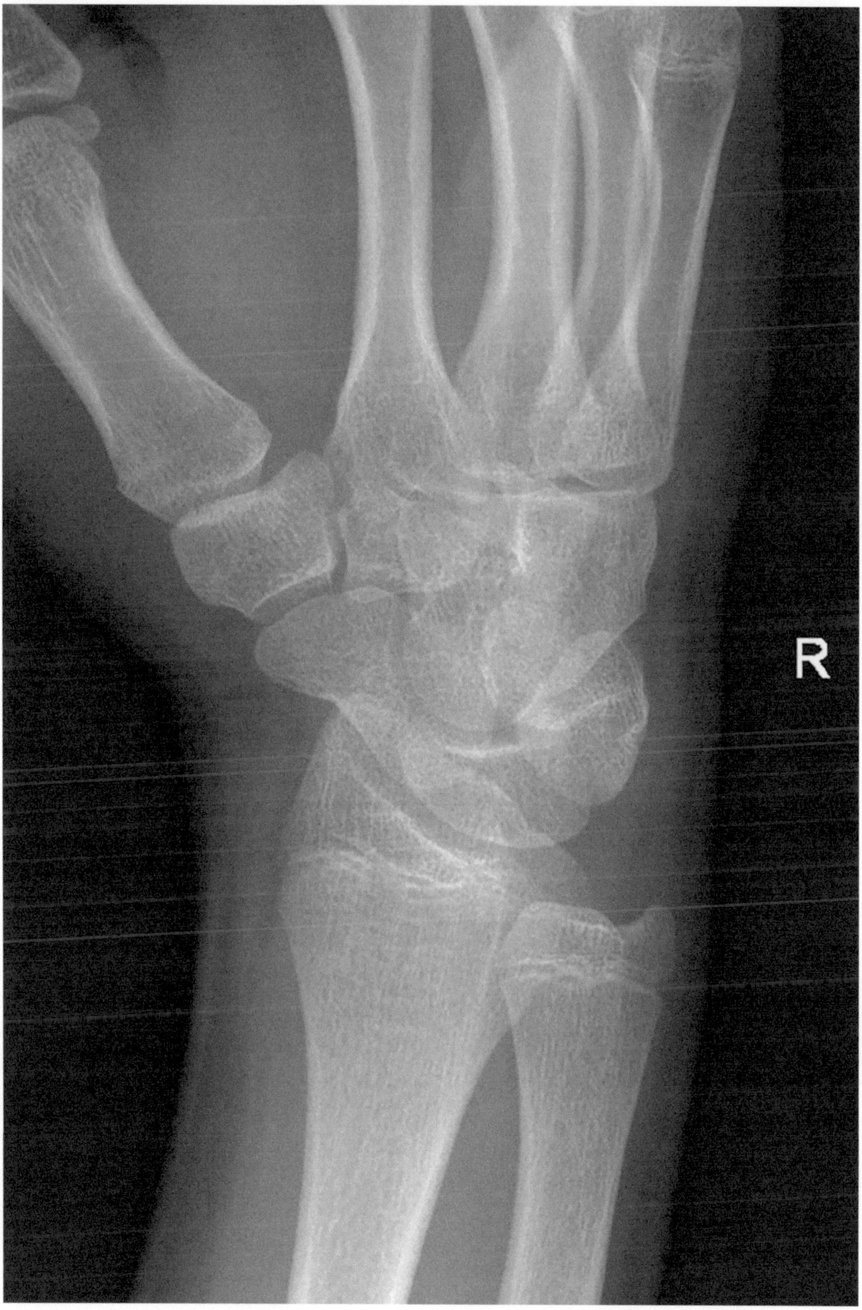

Image 11

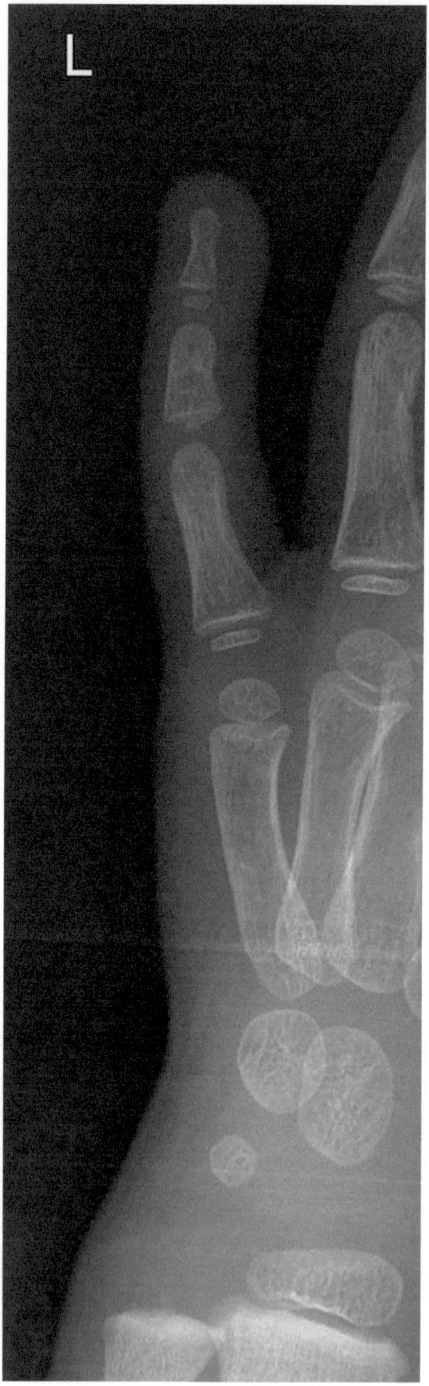

Image 12

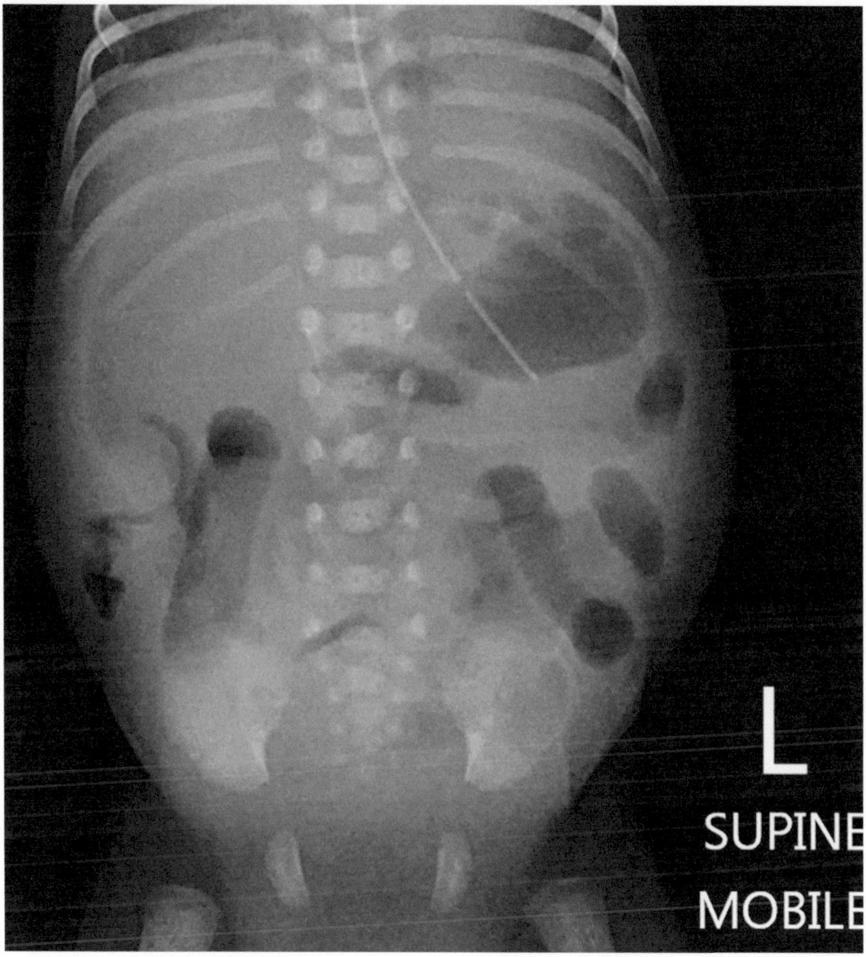

Image 13

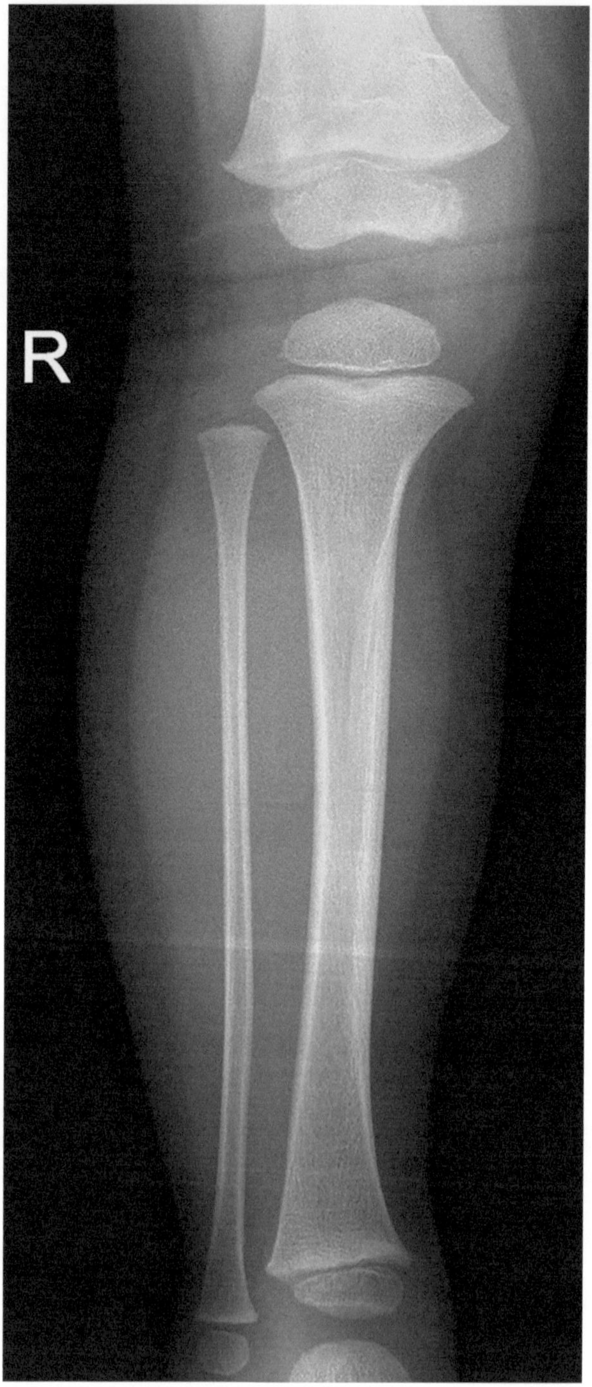

Image 14

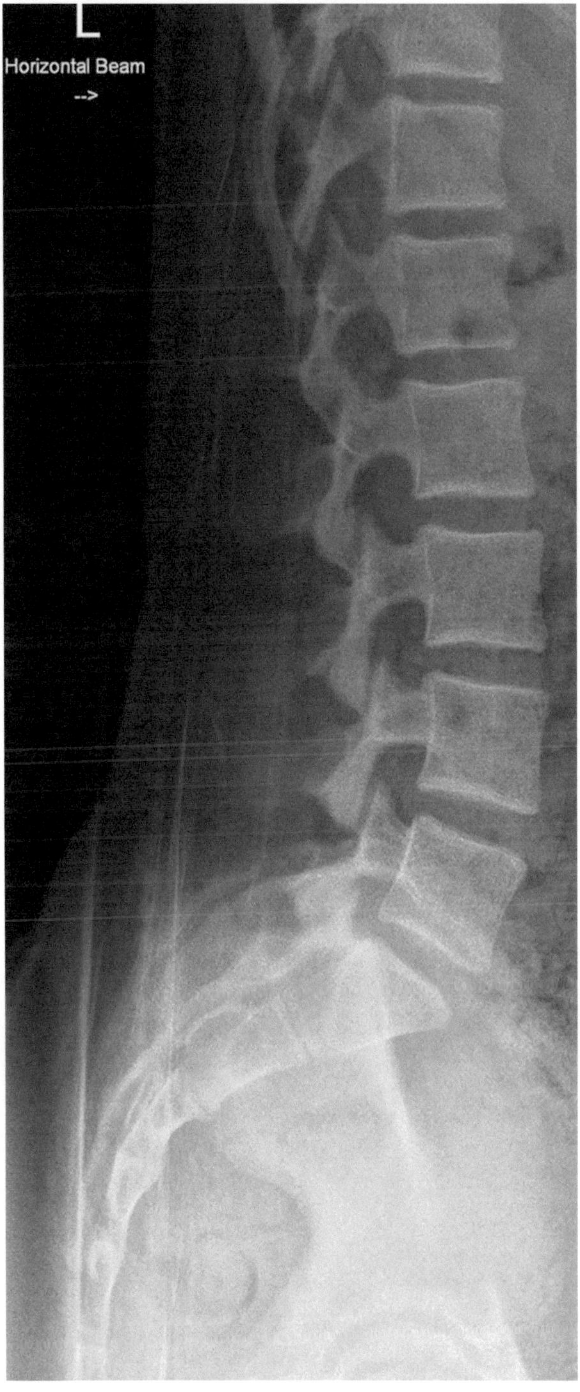

Image 15

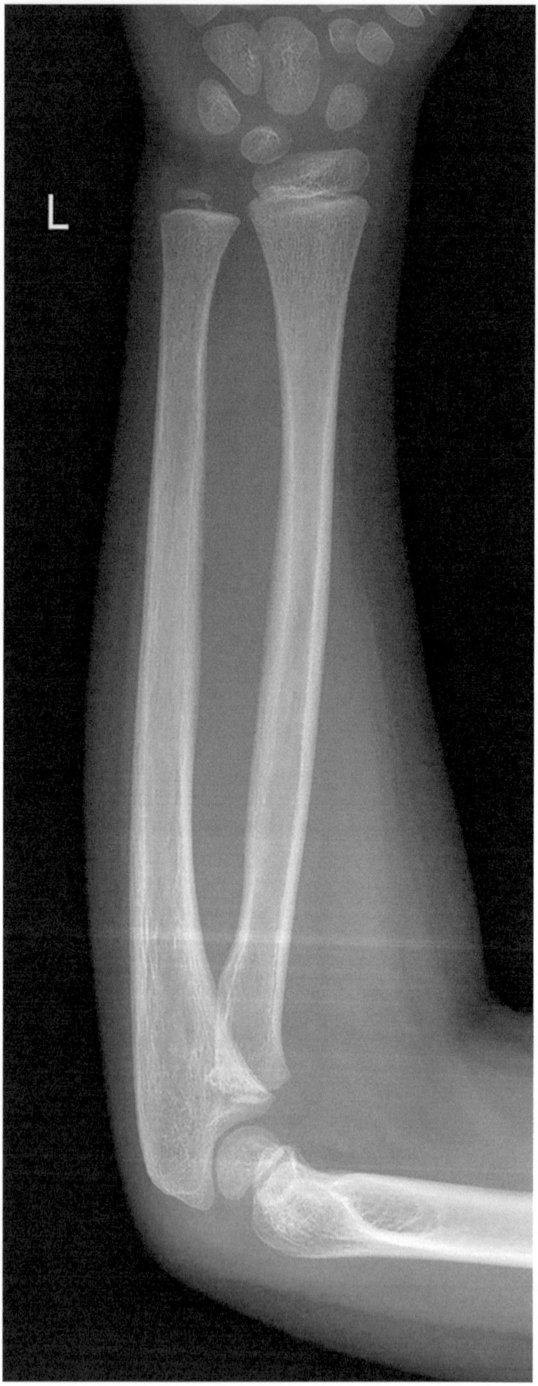

Image 16

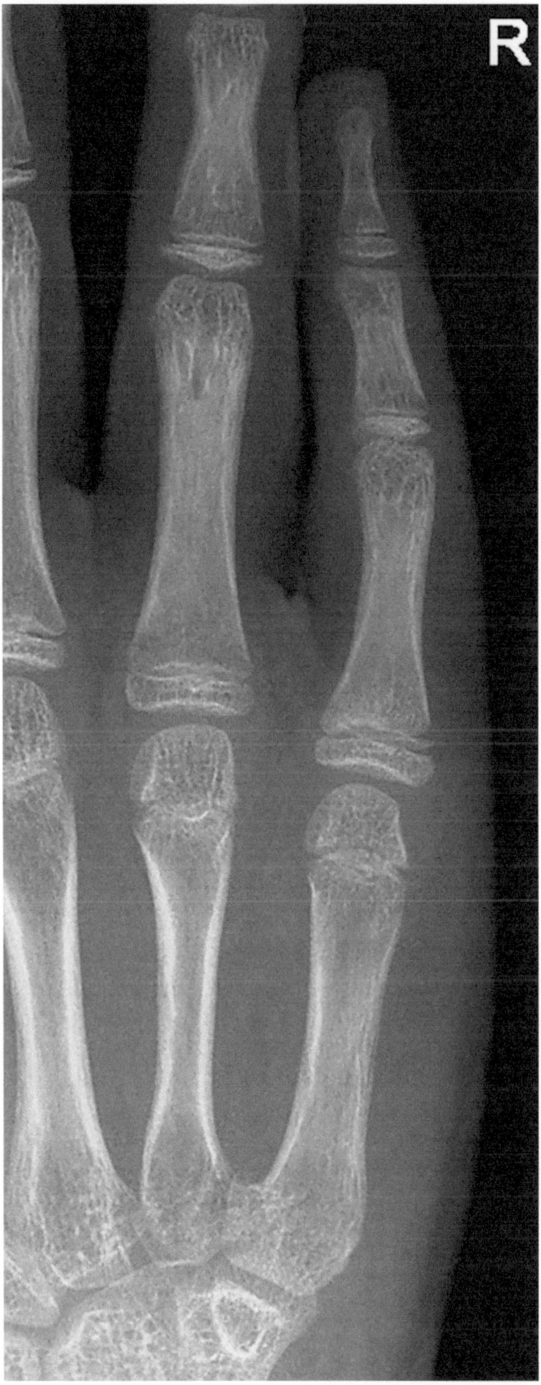

Image 17

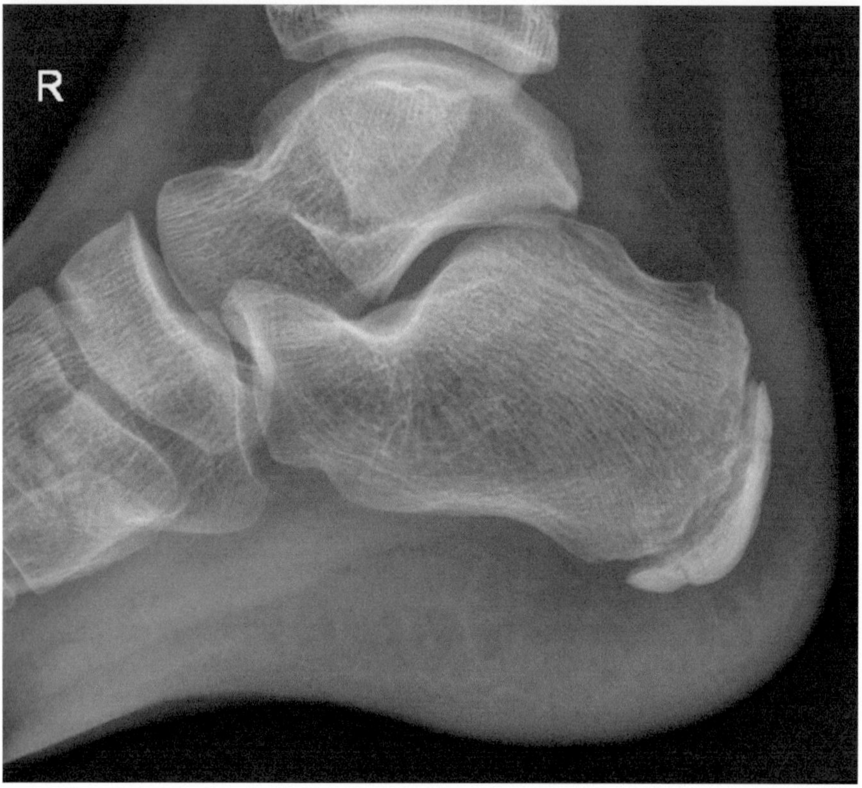

Image 18

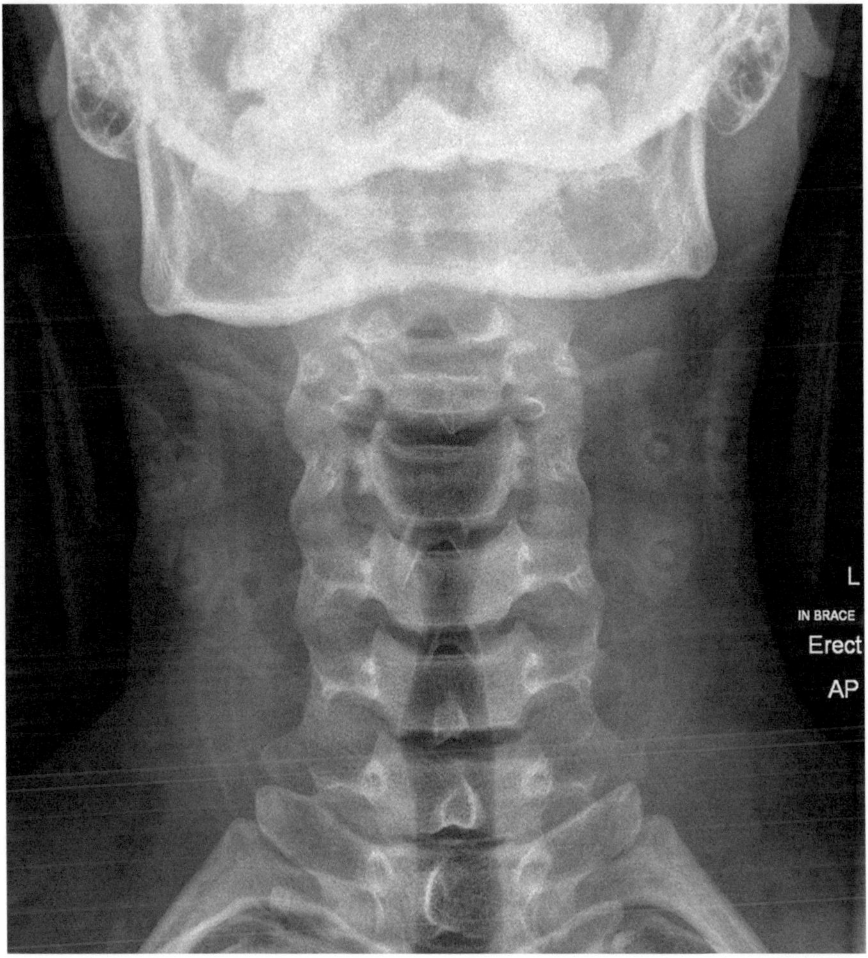

Image 19

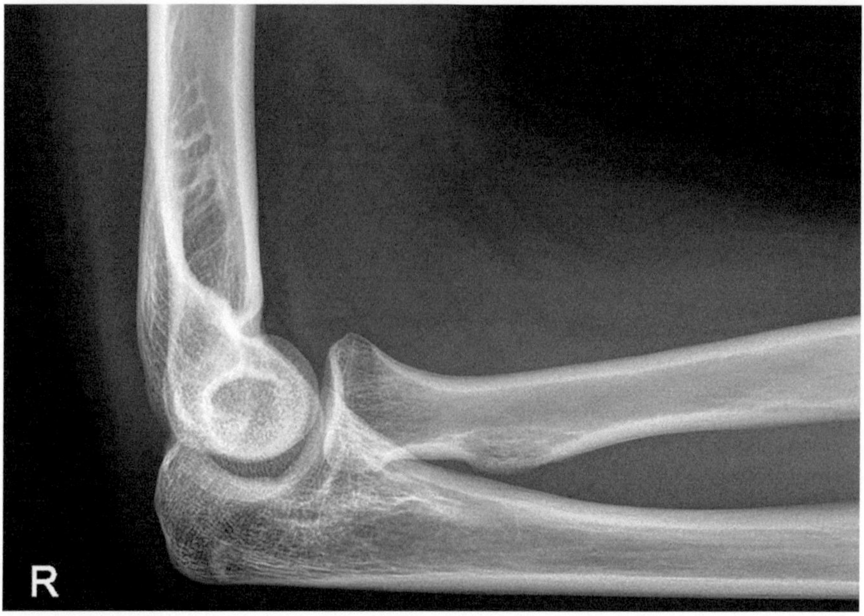

Image 20

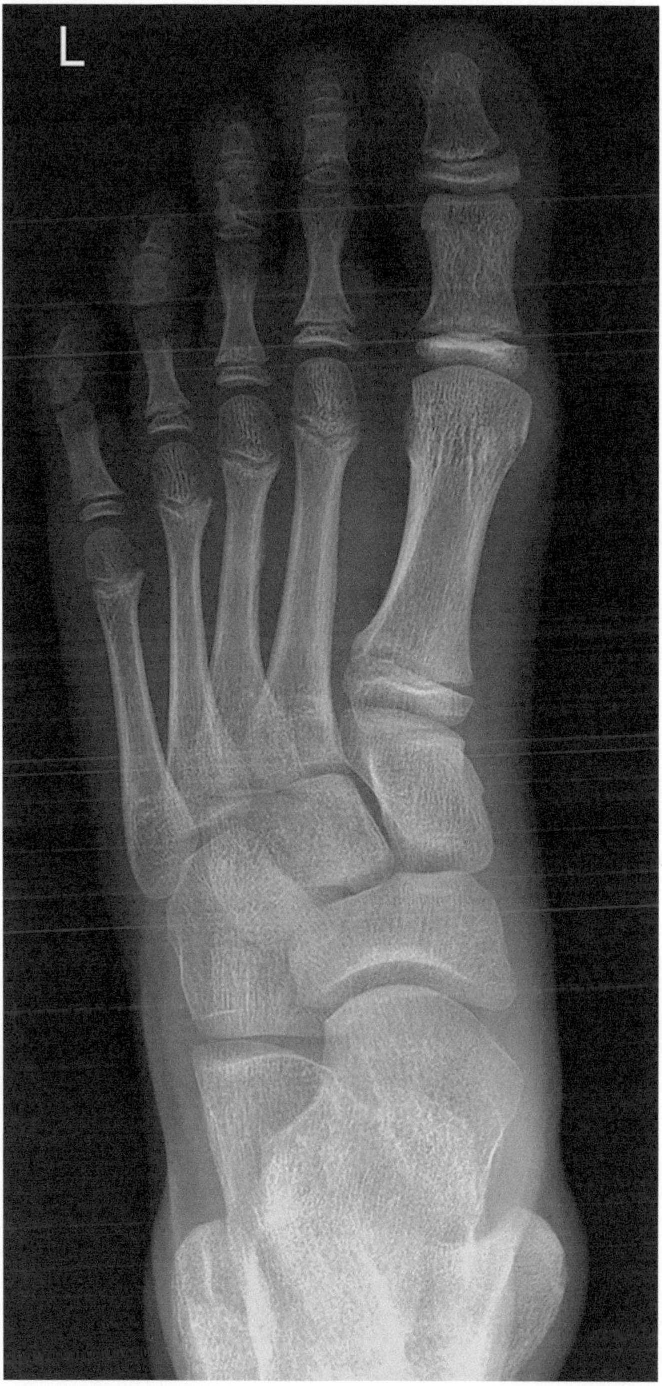

Image 21

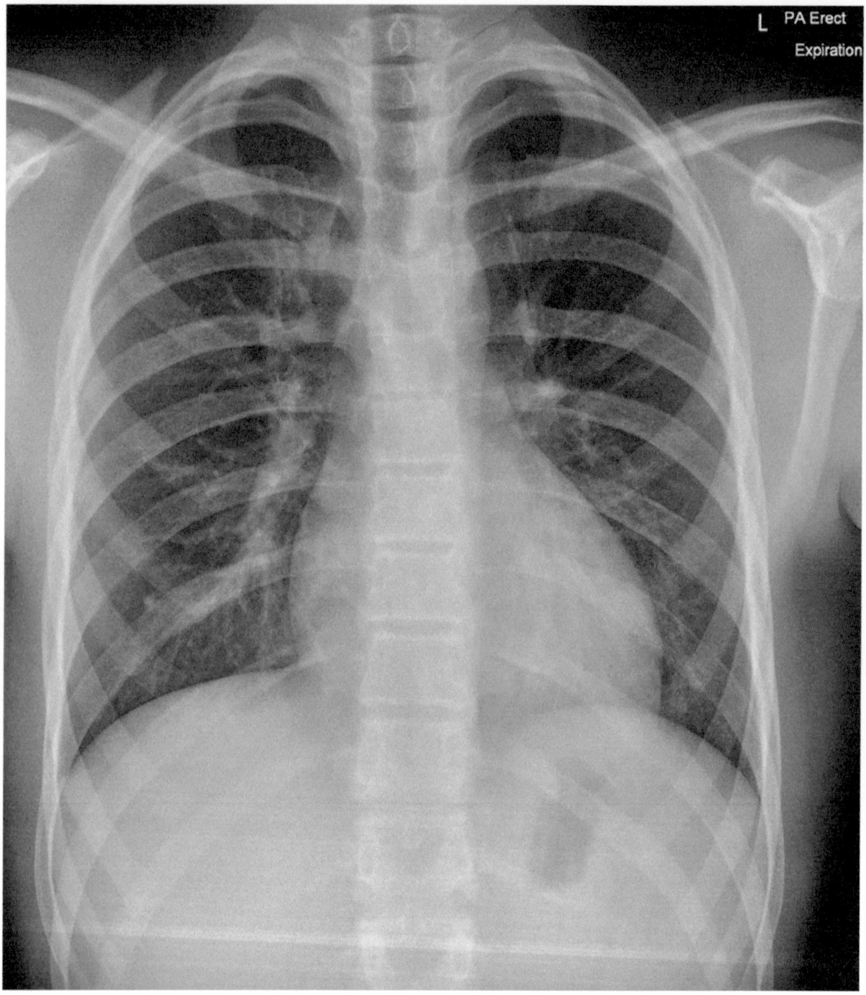

Image 22

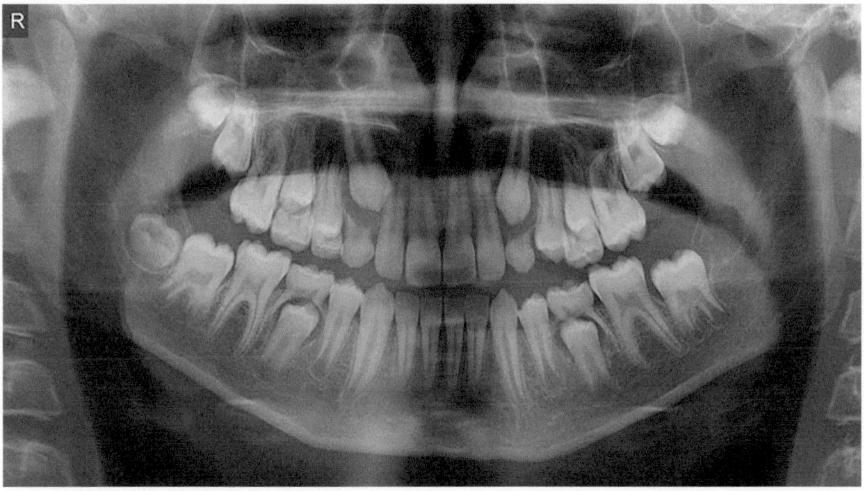

Image 23

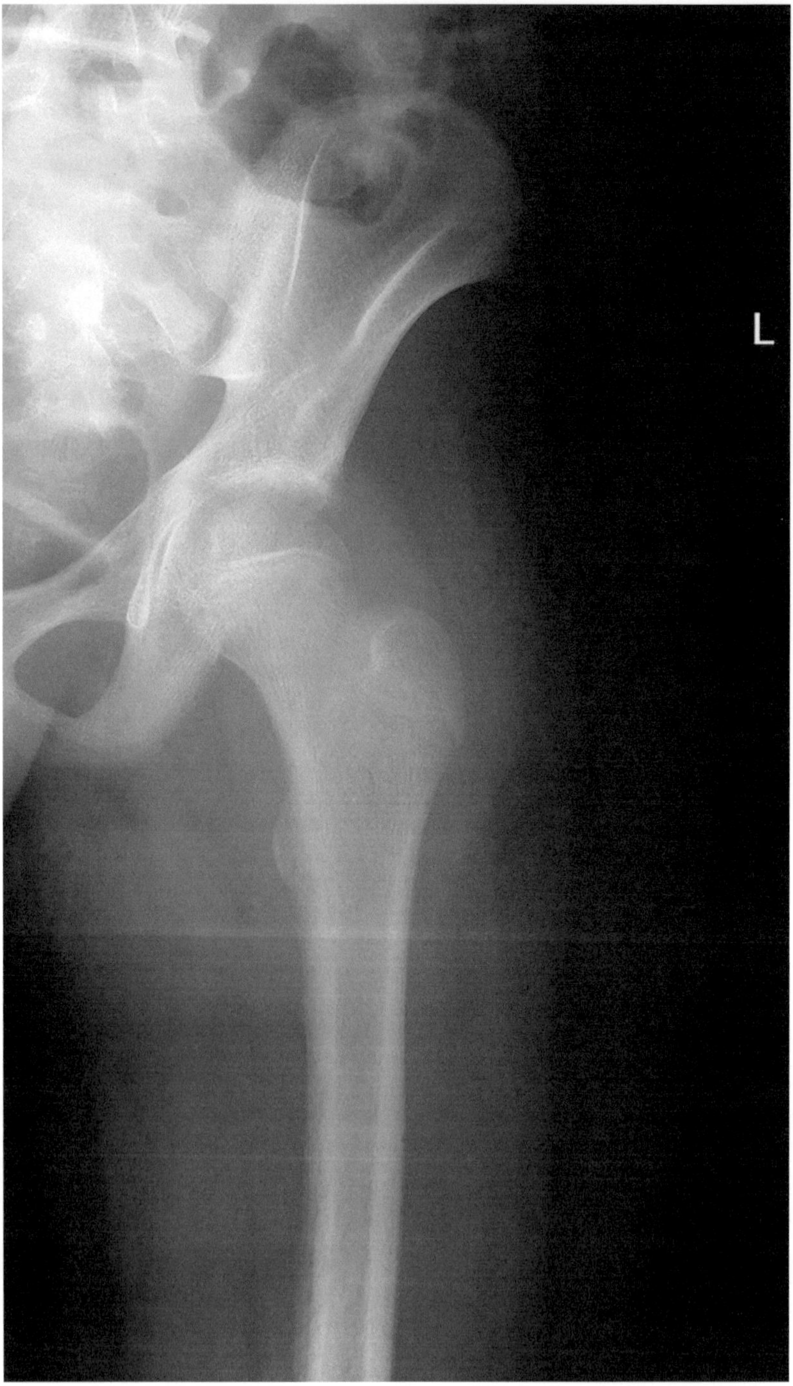

Image 24

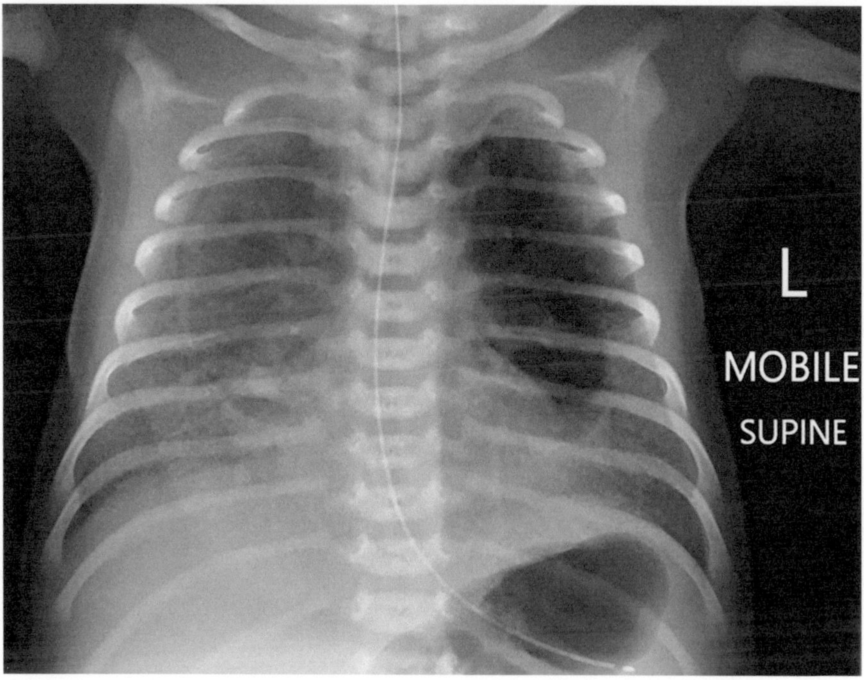

Image 25

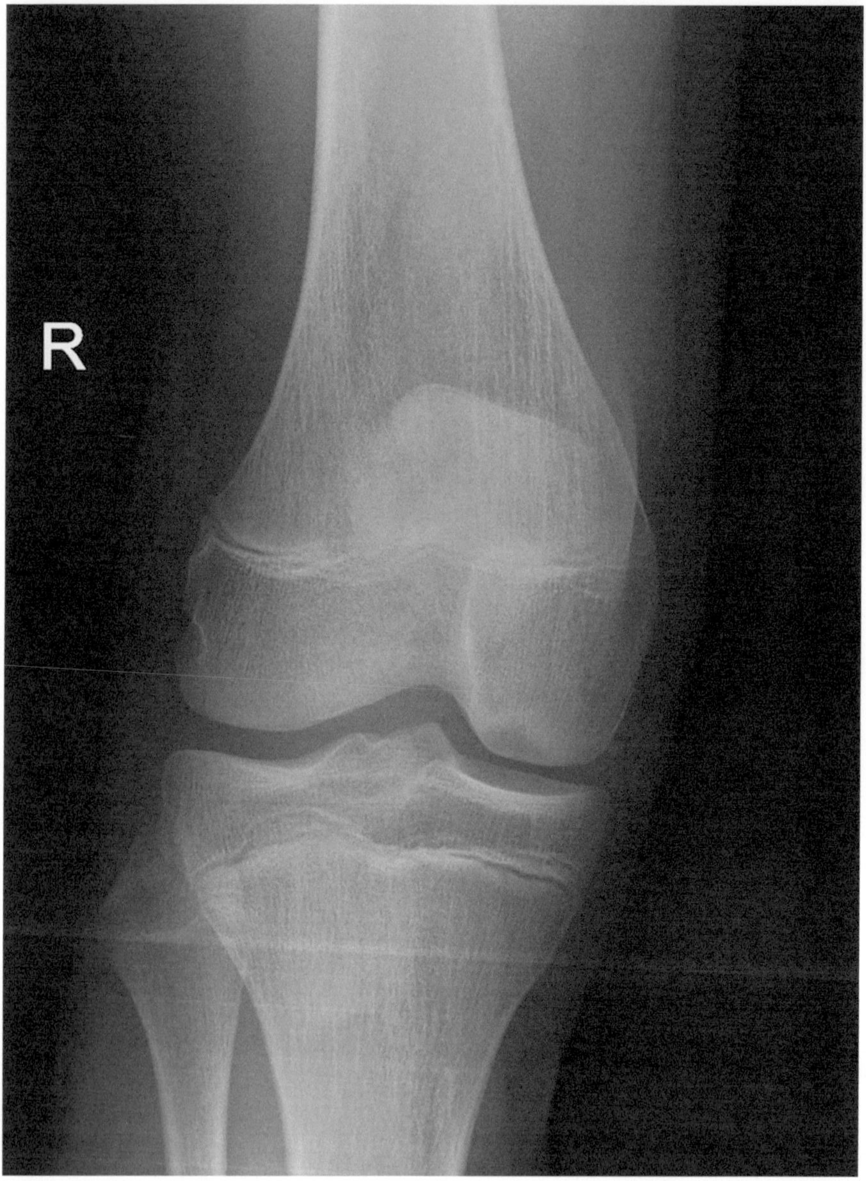

Image 26

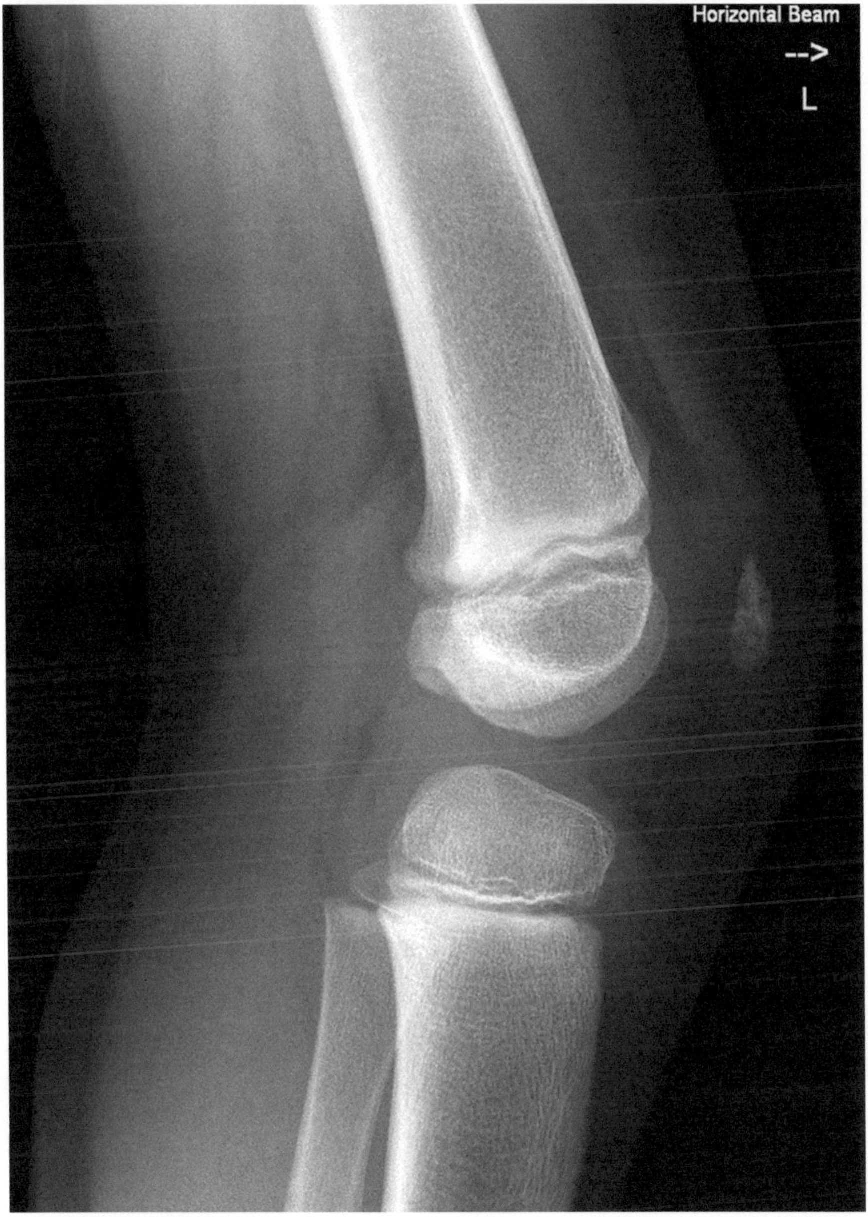

Image 27

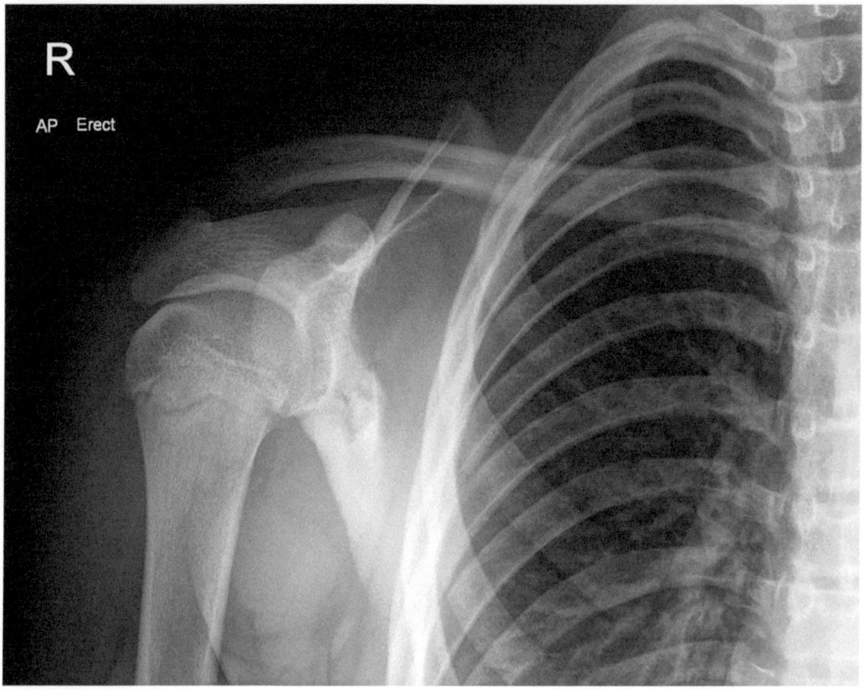

Image 28

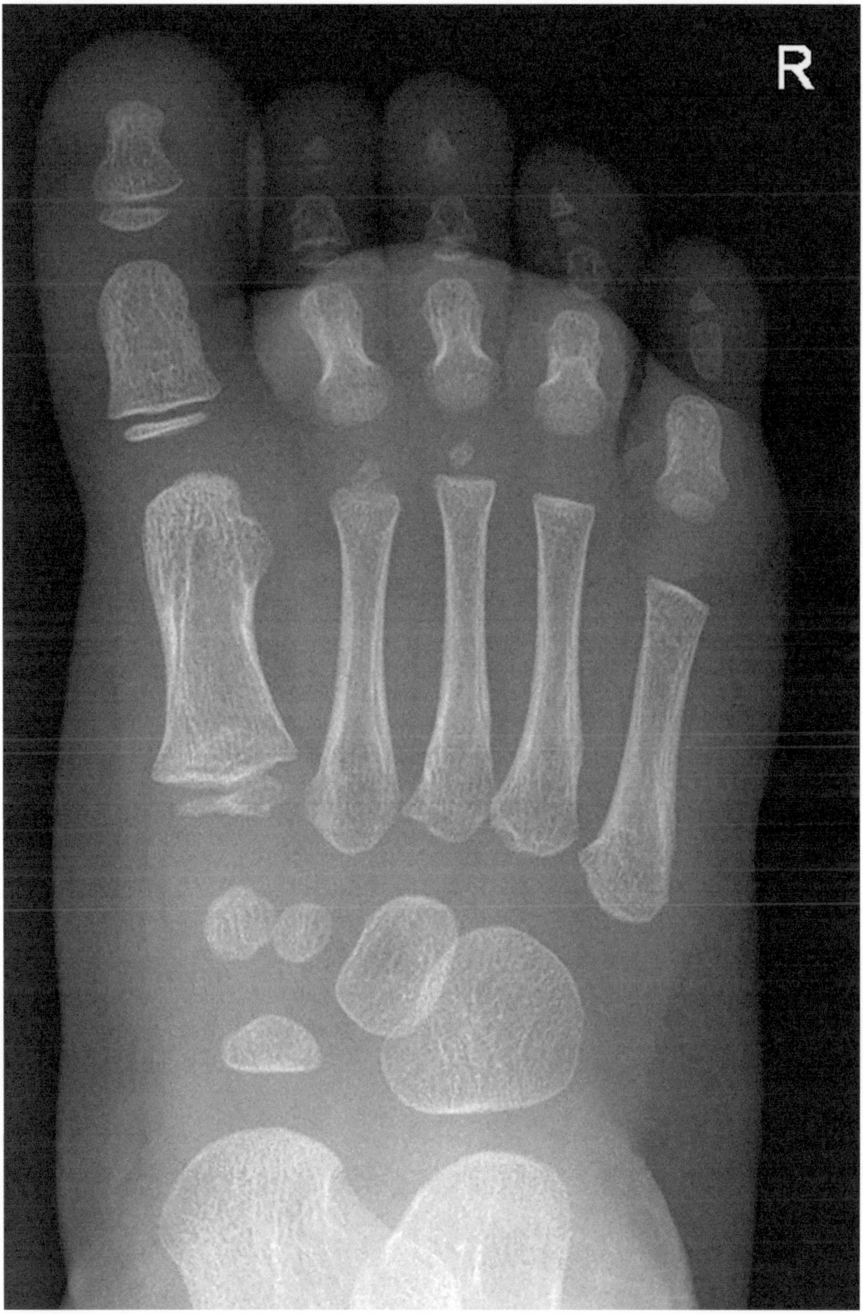

Image 29

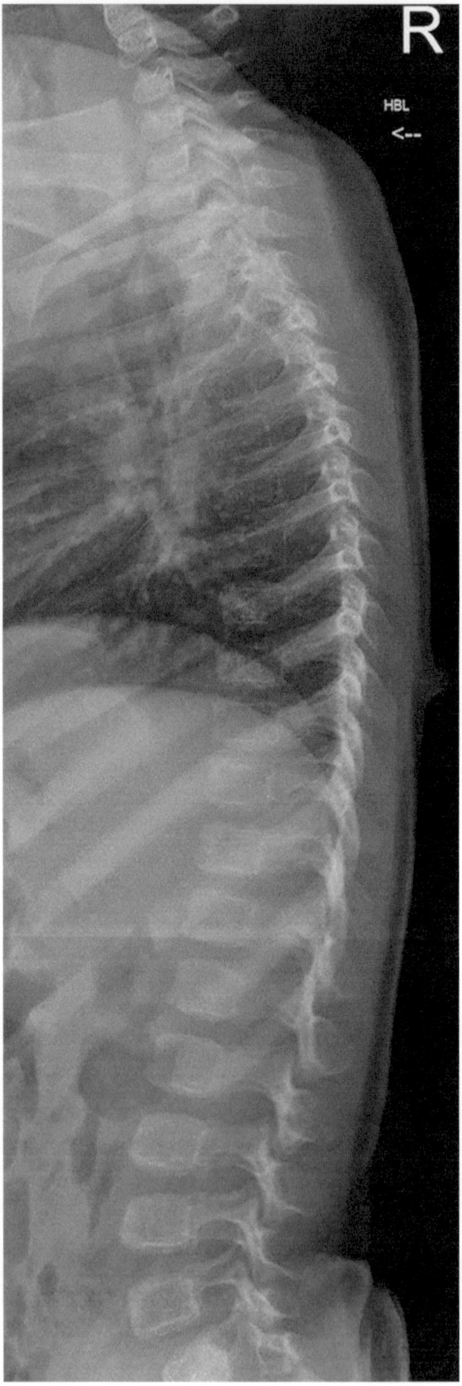

Image 30

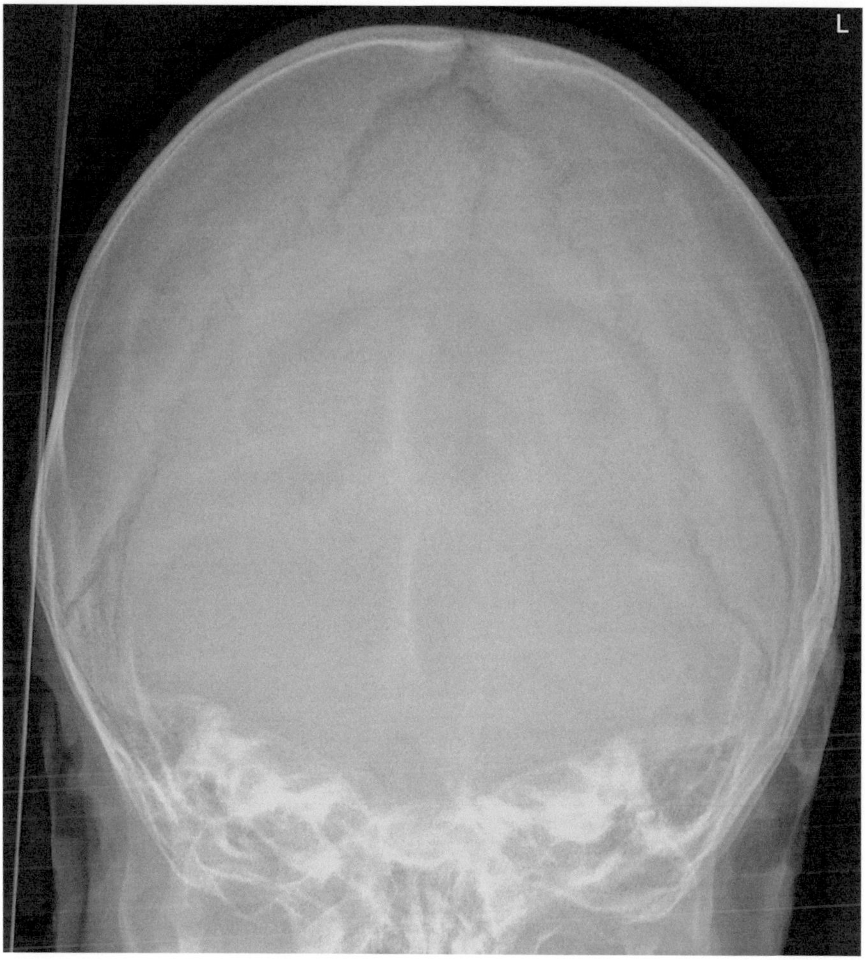

11.2 Answers

Image	Normal	Abnormal	Diagnosis/abnormality (only if abnormal)
1		✓	R abdominal mass
2		✓	Sclerotic R iliac bone
3		✓	OCD L capitellum
4		✓	Hyperlucency R mid and lower zones
5	✓		
6	✓		
7	✓		
8		✓	# R distal tibia
9	✓		
10	✓		
11	✓		
12		✓	NEC
13		✓	# R distal femoral metadiaphysis
14	✓		
15		✓	# L radial neck
16		✓	SH2 # R little finger proximal phalanx
17	✓		
18	✓		
19	✓		
20		✓	Healing stress # L third metatarsal
21	✓		
22		✓	# L mandibular condyle
23		✓	Periosteal reaction L proximal femoral diaphysis
24		✓	Pneumomediastinum
25		✓	OCD R medial distal femoral condyle
26	✓		
27		✓	# R scapula
28	✓		
29	✓		
30	✓		

11.3 Explanations

1. **R abdominal mass**

   There is abnormal soft tissue density in the right abdomen with left and inferior displacement of gas-filled bowel loops. There is no associated calcification. The imaged lungs are clear and the visualised bones appear normal. Following this radiograph, an ultrasound and computed tomography (CT) were performed which confirmed a large right-sided mass of renal origin favoured to represent a Wilms tumour.

   Wilms tumour, also known as nephroblastoma, is the most common malignant renal tumour in children, occurring typically before the age of 5 years. Ultrasound is the initial imaging modality of choice and often demonstrates a large retroperitoneal mass arising from the kidney with a surrounding 'claw' of normal renal parenchyma. This is known as the 'claw sign' and is a useful radiological sign that helps to determine whether a mass arises from solid parenchyma (intrinsic mass) or adjacent to it (extrinsic mass), distorting the parenchyma, and can be visualised on ultrasound, CT, and magnetic resonance imaging (MRI). The renal vein and inferior vena cava should be assessed for tumour thrombus, which is seen in approximately 10% of cases. CT of the thorax, abdomen and pelvis is performed to assess for metastases, which most commonly occur to the lungs: 10–20% of cases have pulmonary metastases at the time of diagnosis.

2. **Sclerotic R iliac bone**

   This lumbar spine radiograph demonstrates abnormal, asymmetric sclerosis of the right iliac bone which extends to the right sacroiliac joint and right acetabulum. Following this radiograph, an MRI was performed which confirmed a large infiltrative mass centred on the right iliac bone: Ewing's sarcoma was subsequently diagnosed on biopsy. See the explanation for Image 20 of Test 3.

3. **Osteochondral defect L capitellum**

   Close inspection of the left capitellum ossification centre reveals the osteochondral defect (OCD), visualised in the magnified image below:

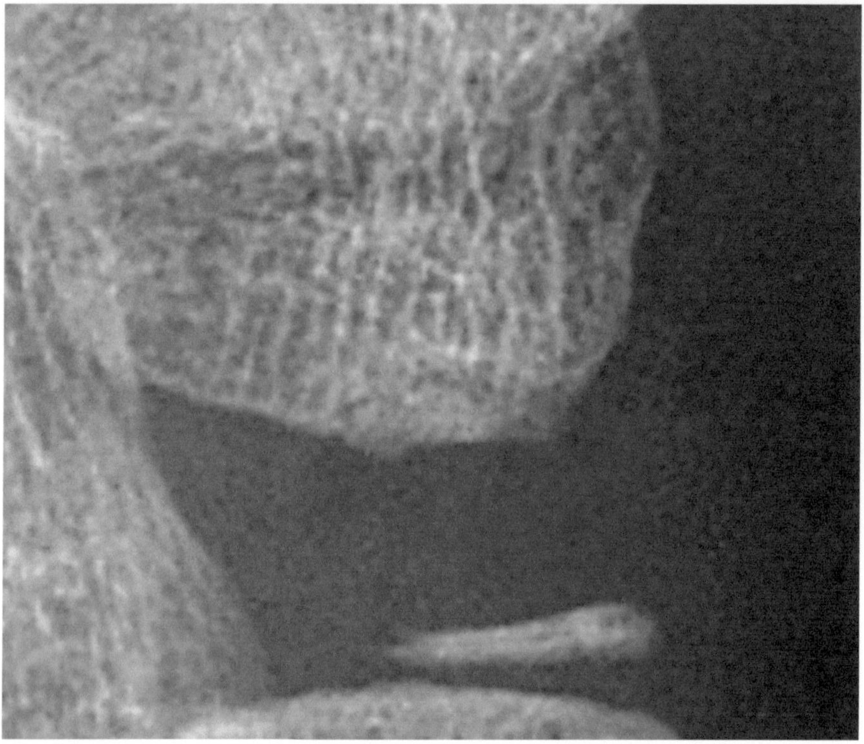

See the explanation for Image 10 of Test 4.

4. **Hyperlucency R mid and lower zones**
This 14-month-old boy was brought to the Emergency Department (ED) with increased work of breathing following a "choking" episode on the previous day. This chest radiograph demonstrates hyperlucency (note the relative absence of bronchovascular markings) from hyperinflation (note the flattening of the right hemidiaphragm on this expiratory image, labelled in the top right of the image) of the right mid and lower zones, suggesting air trapping. There is no radiopaque foreign body, atelectasis or lobar collapse visualised. There is bilateral perihilar peribronchial thickening, which could be reactive or inflammatory and is often visualised on chest radiographs in children of this age. A low-dose chest CT was subsequently performed which confirmed a foreign body in the right lower lobe bronchus. The child proceeded to have a bronchoscopy at which a popcorn kernel was found and removed!

If there is a concern regarding foreign body aspiration and the initial chest radiograph is normal, expiratory (or conversely inspiratory, if an expiratory image has already been obtained) or lateral decubitus projections can accentuate air trapping; the latter can be helpful in younger patients who are unable to follow breathing instructions. CT is more sensitive in the detection of radiolucent inhaled/aspirated foreign bodies.

6. *Normal left tibia/fibula radiograph*
   The cortical undulation at the medial aspect of the left distal fibular metaphysis is normal, reflecting the distal insertion of the interosseous membrane and should not be mistaken for a bony injury (e.g. buckle fracture).

8. **# R distal tibia**
   The right distal tibial fracture is visualised at the bottom of the image and is easy to overlook if a thorough imaging evaluation has not been performed. Do not forget to include the distal tibia and fibula as part of your review of every foot radiograph. The contemporaneous anteroposterior (AP) ankle projection confirmed the presence of a right distal tibial fracture (Salter-Harris 4). The fracture is visualised in the magnified image below:

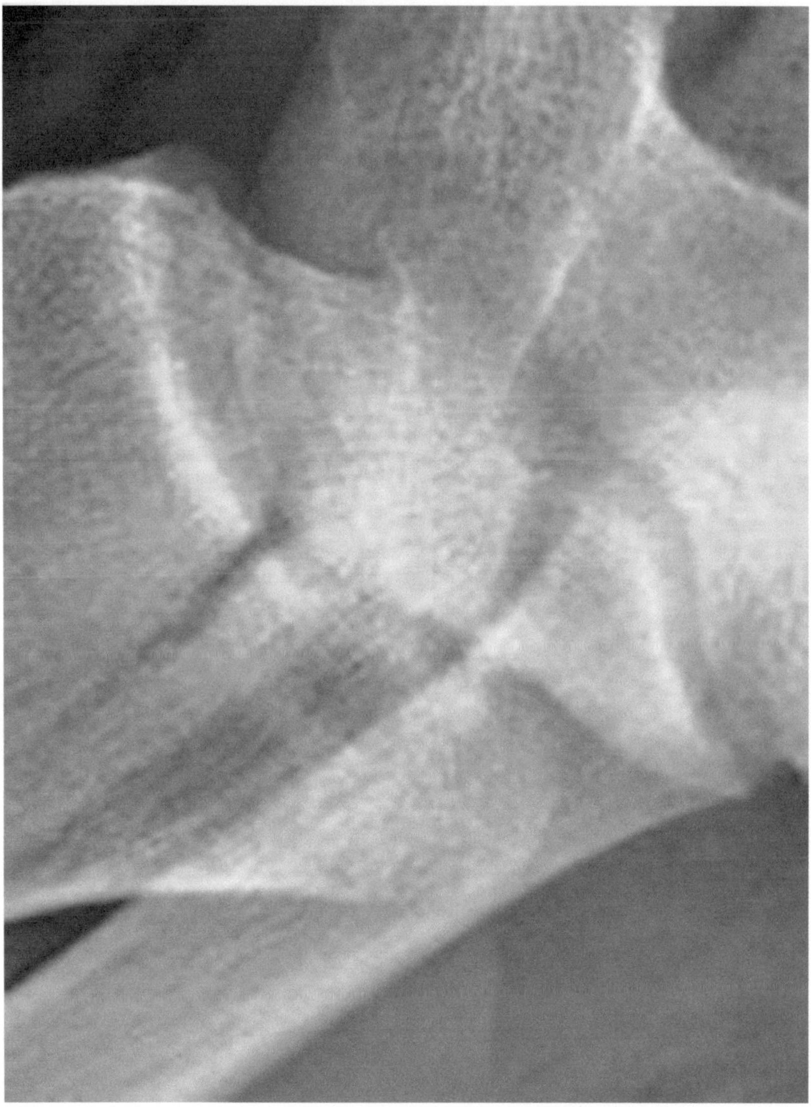

12. **Necrotising enterocolitis**

This image illustrates many of the key radiographic features of necrotising enterocolitis (NEC):

- Dilated, featureless bowel loops in the right and left abdomen.
- Pneumoperitoneum indicated by the abnormal lucency over the liver and central upper abdomen, which was confirmed on the subsequent lateral decubitus radiograph.
- Crescentic lucency in the right flank, indicative of *pneumatosis intestinalis*, which was confirmed on the subsequent ultrasound.

The image quality reflects the low dose parameters used to acquire this portable radiograph in the NICU. See the explanation for Image 10 of Test 8 for a detailed discussion of NEC.

13. **# R distal femoral metadiaphysis**

This radiograph highlights the importance of assessing the edge of the image (previously known as 'edge-of-film', given that radiographic film has been replaced by digital imaging) similar to the right distal tibial fracture in Image 8 of this test. In doing so, one visualises the cortical fracture of the right distal femoral metaphysis.

You must assess every bone that has been imaged, particularly given the absence of clinical information, not only in the examination but also in clinical practice, where radiographs may be obtained for a seemingly unrelated indication (this radiograph was performed for '?toddler's fracture').

Note that the metaphysis is located between the epiphysis and the diaphysis and refers to the wider portion of the long bone (where it flares outward), which is where growth occurs. The fracture in this case is not the same as the metaphyseal fracture resulting from inflicted (abusive) injury, i.e. the classic metaphyseal lesion (CML) with 'corner' and 'bucket handle' configurations. Hence, we prefer to call these fractures "metadiaphyseal" to avoid confusion. Notwithstanding, *any* fracture in a dependent, non-ambulant child is concerning for an inflicted injury. The identification of any fracture in the context of suspected physical abuse (SPA) indicates the application of significant and inappropriate forces. Physical abuse may also be suggested when an injury is inconsistent with the stated mechanism of injury and/or the history proffered by the parent or caregiver.

See the explanation for Image 2 of Test 3 for a discussion of CMLs and the references for Image 14 of Test 2 for further reading regarding the imaging of SPA in infants and young children. Note that metadiaphyseal fractures, but NOT metaphyseal fractures (i.e. CMLs), are common in infants with osteogenesis imperfecta.

15. **# L radial neck**

There is an acute fracture of the dorsal left radial neck but no elbow joint effusion. Remember that elbow joint alignment must be assessed on every radiograph, including any orthogonal projections obtained. See the explanation for

Image 11 of Test 1 for a detailed discussion regarding the radiographic assessment of elbow joint alignment.

16. **Salter-Harris 2 # R little finger proximal phalanx**
Close inspection of the metaphysis of the right little finger proximal phalanx reveals the fracture. See the explanation for Image 30 of Test 1 for a discussion of the Salter-Harris classification.

20. **Healing stress # L third metatarsal**
Note the subtle periosteal reaction along the medial cortex of the third metaphyseal diaphysis in keeping with a healing stress fracture. There is also subtle associated bony sclerosis. See the explanation for Image 10 of Test 2.

22. **# L mandibular condyle**
This 11-year-old boy was presented to the ED with trismus (inability to open his mouth) following a fall from his scooter. The orthopantomogram (OPG) demonstrates an angulated fracture of the left mandibular condylar with anterior subluxation of the left temporomandibular joint (TMJ). Compare this appearance to that of the normally enlocated right TMJ in the magnified images below:

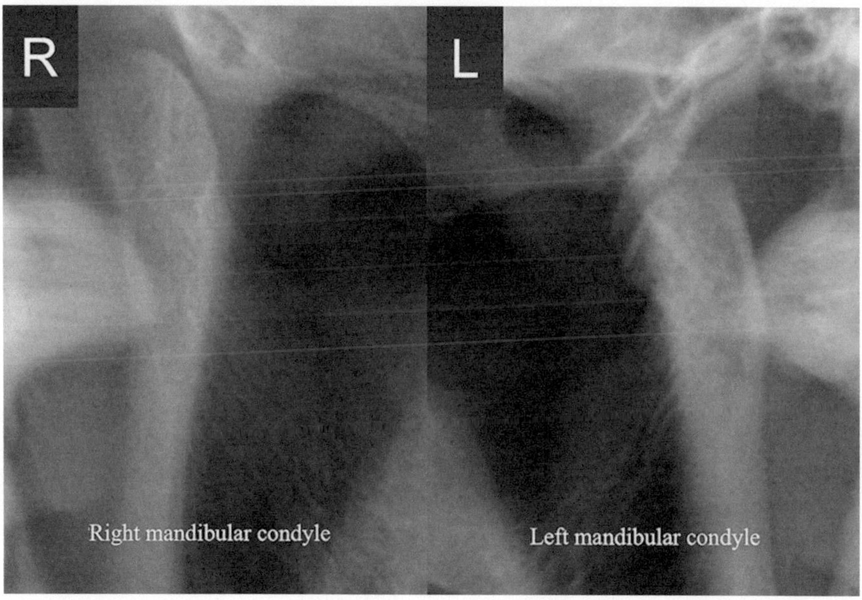

Mandibular fractures are the second commonest type of facial fracture after nasal bone fractures. Traditionally, the mandible and skull base were thought to represent a bony ring (similar to the pelvis), interrupted (but relatively fixed) by the TMJs. As such, one might expect further mandibular fractures in the context of trauma; however, mandibular fractures occur in isolation in 40% of cases. That being said, one should thoroughly assess the mandible for multifocal injury alongside associated TMJ subluxation/dislocation in the context of trauma.

Both deciduous and permanent teeth are present which is reported as mixed dentition. The left mandibular third molar (denoted as 38 using the Fédération Dentaire Internationale [FDI] notation) bud demonstrates delayed development and does not represent a pathological cystic lesion. Note the faint cusp mineralisation which has not yet coalesced. The maxillary right (18) and left (28) third molars demonstrate progressive crown and pulp chamber formation with visible dentinal deposition. The right mandibular third molar (48) demonstrates united cusp mineralisation with well-defined mature coronal morphology. There are no gross caries, periapical lucenices or suspicious osseous lesions.

23. **Periosteal reaction L proximal femoral diaphysis**

This radiograph demonstrates mottled lucency of the medial left proximal femoral diaphyseal cortex with associated cortical thinning/destruction and multilayered/lamellated periosteal reaction visualised at the bottom of the image. The appearances are in keeping with an aggressive process: this 13-year-old girl had left femoral osteomyelitis and staphylococcal bacteraemia.

The radiographic changes of osteomyelitis are often subtle and may not be evident initially. Early changes involve soft tissue swelling with later changes including periostitis, cortical lucency, lysis, and a permeative appearance/texture of the affected bone (in other words, osteomyelitis has the radiographic features of an aggressive bone lesion). MRI is the most useful and sensitive imaging modality in evaluating osteomyelitis and can detect bone marrow signal changes within a few days of the onset of infection. It is also helpful in assessing associated complications such as abscess formation and osteonecrosis. See the explanation for Image 13 of Test 7 for a more detailed discussion of osteomyelitis.

24. **Pneumomediastinum**

This chest radiograph was performed in a premature neonate whose clinical condition had deteriorated after birth with tachypnoea and increasing oxygen requirements. The image demonstrates a large volume pneumomediastinum causing inferior displacement of the heart. The outline of the mediastinum is projected over both lungs with asymmetric distribution of mediastinal gas (the left is more lucent than the right). Whilst not present in this radiograph, one should inspect carefully for an associated pneumothorax (which may be bilateral) once a pneumomediastinum has been identified. See Image 5 of Test 2 for an example of pneumomediastinum in an older child. See the references for further examples of pneumomediastinum in neonates typified by the 'spinnaker sign' and 'angel wing sign'.

The granular opacification throughout the lungs is consistent with hyaline membrane disease (HMD; also known as surfactant deficiency disorder [SDD] or referred to as respiratory distress syndrome [RDS]) and is a common finding on chest radiographs in premature neonates.

Note the appropriately sited nasogastric tube (NGT) tip which is projected over the gas-filled stomach. When present, all lines and tubes should be assessed for satisfactory or malposition.

25. **Osteochondral defect R medial distal femoral condyle**
See the explanation for Image 10 of Test 4.

26. *Normal left knee radiograph*
Note the apparent lucency at the posterior aspect of the medial femoral condyle which is secondary to the overlapping medial and lateral femoral condyles. This is remote from the weight-bearing articular surface and does *not* represent an OCD.

27. **# R scapula**
This radiograph demonstrates a fracture through the body of the right scapula with intra-articular extension to the right glenohumeral joint, as visualised in the magnified image below:

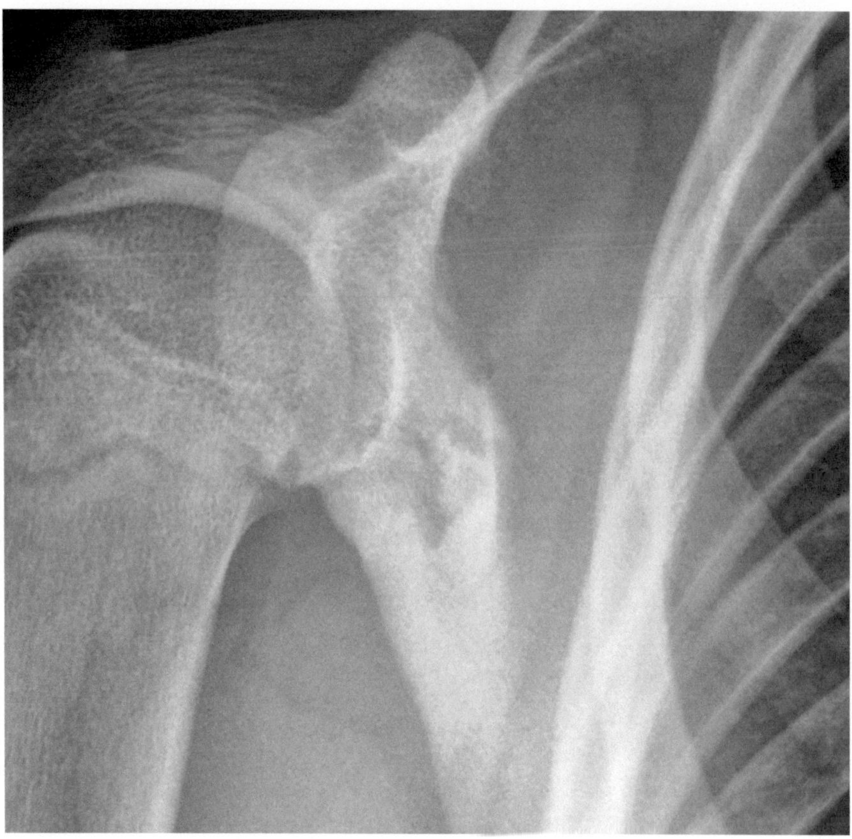

There is no fracture of the right humerus which remains enlocated. This 15-year-old boy was presented to the ED with a right shoulder deformity after being tackled whilst playing rugby.

Scapular fractures are rare in children. They most commonly result from high-energy trauma and are typically associated with other injuries (e.g. rib fractures, pulmonary contusion, haemothorax). They may be overlooked on radiographs resulting in a delayed diagnosis. Most scapular fractures are managed conservatively but intra-articular fractures are more likely to require surgical reduction and fixation.

The undulating lucent line visualised through the anatomical neck of the right proximal humerus (at the level of the inferior aspect of the glenoid fossa), is the projection of the *normal* physis and is *not* a fracture. The proximal humerus is comprised of three separate ossification centres: the head, and the greater and lesser tubercles. The capital (head) ossification centre appears at approximately 3 months of age. The two tuberosity ossification centres appear at approximately 12 months of age and fuse between the ages of 3 and 5 years. The capital and tuberosity ossification centres then fuse into a single proximal epiphysis usually by the age of 6 years. Subsequently, the physis (which separates the proximal humeral epiphysis from the adjacent metaphysis) has a 'double contour' as a result of overlap and projection of the epiphysis over the metaphysis.

The inferior contour of the physis (represented by the undulating lucent line, described above) often has an 'inverted V' or 'tent'-shaped appearance. Again, this appearance is *normal* and should *not* be mistaken for a fracture. That being said, careful examination of the proximal humerus is required given that Salter-Harris 1 injuries (a slip about the physis with associated widening) are the most frequent proximal humeral injury in children aged less than 5 years. Salter-Harris 2 injuries are more common in those aged less than 12 years. See the explanation for Image 30 of Test 1 for a discussion of the Salter-Harris classification of physeal injuries.

Compare this appearance with other proximal humeral radiographs in children of different ages from earlier tests in this book (there are several in every test) alongside the imaged proximal humeri on paediatric chest radiographs in your clinical practice.

Further Reading

Image 1

Rizk MS et al (2023) Claw sign (mass). https://radiopaedia.org/articles/claw-sign-mass. Accessed Jul 2023

Servaes SE, Hoffer FA, Smith EA et al (2019) Imaging of Wilms tumor: an update. Pediatr Radiol 49(11):1441–1452

Image 4

Niknejad M et al (2023) Airway foreign bodies in children. https://radiopaedia.org/articles/airway-foreign-bodies-in-children. Accessed Mar 2023

Tseng HJ, Hanna TN, Shuaib W et al (2015) imaging foreign bodies: ingested, aspirated, and inserted. Ann Emerg Med 66(6):570–582.e5

Image 22

Heffernan E (2023) Mandibular fractures—OPG. http://www.svuhradiology.ie/case-study/mandibular-fractures-opg. Accessed Mar 2023

Jung YH, Cho BH (2014) Radiographic evaluation of third molar development in 6- to 24-year-olds. Imaging Sci Dent 44(3):185–91.

Weerakkody Y et al (2022) Mandibular fracture. https://radiopaedia.org/articles/mandibular-fracture. Accessed Mar 2023.

Weerakkody Y et al (2021) Fédération Dentaire Internationale (FDI) notation. https://radiopaedia.org/articles/federation-dentaire-internationale-fdi-notation. Accessed Mar 2024.

Image 24

Akin K, Cizmeci MN, Kanburoglu MK et al (2013) Angel wing sign in a neonate with pneumomediastinum. J Pediatr 163(1):296

Alhudhaif JM, Almusallam AY, Alfayez AA et al (2022) Benign spontaneous pneumomediastinum in a late preterm newborn. Cureus 14(11):e31413

Altamimi T, Read B, da Silva O et al (2021) Airway injury and pneumomediastinum associated with less invasive surfactant administration in a premature neonate: a case report. BMC Pediatr 21(1):500

Correia-Pinto J, Henriques-Coelho T (2010) Images in clinical medicine. Neonatal pneumomediastinum and the spinnaker-sail sign. N Engl J Med 363(22):2145

Molinari A et al (2022) Spinnaker sign (mediastinum). https://radiopaedia.org/articles/spinnaker-sign-mediastinum. Accessed Mar 2023.

Image 27

Ropp AM, Davis DL (2015) Scapular fractures: what radiologists need to know. Am J Roentgenol 205(3):491–501

Whooley PJ (2021) Proximal humeral fractures. https://dontforgetthebubbles.com/proximal-humeral-fractures/. Accessed Mar 2023

Whooley PJ, Foley J (2022) Shoulder X-ray interpretation. https://dontforgetthebubbles.com/shoulder-x-ray-interpretation/. Accessed Mar 2023

Test 12

12

M. Paddock et al., *Paediatric Radiology Rapid Reporting*,
https://doi.org/10.1007/978-3-031-48255-7_12

12.1 Images

Image 1

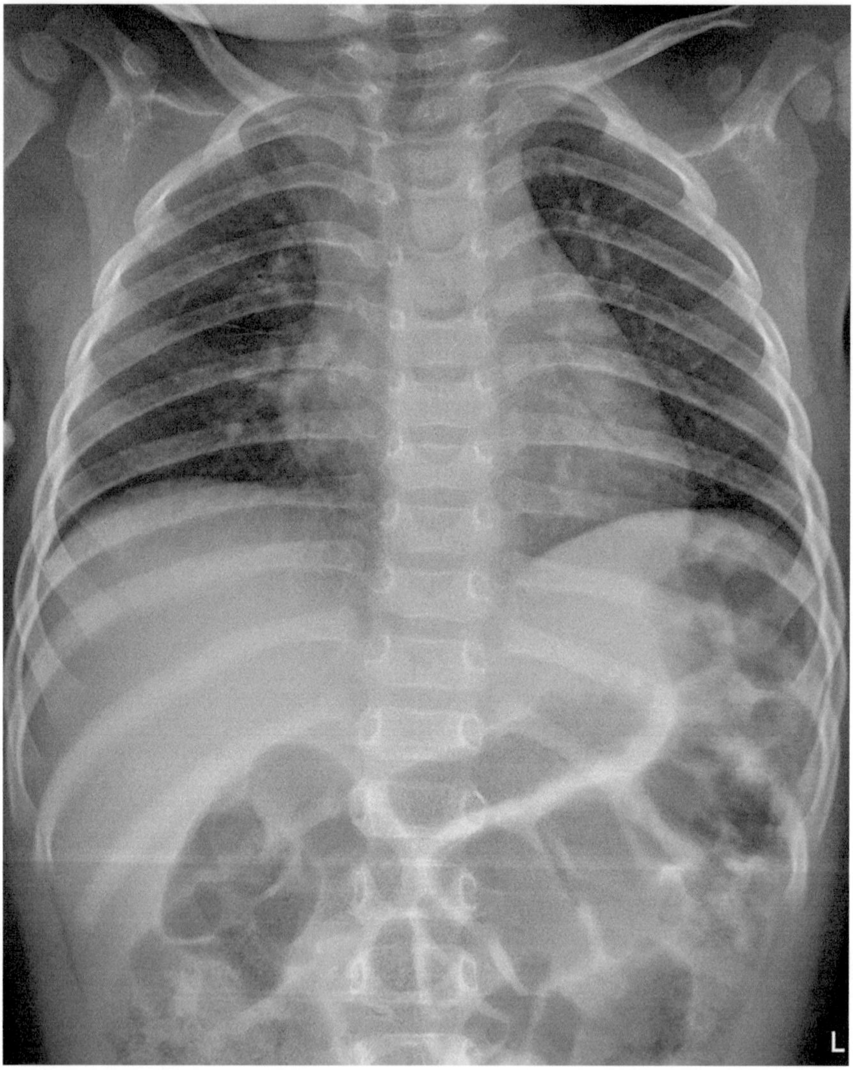

Image 2

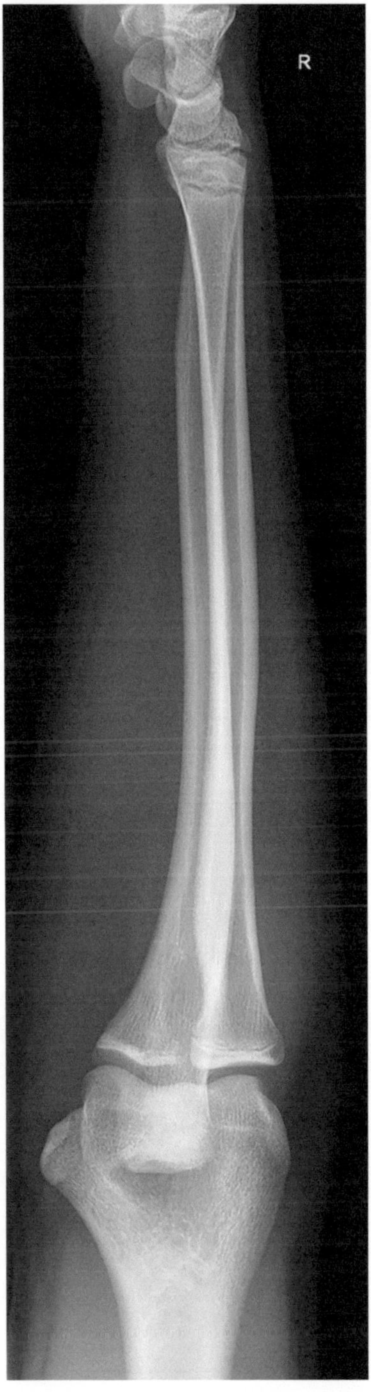

Image 3

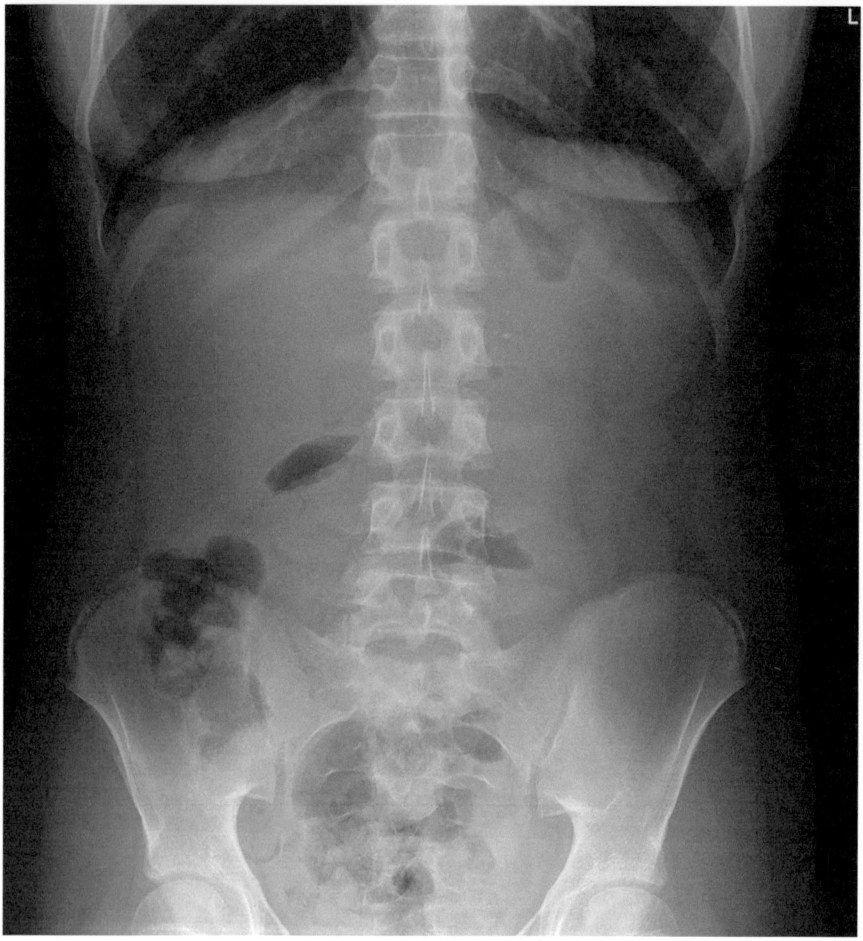

Image 4

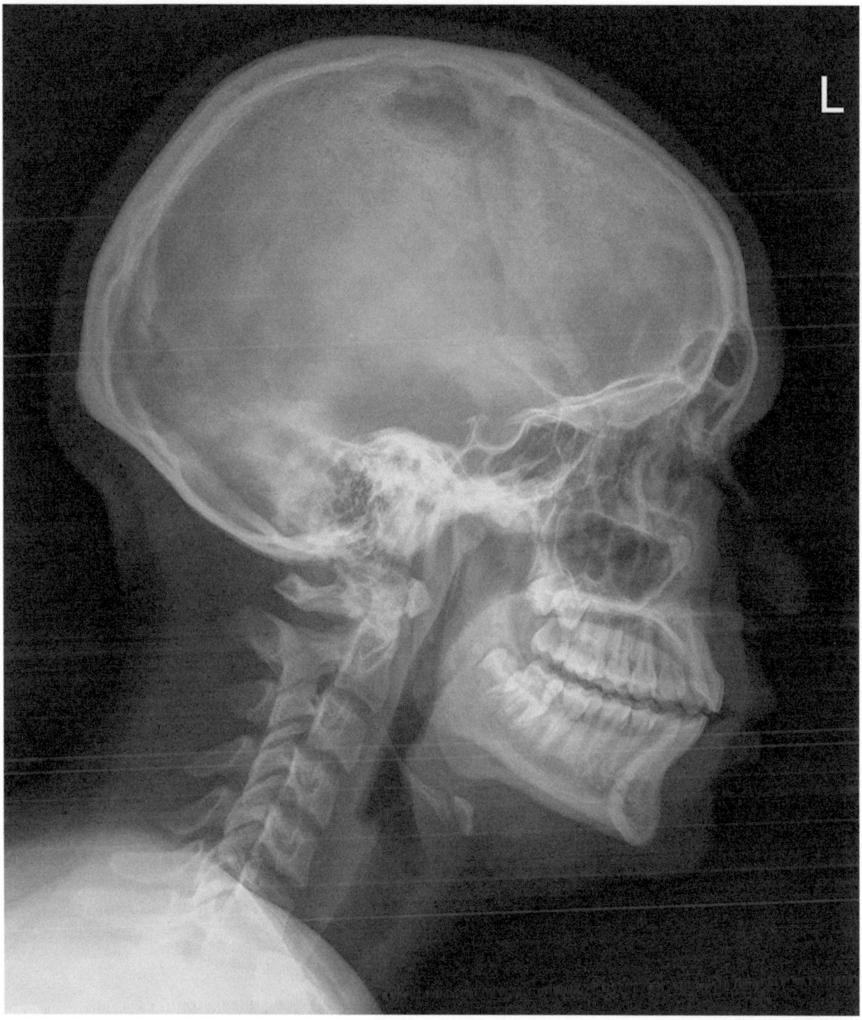

Image 5

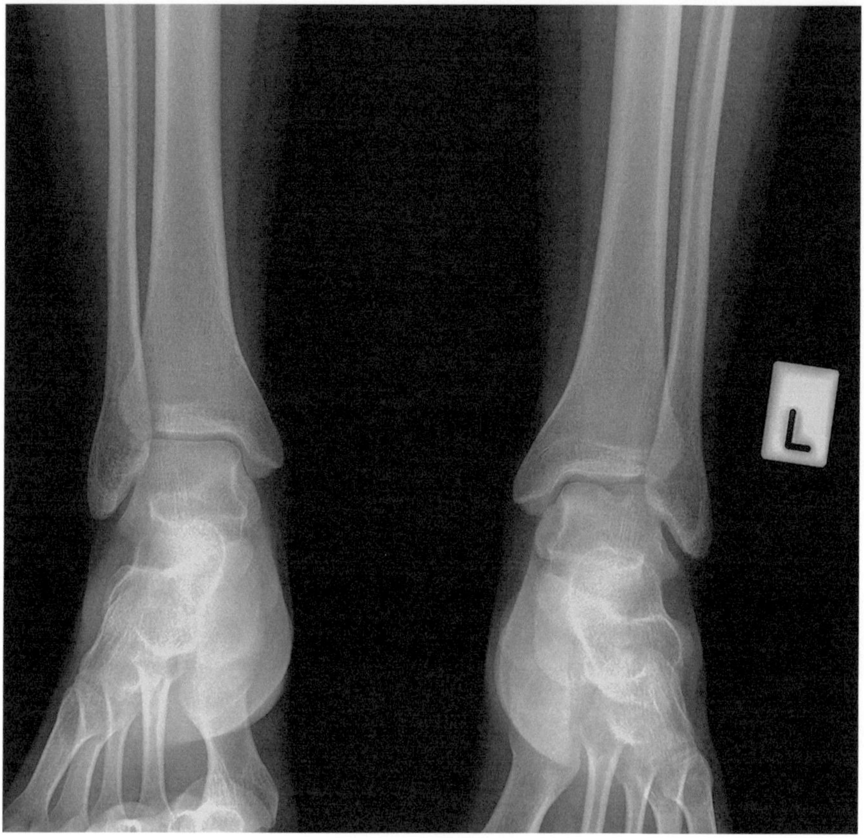

Image 6

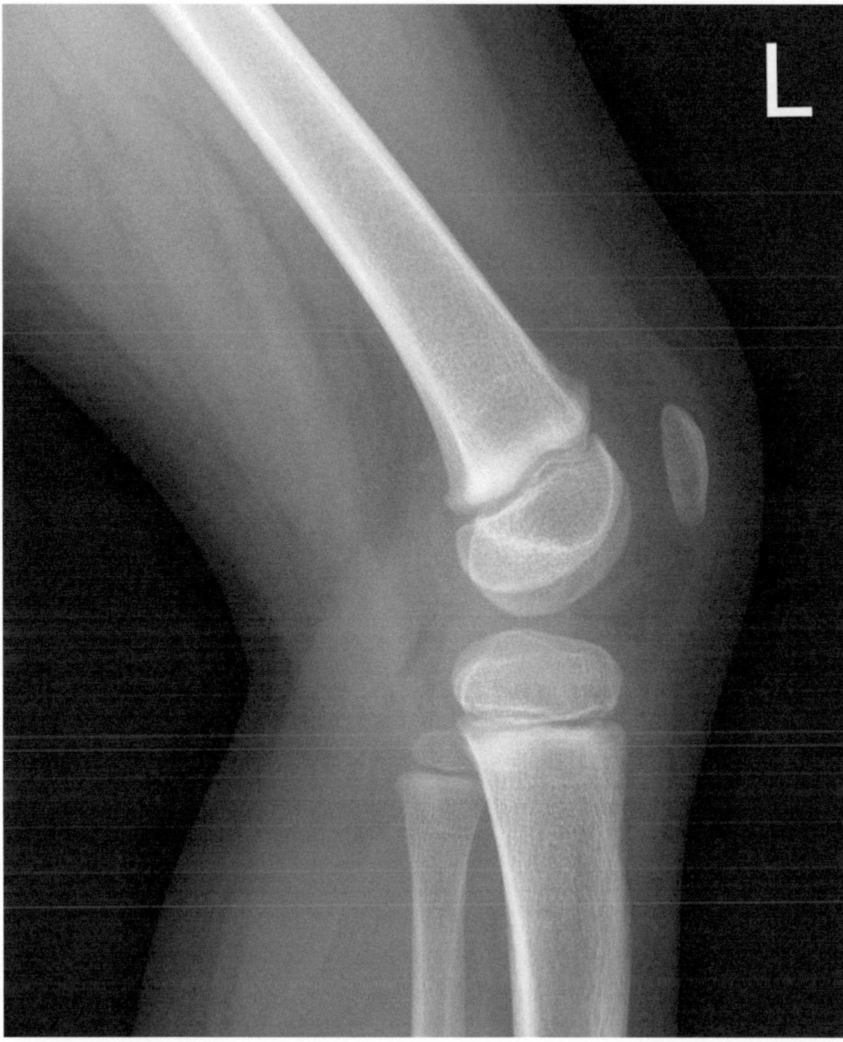

Image 7

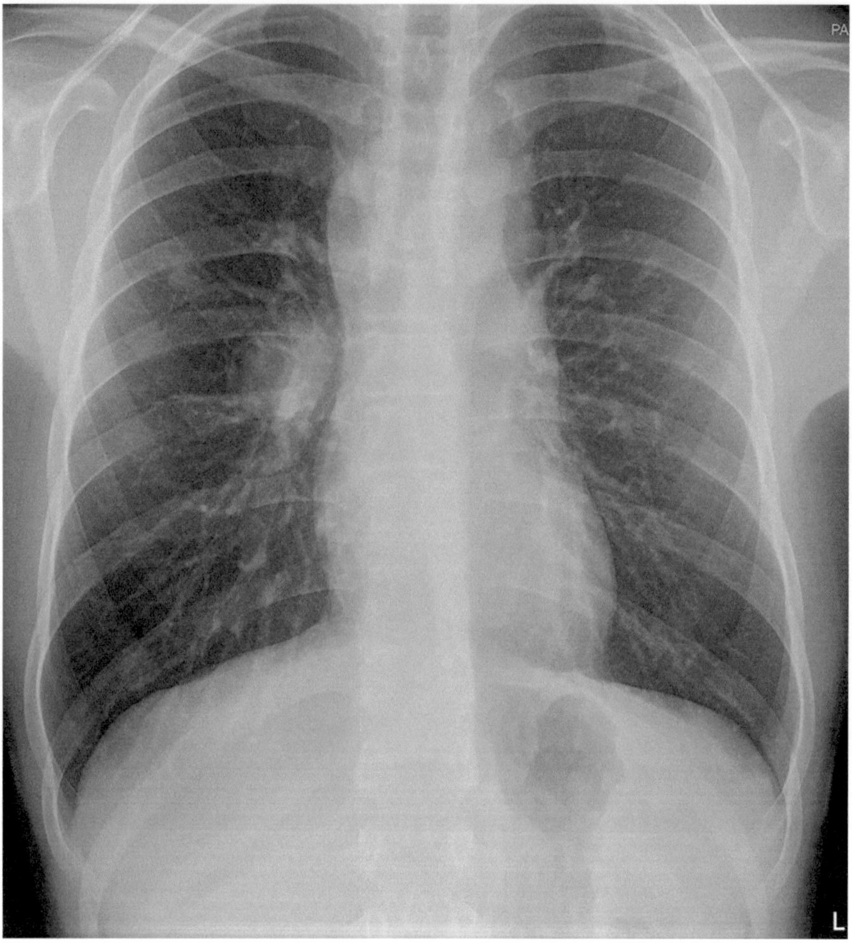

Image 8

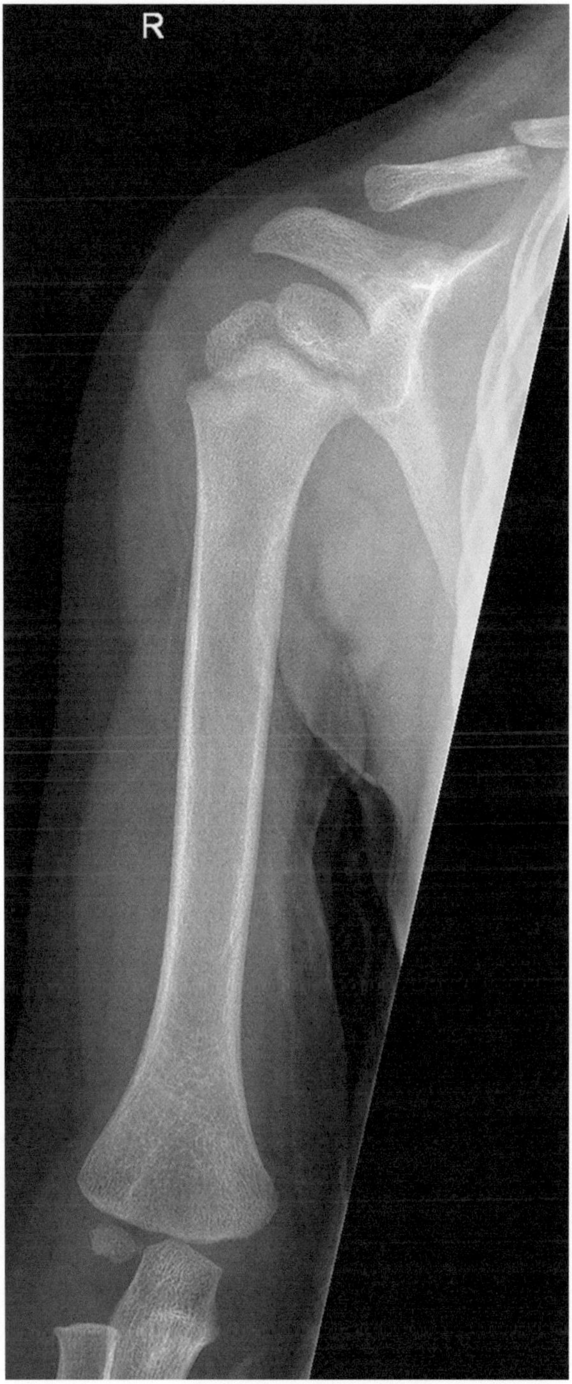

Image 9

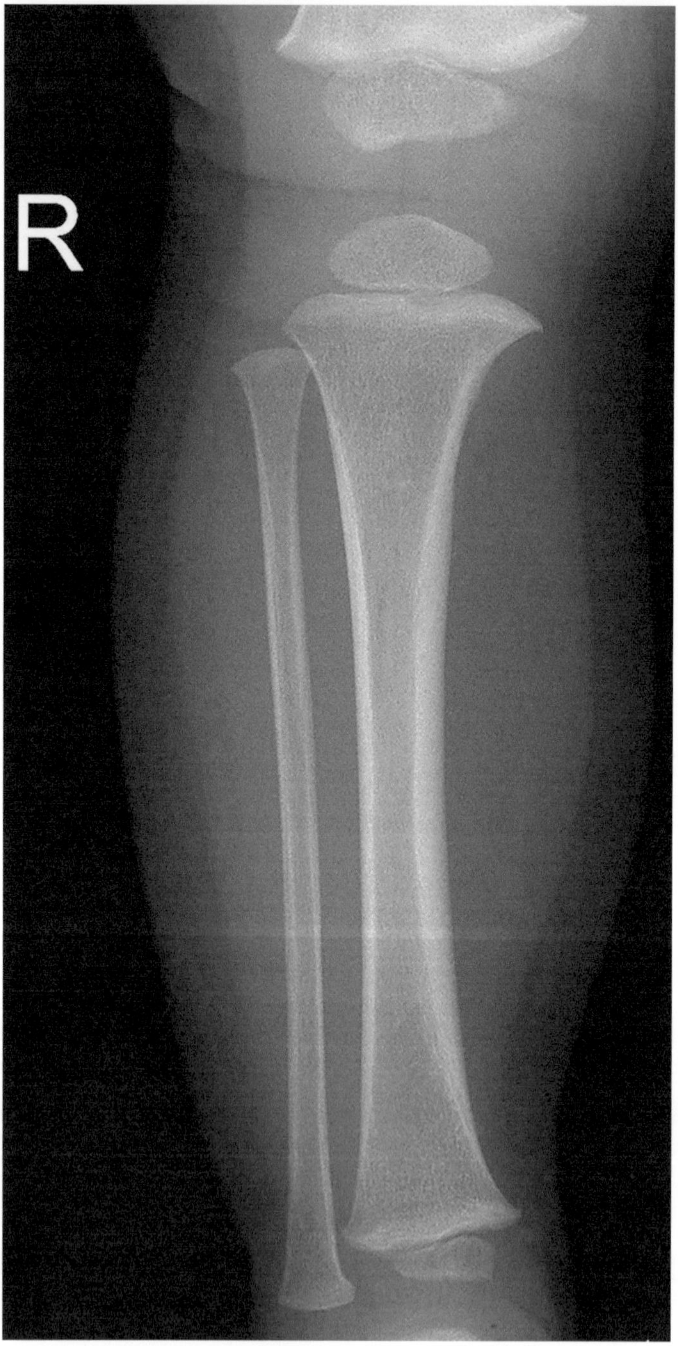

Image 10

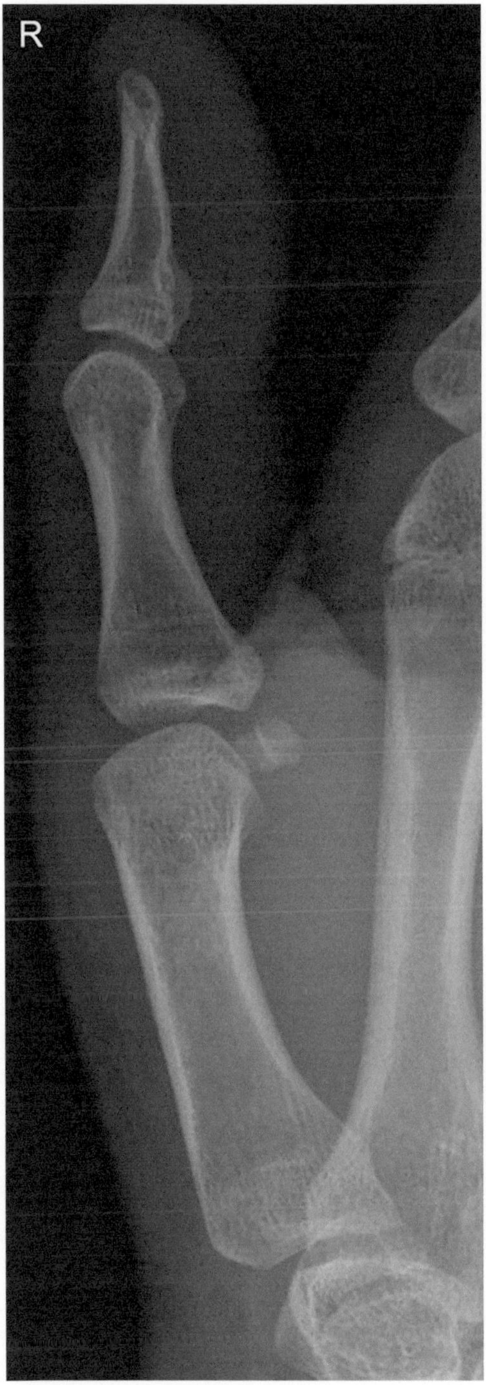

Image 11

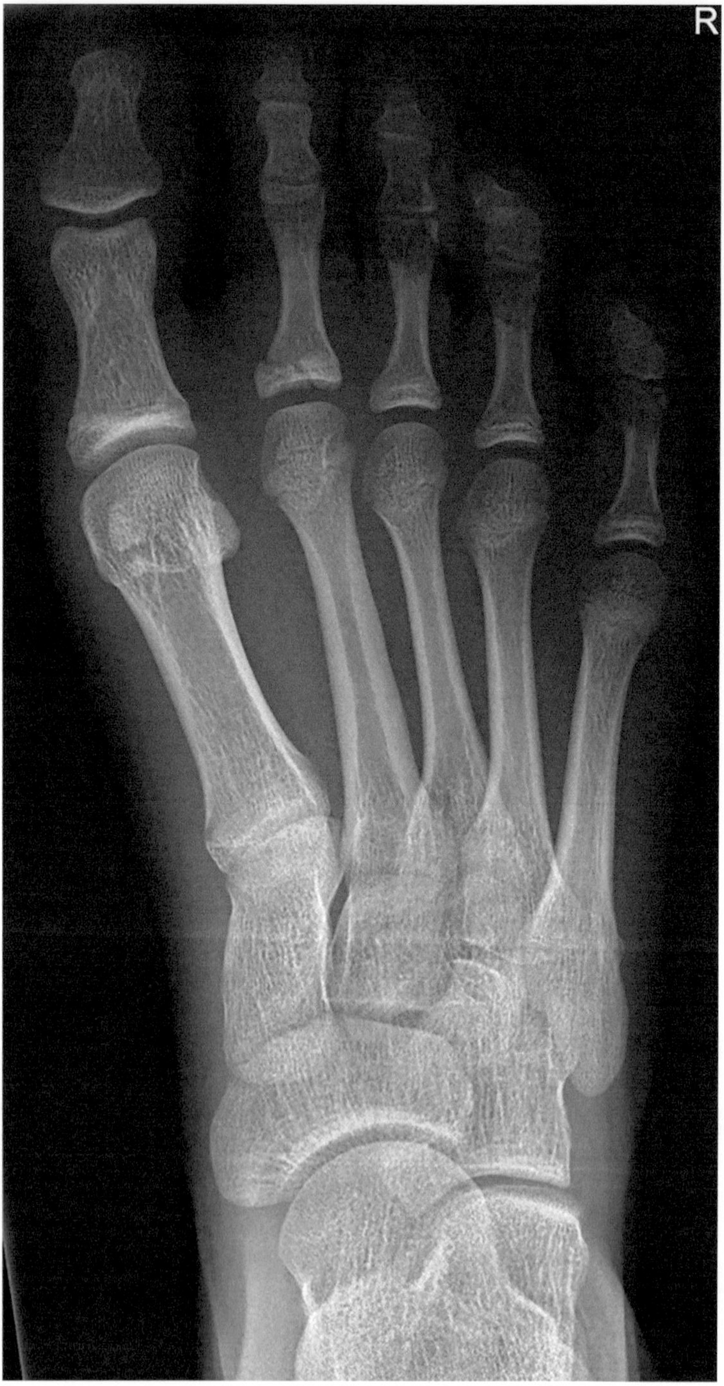

Image 12

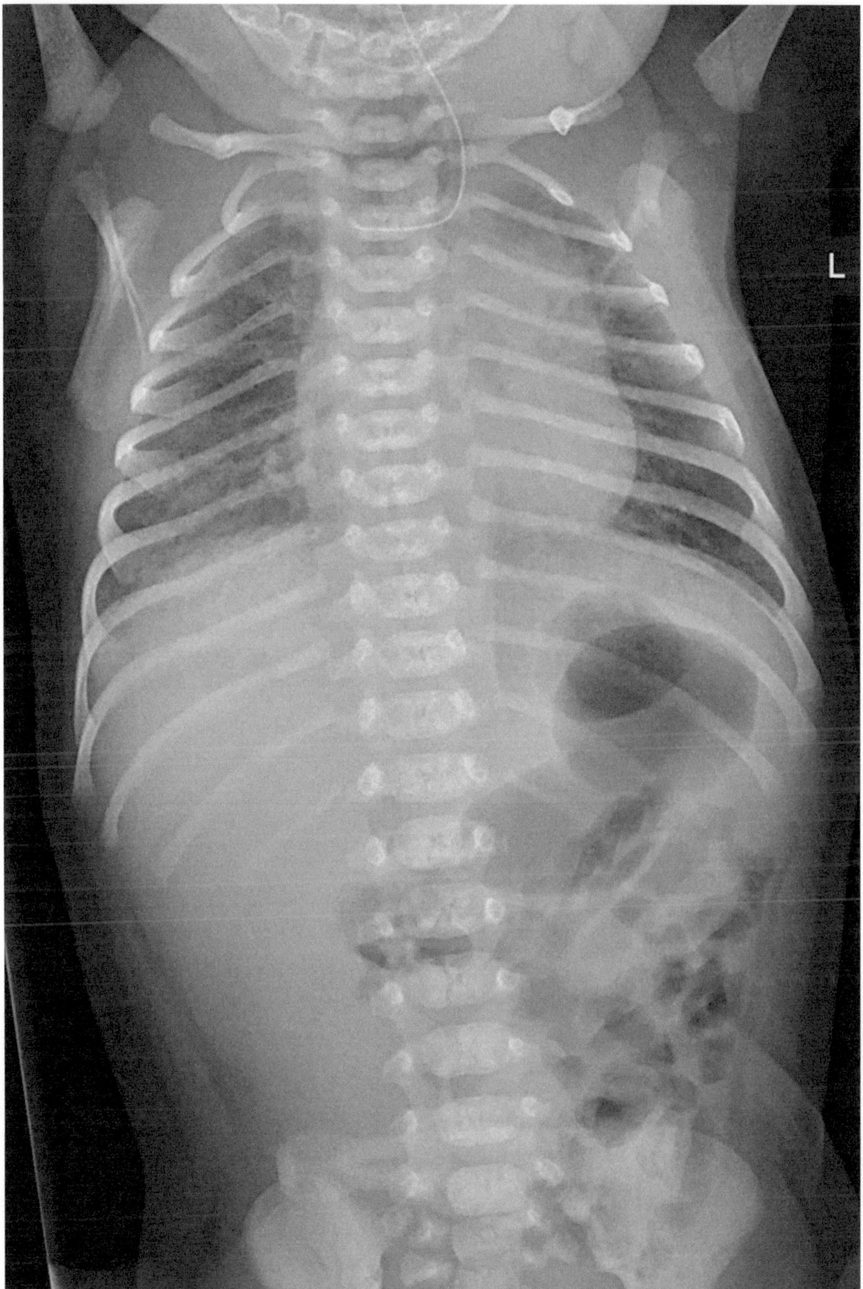

Image 13

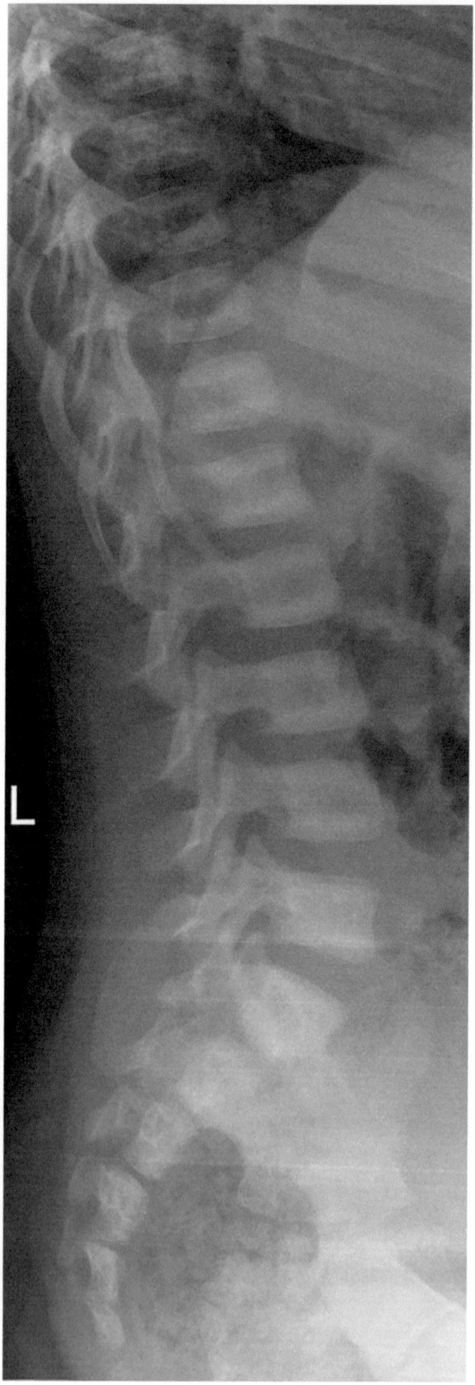

Image 14

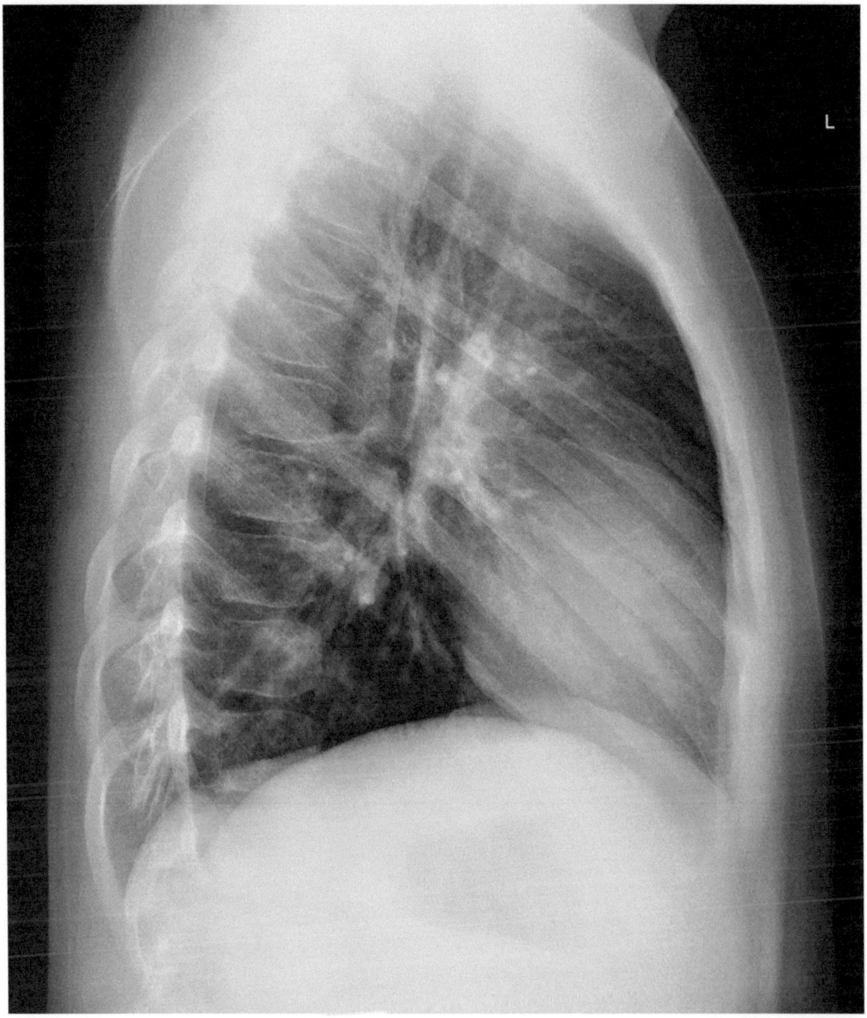

Image 15

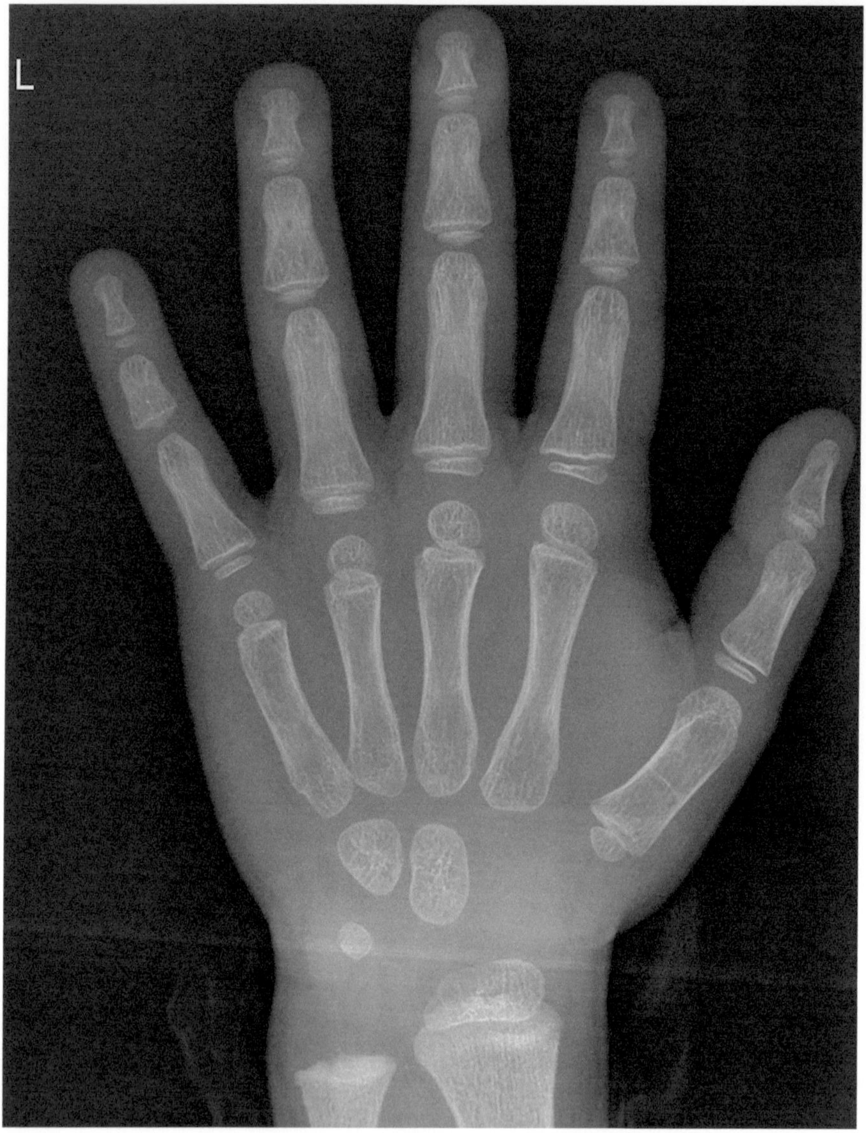

Image 16

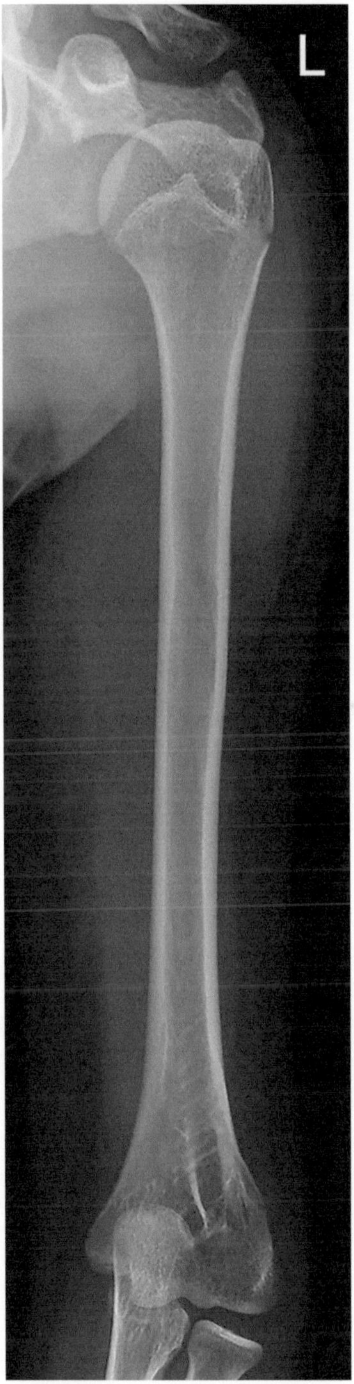

Image 17

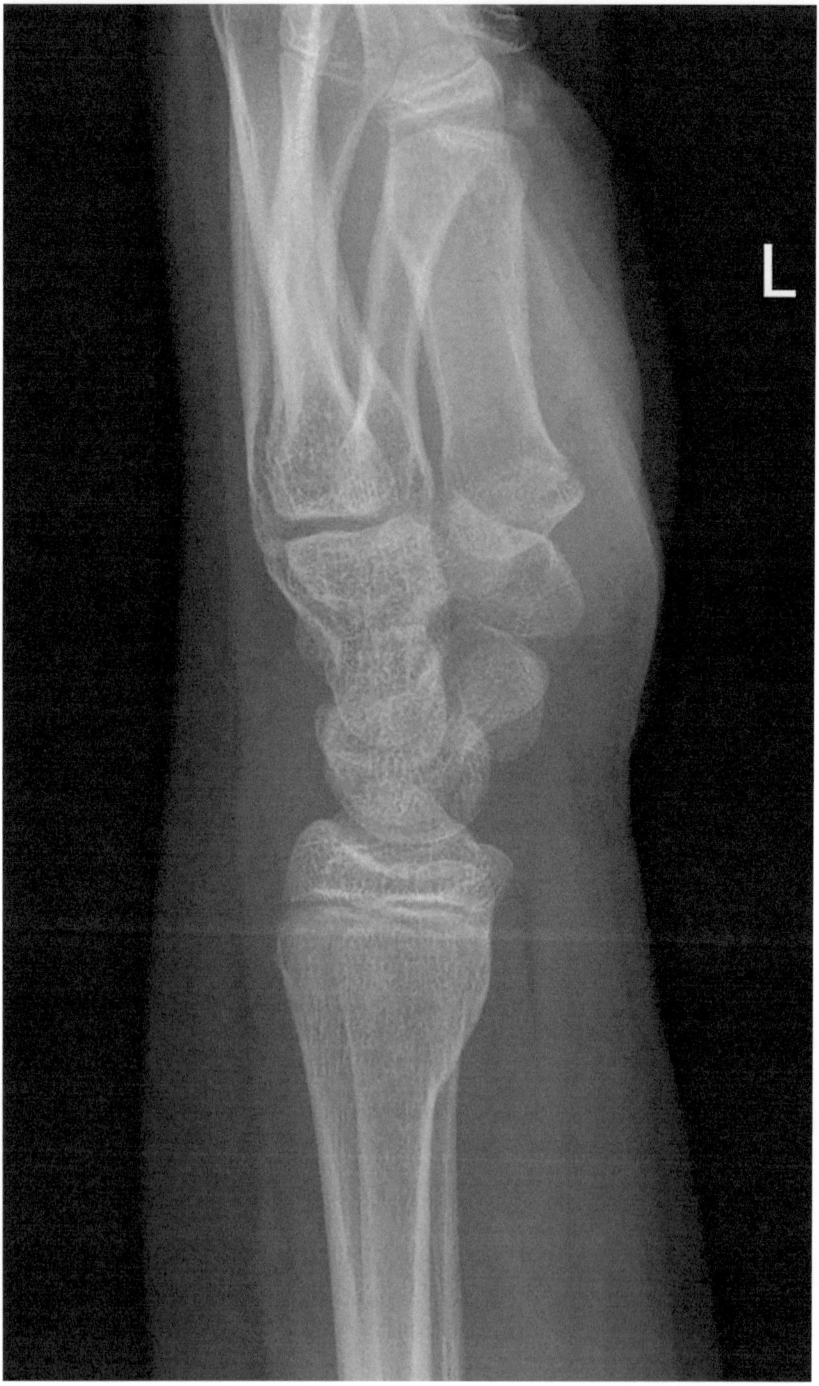

Image 18

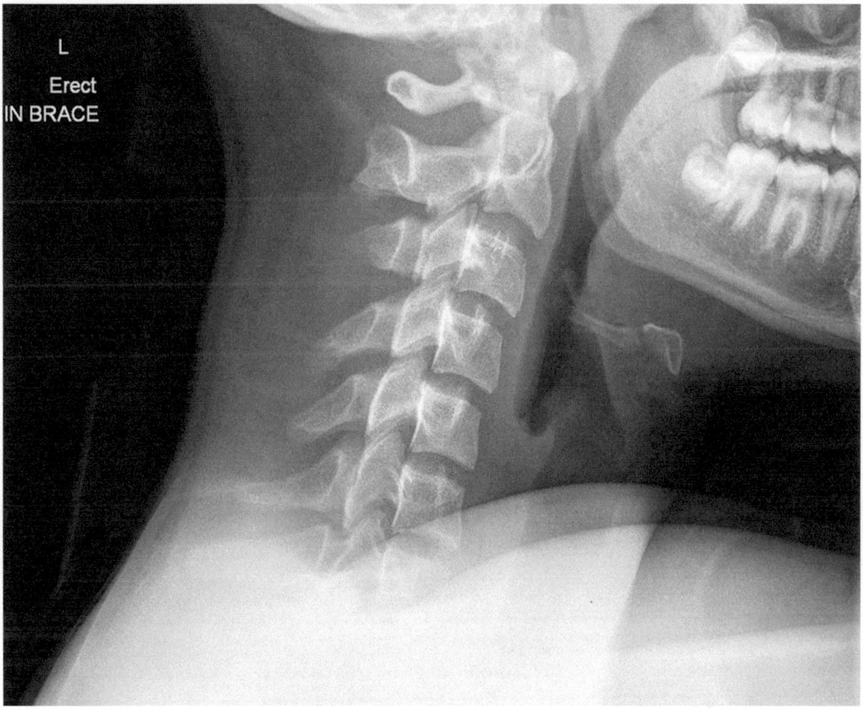

Image 19

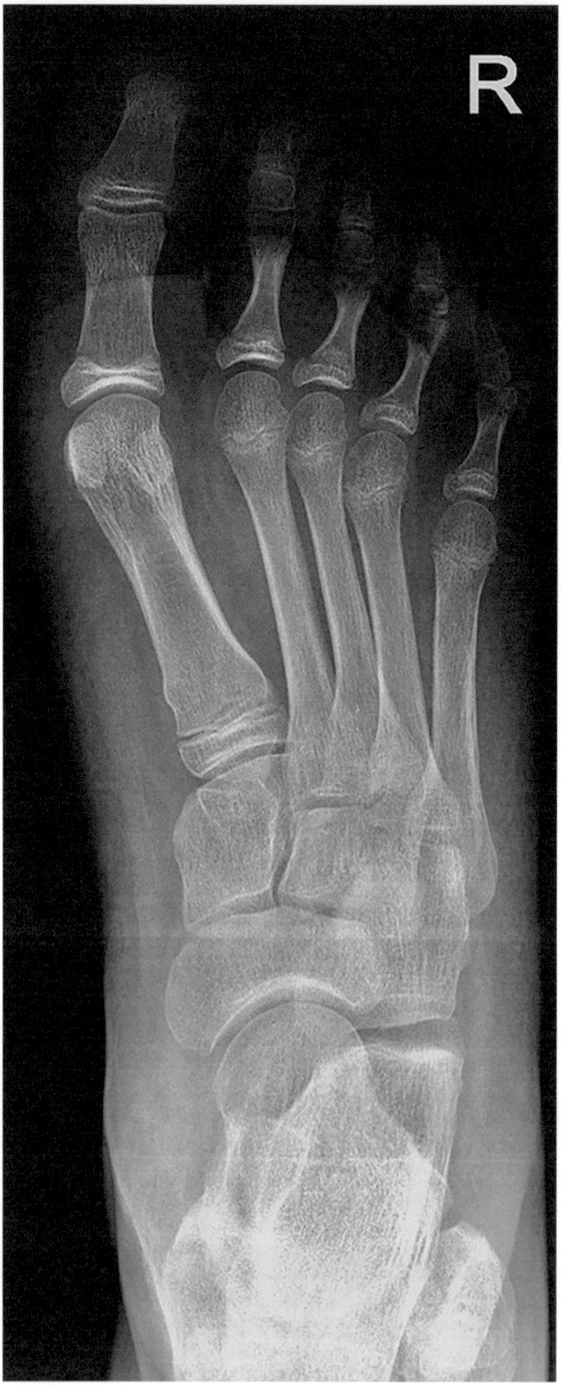

Image 20

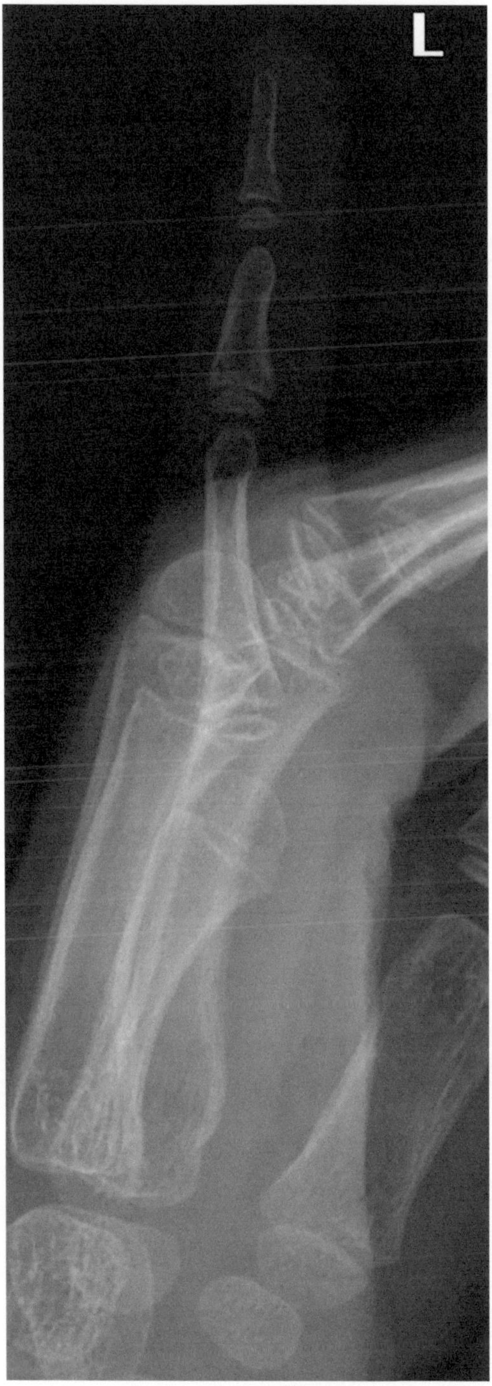

Image 21

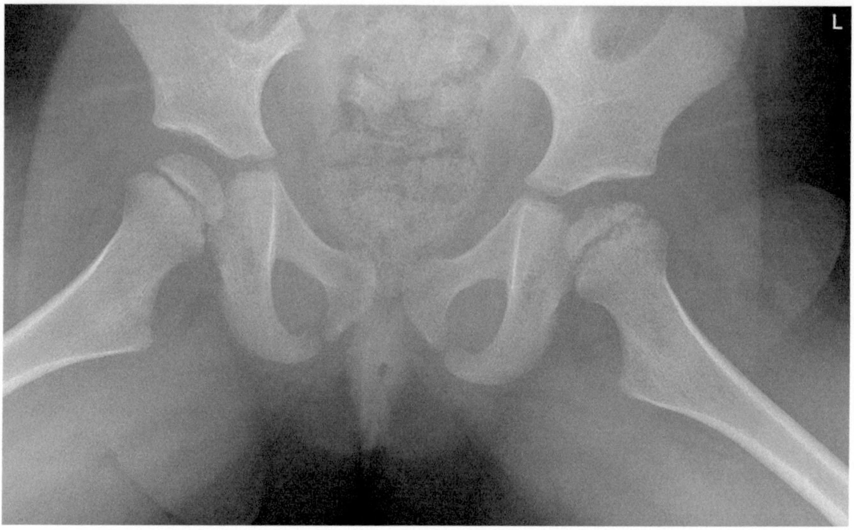

Image 22

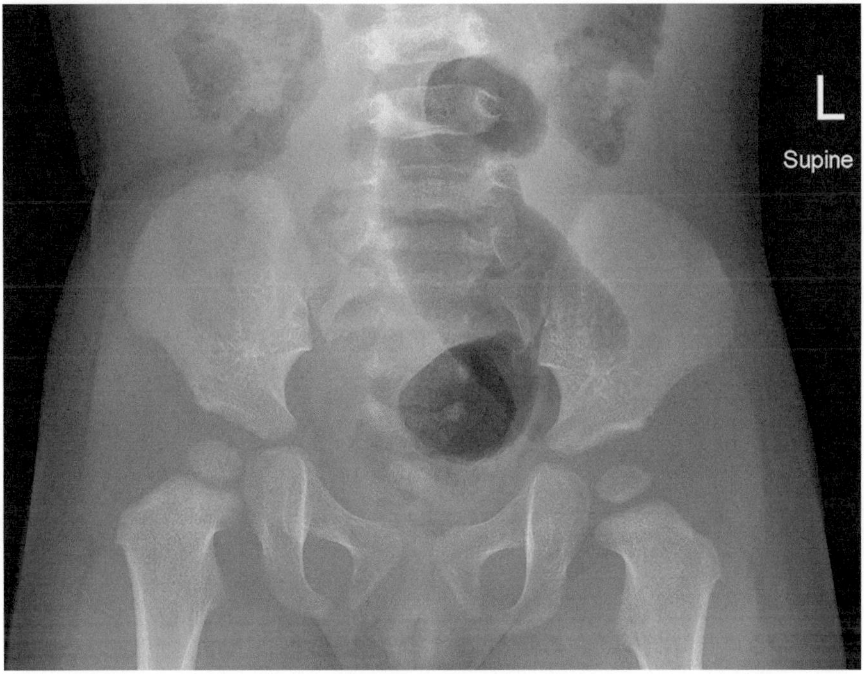

Image 23

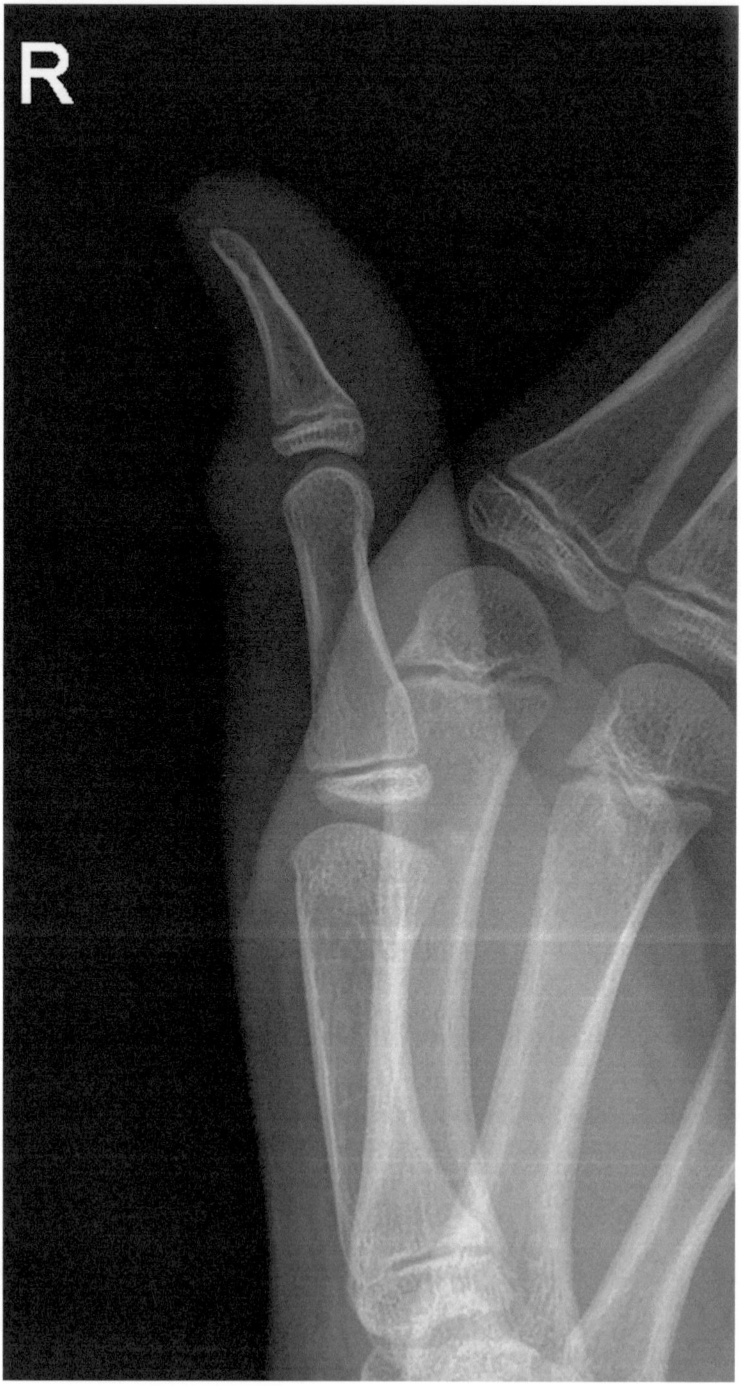

Image 24

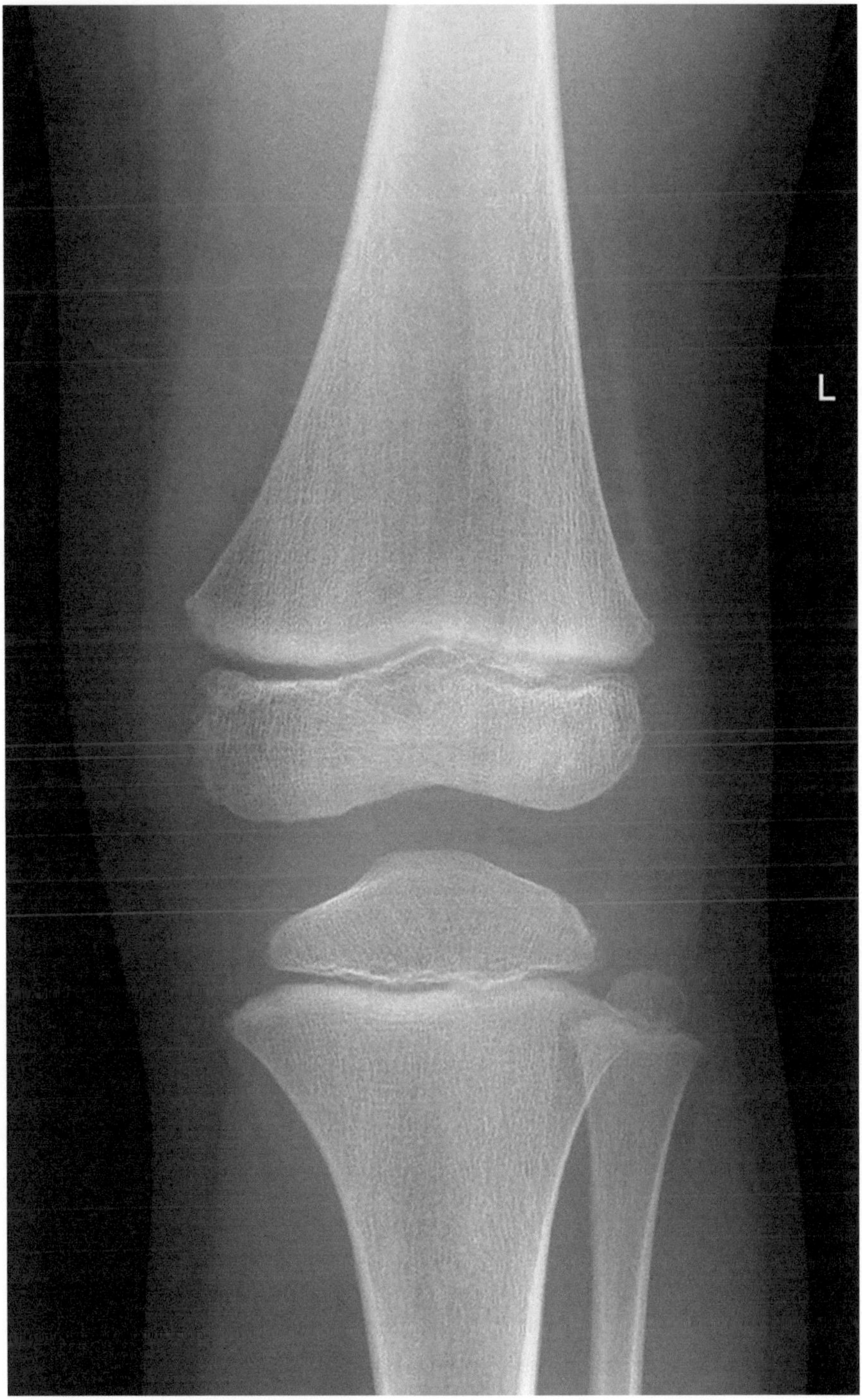

Image 25

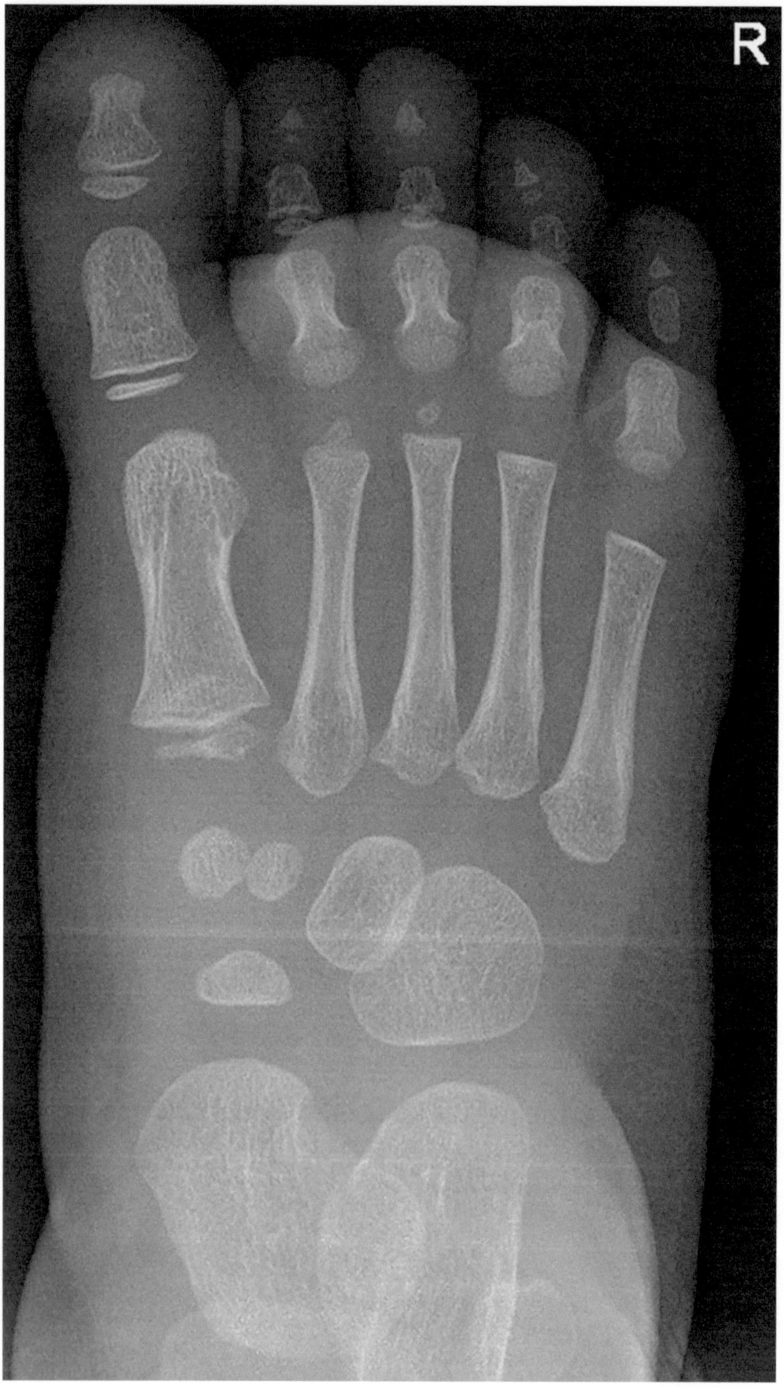

Image 26

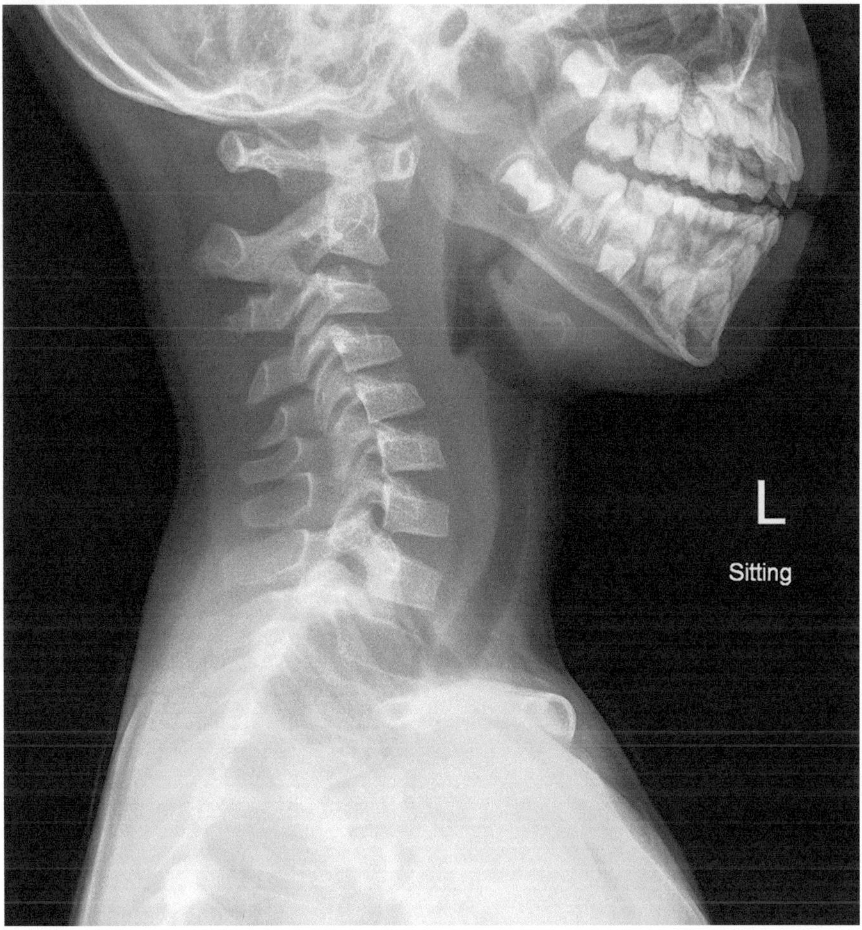

Image 27

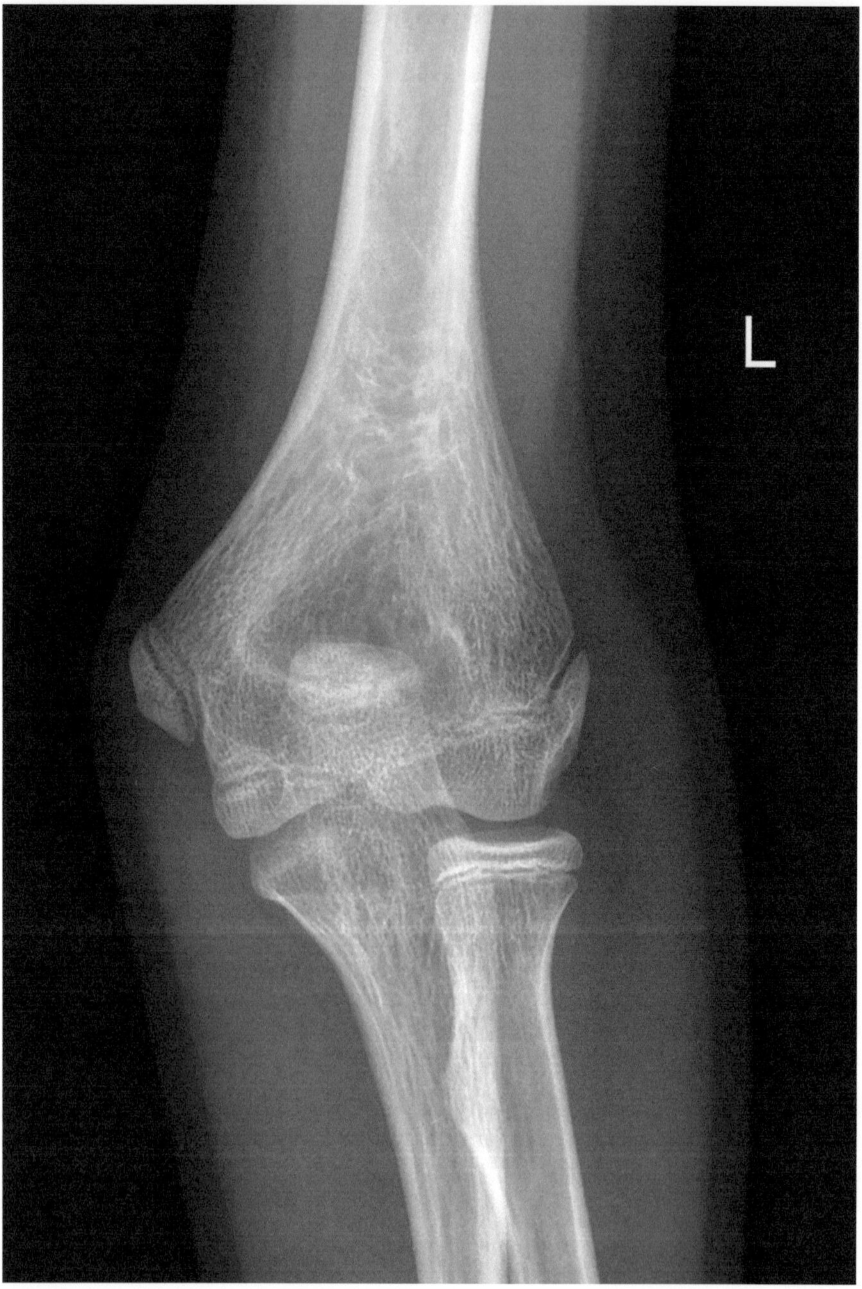

Image 28

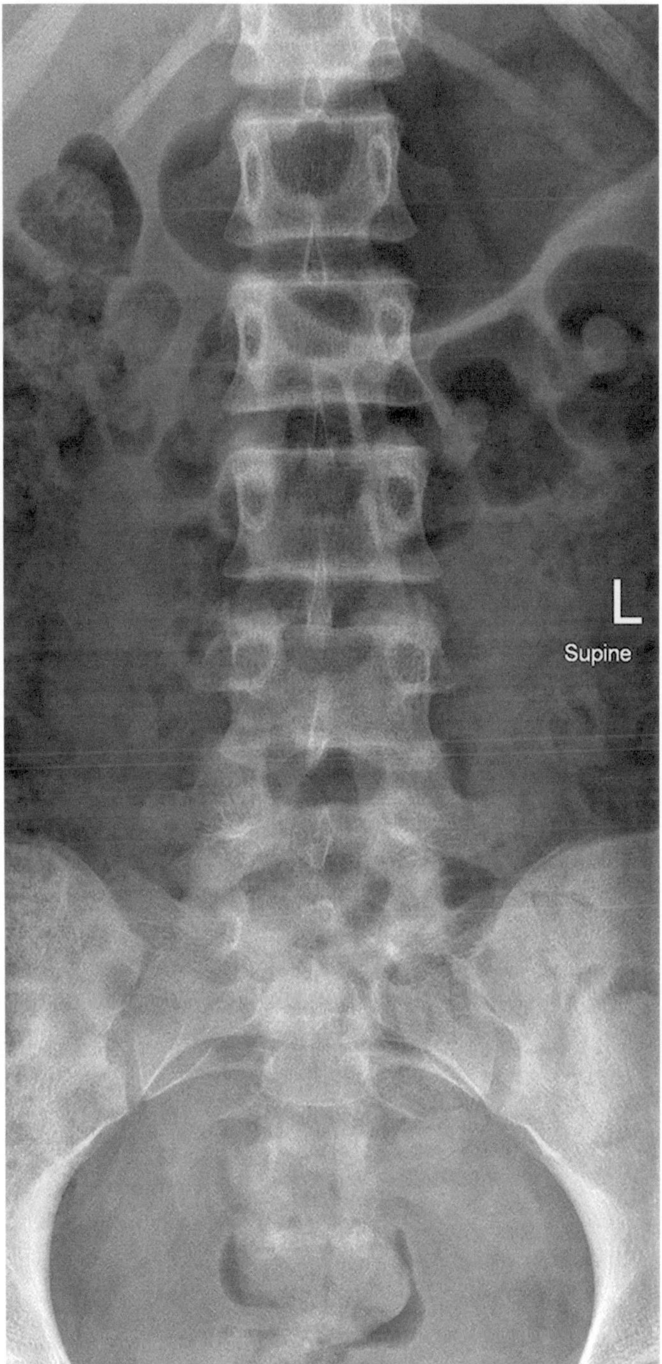

Image 29

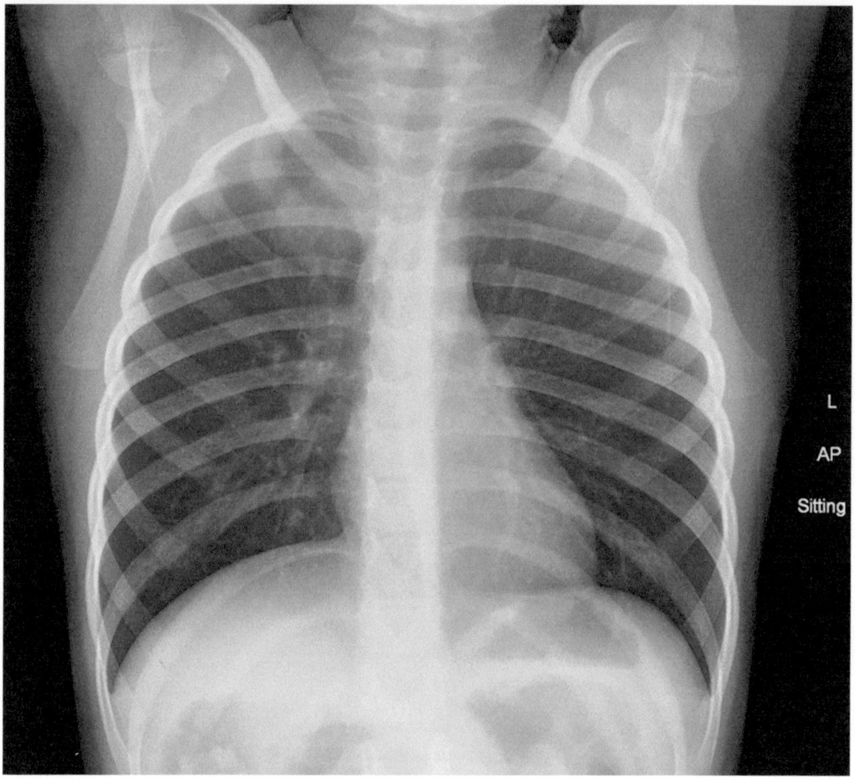

Image 30

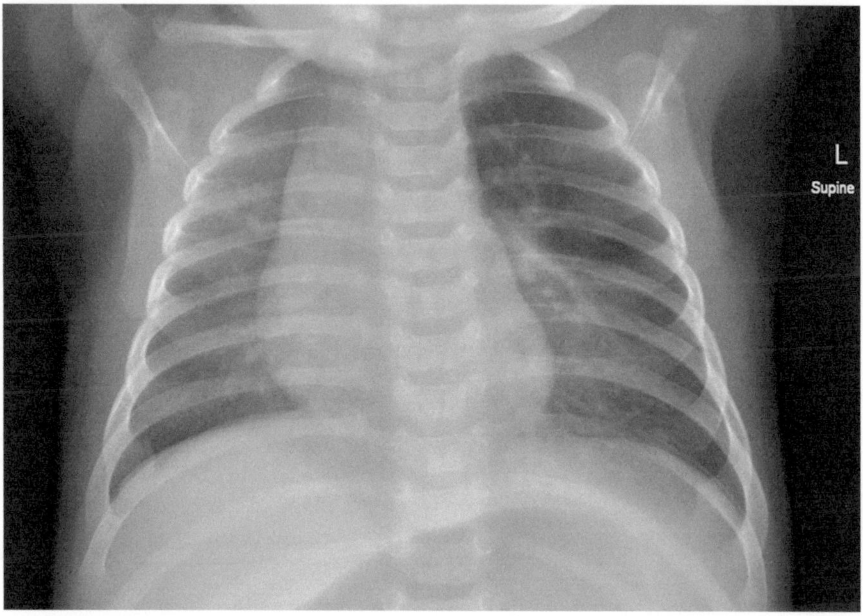

12.2 Answers

Image	Normal	Abnormal	Diagnosis/abnormality (only if abnormal)
1	✓		
2	✓		
3		✓	Pancreatic calcification
4		✓	Lucent lesion parietal skull
5		✓	OCD L talar dome
6	✓		
7		✓	Mediastinal and hilar lymphadenopathy/R hilar mass
8		✓	# R clavicle
9	✓		
10	✓		
11		✓	SH3 # R second toe proximal phalanx
12		✓	Coiled enteric tube in the proximal oesophagus
13		✓	Rugger jersey spine
14	✓		
15	✓		
16	✓		
17		✓	Buckle # L distal radial metaphysis
18	✓		
19		✓	Buckle # R first metatarsal proximal metaphysis
20	✓		
21		✓	AVN L proximal femoral epiphysis
22	✓		
23		✓	Buckle # R thumb proximal phalanx
24	✓		
25	✓		
26		✓	Prevertebral soft tissue thickening
27	✓		
28	✓		
29		✓	R upper lobe round pneumonia
30		✓	L upper lobe hyperinflation/lucency

12.3 Explanations

3. **Pancreatic calcification**

This 14-year-old girl with cystic fibrosis (CF) was presented to the Emergency Department (ED) with abdominal pain and distention. Note the calcific densities projected to the left of the L2 vertebral body in keeping with pancreatic calcification from chronic pancreatitis. Also note the faeculent content within the bowel loops in the lower right iliac fossa. A subsequent computed tomography (CT) abdomen/pelvis demonstrated distal intestinal obstruction syndrome (DIOS) in the context of CF.

Unlike adults, in whom calcification may be incidental/insignificant, abdominal calcification in children is frequently pathological. It can be seen in the context of benign conditions (e.g., renal calculi) but also malignant conditions (e.g. neuroblastoma). It almost always requires further investigation, typically with ultrasound in the first instance.

CF is an inherited condition which results in abnormally viscous mucus and secretions. Whilst the lungs are the most severely affected organ, abdominal complications are common. DIOS is characterised by mucofaeculent material in the distal small bowel with a 'bubbly soft tissue mass' often described in the right lower quadrant on radiography, alongside clinical and radiographic features of small bowel obstruction. Other abdominal radiographic findings in patients with CF include gallstones (in up to 25% of patients) and renal calculi (in which symptomatic disease is twice as common in patients with CF than in the general population).

4. **Lucent lesion parietal skull**

This 13-year-old girl presented with scalp swelling. This lateral skull radiograph demonstrates a lucent lesion in the (right) parietal bone lesion (posterior to the coronal suture which localises the lesion to the parietal bone) with minor thickening of the overlying scalp. Magnetic resonance imaging (MRI) confirmed a transcalvarial right parietal bone tumour which was confirmed to be Langerhans cell histiocytosis (LCH) on subsequent biopsy.

LCH is one of a number of disorders caused by the uncontrolled proliferation of histiocytes accumulating in various organs. LCH predominantly affects children: lesions can be single or multiple and can involve one or multiple body systems. Bone lesions are the most common radiological manifestation of LCH and are seen in approximately 80% of affected patients. The 'classic' bone manifestations include: a lucent skull lesion with a 'bevelled' edge due to asymmetric involvement of the inner and outer tables of the skull; and flattening of a single vertebral body known as 'vertebra plana' (cf. platyspondyly which refers to the near complete loss of vertebral body height in the context of skeletal dysplasia, e.g. thanatophoric dysplasia, achondroplasia, spondyloepiphyseal dysplasia, and autosomal recessive mucopolysaccharidosis [MPS] type IV [Morquio syndrome]). Other locations for bony disease include the mandible, ribs, and pelvis.

Common extraskeletal sites of disease include the liver, spleen and lymph nodes, central nervous system (where loss of the pituitary bright spot alongside infundibular thickening and enhancement on MRI are characteristic), and the lungs (centrilobular nodules and, later in the disease, multiple irregular thin-walled cysts which may spare the extreme lung bases. The pulmonary manifestations of LCH may be seen as part of disseminated disease or a distinct entity in young adult smokers). The treatment depends on the extent and severity of disease. Bone lesions can be treated with curettage, intralesional steroids, and/or radiation. Systemic treatment options include chemotherapy, steroids, retinoic acid, and intravenous immunoglobulins. See the explanations for Images 5 and 14 of Test 6.

5. **Osteochondral defect L talar dome**
   See the explanation for Image 10 of Test 4.

7. **Mediastinal and hilar lymphadenopathy/R hilar mass**
   This 15-year-old boy was presented with a mass in his right anterior neck. The chest radiograph demonstrates: abnormal mediastinal and bilateral hilar soft tissue consistent with lymphadenopathy; a large rounded soft tissue mass in the right hilar region; and a smaller opacity projected over the right third anterior rib. The patient underwent staging chest, abdomen, and pelvis CT which demonstrated cervical, supraclavicular, mediastinal and hilar lymphadenopathy, and bilateral pulmonary nodules which were all fluorodeoxyglucose (FDG) avid on positron emission tomography-computed tomography (PET-CT). Histopathology from the biopsy revealed Hodgkin's lymphoma.

   The differential for mediastinal lymphadenopathy in children includes:
   - Primary (e.g. haematological or lymphatic) or metastatic malignancy.
   - Castleman disease (an uncommon B-cell lymphoproliferative condition also known as angiofollicular or giant lymph node hyperplasia).
   - Infection (e.g. tuberculosis and mycoplasma).
   - Sarcoidosis (rare).

8. **# R clavicle**
   Edge of the image review demonstrates this displaced complete fracture of the distal 1/3 of the right clavicle. See the explanation for Image 26 of Test 4.

11. **Salter-Harris 3 # R second toe proximal phalanx**
   As the physes have almost, but not quite, completely fused, the appearances are consistent with a minimally displaced Salter-Harris 3 fracture (which involves the physis and epiphysis) of the right second toe proximal phalanx. Note the intra-articular extension to the second metatarsophalangeal joint. See the explanation for Image 30 of Test 1 for a discussion regarding the Salter-Harris classification.

12. **Coiled enteric tube in the proximal oesophagus**
An enteric tube (which could be naso- or oro-gastric) is coiled within a gas-filled structure (the oesophagus) at the level of the upper thoracic spine. These appearances suggest oesophageal atresia as the tube is unable to pass further inferiorly. There must be an associated tracheo-oesophageal fistula as there is gas in the stomach.

Oesophageal atresia is the most common congenital oesophageal anomaly and is characterised by a blind-ending oesophagus. In the vast majority of cases (approximately 85%), there is proximal oesophageal atresia with a distal tracheo-oesophageal fistula (type C). In 8% of cases, there is isolated oesophageal atresia (i.e. without tracheo-oesophageal fistula), whereas isolated tracheo-oesophageal fistula (without oesophageal atresia) is seen in approximately 4%. The latter cases are rare and are characterised by an abnormal communication between the posterior wall of the trachea and the anterior wall of the oesophagus. The orientation of the fistula (an abnormal connection between two structures, in this case, epithelial surfaces) between the trachea and the oesophagus determines how they are classified, i.e. a transversely oriented fistula is described as H-type and an obliquely oriented fistula is described as N-type.

Oesophageal atresia is often diagnosed clinically by the inability to successfully pass an enteric tube into the stomach. This is confirmed radiographically with a coiled enteric tube projected over the superior mediastinum, often within a distended air-filled oesophageal pouch. Gas visualised in the stomach and bowel radiographically confirms that a trachea-oesophageal fistula must be present, whereas the absence of gastrointestinal gas indicates an isolated oesophageal atresia. A contrast oesophagogram can be performed to assess for tracheo-oesophageal fistula, if required. Oesophageal atresia with tracheo-oesophageal fistula requires surgical repair with disconnection of the tracheo-oesophageal fistula, closure of the tracheal defect and primary anastomosis of the oesophagus.

Tip for the viva:

- In the presence of a coiled enteric or Repogle tube suggesting oesophageal atresia +/− tracheo-oesophageal fistula, search for any additional abnormalities such as the 'double bubble' sign of duodenal atresia, and vertebral (segmentation or fusion) and/or rib abnormalities which may form part of VACTERL syndrome. In the context of oesophageal atresia and tracheo-oesophageal fistula, patients are usually screened for these associated abnormalities. Discuss the process with your local paediatric radiologists and see the explanation for Image 30 of Test 5.

13. **Rugger jersey spine**
All of the imaged vertebral bodies demonstrate increased endplate density giving them an alternating sclerotic-lucent-sclerotic appearance analogous to the stripes on a rugby jersey, the so-called 'rugger jersey spine'.

This patient has chronic renal failure and resultant renal osteodystrophy (osteomalacia and secondary hyperparathyroidism). When presented with one imaging feature of hyperparathyroidism, search for further abnormalities which, if present, may include:

- Osteopenia.
- Subchondral resorption of the lateral clavicles and sacroiliac joints.
- Subperiosteal resorption of the radial margins of the proximal and intermediate phalanges of the index and the middle fingers.
- Brown tumours: these are the result of cellular repair, *not neoplasia*, and are so named for their haemosiderin content. In the setting of chronic renal disease, repeated and excessive urinary calcium excretion results in decreased serum calcium levels and an elevated parathyroid hormone level. This promotes osteoclastic bone turnover (these tumours were previously termed osteoclastomas) by liberating skeletal calcium in an attempt to maintain normal serum calcium levels. At sites where bone loss occurs particularly rapidly, there may be haemorrhage (and ensuing haemosiderin deposition) with granulation tissue and proliferating fibrosis as a part of the cellular healing response: this replaces the normal marrow and results in 'brown tumour' formation. Histologically, these tumours are identical to giant cell tumours (GCT) and may be misdiagnosed as such if serum calcium and/or parathyroid hormones levels are not assessed. If you are considering a GCT in a differential diagnosis, consider Brown tumour if there is a supportive clinical history of chronic renal failure or renal osteodystrophy.

Tip for the viva:

- Consider the different types of abnormal vertebral endplate density:

Radiographic finding	Descriptor	Diagnosis
Prominent endplate densities/sclerosis at multiple contiguous vertebral levels	Rugger jersey spine	Hyperparathyroidism (there is some overlap with osteopetrosis)
Densely sclerotic endplates (which appear denser and more sharply defined than in rugger jersey spine)	Sandwich vertebrae	Osteopetrosis (benign adult autosomal dominant)
Increased cortical density of all sides of the vertebral body	Picture-frame vertebrae	Paget's disease

Compare the appearances of the abnormal rugger jersey spine with that of normal vertebral endplates in a different patient in the image below:

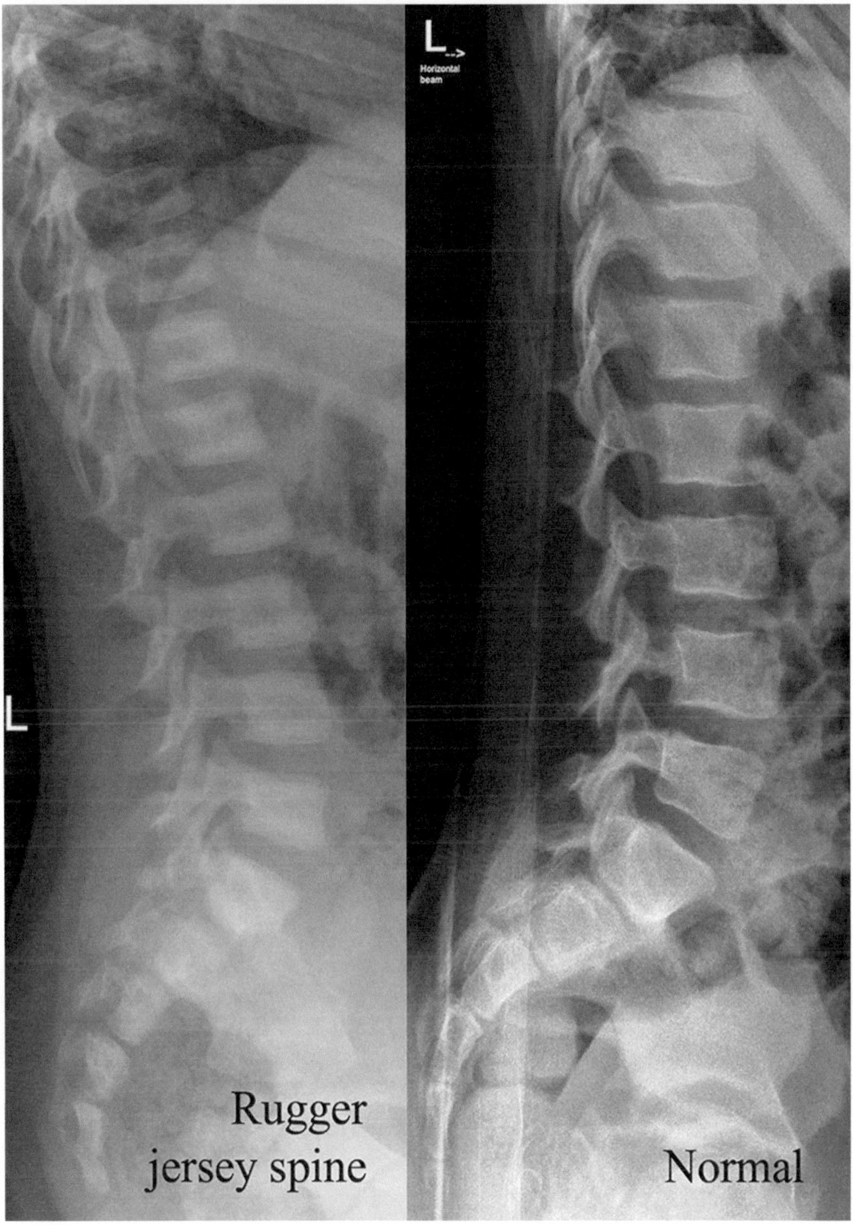

17. **Buckle # L distal radial metaphysis**
Note the cortical 'step' at the volar aspect of the left distal radial metaphysis consistent with a buckle fracture. There is associated soft tissue swelling in keeping with an acute injury.

19. **Buckle # R first metatarsal proximal metaphysis**
There is a cortical buckle of the medial aspect of the right first metatarsal proximal metaphysis consistent with an acute fracture.

21. **Avascular necrosis L proximal femoral epiphysis**
The left proximal femoral epiphysis is flatter and more sclerotic than the right with crescentic subchondral lucency i.e. the crescent sign of avascular necrosis (AVN) suggesting imminent articular collapse. See the explanation for Image 1 of Test 1.

22. *Normal pelvic radiograph*
Both hips are enlocated. The proximal femoral epiphyses are similar in size and radiographic density. The left appears marginally smaller and is slightly more inferiorly postioned than the right but this is secondary to patient positioning. The acetabular morphology is normal and there is no lateral uncovering of either proximal femoral epiphysis, i.e. there are no features to suggest developmental dysplasia of the hip.
The rectosigmoid colon is distended with gas and there is faecal loading of the ascending and descending colon and rectum. This may be a common finding on abdominal and pelvic radiographs and would not constitute an abnormality in the examination.

23. **Buckle # R thumb proximal phalanx**
There is a cortical 'step' at the dorsal aspect of the right thumb proximal phalanx consistent with a buckle fracture. Close inspection of the cortex is required as this finding could be easily overlooked given that the contour of the bony injury aligns perfectly with that of the overlapping dorsal soft tissue of the right index finger metacarpal. The fracture is visualised in the magnified image below:

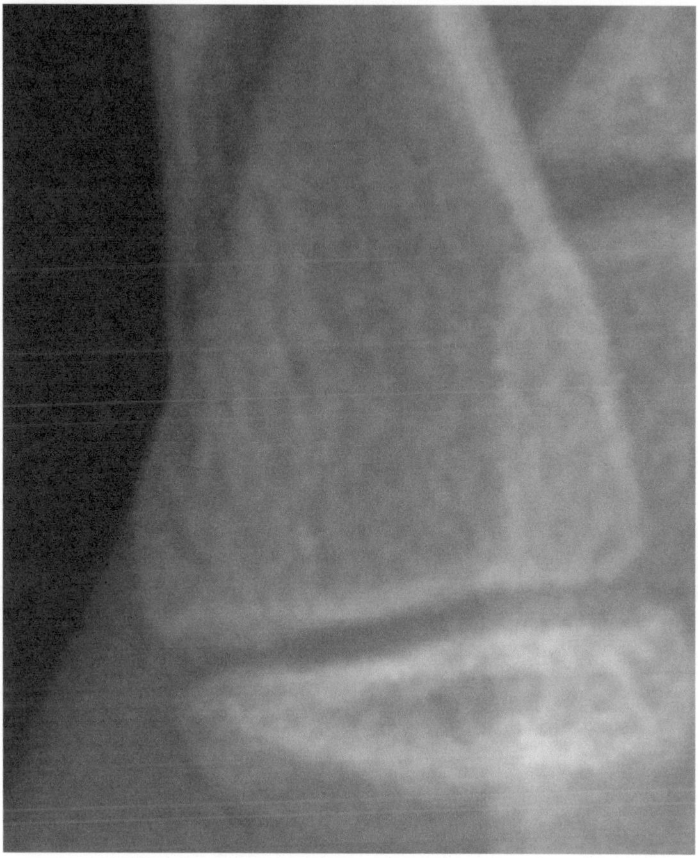

26. **Prevertebral soft tissue thickening**
This 7-year-old boy was presented to the ED with fever, a right-sided neck swelling and torticollis. The lateral neck radiograph demonstrates marked prevertebral soft tissue swelling with no associated gas. The normal thickness of prevertebral soft tissue increases with age and varies according to the cervical spine level. The C2 and C6 vertebral levels are the least variable and are therefore considered to be the most reliable when determining whether there is soft tissue thickening or abnormality. However, it is important to remember that cervical spinal imaging is often obtained with obliquity (rather than true lateral), which hinders an accurate assessment of prevertebral soft tissue thickness.

This patient went on to have post-contrast CT imaging of the neck which demonstrated large peripherally enhancing abscesses in the right parapharyngeal and retropharyngeal spaces with resultant oropharyngeal narrowing and displacement. See the explanation for Image 8 of Test 3 for a more detailed discussion of prevertebral soft tissue thickening and assessment of cervical spine alignment.

29. **R upper lobe round pneumonia**
This 4-year-old girl was presented to the ED with fever and cough. Note the round, mass-like opacity in the right upper zone projected over the posteromedial third to fifth ribs within which are air bronchograms, i.e. visible air-filled bronchi due to surrounding alveolar/airspace opacification. There is no associated cavitation, calcification or additional opacity (nodular or otherwise) in the remainder of the lungs. The adjacent ribs are normal with no splaying or bony destruction. See the explanation for Image 21 of Test 1.

30. **L upper lobe hyperinflation/lucency**
This chest radiograph was obtained in a 9-week-old infant who had an echogenic lesion detected in the left hemithorax on antenatal ultrasound. There is asymmetric lucency in the left upper and mid zones and associated mass effect with mediastinal shift to the right. The differential for this appearance includes congenital pulmonary airway malformation (CPAM; previously known as congenital cystic adenomatoid malformation [CCAM]) and congenital lobar overinflation (CLO; previously referred to as congenital lobar emphysema [CLE]). See the explanation for Image 28 of Test 9 for a more detailed discussion on CLO.

CPAMs are congenital lung lesions that arise due to airway maldevelopment. They are most commonly seen in the lower lobes and usually consist of one or more cysts that range from large/macrocystic to very small/microcystic, and are therefore solid-appearing. They typically receive their blood supply from the pulmonary arterial system and drain via pulmonary veins (unless the lesion is hybrid, i.e. mixed CPAM/bronchopulmonary sequestration with systemic blood supply). CPAMs are the most common fetal lung lesions and are typically visualised as hyperechoic lesions on fetal ultrasound and T2 hyperintense on in utero MRI. Hydrops fetalis (from Latin meaning oedema of the fetus) and polyhydramnios (excessive accumulation of amniotic fluid) may also be present. Postnatal radiographs may demonstrate a multicystic (air-filled) lesion with associated mass effect. CT thoracic angiography is helpful in delineating the type of CPAM, its location, extent, and vascular supply.

The commonest type of CPAM is type 1 (approximately 70% of cases) in which the cysts are large, often with a variable sized dominant cyst (2–10 cm) surrounded by smaller cysts. These lesions have the best prognosis. Type 2 is less common (approximately up to 20% of cases) with smaller diameter cysts (<2 cm) but which may be associated with other abnormalities such as renal agenesis or dysgenesis, bronchopulmonary sequestration (hybrid lesion), and congenital cardiac anomalies. Type 4 CPAM is rare. Type 1 and type 4 CPAM are indistinguishable from pleuropulmonary blastoma (PPB) on imaging. PPBs are more often right-sided pleural lesions without chest wall invasion and may present with pneumothorax. PPBs are classified as:

- Type 1 cystic: fetal, up to approximately 12 months of age; less malignant.
- Type 2 mixed cystic-solid: up to approximately 36 months of age.
- Type 3 solid: up to approximately 48 months; more malignant.

Type 2 and 3 PPB may be associated with bony and central nervous system metastases. Patients with PPB may have the *DICER1* gene mutation (a tumour suppressor gene) and the associated autosomal dominant DICER1 syndrome which predisposes them to developing multiple tumour types, including (but not limited to):

- Wilms tumour.
- Multilocular cystic nephroma: which may be present in up to 10% of cases of PPB.
- Pineoblastoma: the combination of pineoblastoma and bilateral retinoblastoma is referred to as trilateral retinoblastoma. Whilst it may only affect a small number of patients with bilateral retinoblastoma (<5%), it serves as a reminder that the pineal gland should be scrutinised on cross-sectional neuroimaging in the presence of known retinoblastoma.
- Pituitary blastoma.
- Rhabdomyosarcoma.

CPAM is more likely to be detected on a second trimester ultrasound examination, whereas PPB is usually a postnatal diagnosis. CPAMs may spontaneously regress, but if persistent and the patient is symptomatic, surgical resection is the treatment of choice, primarily due to the risk of recurrent infection but also the questionable/potential risk of malignancy (which may be more likely due to the underlying genetic predisposition as discussed, rather than malignant transformation).

Further Reading

Image 3

Bell DJ et al (2022) Distal intestinal obstruction syndrome. https://radiopaedia.org/articles/distal-intestinal-obstruction-syndrome-1. Accessed Mar 2023

Lavelle LP, McEvoy SH, Ni Mhurchu E et al (2015) Cystic fibrosis below the diaphragm: abdominal findings in adult patients. Radiographics 35(3):680–695

Menashe SJ, Iyer RS, Parisi MT et al (2017) Pediatric abdominal radiographs: common and less common errors. Am J Roentgenol 209(2):417–429

Skalina T et al (2022) Cystic fibrosis. https://radiopaedia.org/articles/cystic-fibrosis. Accessed Mar 2023

Image 4

Rock PJ et al (2021) Platyspondyly. https://radiopaedia.org/articles/platyspondyly. Accessed Mar 2023

Zaveri J, La Q, Yarmish G et al (2014) More than just Langerhans cell histiocytosis: a radiologic review of histiocytic disorders. Radiographics 34(7):2008–2024

Image 7

Biko DM, Lichtenberger JP III, Rapp JB et al (2021) Mediastinal masses in children: radiologic-pathologic correlation. Radiographics 41(4):1186–1207

Image 12

Ayaz E, Haliloglu M (2022) Radiologic diagnosis of tracheoesophageal fistula in children. Curr Chall Thorac Surg 4:25

Image 13

Anan RA et al (2023) Brown tumour. https://radiopaedia.org/articles/brown-tumour. Accessed Jul 2023

Bell DJ et al (2021) Picture frame vertebral body. https://radiopaedia.org/articles/picture-frame-vertebral-body. Accessed Mar 2023

Bennett J, Suliburk JW, Morón FE (2020) Osseous manifestations of primary hyperparathyroidism: imaging findings. Int J Endocrinol 21(2020):3146535

Chang CY, Rosenthal DI, Mitchell DM et al (2016) Imaging findings of metabolic bone disease. Radiographics 36(6):1871–1887

Mihelčič K, Cruz M, Caseiro-Alves F (2018) Rugger jersey spine. https://www.eurorad.org/case/15374. Accessed Mar 2023

Panda A, Gamanagatti S, Jana M et al (2014) Skeletal dysplasias: a radiographic approach and review of common non-lethal skeletal dysplasias. World J Radiol 6(10):808–825

Qureshi PAAA et al (2021) Sandwich vertebral body. https://radiopaedia.org/articles/sandwich-vertebral-body. Accessed Mar 2023

Sharma R et al (2023) Rugger jersey spine (hyperparathyroidism). https://radiopaedia.org/articles/rugger-jersey-spine-hyperparathyroidism-1. Accessed Mar 2023

Image 26

Vermess D, Rojas CA, Shaheen F et al (2012) Normal pediatric prevertebral soft-tissue thickness on MDCT. Am J Roentgenol 199(1):W130–W133

Image 29

Murphy A et al (2023) Air bronchogram. https://radiopaedia.org/articles/air-bronchogram. Accessed Mar 2023

Image 30

Adams NC, Victoria T, Oliver ER et al (2020) Fetal ultrasound and magnetic resonance imaging: a primer on how to interpret prenatal lung lesions. Pediatr Radiol 50(13):1839–1854
Durhan G, Ardali Duzgun S, Akpınar MG et al (2021) Imaging of congenital lung diseases presenting in the adulthood: a pictorial review. Insights Imaging 12(1):153
El-Ali AM, Strubel NA, Lala SV (2022) Congenital lung lesions: a radiographic pattern approach. Pediatr Radiol 52(4):622–636
Iqbal S et al (2020) Trilateral retinoblastoma. https://radiopaedia.org/articles/trilateral-retinoblastoma. Accessed Jul 2023
Jin TY et al (2023) Congenital pulmonary airway malformation. https://radiopaedia.org/articles/congenital-pulmonary-airway-malformation. Accessed Mar 2023
Jones J et al (2021) Pleuropulmonary blastoma. https://radiopaedia.org/articles/pleuropulmonary-blastoma. Accessed Mar 2023
Jones J et al (2023) DICER1 syndrome. https://radiopaedia.org/articles/dicer1-syndrome-1. Accessed Mar 2023

Test 13

13

M. Paddock et al., *Paediatric Radiology Rapid Reporting*,
https://doi.org/10.1007/978-3-031-48255-7_13

13.1 Images

Image 1

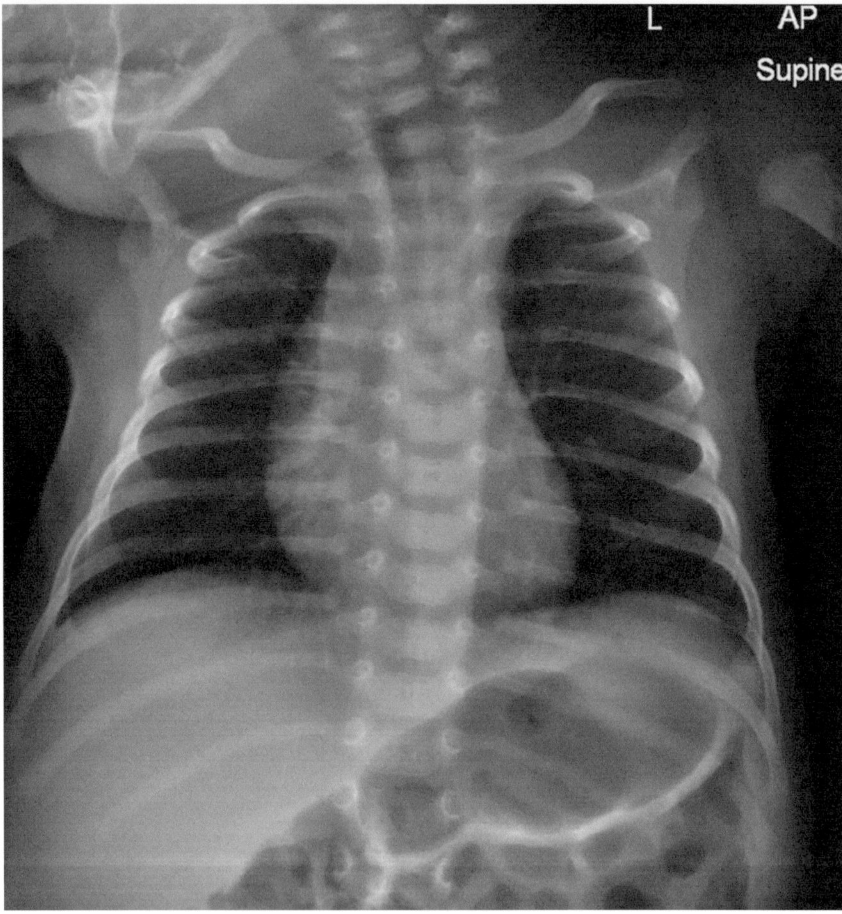

Image 2

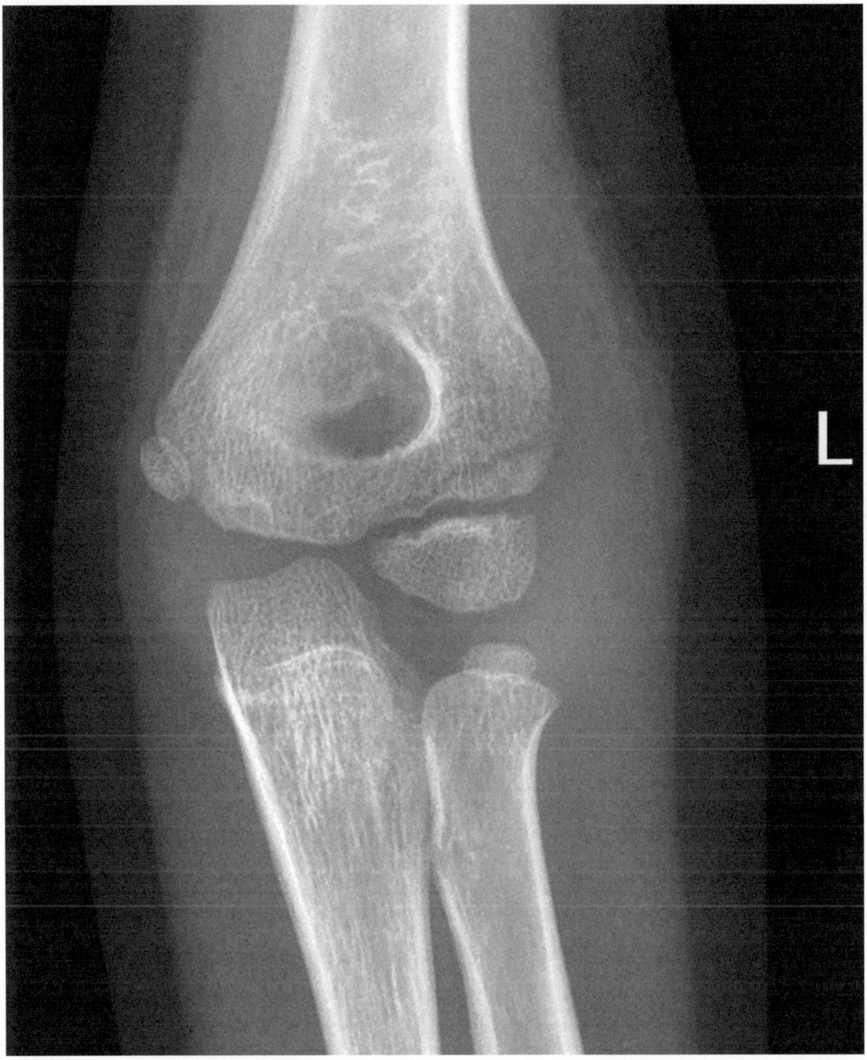

Image 3

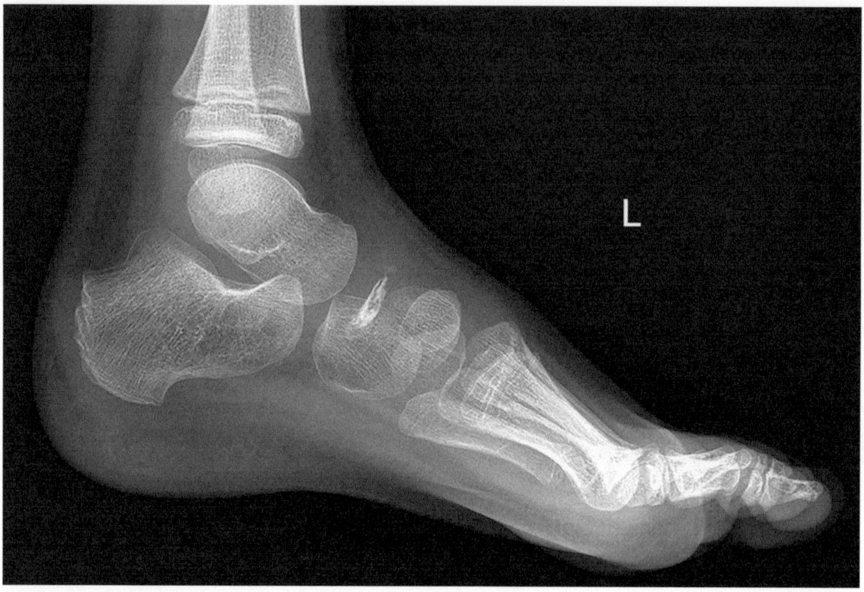

Image 4

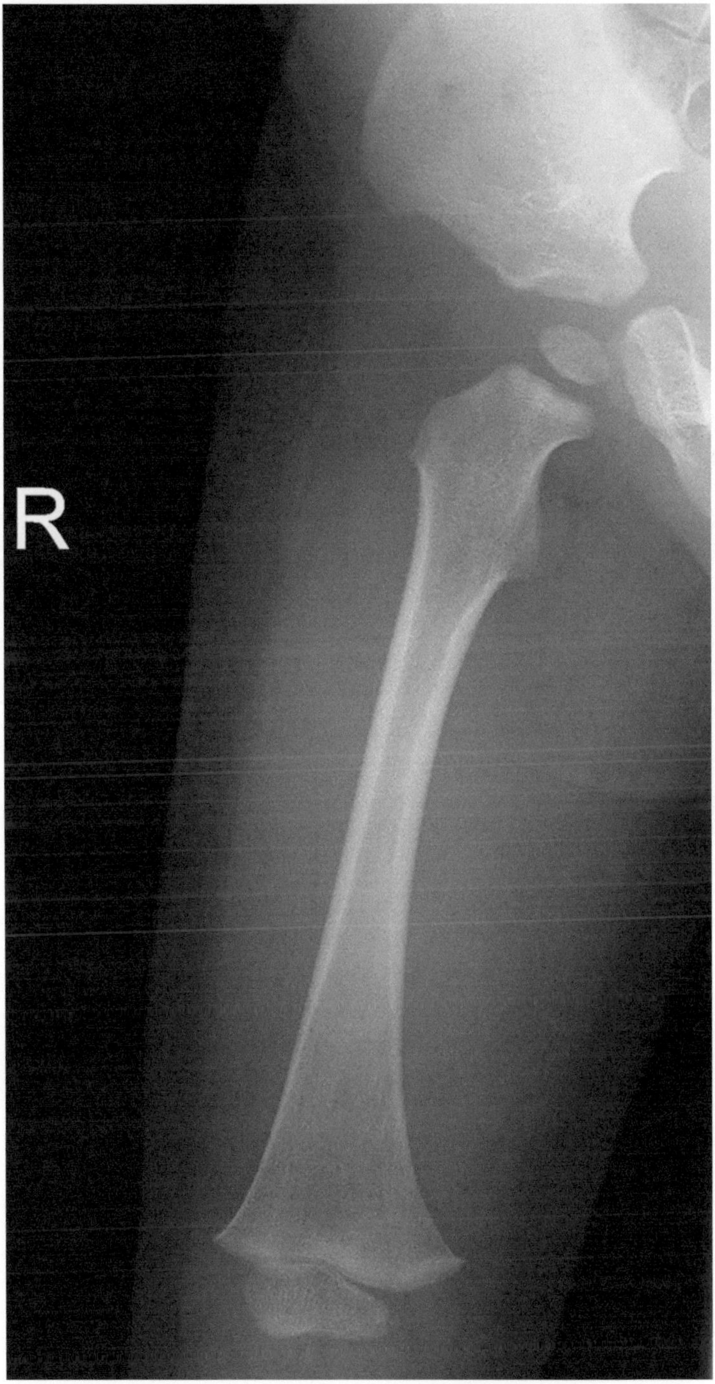

Image 5

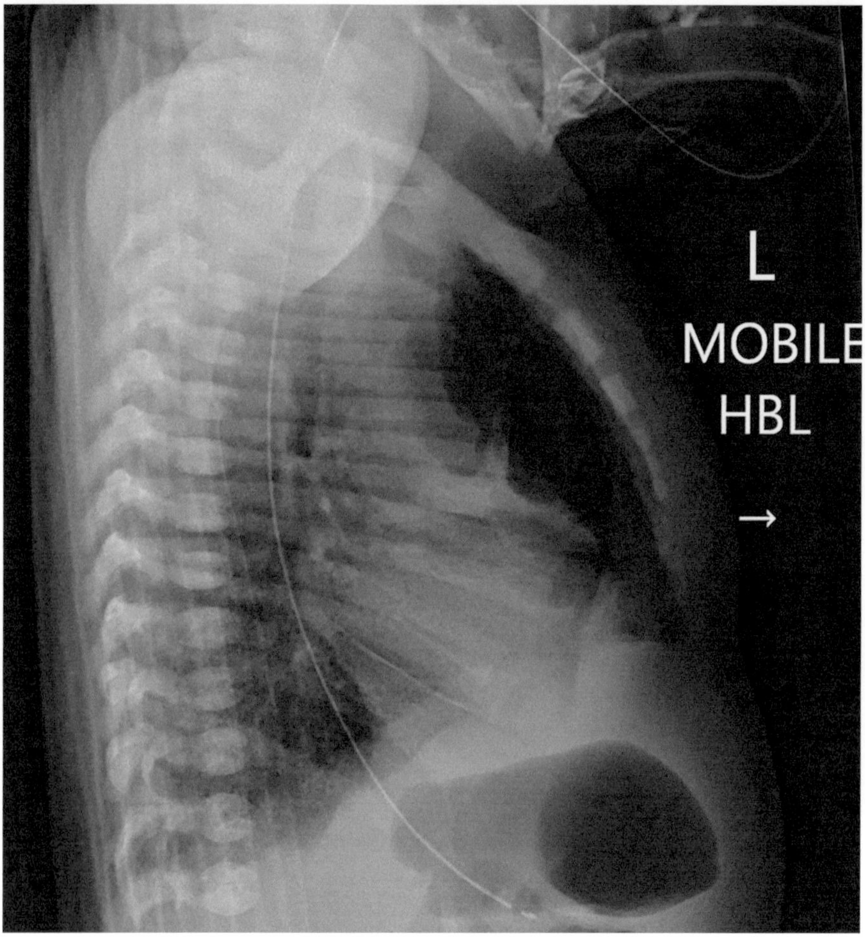

Image 6

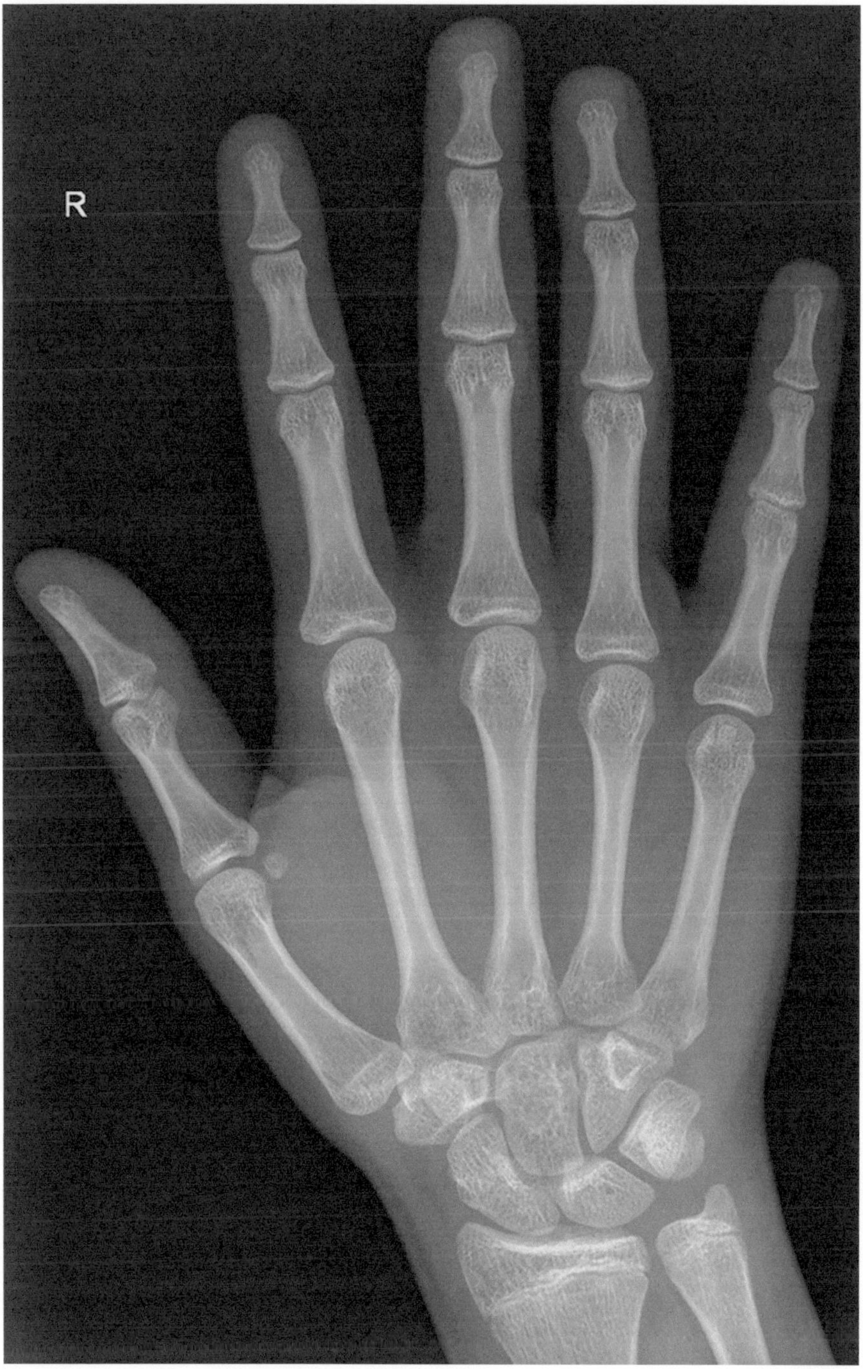

Image 7

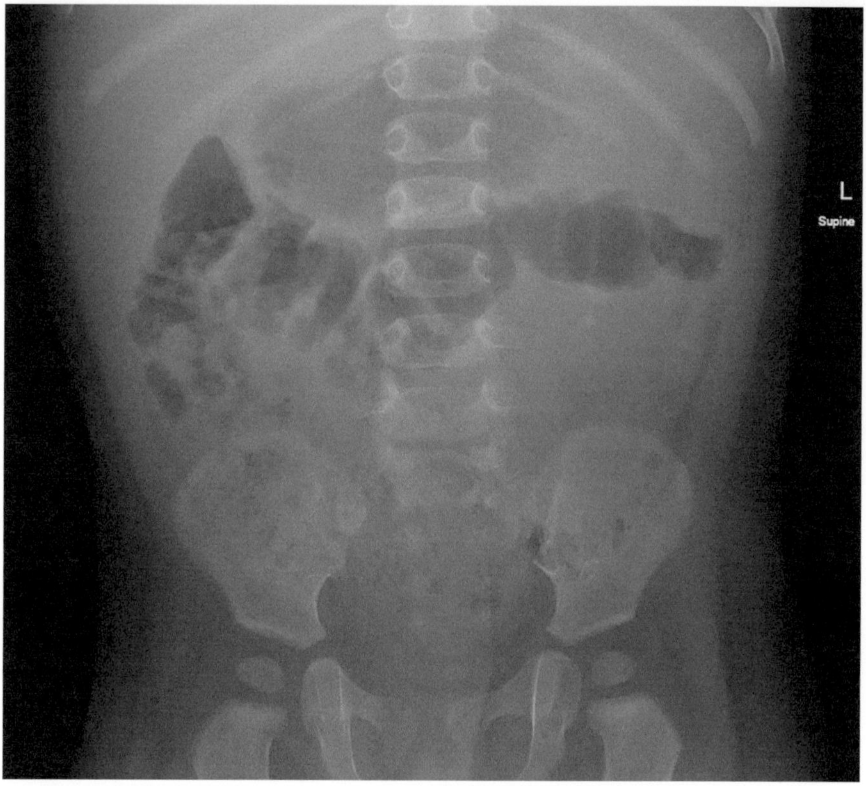

Image 8

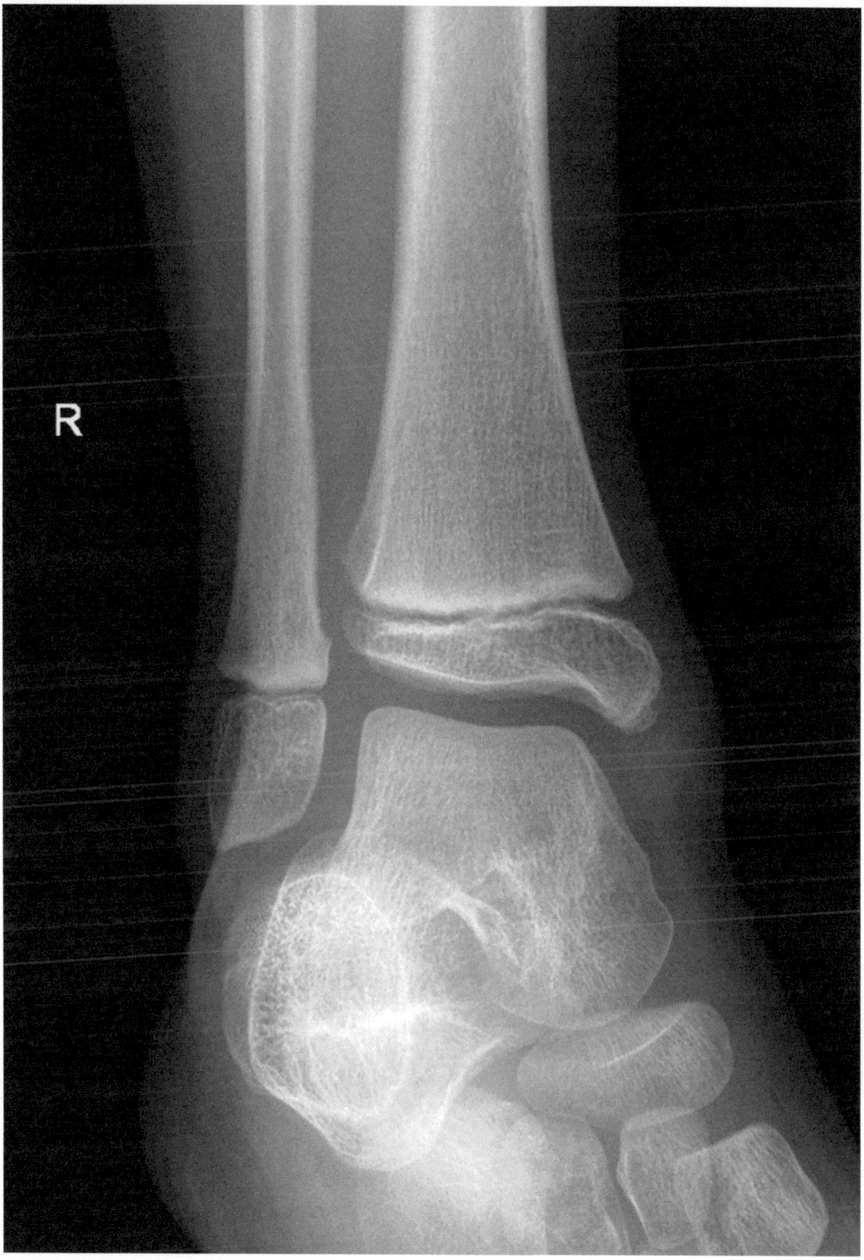

Image 9

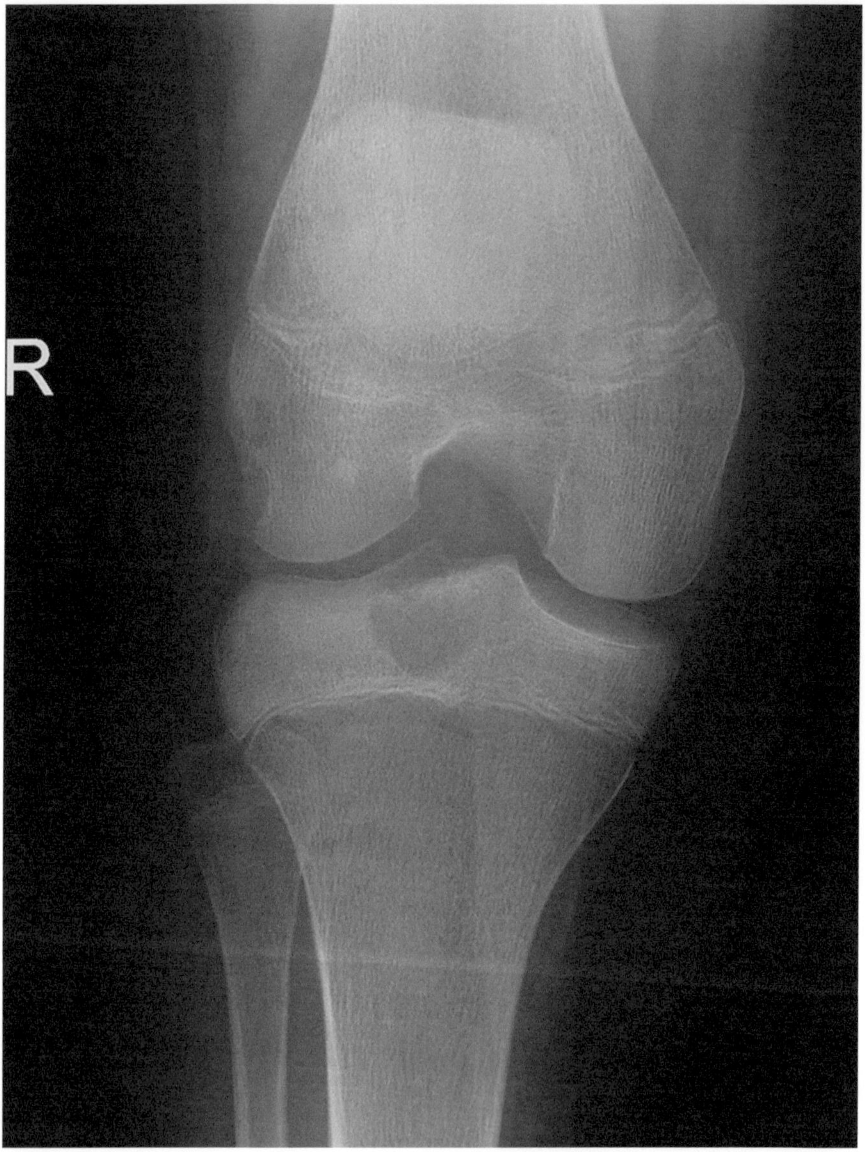

Image 10

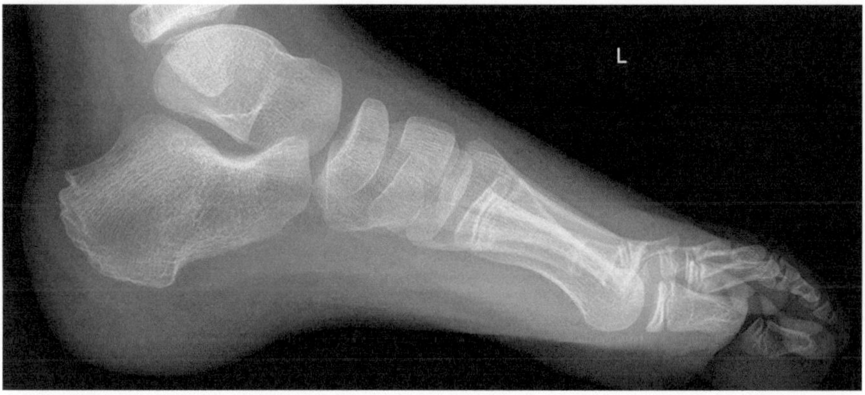

Image 11

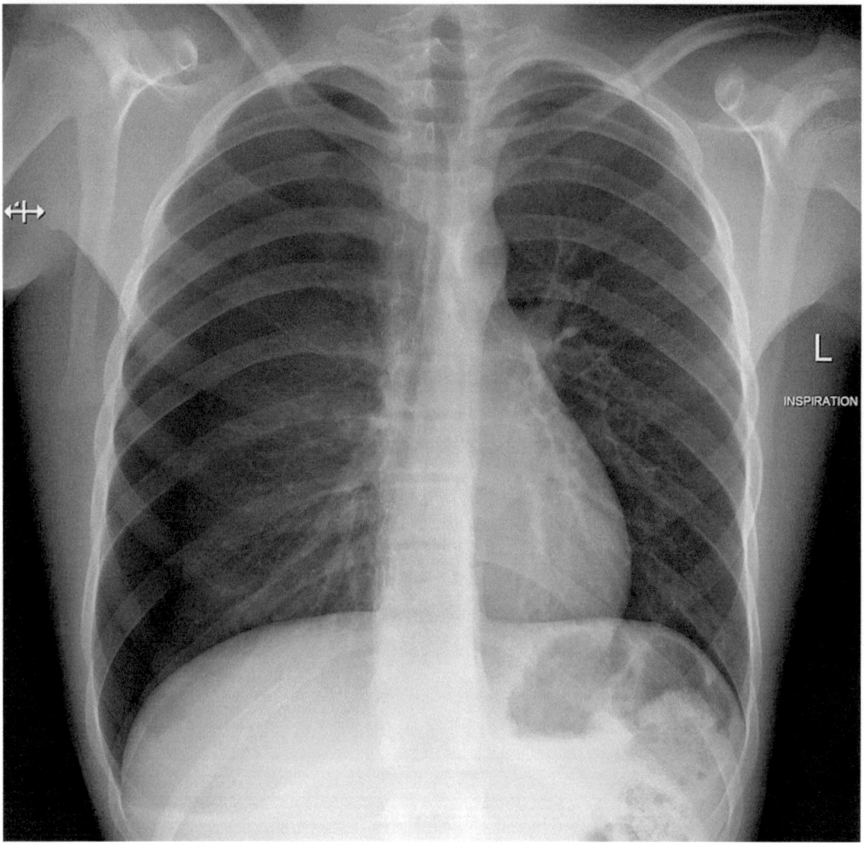

Image 12

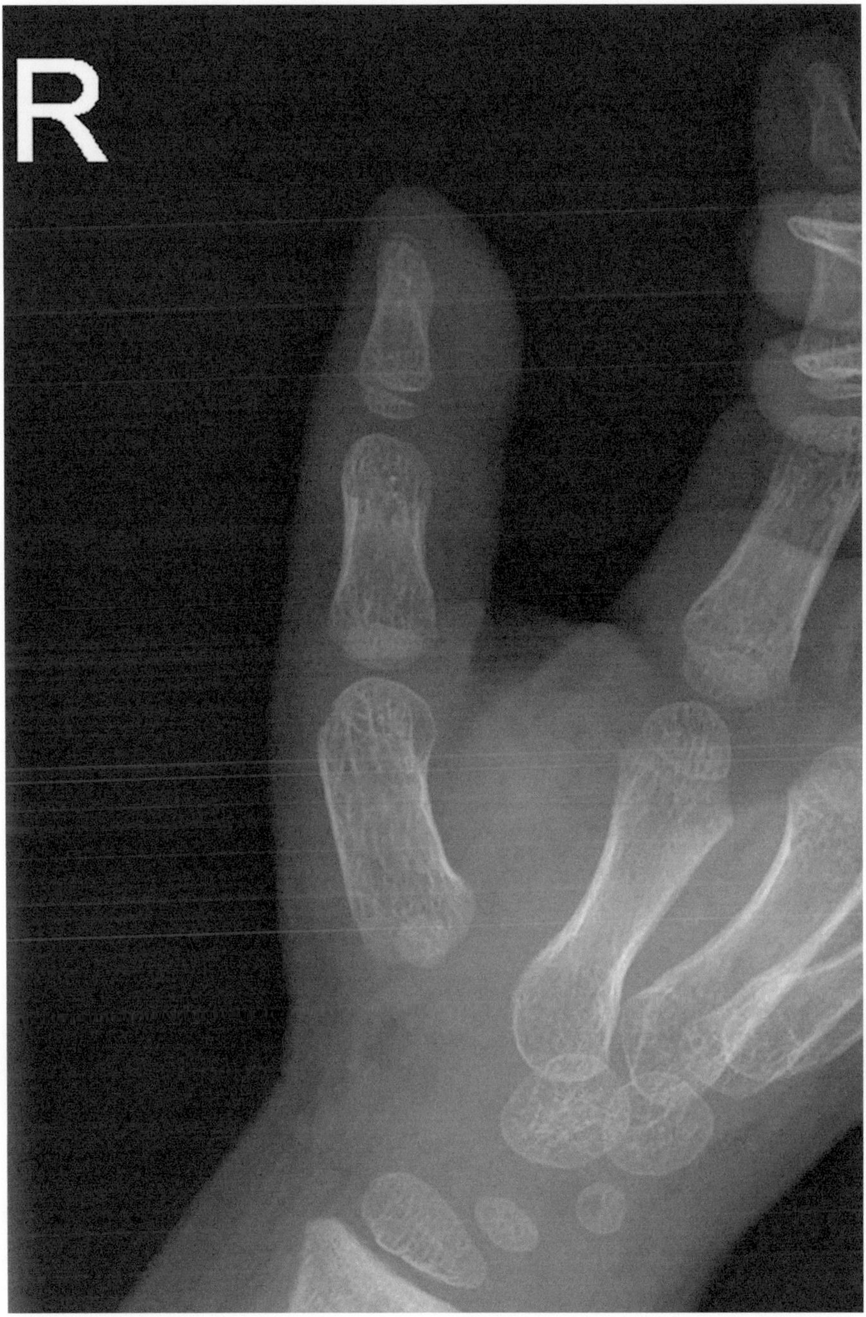

Image 13

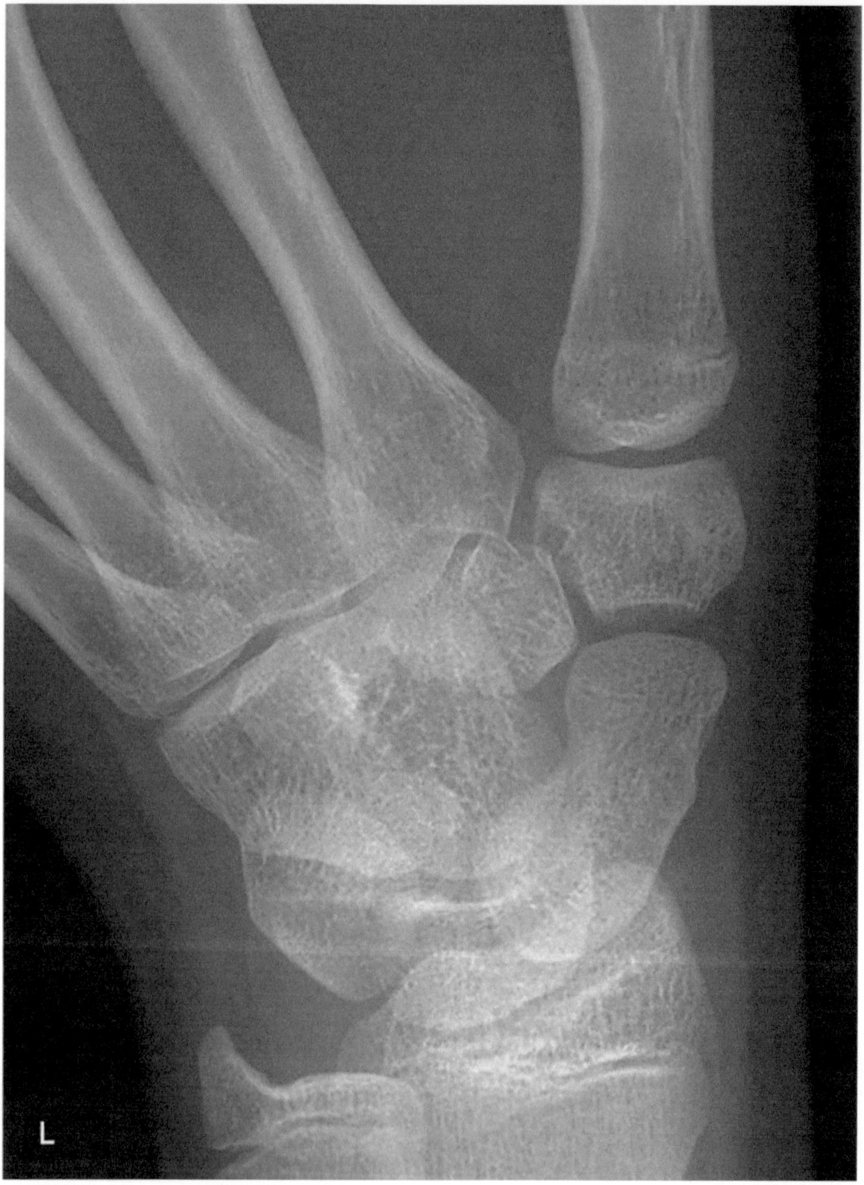

Image 14

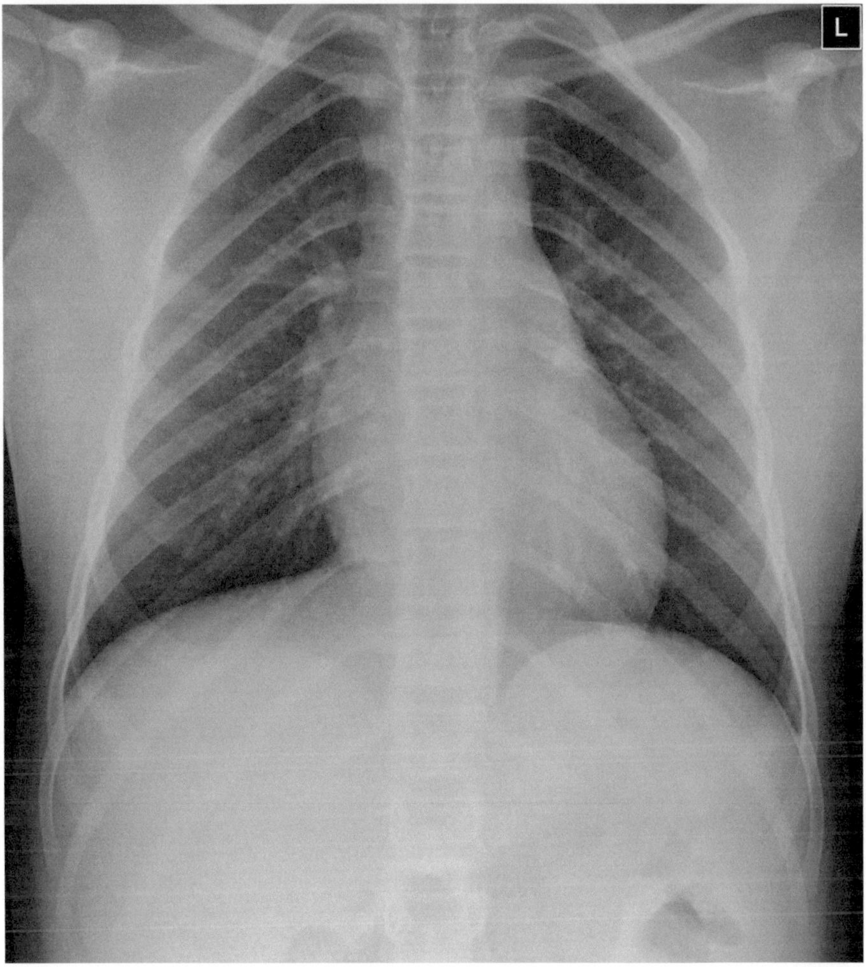

Image 15

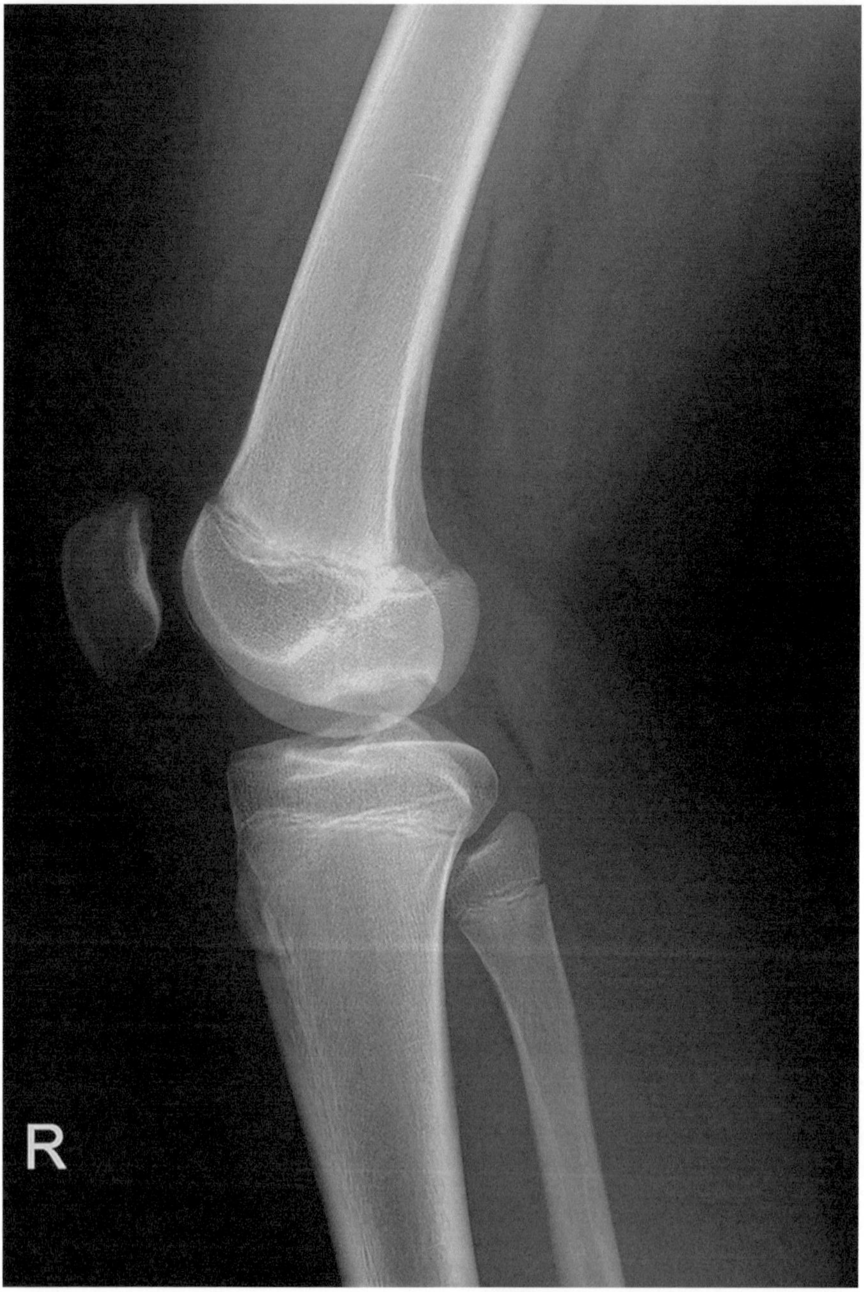

Image 16

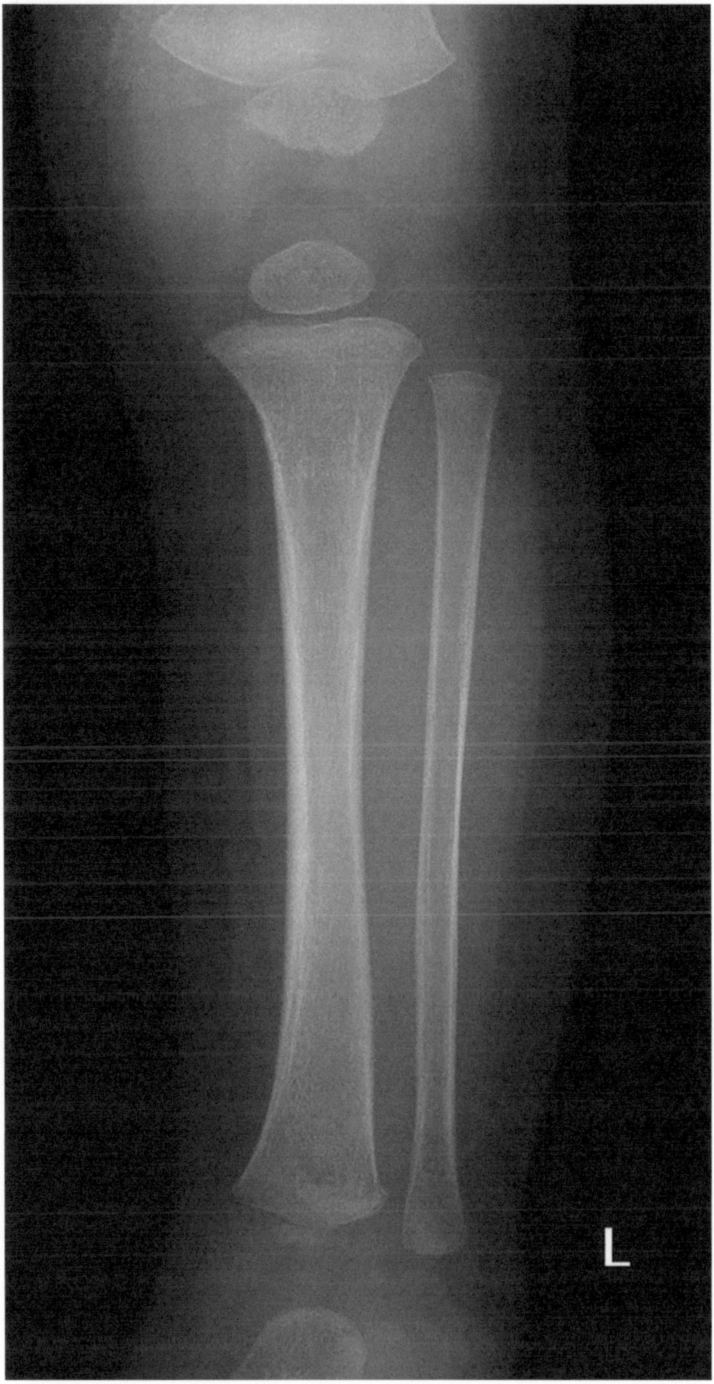

Image 17

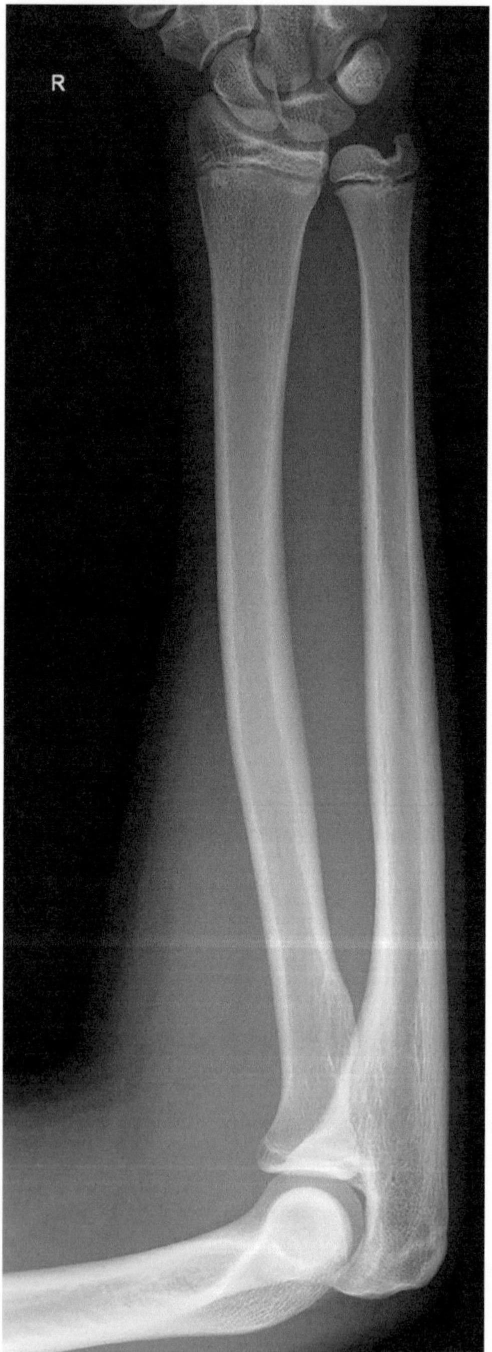

Image 18

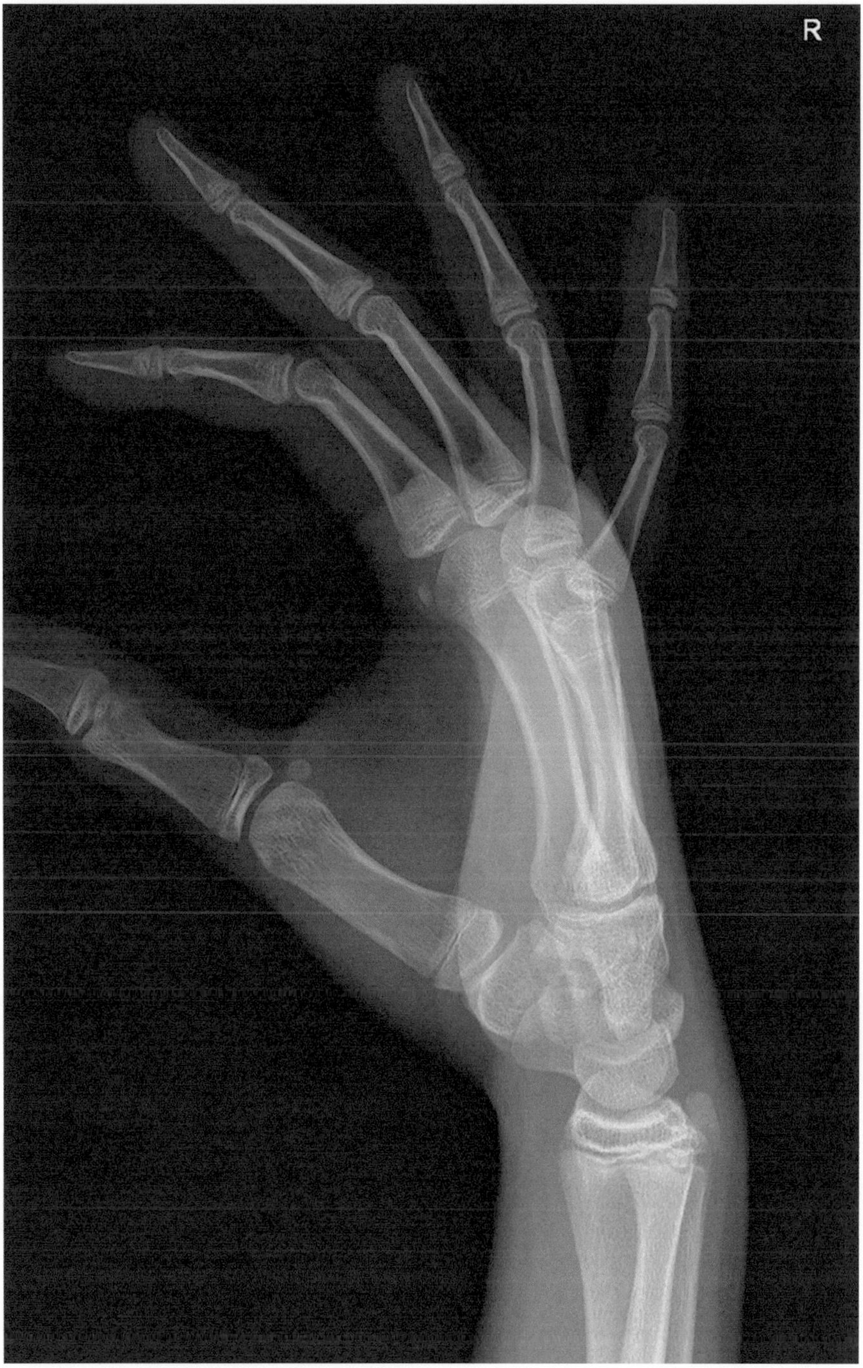

Image 19

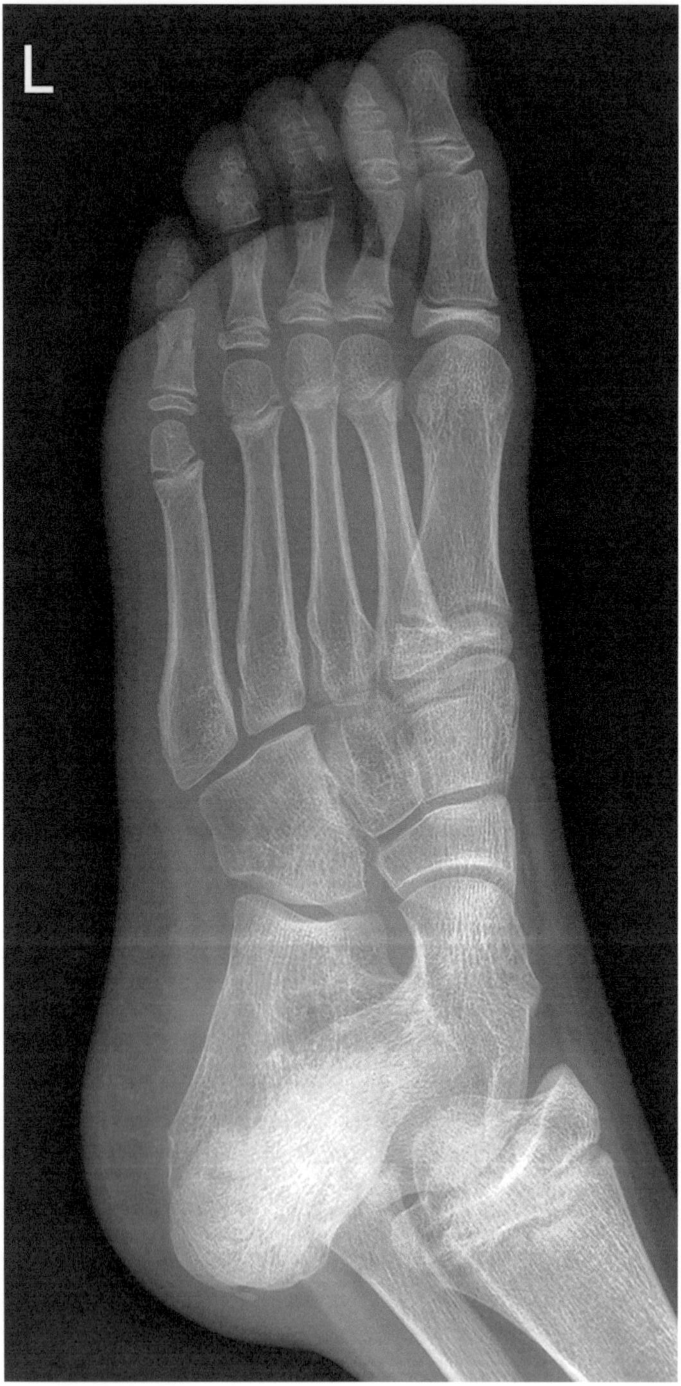

Image 20

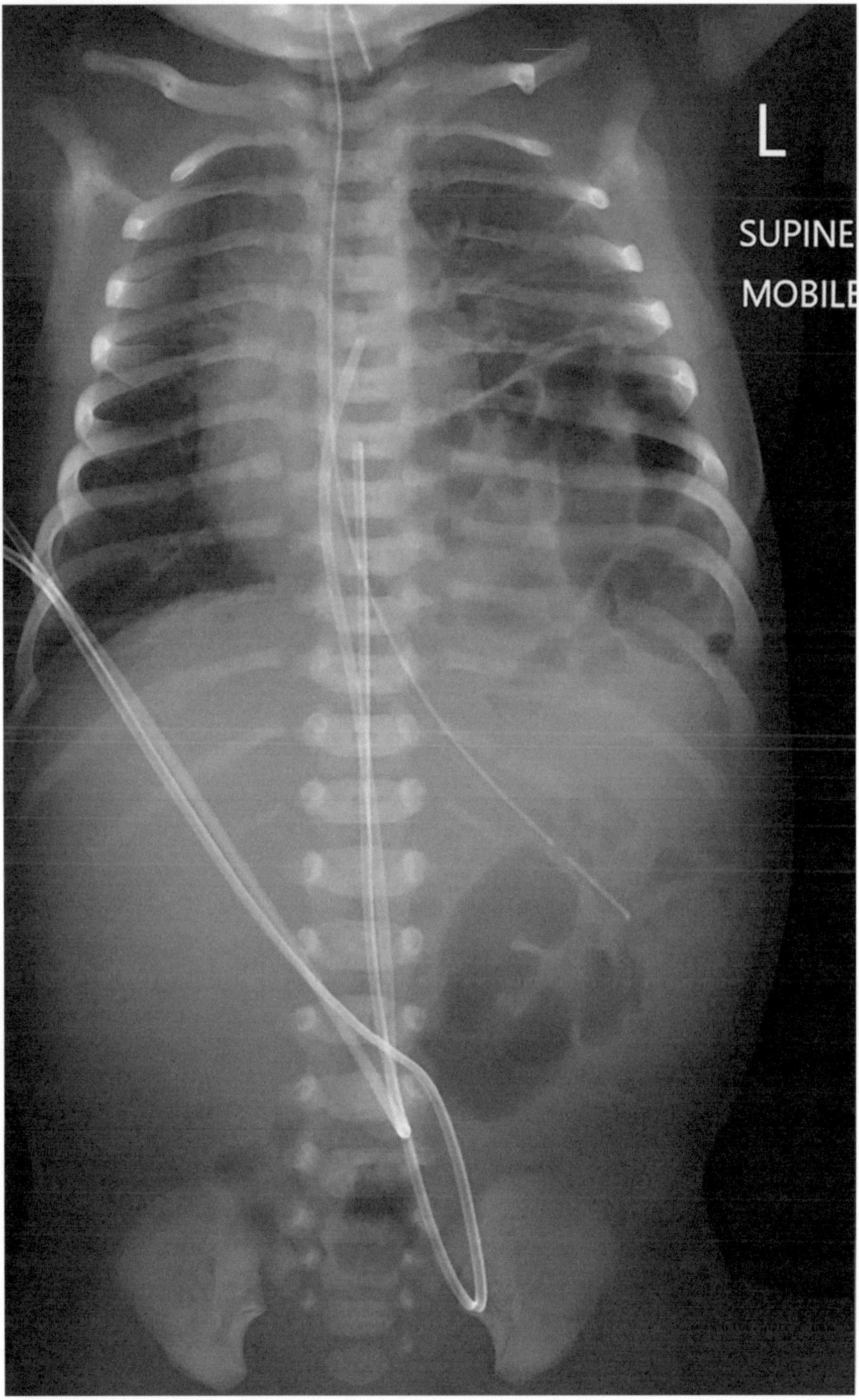

Image 21

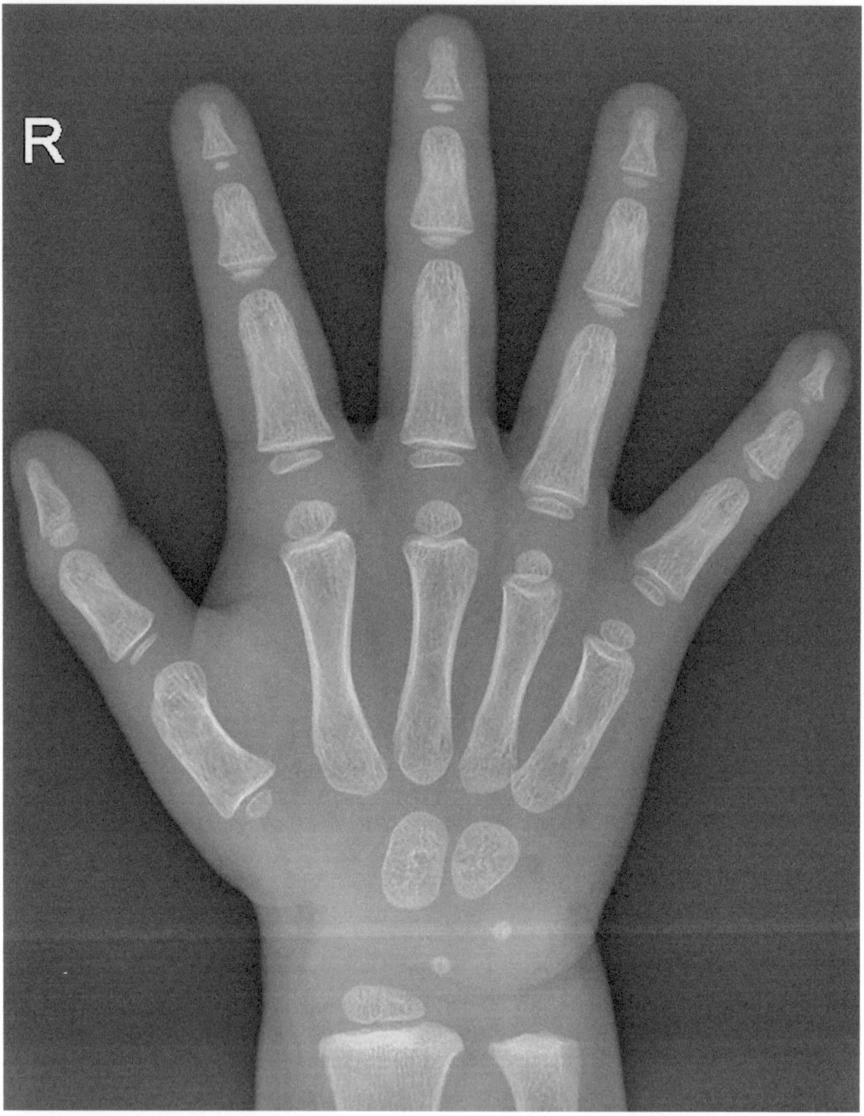

Image 22

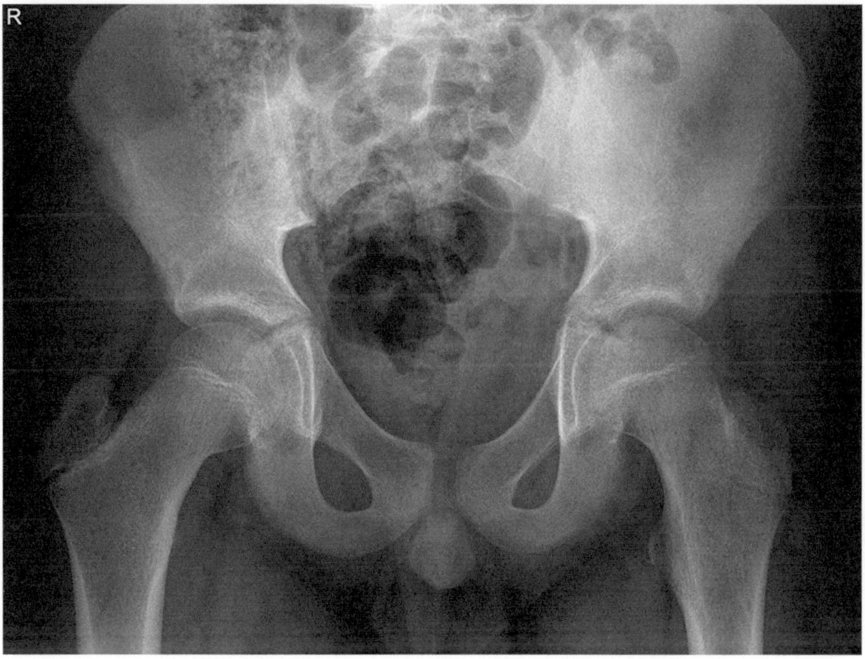

Image 23

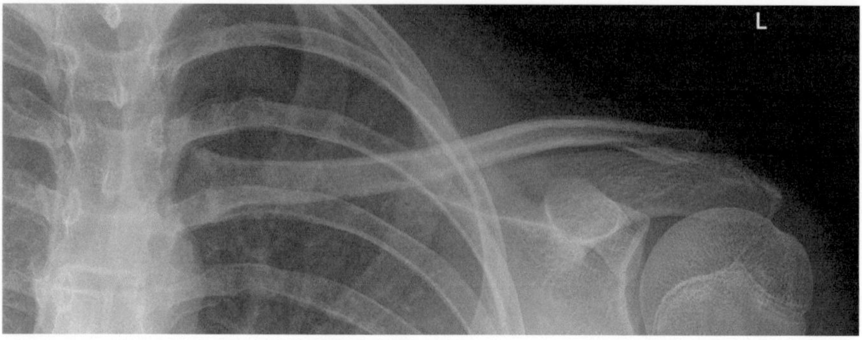

Image 24

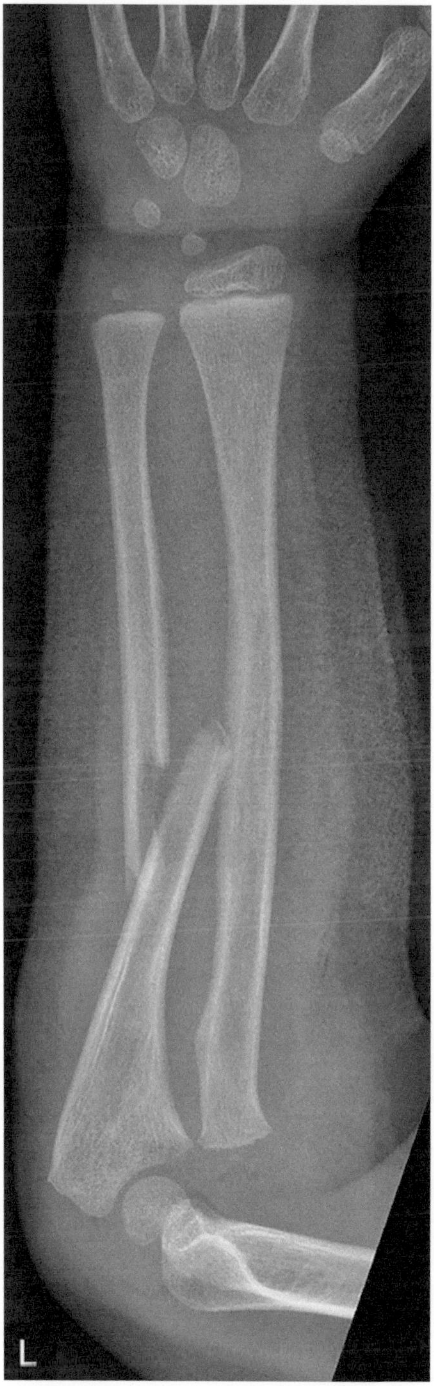

Image 25

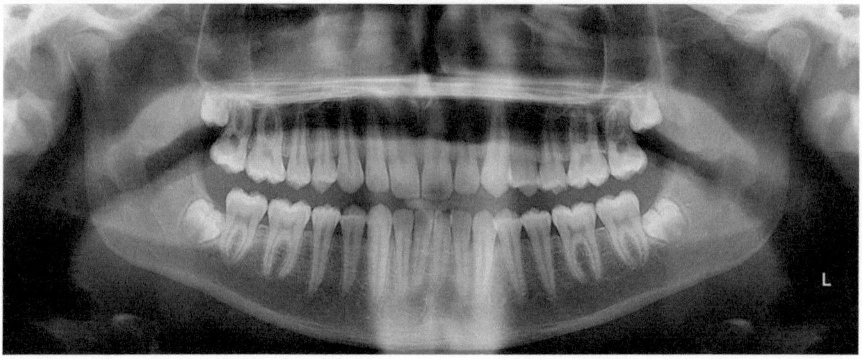

Image 26

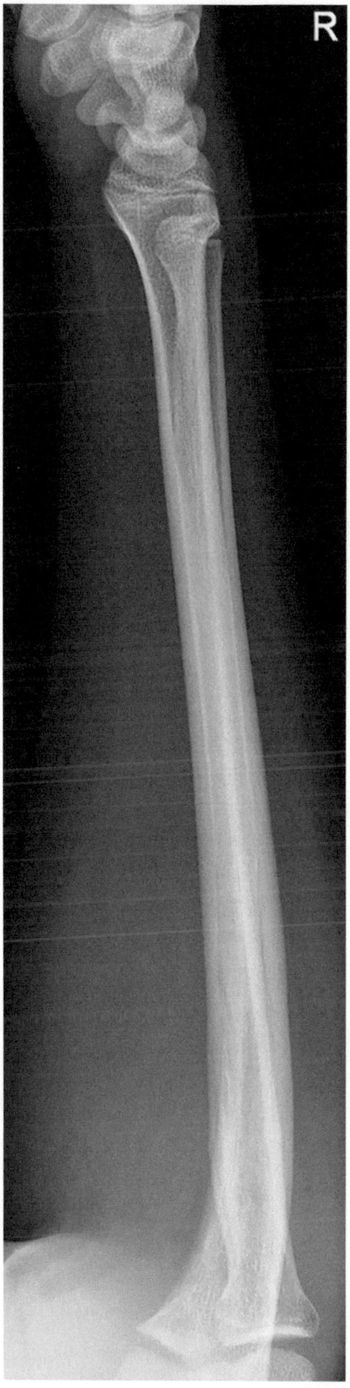

Image 27

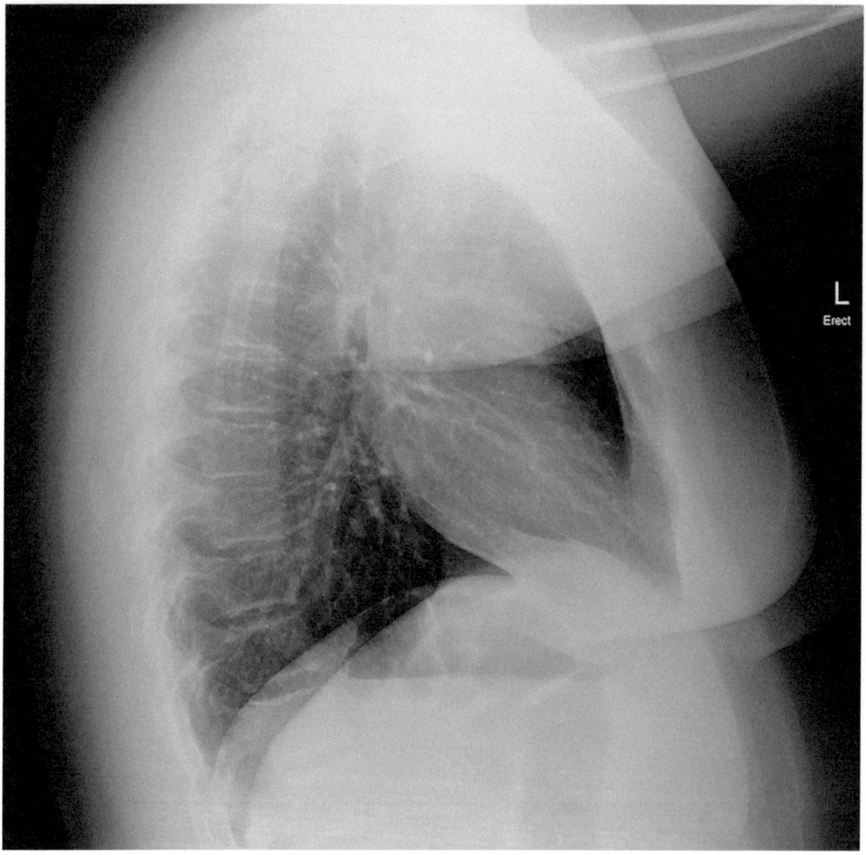

Image 28

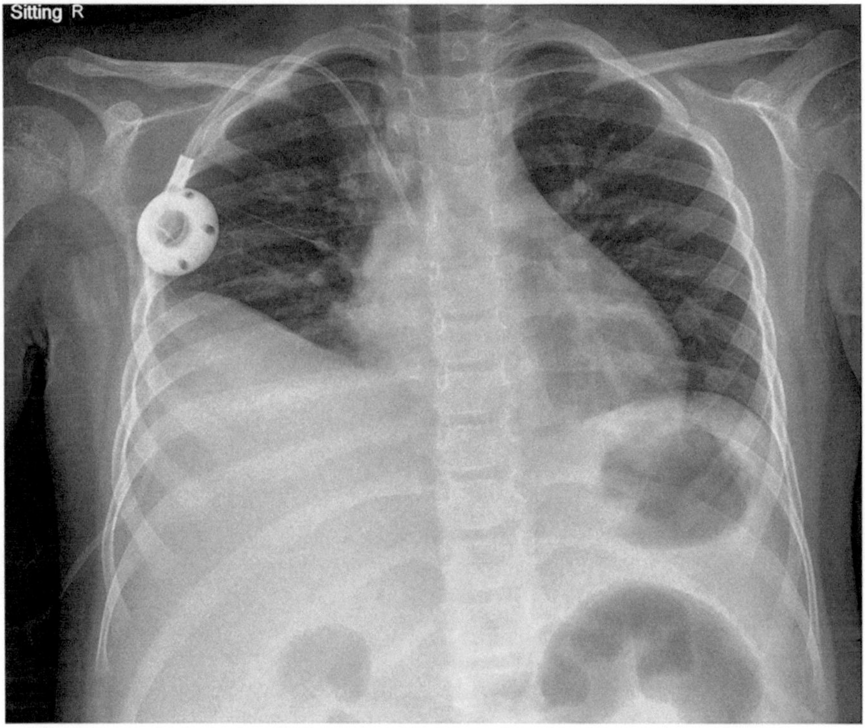

Image 29

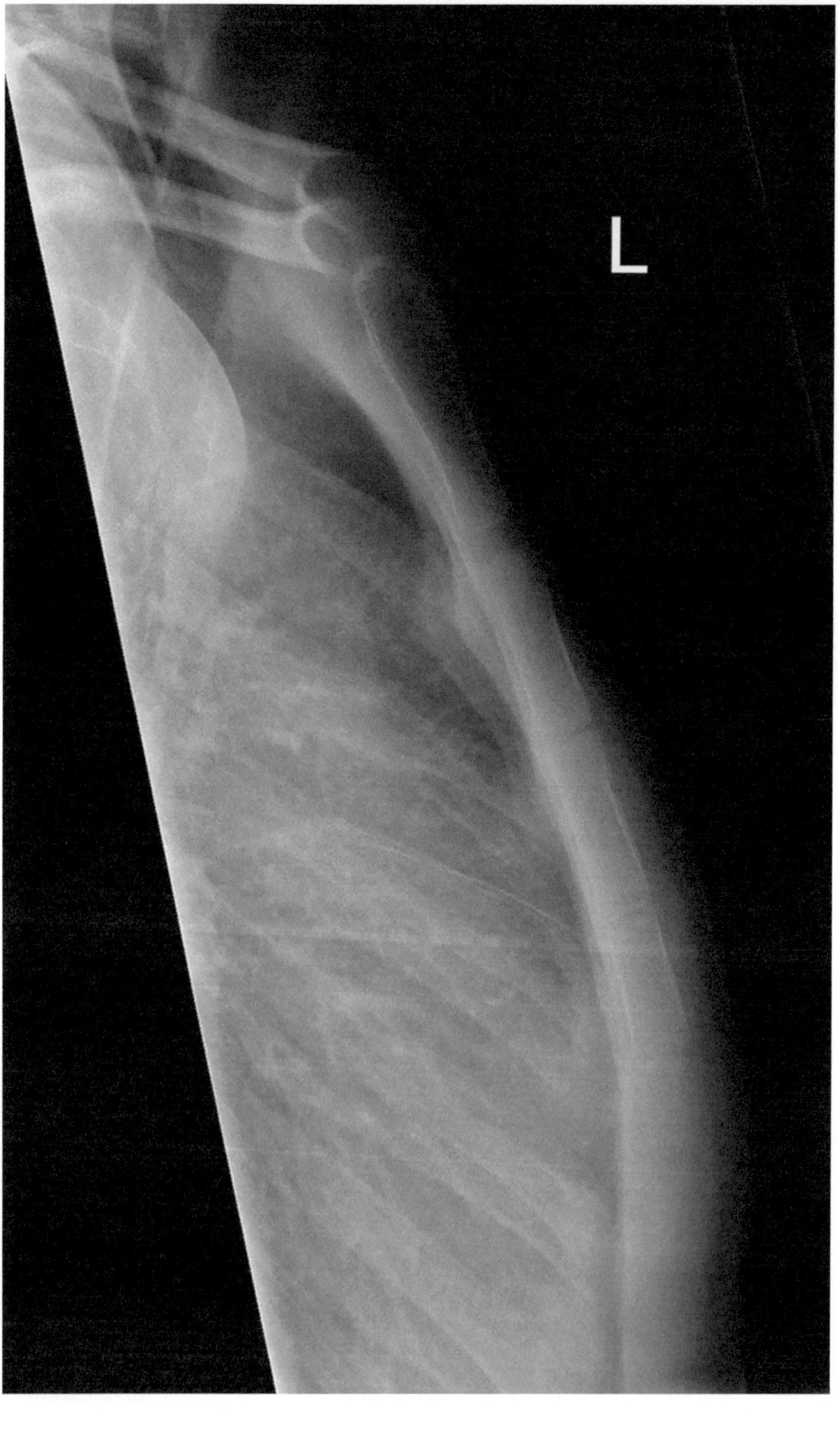

Image 30

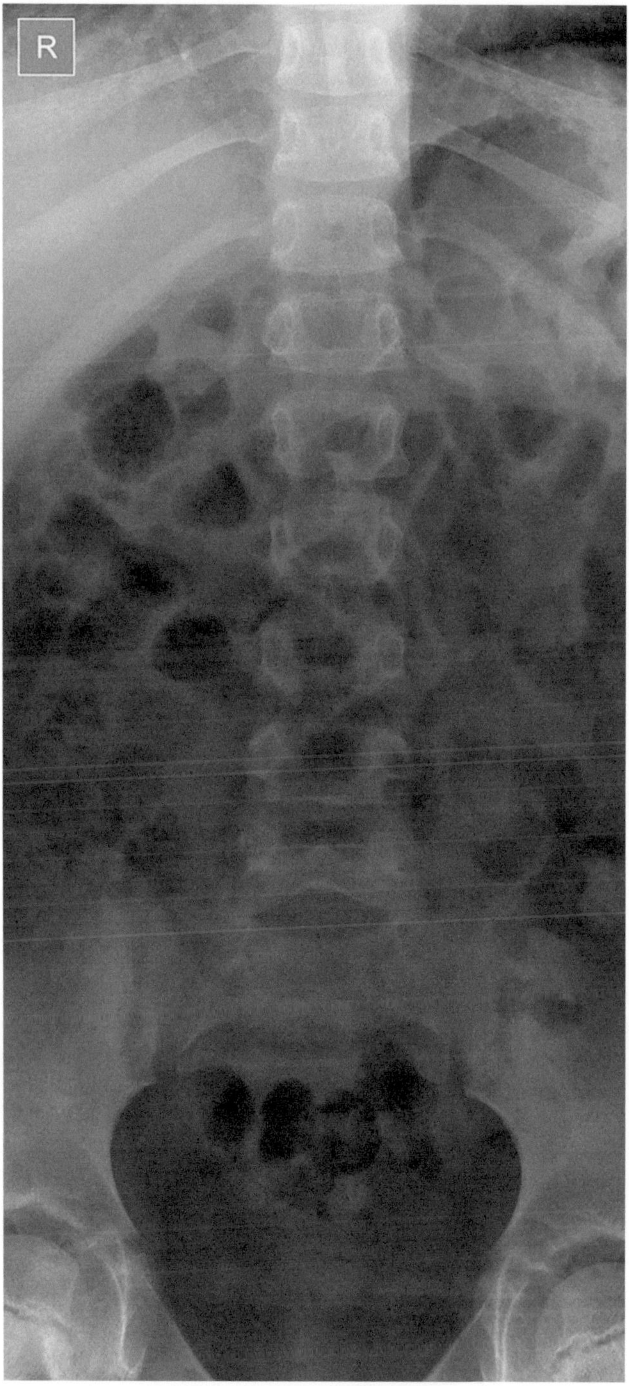

13.2 Answers

Image	Normal	Abnormal	Diagnosis/abnormality (only if abnormal)
1	✓		
2		✓	# L lateral humeral condyle
3		✓	Osteonecrosis L navicular
4	✓		
5		✓	Pneumomediastinum
6	✓		
7		✓	L renal calculi
8	✓		
9		✓	Lucent lesion R proximal tibial epiphysis
10	✓		
11		✓	R pneumothorax
12		✓	# R thumb distal phalanx terminal tuft
13	✓		
14	✓		
15		✓	OCD R distal femoral condyle
16		✓	Lucent/aggressive lesion L distal tibial metaphysis
17	✓		
18	✓		
19		✓	# L little toe proximal phalanx
20		✓	L CDH
21	✓		
22		✓	Periosteal reaction L iliac and pubic bones
23	✓		
24		✓	L Monteggia #-dislocation
25	✓		
26		✓	Buckle # R distal radial metaphysis
27	✓		
28		✓	R subpulmonic effusion
29		✓	# anterior sternal cortex
30	✓		

13.3 Explanations

2. **# L lateral humeral condyle**

   There is an obliquely oriented minimally displaced left lateral humeral condyle fracture with soft tissue swelling over the lateral left elbow. Lateral condylar fractures are the second commonest type of elbow fracture in children after supracondylar humeral fractures. They can be classified using the Milch classification:

   - Type 1: stable fractures which pass *lateral to* the trochlear groove through to the radiocapitellar joint space; less common.
   - Type 2: unstable fractures which pass *through* the trochlear groove, as in this case; more common.

   Whilst these fractures may appear as Salter-Harris 2 fractures radiographically, they are actually Salter-Harris 4 injuries because the fracture extends through the cartilaginous portion of the ossification centre which is not visible on radiographs. Displaced and unstable lateral condylar fractures require open reduction and internal fixation (ORIF).

   The Weiss classification may also be used to assess the degree of fracture displacement on internal oblique projections to determine which patients are at increased risk of further displacement and require operative management. Weiss type 1, 2, and 3 fractures correspond to <2, 2–4 and >4 mm displacement, respectively, with increasing complications associated with type 3 injuries.

   Note that the lateral humeral condylar fractures described above are different from the lateral epicondyle avulsion fractures in which the lateral epicondyle ossification centre has been avulsed.

3. **Osteonecrosis L navicular**

   This lateral left foot radiograph in a 7-year-old boy demonstrates a flattened, irregular, fragmented, and sclerotic navicular bone in keeping with osteonecrosis, which was confirmed on the subsequent magnetic resonance imaging (MRI). Navicular osteonecrosis (eponymously known as Köhler's disease) is an uncommon condition whereby mechanical compression of the developing navicular is thought to result in ischaemia, osteonecrosis, and osteochondrosis (defined as aseptic ischaemic necrosis from focal disruption of endochondral ossification, which usually involves epiphyseal ossification centres). It is typically visualised between the ages of 3 and 7 years and affects boys more often than girls. Radiographs may demonstrate sclerosis, rarefaction (thinner, reduced density), collapse or fragmentation of the navicular, as in the case above. Management is usually conservative. See the explanation for Image 22 of Test 7.

5. **Pneumomediastinum**

   This is the contemporaneous lateral chest radiograph of the same patient from Image 24 of Test 11. There is increased lucency in the retrosternal space causing posterior displacement of cardiomediastinal structures. There are lung markings in the anteroinferior thorax indicating that this is a pneumomediastinum and not a pneumothorax. See the explanations for Image 5 of Test 2 and Image 24 of Test 11.

7. **L renal calculi**
   There are two radiopacities projected over the expected anatomical position of the lower pole of the left kidney in keeping with renal calculi. No calculus is visualised in the expected anatomical position of either ureter. This 8-month-old girl had a complex history of right hydroureteronephrosis with ectopic ureteral insertion and recurrent urinary tract infections.

   Children with renal calculi usually have associated metabolic abnormalities (such as hypercalciuria or hyperoxaluria) with infection playing a contributory role. Ultrasound is the initial imaging modality of choice in children with suspected renal calculi. Once the underlying cause of stone disease has been identified, treatment is initiated to prevent recurrence. Medical expulsive therapy and/or surgery may be required for clearance of calculi. See the explanation for Image 26 of Test 5.

8. *Normal right ankle radiograph*
   The fragmented epiphyseal ossification at the right medial malleolus is normal: remember that epiphyseal ossification can have variable appearances at all ages. The undulating appearance of the distal medial fibular cortex is a normal developmental appearance which results from the accommodation of the adjacent distal tibial epiphyseal cartilage, which has yet to ossify and is not visualised radiographically.

9. **Lucent lesion R proximal tibial epiphysis**
   There is a lucent lesion in the lateral right tibial spine and right proximal tibial epiphysis. It is well-defined with a narrow zone of transition and the surrounding proximal tibial epiphysis is diffusely sclerotic. There is no associated pathological fracture, periosteal reaction, or soft tissue mass. These features are in keeping with a non-aggressive lesion and the subsequent MRI demonstrated findings consistent with chondroblastoma.

   Chondroblastoma is a benign cartilaginous tumour that most commonly occurs in the epiphyses of long bones. It is typically visualised as a lucent lesion with well-defined borders on radiographs. MRI demonstrates corresponding high T2- and low T1-weighted signal with marked perilesional oedema: it is this perilesional oedema that accounts for the diffuse proximal tibial epiphyseal sclerosis visualised radiographically. Treatment is with curettage and bone grafting.

Tip for the viva:

- The commonest epiphyseal lesions can be best remembered using the phrase/mnemonic, **Chrondoblastoma IS AGE(-related)**
  - **Chondroblastoma.**
  - **I**nfection.
  - **S**imple/unicameral bone cyst, **S**ubchondral cyst.
  - **A**neurysmal bone cyst, **A**vascular necrosis.
  - **G**iant cell tumour.
  - **E**nchondroma.
- Do not forget to consider the 'epiphyseal equivalents', i.e. the patella, the calcaneus, the greater and lesser trochanters, and most apophyses (ossification centres which are the site of ligamentous attachment or tendinous insertion) for the purposes of the above differential diagnosis of lucent bone lesions.

11. **R pneumothorax**
    There is a large right-sided pneumothorax without significant mediastinal tension. Do not forget to assess for evidence of mediastinal tension, i.e. contralateral shift of the mediastinum, flattening of the ipsilateral hemidiaphragm, and increased width of the ipsilateral intercostal spaces. See the explanations for Image 10 of Test 1, Image 1 of Test 4 and Image 30 of Test 8.

12. **# R thumb distal phalanx terminal tuft**
    There is a thin bony fragment paralleling the right thumb distal phalanx terminal tuft consistent with a minimally displaced fracture.

15. **Osteochondral defect R distal femoral condyle**
    We have included this case as a reminder that assessment of the distal femoral condyles on lateral projections should not be overlooked. The magnified image below better visualises the osteochondral defect (OCD):

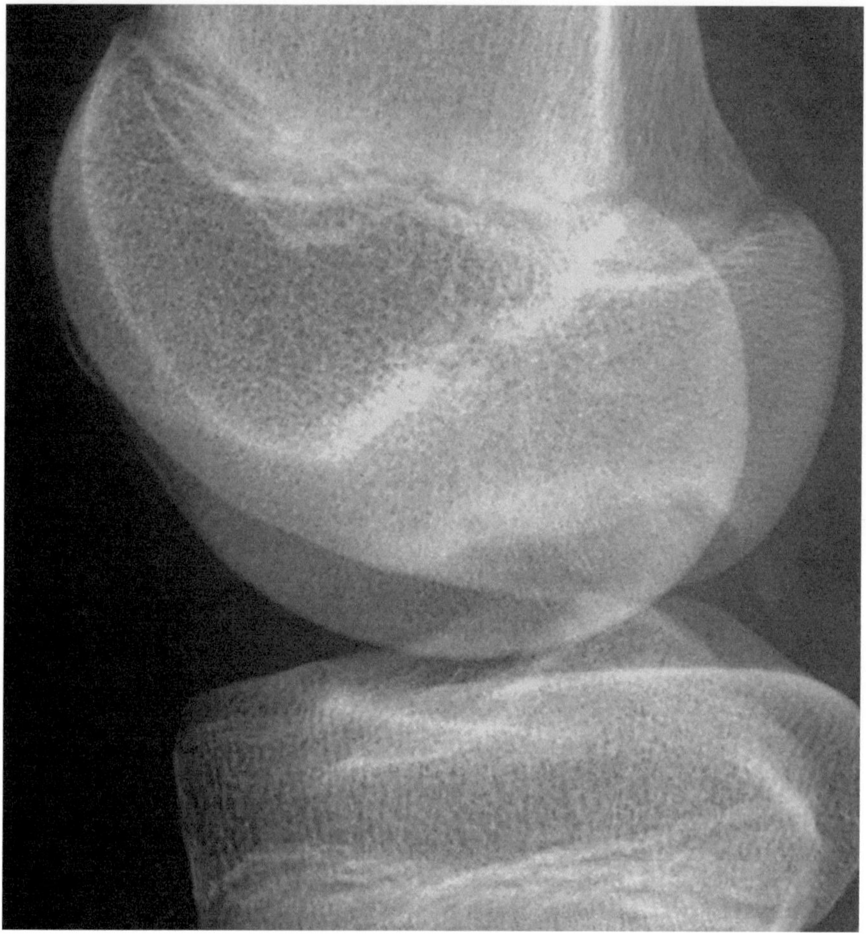

See the explanation for Image 10 of Test 4.

16. **Lucent/aggressive lesion L distal tibial metaphysis**
There is ill-defined lucency within the central and lateral left distal tibial metaphysis with a wide zone of transition and associated irregularity and lucency of the left distal tibial lateral metaphyseal cortex. There is also a small amount of adjacent periosteal reaction along the medial metaphysis. The features are in keeping with an aggressive process. The findings are better visualised in the magnified image below:

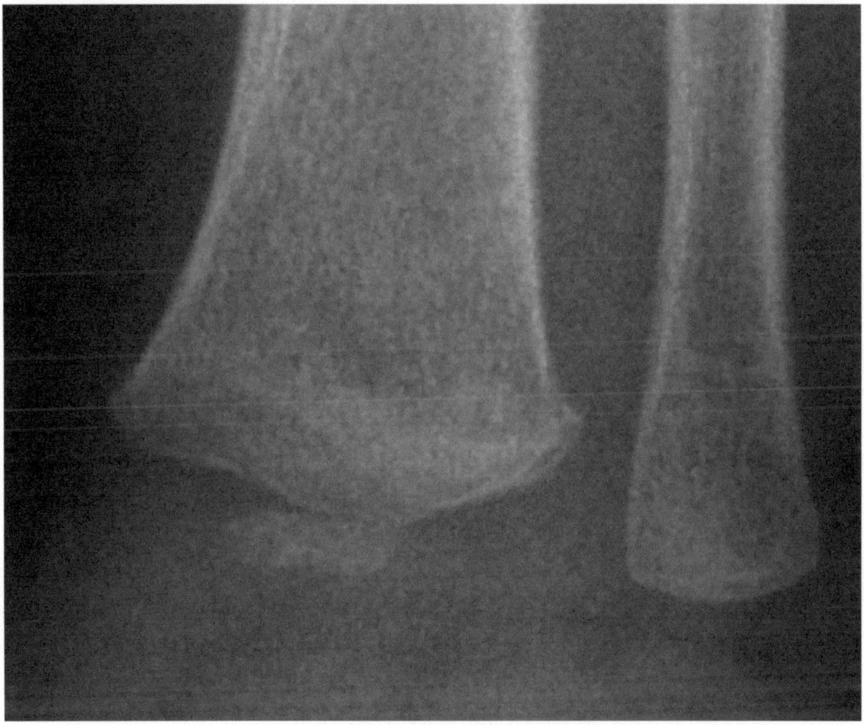

This 8-month-old boy was brought to the Emergency Department (ED) with left leg swelling and had clinically suspected left ankle septic arthritis/osteomyelitis. This case is challenging but demonstrates the importance of a thorough radiographic assessment in the absence of a relevant clinical history, and reinforces that early changes of aggressive pathology can be subtle on radiography. Any focal lucency, especially within the metaphysis, should be considered suspicious for infection. See the explanations for Image 13 of Test 7 and Image 23 of Test 11.

19. **# L little toe proximal phalanx**
    There is an oblique lucency traversing the left little toe proximal phalanx with an associated step in the medial cortex consistent with a minimally displaced fracture.

20. **L congenital diaphragmatic hernia**
    The multiple tubular lucencies in the lower left hemithorax represent bowel loops and there is associated mass effect with mediastinal shift to the right. The absence of the proximal humeral ossification centres indicates that the patient is a neonate. Appearances are consistent with a left congenital diaphragmatic hernia (CDH).

    The most common type of CDH is the Bochdalek hernia in which there is a defect in the left posterolateral diaphragm due to a failure of the pleuroperitoneal membrane to close *in utero* (as such, these hernias may also be referred to as pleuroperitoneal) through which the abdominal contents herniate. Morgagni hernias (through the foramen of Morgagni) are less common and result in right-sided CDH.

CDH is often identified on antenatal ultrasound and can be characterised further with MRI, which is helpful in assessing the degree/extent of intrathoracic herniation of abdominal viscera and/or bowel (intraluminal meconium demonstrates high T1-weighted signal). Both antenatal ultrasound and MRI can be used to assess for lung hypoplasia and future risk of respiratory failure. Chest radiography is usually used for diagnosis in the postnatal period, as in this case.

There is significant morbidity and mortality associated with CDH with important prognostic factors including: hernia size; presence or absence of liver and/or stomach herniation; degree of mediastinal shift; degree of pulmonary hypoplasia (and pulmonary hypertension); and the presence or absence of other congenital anomalies.

Tip for the viva:

- Remember that Bochda**L**ek hernias more commonly occur on the **L**eft, whereas Mo**R**gagni hernias are more commonly **R**ight-sided.
- The features of Bochdalek herniae can be remembered with the mnemonic:
  - **B**ochdalek.
  - **B**ig.
  - **B**ack (i.e. posterior) and lateral, usually left-sided.
  - **B**aby.
  - **B**ad (associated with pulmonary hypoplasia).
- Do not forget to scrutinise all lines and tubes on every neonatal chest radiograph for correct or malposition. In this image:
  - The endotracheal tube (ETT) lies above the level of the thoracic inlet which is too high. The ideal position of the ETT lies between the thoracic inlet and the carina, usually 1 cm above the level of the carina.
  - The tip of the enteric tube is projected over the stomach having descended in the midline, bisected the carina, and passed beneath the left hemidiaphragm.
  - The tip of the umbilical arterial catheter (UAC) is satisfactorily positioned at the level of the T6 vertebral body. The UAC demonstrates its characteristic inferior loop as it passes from the umbilical artery into the internal iliac artery before ascending in the aorta. Its tip may be positioned in the high position between the T6 and T9 vertebral levels (preferable) or in the low position between the L3 and L5 vertebral levels, thereby avoiding the origins of the renal arteries (approximately at the L1/L2 level, immediately inferior to the origin of the superior mesenteric artery) and the inferior mesenteric artery (which arises from the left anterior surface of the aorta at the L3 level).
  - The tip of the umbilical venous catheter (UVC) lies within the right atrium which is too high. The ideal position is at the cavoatrial junction, i.e. the junction of the right atrium and inferior vena cava (IVC) at the level of the hemidiaphragm. The UVC passes from the umbilical vein into the left portal vein, the ductus venosus, the middle of the left hepatic vein, and then finally into the IVC.

22. **Periosteal reaction L iliac and pubic bones**
This is another challenging radiograph with a subtle but genuine finding. The left iliac ala is sclerotic relative to the right and there is associated periosteal reaction along the left iliac bone which involves the greater sciatic notch and the inferior aspect of the left superior pubic ramus. It is always helpful to compare left and right, where possible, with the caveat that certain pathologies can be bilateral and/or symmetrical. The periosteal reaction is more readily appreciated in the magnified image below:

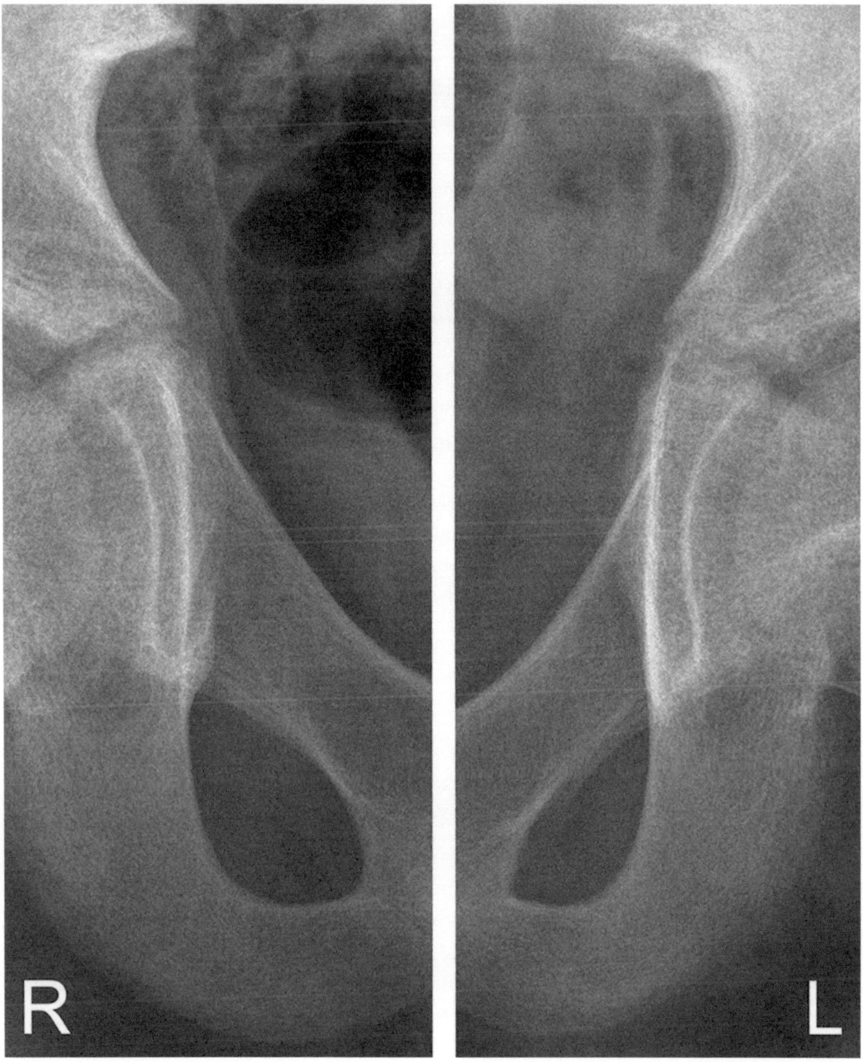

This 11-year-old boy was presented to the ED with a 4-week-history of left hip and groin pain. This finding was detected on his initial presentation radiograph, which reinforces the responsibility we have as radiologists to detect subtle pathologies so that appropriate further investigations and management can be instigated promptly. The differential diagnosis for this appearance includes infection and malignancy (e.g. Ewing's sarcoma). The diagnosis of osteomyelitis was subsequently made following MRI alongside correlation with biochemical markers. See the explanations for Image 13 of Test 7, Image 23 of Test 11 and Image 16 of this test.

24. **L Monteggia #-dislocation**

Whilst the left proximal ulnar diaphyseal fracture is easy to spot, do not miss the associated radial head dislocation—this can be easily overlooked and can have significant functional complications, if missed. As discussed throughout this text, alignment should be assessed on *every* radiograph. Remember that radiocapitellar alignment is normal if a line drawn through the radial neck intersects the capitellum; if not, there is radial head dislocation, as in this case.

Monteggia fracture-dislocation complexes commonly result from a fall on an outstretched hand (FOOSH). They are classified depending on the radial component of the complex (using the Bado classification) and, in general, relate to the direction of the dislocation being the same direction as the apex of the ulnar fracture. Type 1 is the commonest type and thought of as the 'classic' Monteggia fracture-dislocation pattern with anterior dislocation of the radial head and apex anterior ulnar shaft fracture, as in this case. Do not forget that in children, the ulnar fracture component can include the spectrum of bony injuries seen in paediatric bones (i.e. plastic deformation, greenstick fractures, and buckle/torus fractures) as opposed to the often complete fractures seen in adults. As such, in the context of an 'isolated' dislocation of the radial head, close scrutiny of the ulna for an acute bony injury is required. In children, an isolated closed reduction may be possible given that anatomical reduction of the ulna facilitates a closed reduction of the radial head. Where this is not possible, an open reduction and internal fixation (ORIF) is indicated.

BUM BRaG is a useful mnemonic to help you remember which bone is fractured in either the Monteggia or Galeazzi fracture-dislocation complexes:

- **B**roken **U**lna = **M**onteggia.
- **B**roken **Ra**dius = **G**aleazzi.

Once you have remembered which bone is fractured, it is the *other* bone which accounts for the dislocation component, i.e.

- Rad**IA**l head dislocation = Montegg**IA.**
- Distal radioulnar joint dislocation/dissociation = **G**aleazzi: a way to remember this is that Galea**zz**i contains two letters from the *end* of the alphabet and so it is the **end** of the two bones of the wrist which are dislocated.

Galeazzi fracture-dislocations are unstable injuries which often require ORIF of the radial fracture, assessment and reduction/stabilisation of the distal radioulnar joint, and exploration of the triangular fibrocartilage complex (TFCC). In children, remember that Galeazzi-equivalent fractures are those in which there is a distal radius fracture alongside a concomitant (Salter-Harris) fracture of the distal ulna physis. Recovery may be complicated by physeal arrest of the ulna.

26. **Buckle # R distal radial metaphysis**
There is acute angulation of the dorsal cortex of the distal radial metaphysis on this lateral forearm projection, which is better visualised in the magnified image below:

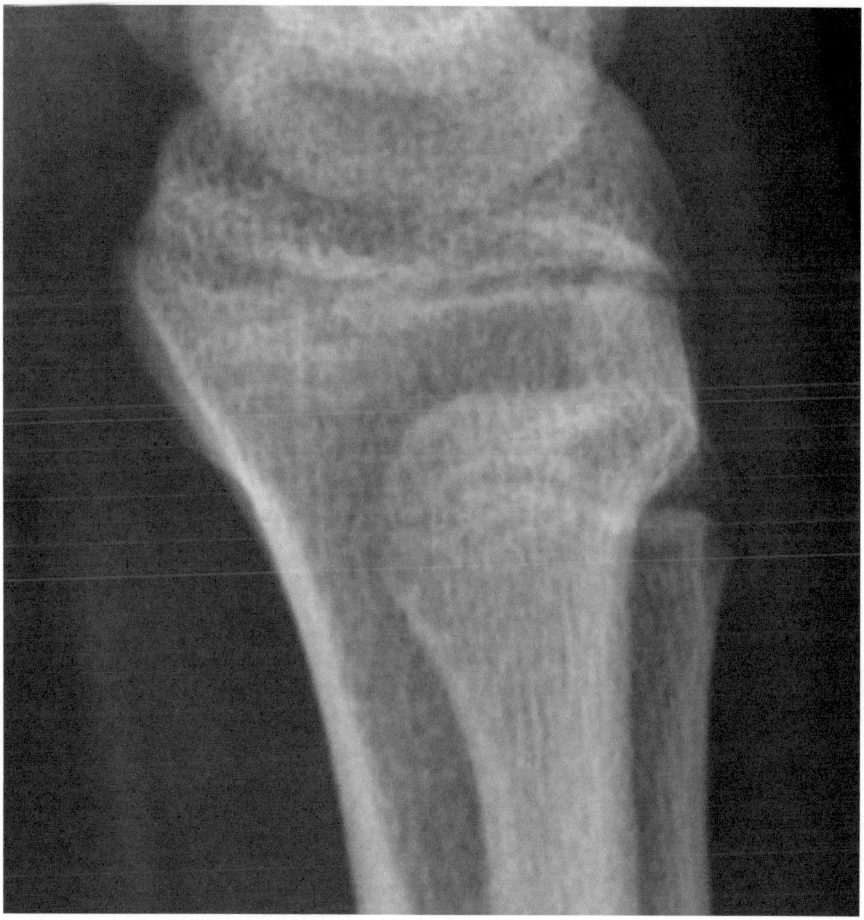

Overlapping structures (such as the distal ulna overlapping the dorsal cortex of the distal radius in the image above) can make visualisation of buckle fractures more difficult, so it is important that the outline of every bony structure is carefully assessed. There is also a small amount of associated soft tissue swelling, which helps to localise/identify the acute injury. See the explanation for Image 18 of Test 1.

28. **R subpulmonic effusion**

The right hemidiaphragm is elevated with a lateral diaphragmatic peak, typical of a right subpulmonic effusion. This radiograph was obtained in a 6-year-old girl with a history of acute lymphoblastic leukaemia (ALL) and desaturations.

Subpulmonic effusions occur when pleural fluid accumulates in the subpulmonic space, i.e. the potential space between the lung base and the diaphragm. The fluid displaces the lung superiorly and the diaphragm inferiorly. Thus, what appears to be the diaphragm is the *visceral pleura* of the superiorly displaced lung: the true diaphragm is obscured by fluid (opacity). Subpulmonic effusions have this characteristic appearance on erect chest radiographs (indicated by 'Sitting' in the top left corner of the image) with elevation of the 'pseudo-diaphragm' along with lateralisation of the hemidiaphragmatic peak, as visualised in this case.

29. **# anterior sternal cortex**

There is a step in the anterior cortex of the second sternal body segment with significant overlying soft tissue swelling in keeping with a minimally displaced sternal fracture. These features are better appreciated in the magnified image below:

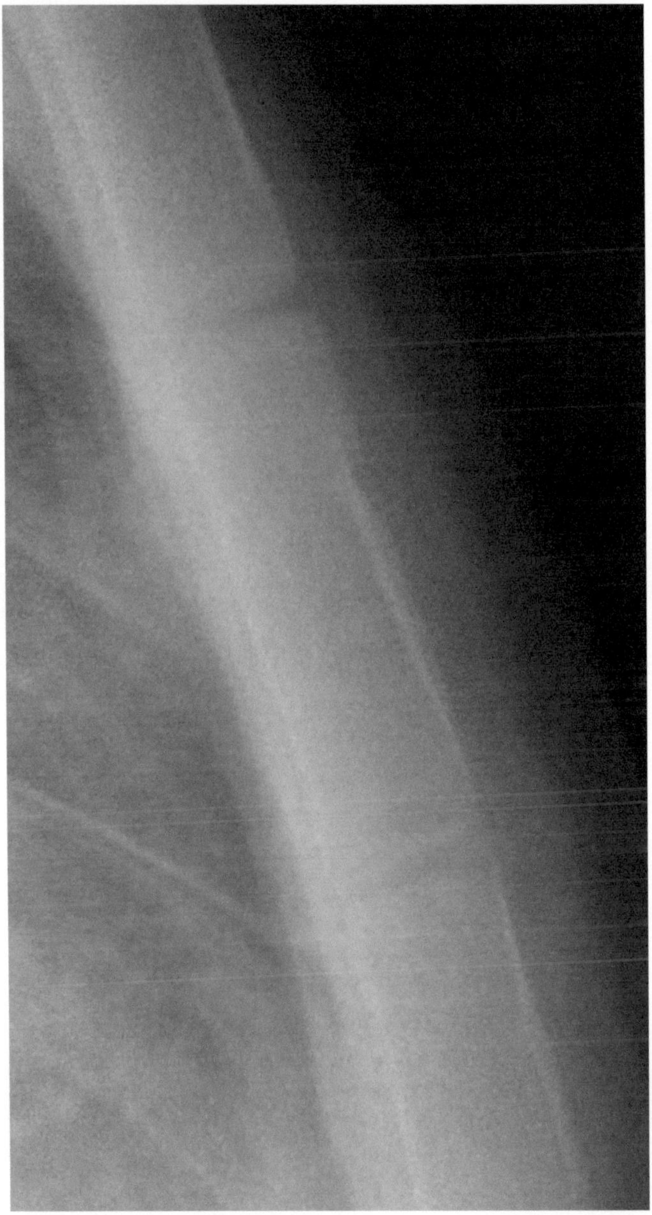

Sternal fractures are uncommon in children and occur mostly due to direct trauma to the anterior chest, as in this case. They are usually isolated and involve the anterior cortex of the first or second segments of the sternal body. Remember that the sternal body comprises four sternal segments (also known as sternebrae), which progressively ossify and fuse to form the sternal body proper. Stable patients with isolated, undisplaced anterior cortical fractures can be safely discharged from the ED.

Further Reading

Image 2

El-Feky M et al (2022) Lateral humeral condyle fractures. https://radiopaedia.org/articles/lateral-humeral-condyle-fracture-1. Accessed Mar 2023

Saber M et al (2021) Weiss classification of lateral humeral condyle fractures. https://radiopaedia.org/articles/weiss-classification-of-lateral-humeral-condyle-fractures. Accessed Mar 2023

Smithus R (2008) Elbow fracture in children. https://radiologyassistant.nl/pediatrics/hip/fractures-in-children-1. Accessed Mar 2023

Yap J et al (2023) Milch classification of lateral humeral condyle fractures. https://radiopaedia.org/articles/milch-classification-of-lateral-humeral-condyle-fractures. Accessed Mar 2023

Image 3

Shanley J, James DR, Lyttle MD et al (2017) Kohler's disease: an unusual cause for a limping child. Arch Dis Child 102(1):109

Image 7

Moore CL, Carpenter CR, Heilbrun ME et al (2019) Imaging in suspected renal colic: systematic review of the literature and multispecialty consensus. J Am Coll Radiol 16(9 Pt A):1132–1143

Penido MG, Tavares Mde S (2015) Pediatric primary urolithiasis: symptoms, medical management and prevention strategies. World J Nephrol 4(4):444–454

Image 9

Badar Z, Yegorov A, Rachun M et al (2017) "Chondroblastoma IS AGE-related": a novel approach for epiphyseal bone lesions, with focus on prevalence, management and clinical relevance. https://epos.myesr.org/poster/esr/ecr2017/C-0956. Accessed Apr 2023

El-Ali AM, Coblentz A, Degnan AJ (2020) Solitary long-bone epiphyseal lesions in children: radiologic-pathological correlation and epidemiology. Pediatr Radiol 50(12):1724–1734

Jones J et al (2021) Epiphyseal lesions (mnemonic). https://radiopaedia.org/articles/epiphyseal-lesions-mnemonic. Accessed Apr 2023

Image 20

Amodeo I, Borzani I, Raffaeli G et al (2022) The role of magnetic resonance imaging in the diagnosis and prognostic evaluation of fetuses with congenital diaphragmatic hernia. Eur J Pediatr 181(9):3243–3257

Marlow J, Thomas J (2013) A review of congenital diaphragmatic hernia. Australas J Ultrasound Med 16(1):16–21

Niknejad M et al (2023) Bochdalek hernia. https://radiopaedia.org/articles/bochdalek-hernia. Accessed May 2023

van Schuppen J, Onland W, van Rijn R (2013) Lines and tubes in neonates. https://radiologyassistant.nl/pediatrics/abdominal-masses/lines-and-tubes-in-neonates. Accessed Mar 2023
Vikas S et al (2020) Bochdalek hernia features (mnemonic). https://radiopaedia.org/articles/bochdalek-hernia-features-mnemonic. Accessed May 2023

Image 24

El-Feky M et al (2023) Galeazzi fracture-dislocation. https://radiopaedia.org/articles/galeazzi-fracture-dislocation. Accessed Jul 2023
Lustosa L et al (2022) Bado classification of Monteggia fracture-dislocations. https://radiopaedia.org/articles/bado-classification-of-monteggia-fracture-dislocations-1. Accessed Jul 2023
Yap J et al (2023) Monteggia fracture-dislocation. https://radiopaedia.org/articles/monteggia-fracture-dislocation. Accessed Jul 2023

Image 28

Weerakkody Y et al (2022) Subpulmonic effusion. https://radiopaedia.org/articles/subpulmonic-effusion. Accessed May 2023

Image 29

Chalphin AV, Mooney DP (2020) Pediatric sternal fractures: a single center retrospective review. J Pediatr Surg 55(7):1224–1227

MIX
Papier aus verantwortungsvollen Quellen
Paper from responsible sources
FSC® C105338
FSC
www.fsc.org

If you have any concerns about our products,
you can contact us on
ProductSafety@springernature.com

In case Publisher is established outside the EU,
the EU authorized representative is:
Springer Nature Customer Service Center GmbH
Europaplatz 3, 69115 Heidelberg, Germany

Printed by Libri Plureos GmbH
in Hamburg, Germany